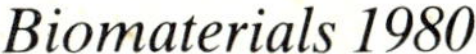

Biomaterials 1980

ADVANCES IN BIOMATERIALS

Edited by

George D. Winter,†
Central Research Laboratories,
3M Company, St. Paul,
Minnesota, USA

Assistant Series Editor

Jenny Upton,

Central Research Laboratories,
3M Company, St. Paul,
Minnesota, USA

Volume 1: *Evaluation of Biomaterials*

Volume 2: *Mechanical Properties of Biomaterials*

Volume 3: *Biomaterials 1980*

† Deceased 1st April 1981

Biomaterials 1980

Edited by

George D. Winter
Central Research Laboratories,
3M Company, St. Paul, Minnesota, USA

Donald F. Gibbons
Case Western Reserve University,
Cleveland, USA

Hanns Plenk Jr
Histological-Embryological Institute,
University of Vienna, Austria

Proceedings of the First World Biomaterials Congress held in Baden, Vienna, Austria, in April 1980, in conjunction with the 12th International Biomaterials Symposium and the 6th Annual Meeting of the Society for Biomaterials, USA.

A Wiley–Interscience Publication

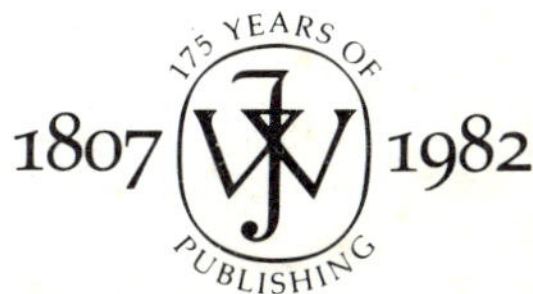

JOHN WILEY & SONS
Chichester . New York . Brisbane . Toronto . Singapore

Library of Congress Cataloguing in Publication Data:

World Biomaterials Congress (1st: 1980: Baden, Austria)
    Biomaterials 1980.
    (Advances in biomaterials; v. 3)
    'A Wiley–Interscience publication.'
    1. Biomedical materials—Congresses. I. Winter, George D.
    II. Gibbons, Donald F. III. Plenk, Hanns. IV. Society for
    Biomaterials. V. International Biomaterials Symposium
    (12th: 1980: Baden, Austria) VI. Title. VII. Series. [DNLM:
    1. Biocompatible materials—Congresses. 2. Biomedical
    engineering—Congresses. 3. Prosthesis—Congresses. 4.
    Dental materials—Congresses.
    W3 AD23 v. 2 1980/QT 34 W9265 1980b]
    R857.M3W67 1980   610′.28   81-15923
                                           AACR2

ISBN 0 471 10126 5

British Library Cataloguing in Publication Data:

World Biomaterials Congress *(1st: 1980: Baden)*
    Biomaterials 1980—(Advances in biomaterials; v. 3)
    1. Biomedical materials—Congresses
    I. Title II. Winter, George D. III. Gibbons, Donald F. IV.
    Plenk, Hanns V. Series
    574.19′2   R857.M3

ISBN 0 471 10126 5

Printed in Great Britain

CONTENTS

Artificial heart valves and devices

PART 3.   SPECIAL APPLICATIONS OF BIOMATERIALS

Dressings and sutures

Adhesives

Biomaterials in tissue and organ reconstruction

FOREWORD

The First World Biomaterials Congress was held in Baden, Vienna,
Austria, on April 12th 1980, in conjunction with the 12th
International Biomaterials Symposium and the 6th Annual Meeting of
the Society for Biomaterials, USA.

For many it was a dream come true. The Congress brought together
members of the European Society for Biomaterials, the Society for
Biomaterials, USA, the Biomaterials Group of the Biological
Engineering Society, UK, the Canadian Society for Biomaterials and
the Japanese Society for Biomaterials.

The quality of the papers was outstanding. The plenary sessions
served to review the state of the art of biomaterials. The poster
section and the exhibits were exceptionally good. Perhaps, more
important than the technical quality of the papers was the chance
for biomaterials researchers around the world to meet and exchange
ideas. All of the social functions were well attended. Although
the participants enjoyed socializing the conversations usually
quickly turned to some aspect of biomaterials research. There is
no question but that the First World Biomaterials Congress is
going to serve as a major catalyst for the development of new and
important biomaterials. The end result of this Congress will be
improved health care for citizens of our planet.

What follows is a printing of the papers that were submitted for
publication. I am sure that this collection of papers will become
a classic and the biomaterials research community will use this
publication as a major reference text for many years to come.

There is a particularly sad note, however, and that is that two of
the major organizers of the First World Biomaterials Congress have
recently died. Dr. George D. Winter, President of the Congress,
died of a heart attack on the very day he learned that the Secretary
General of the Executive Committee, Dr. Jean L. Leray, had been
killed by an avalanche whilst skiing in France.

George Winter served as the first President of the European Society
for Biomaterials and Jean Leray was serving as the Society's second
President. The biomaterials research community has suffered a
great loss. I would propose that we dedicate the publication of
the First World Congress to our good friends George D. Winter and
Jean L. Leray. I would also propose that each of us rededicate our
commitment to biomaterials research in order to attempt to make up
for the loss of two of the world's foremost biomaterials researchers.
In final tribute to George and Jean, I would like to paraphrase John
Doone's "Holy Sermon XV11."

xvii

"The Church is catholic, universal, so are all her
actions; all that she does belongs to all. When
she baptizes a child, that action concerns me;
and when she buries a man, that action concerns me;
all mankind is of one author, and is one volume;
when one man dies, one chapter is not torn out of
the book, but translated into a better language;
and every chapter must be so translated...

No man is an island, entire of itself; every man
is a piece of the continent, a part of the main;
any man's death diminishes me, because I am involved
in mankind; and therefore never ask to know for
whom the bell tolls; it tolls for you and it tolls
for me."

Samuel F. Hulbert
A friend of Jean and George

Biomaterials is that branch of biomedical engineering that is concerned with the materials aspects of medical devices. Any material, metal, ceramic, plastics or organic, brought into contact with the fluids, cells, and tissues of the living body comes within the domain of biomaterials science. Included are surgical implant and dental materials, dressings, orthotics, prosthetics materials, and those used in extracorporeal circulation devices. Biomaterials scientists are concerned with the physical and chemical properties of materials and their suitability for a particular device. They are concerned how these properties are altered by the biological environment and how the materials may affect the body. The subject spans the physical and life sciences.

Biomaterials science has expanded rapidly in the last few years, nurtured by enthusiasts in the medical profession, in universities, commerce, and government agencies. Many universities now offer undergraduate and post-graduate teaching courses. Among the societies that exist to promote the safe and efficient use of biomaterials and to encourage the development of a sound rational basis for this discipline are: The Society for Biomaterials (USA) founded in 1974, the Biological Engineering Society (UK) founded in 1960 and which established a specialist topic group in biomaterials in 1974, and the European Society for Biomaterials founded in 1976. Japanese and Canadian Societies were inaugurated in 1979. These societies play a major part in the development of our subject by organizing international meetings which provide a forum for the exchange of ideas in clinical and basic research. Special mention should be made of the International Biomaterials Symposia inaugurated at Clemson University, South Carolina, 11 years ago. This series of annual meetings, sponsored by the Society for Biomaterials (USA) is held in high esteem by the biomaterials fraternity. Other regular conferences are the series entitled "Materials for Use in Medicine and Biology", organized by the Biological Engineering Society (UK), the Gordon Conferences on Biomaterials, and the European International Conferences. The First World Biomaterials Congress was held in Austria in the Spring of 1980 and this volume represents contributions presented at that meeting.

Many other meetings having a biomaterials content are held each year, such as the Annual Conference on Engineering in Medicine and Biology and meetings organized by associations of biomechanics, artificial organs, orthopaedics, dentistry, cardiovascular surgery, plastic and reconstructive surgery, etc.

It was to complement the valuable activities of these societies that the idea for this series on "Advances in Biomaterials" was born. It is intended to provide a vehicle for the publication of the proceedings of meetings on biomaterials which will grow into a valuable reference library. Volumes dealing with special topics may be commisioned as

as appropriate. It is inevitable that in an inderdisciplinary field
such as this data are rather widely scattered in the literature. The
series will fulfill its purpose if it succeeds in building a coherent
body of knowledge for the use of students and practitioners in
biomaterials, for the ultimate benefit of patients.

March 1981   George D. Winter

Addendum to Series Preface

It is with great regret that we acknowledge the sudden death of Dr.
George D. Winter on April 1st, 1981. Dr. Winter was an international
authority on the biological responses of tissues to implants, and
particularly that of materials for burn dressings. In 1979 he was the
recipient of the Clemson Award for Technical Literature on Biomaterials
in recognition of his contributions. Dr. Winter recognised the need
to exchange ideas and information between scientists of the diverse
disciplines actively engaged in the relatively new field of biomedical
materials. He unselfishly contributed considerable time and much
energy towards the development of such opportunities. Dr. Winter was
a significant force in the development of the Biomaterials Section
of the Biological Engineering Society (UK) and the formation and
organisation of the European Society for Biomaterials in 1976, of
which he was the first President. It is appropriate that his last
contribution as a service to the field of biomaterials should have
been as proponent, initiator, organiser and President of the First
World Biomaterials Congress.

Dr. George Winter was the primary force in initiating the series
"Advances in Biomaterials" and had completed the editing of the
scientific papers contained in Volume 3 of the series only two weeks
prior to his untimely death.

It is sad that Volume 3 of "Advances in Biomaterials" has also to
include the announcement of another untimely death, that of Professor
Jean L. Leray, President of the European Society for Biomaterials and
Secretary General for the First World Biomaterials Congress.

May 1981   Jenny Upton
                                               Donald F. Gibbons
                                                  Hanns Plenk

VOLUME PREFACE

The First World Biomaterials Congress, which was held in Baden, near
Vienna, Austria, in April 1980, marked the first time that the members
of international biomaterials societies joined together to present
scientific papers on topics which represented the state of knowledge
of biomaterials in the world at that time. Over 500 biomaterials
research scientists from around the world joined together to either
present original papers, reviews, poster sessions or to attend the
lectures. The European Society for Biomaterials was the host Society
with representatives from the Society for Biomaterials (USA), the
Biomaterials Group of the Biological Engineering Society (UK), the
Canadian Society for Biomaterials and the Japanese Society for
Biomaterials all participating.

Two hundred and seventy papers were either presented in lectures or
poster sessions. Volume 3 contains 116 papers which were submitted
to the editors for inclusion in this volume and which were accepted
after scientific peer reviews. These papers represent contributions
from sixteen countries and are an overview of the areas in biomaterials
in which active research was flourishing at the time of the Congress.

Volume 3 has been organised into four principle sections: Bone
Implant Applications, Cardiovascular Applications of Biomaterials,
Special Applications of Biomaterials and, finally, Characterisation
and Specific Tissue Responses to Polymers. The first section is
concerned with orthopaedic and dental applications of materials for
bone implants and their response. It includes the methods being
used and data obtained on implant design, analysis and evaluation,
both experimental and clinical. The second section includes papers
concerned with the methods used to analyse the effect of materials
on thrombogenicity, protein and cellular interactions, as well as
the evaluation and clinical experience with vascular grafts and tissue
valves. The third section includes contributions which characterise
and evaluate the special problems associated with wound closure, wound
dressings and the use of biomaterials in organ and tissue reconstruction.
The fourth section concerns material characterisation as well as the
evaluation of degredation, and _in vivo_ cytotoxic and neoplastic
responses of materials in soft tissue.

The wide range of studies incorporated in this volume, together with
the detailed considerations appropriate to particular tissues and
organs, has made some of the decisions regarding the organisation of
this volume arbitrary. However, the editors hope that the format
will allow the basic research scientists and clinicians to appreciate
the state of the art in biomaterials as represented at the Congress.

The editors extend their appreciation to the authors for the splendid
way in which they responded to the request for camera-ready copy.

xxi

A debt of gratidue is owed to the reviewers, their criticisms
and suggestions have been instrumental in maintaining the high
scientific quality represented by the papers included in this
volume. The editors wish to publicly recognise the work of the
reviewers and a list of their names follows immediately after
this preface.

In conclusion, the work of the Scientific Programme Committee must
be acknowledged. During a short weekend at Baden in November,
1979, they undertook the monumental task of assembling and
reviewing the abstracts submitted for the Congress and then
organised the final selection of papers into an excellent
programme of scientific sessions. The editors are truly grateful.

Jenny Upton.
Donald F. Gibbons.
Hanns Plenk.

List of Reviewers

Anderson, B.S.	Hammar, W.J.	Pawluk, R.
Anderson, J.M.	Heinecke, S.B.	Picha, G.J.
Bantli, H.	Heiple, K.	Placheta, P.
Barenburg, S.	Hench, L.L.	Plitz, W.
Barrows, T.H.	Hoffman, A.S.	Pollack, S.
Blackshear, P.	Hottel, T.L.	Rahn, B.A.
Brand, G.K.	Hulbert, S.	Rice, T.K.
Brand, I.	Jameison, A.	Rose, R.M.
Brown, R.	Jones, R.D.	Salthouse, T.
Bunker, J.E.	Kemmetmüller, H.	Sonstegard, D.A.
Cooke, F.W.	Kent, J.	Sudilovsky, O.
Devore, D.P.	King-Smith, E.A.	Unger, F.
Driskell, T.	Kraft, D.	Van Kampen, C.L.
Ducheyne, P.	Lautenschlager, E.	Vigdahl, R.L.
Ebbens, K.L.	Lee, A.J.C.	Weinstein, A.
Feijen, J.	Luckey, H.A.	Williams, D.F.
Frisch, E.	McMillin, C.R.	Wollner, E.
Galante, J.	McPherson, G.K.	Zechner, G.
Gilding, K.	Mendenhall, H.V.	Zingg, W.
Gottlob, E.	Mjör, I.A.	Zitter, H.
Greenwald, S.	Ofstead, R.F.	
Griss, P.	Parks, P.J.	

PART 1

BONE IMPLANT APPLICATIONS

Material for hard tissue implants

ELECTRICAL AND MATHEMATICAL MODEL OF THE AXIAL PROPAGATION OF THE CURRENT IN HARD BIOMATERIALS

Y.K. VILKS and A.V. JAUNZEMS

Department of Biomechanics and Biomaterials

Riga Scientific Research Institute of Traumatology and Orthopaedics, USSR

SUMMARY

To determine real current flow in the hard biomaterials it is necessary to know numeral values of the complex resistence, which are obtained by using special multipoint measuring method and following mathematical approximation. These results allows to build-up a system of mathematical equations, solution of which gives the distribution of current (on amplitudes and phase) in electrical stimulation or diagnostic process.

INTRODUCTION

Optimization of the current and voltage is regarded as an initial precondition for an effective use of electric fields to stimulate the ingrowth of the bony tissue into the surface layer of the natural or artificial biomaterial. The problem can be solved by determining the propagation of current and the resultant distribution of potentials in both types of biomaterials. The application of the usual electrical probe is neither advisable nor practical clinicaly since the method requires multipoint access not only to the skin surface but also to the deepmost lying layers of bony tissue or callus. However the problem can be easily solved theoretically. The application of electrical and mathematical models enables the determination of the distribution of the electric pulse field both in space and time. Bony tissue electrical parameters served as bases for the construction of the respective models. Precision of measurements of the respective parameters depends to a considerable degree on the possibility of excluding the influence of contact resistance, the latter arising from the change of the electronic into ionic conduction and vice versa.

1

<u>METHODS</u>

The middle third of diaphyses of eight rabbit radii was
experimentally investigated in vivo, and six pig femurs
in situ immediately after the animals were sacrificed.
Measurements were performed according to a four point
method (FPM). The electrodes of the measuring probe are
made of insulated platinum wire of diameter 0.70 mm,
with a contact surface of 0.39 mm^2 on the end portion.
Volt-ampere curves were determined between all electrodes in pairs, to enable exclusion in the subsequent evaluations of the value of contact resistance in the voltage range between 0 and 0.70 V, where electrochemical
phenomena which cause changes in conductivity are not
considered to take place. Measurements were made at frequencies between 0 and 20 kHz, corresponding to the frequencies used for local electric influence in traumatology.

<u>CONSTRUCTION OF THE ELECTRICAL MODEL</u>

The results obtained by means of the FPM were used to determine the parameters of the corresponding equivalent
circuit schematic (Fig. 1). The circuit element Z_3 represents bulk impedance of the section of biomaterial under
study, but Z_2 and Z_4 stand for contact resistance. The
equivalent schematic is described by a system of equations.

$$AZ = B$$

where

$$A = \begin{Vmatrix} 1 & 0 & 1 & 1 & 0 \\ 1 & 1 & 0 & 0 & 0 \\ 1 & 0 & 1 & 0 & 1 \\ 0 & 0 & 0 & 1 & 1 \\ 0 & 1 & 1 & 0 & 1 \end{Vmatrix} \qquad B = \begin{Vmatrix} \dfrac{U_{1,3}}{J_{1,3}} \\[2mm] \dfrac{U_{1,2}}{J_{1,2}} \\[2mm] \dfrac{U_{1,4}}{J_{1,4}} \\[2mm] \dfrac{U_{3,4}}{J_{3,4}} \\[2mm] \dfrac{U_{2,4}}{J_{2,4}} \end{Vmatrix} \qquad (1)$$

and

$$U_{ij} = \Psi_i - \Psi_j \ ,$$

where Ψ_i are the potentials at the ptactically accessible
points of the measuring scheme. Solution of the equation
system (1) for Z_3 (biomaterials bulk impedance) at different current frequencies demonstrated that the bony tissue impedance displayed a nonlinear dependence with frequency (Fig. 2). With the increase of measurement frequency, impedance Z_3 tends to a constant value. The equivalent schematic (Fig. 3) consisting of series-connected

resistances, across one of which is a parallel capacitance, displays analogous frequency dependence. The modulus of the impedance vector of the given scheme under different frequencies was derived from equations

$$Z_k = \sqrt{\left(\frac{r_i + R_i + \omega_k^2 r_i R_i^2 C_i^2}{1 + \omega_k^2 R_i^2 C_i^2} \right)^2 + \left(\frac{\omega_k R_i^2 C_i}{1 + \omega_k^2 R_i^2 C_i^2} \right)^2} \tag{2}$$

Satisfactory results of the mathematical approximation of the experimentally obtained data by means of the equation gave possibility of identifying the scheme (Fig. 3) as the bony tissue electrical model. The values of all circuit elements for the elementary part of the biomaterial under study could be determined by means of the solution (2) as a system of equations at different frequencies. Values of the circuit elements of the uninjured bony tissue model in the longitudinal direction, are determined as

$$R_i = 375 \pm 2 \text{ kOhm/cm};$$
$$r_i = 5.6 \pm 1.2 \text{ kOhm/cm};$$
$$C_i = 1.2 \pm 0.2 \times 10^{-7} \text{ F}.$$

CONSTRUCTION OF MATHEMATICAL MODEL

The complete electrical model is developed as a series of Figs 3. Presenting the scheme of the model as a definite "i" elementary circuit section (Fig. 4), potentials φ on the end portions of the respective sections were determined by means of equation system solution

$$\tag{3}$$

$$\begin{cases} \dfrac{\varphi_{i-1} - \varphi'}{r_i} = C_i \dfrac{d(\varphi' - \varphi_i)}{dt} + \dfrac{\varphi' - \varphi_i}{R_i} \\[2em] \varphi_{i-1} - \varphi' = \varphi_i - \varphi'' \\[2em] \dfrac{\varphi_i - \varphi''}{r_i} = C_i \dfrac{d(\varphi'' - \varphi_{i+1})}{dt} + \dfrac{\varphi'' - \varphi_{i+1}}{R_i} \end{cases}$$

The distribution of electrical potentials, along the biomaterial under study (one-dimensional) and the dynamics
of these potentials with time were established for any
number of elementary sections forming the complete model.
In the constant-current (DC) case, electrical potential
is distributed along the circuit proportionally to the
value of impedance active component of separate circuit
sections. In time-varying case, the distribution of potentials is determined by the dynamic processes depending on the rate of the reactive element charge or discharge. The phase shift between current and voltage of
stimulation signal in separate circuit elements, which
is dependent on the biomaterial studied, was determined
by means of the model.

RESULTS

The evaluation of the model was performed by comparing
the results obtained in the impedance measurements of
the biomaterial, on the electrical model (Fig. 3) of the
bony tissue under study and by means of the mathematical
model (3).
It was determined that:
1. Voltage difference on the elementary section of the
biocomposits, caused by square pulse of current, increases exponentionally with time (Fig. 5).
2. Phase shift between current and voltage appears in
the presence of sine wave signal.
3. Frequency-dependent amplitude changes of the recorded
signal are observed (Fig. 5).
4. Change of electrical parameters of biomaterial causes
redistribution of potentials and waveform changes of the
signal.
5. The necessary values of both the waveform and amplitude parameters of the influence signals, can be determined by means of models according to the electrical parameters of the biomaterials.
6. Plane and spatial models provide for the investigation of individual effect of each type of bony or surrounding tissues, and determine the influence of changing of different parameters on the spatial, as well as
the temporal dependence of the electrical signal of influence.

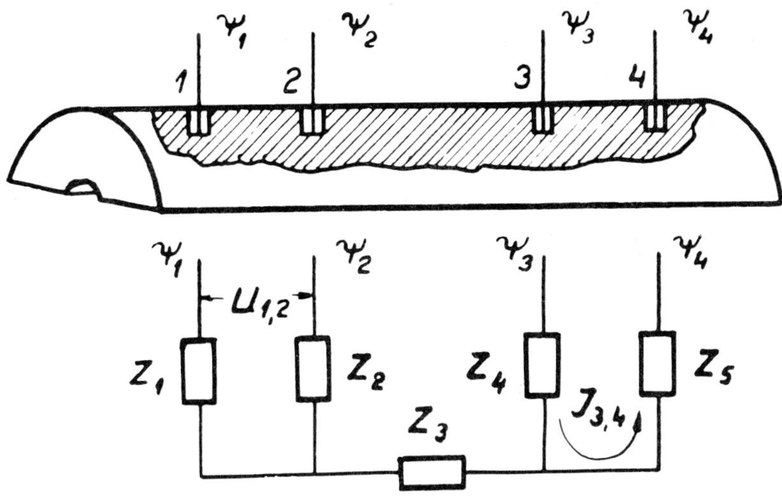

Fig. 1. Equivalent scheme of the four point measurement method.

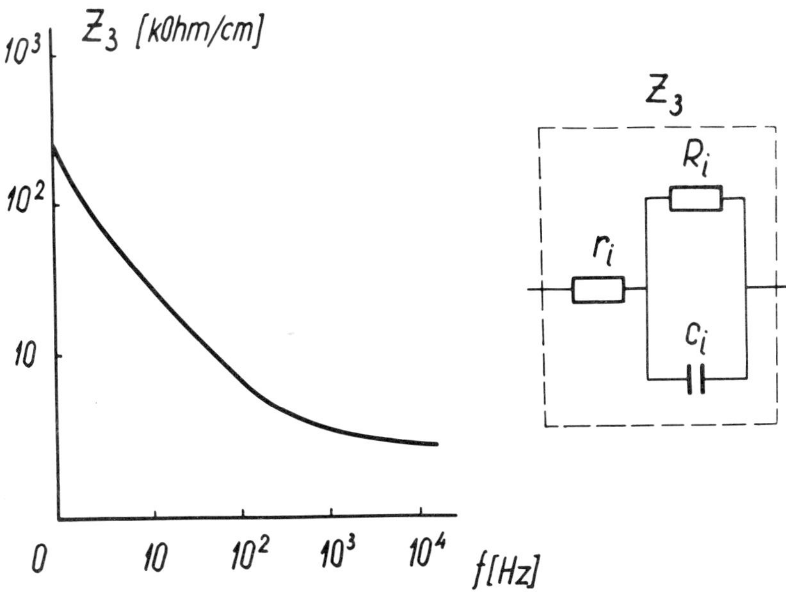

Fig. 2. Dependence of bony tissue impedance from the frequence in current measurements.

Fig. 3. Bony tissue electrical model.

                    Y.Vilks and A.Jaunzems

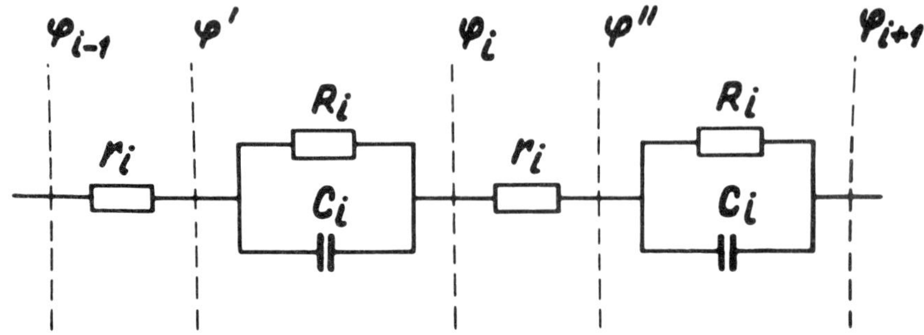

Fig. 4. Electrical circuit for the formation of
the bony tissue mathematical model.

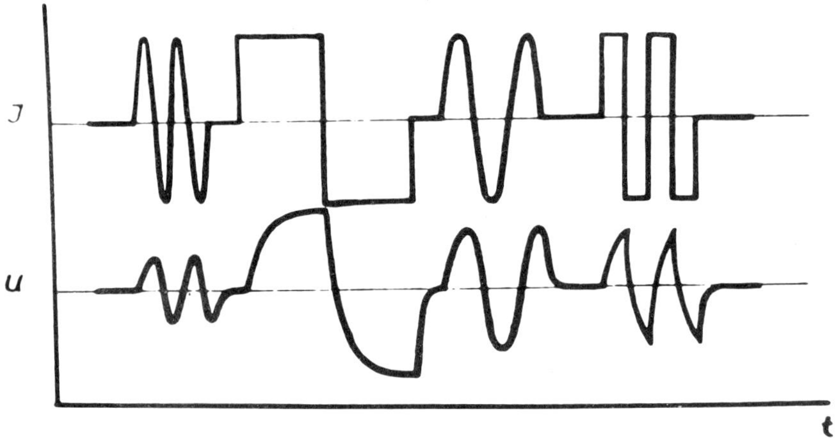

Fig. 5. Frequency dependence of voltage discharge
in the segment of biomaterial.

Biomaterials 1980
Edited by G. D. Winter, D. F. Gibbons, and H. Plenk, Jr.
© 1982 John Wiley and Sons Ltd.

A NEW ALLOY SYSTEM WITH POSSIBLE DENTAL AND ORTHOPAEDIC APPLICATIONS

J.M. Meyer, R. Barraud, C.P. Susz and J.N. Nally

University of Geneva, School of Dentistry,
Geneva, Switzerland

SUMMARY

Starting from the binary nickel-vanadium system, the present investigation has led to the selection of ternary Ni-V-Cr alloys, and then of the 68Ni 13V 17Cr 2Nb alloy, which exhibits properties meeting the basic requirements for a dental use. It is castable, its corrosion resistance is high, its mechanical properties can be improved by age hardening, porcelain adheres to its surface, and preliminary results have indicated a tissue tolerance similar to that of gold alloys. Improvements are still needed, however, e.g. melting by an ordinary torch instead of an induction centrifugal casting machine, and elimination of occasional casting defects.
The high yield strength (up to 800 MPa when fully age hardened), the relatively high elongation (44 % cast), and the excellent corrosion resistance (polarization resistance 600 kΩ), should encourage further investigations for a possible orthopaedic application.

INTRODUCTION

A search was initiated to develop a better alternative to the dental gold casting alloys than the existing nickel-chromium alloys. Any new alloy must meet the following requirements: good castability with dental laboratory equipment, high corrosion resistance, high mechanical properties, response to thermal treatments, possibility of porcelain veneering, and absence of toxicity. Preliminary investigations led to the selection of the nickel-vanadium system because of the numerous possibilities of producing relatively low-fusing alloys with greatly varying mechanical properties. In order to improve the corrosion and mechanical properties of the nickel-vanadium system, further alloying additions were necessary.

MATERIALS AND METHODS

The alloys were synthetized from pure metals in an argon arc furnace. Tensile bars and disks were prepared by use of the dental lost wax technique. The mechanical properties were evaluated by tensile and hardness tests. The electrochemical properties were studied in an artificial saliva, using potentiodynamic polarization curves and li-

                            J.M. Meyer et al.

near polarization plots (Mansfeld, 1973). Their potential for porcelain veneering was evaluated by coefficient of thermal expansion measurements and by testing the porcelain bond strength (Asgar and Giday, 1978).

RESULTS

Nickel-Vanadium System. Preliminary results (Susz, Meyer, Nally,
1977) indicated that the alloy 67Ni 33V was a suitable base composition (hardness 534 HVN, tensile strength 1100 MPa) for further studies aimed at improving its corrosion resistance (polarization resistance 55 kΩ).

Nickel-Vanadium-Chromium-System. Addition of chromium led to a considerable increase in the polarization resistance (Barraud et al.,
1977; Meyer et al., 1977). Further research therefore was concentrated on the Ni-V-Cr system. All the 33 alloys prepared and tested in
this system are indicated in Fig. 1 (Barraud et al., 1978).

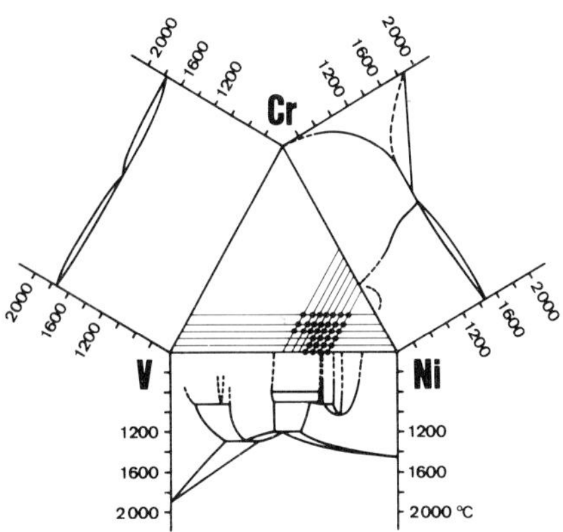

Fig. 1 Alloys prepared and tested in the Ni-V-Cr system.

Two alloys: 60Ni 23V 17Cr and 70Ni 13V 17Cr were selected for additional testing. Their main properties are given in Fig. 2. The differences are chiefly mechanical, with an increase in ductility accompanying an increase in nickel concentration.

The microstructure of these alloys (Fig. 3) shows that the annealed
"equilibrium" state is two phase for the 60Ni 23V 17Cr, and a solid
solution for the 70Ni 13.5V 16.5Cr composition. Increasing the nickel-
content therefore eliminated the brittle and hard σ phase, which is
also responsible for an inconsistant electrochemical behavior.

Nickel-Vanadium-Chromium-Niobium System. Minor amounts (up to 2 atomic per cent) of niobium were added to the 70Ni 13V 17Cr base (Barraud et al., 1979). The alloy 68Ni 13V 17Cr 2Nb showed improved me-

chanical properties and a highly satisfactory resistance to corrosion. Moreover, it retains the favorable solid solution structure in
the near equilibrium state, as exhibited by the parent alloy 70Ni 13V
17Cr (Fig. 3).

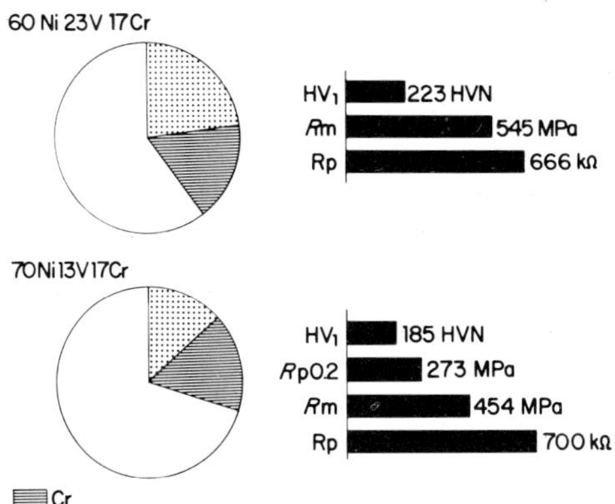

Fig. 2. Main properties of the two alloys selected in the
Ni-V-Cr system. HV_1 = Vickers hardness. $R_{p0.2}$ = yield
strength. R_m = tensile strength. R_p = polarization resistance.

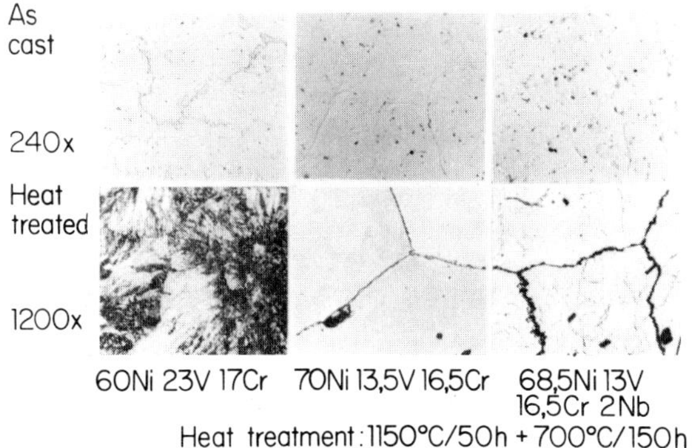

Fig. 3. Microstructures of the two Ni-V-Cr alloys and the
Ni-V-Cr-Nb alloy, in the as cast condition and after a heat
treatment (annealed near equilibrium). 70Ni 13.5V 16.5Cr and
68.5Ni 13V 16.5Cr 2Nb retain a solid solution structure in
the near equilibrium state.

DISCUSSION

A comparison of the characteristic properties of the 68Ni 13V 17Cr
2Nb alloy with those of a commercial dental casting Ni-Cr alloy (Wiron S) (Fig. 4) shows that the experimental alloy is softer, more ductile, and has a lower proof stress ($R_{p0.2}$); however, its properties
are comparable with the corresponding data given for a wrought, soft
annealed Co-Ni-Cr-Mo-Ti alloy intended for orthopaedic applications
(Süry and Semlitsch, 1978).

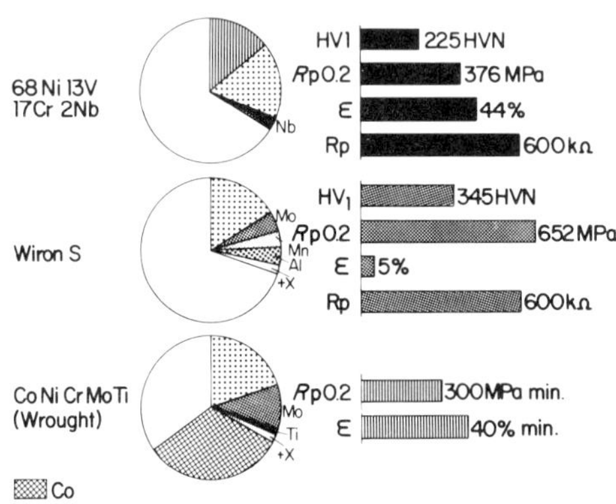

Fig. 4. Comparison of the properties of an experimental Ni-
V-Cr-Nb alloy, a commercial Ni-Cr alloy (Wiron S), and a
commercial alloy for orthopaedic applications (Co-Ni-Cr-Mo-
Ti). HV_1 = Vickers hardness. $R_{p0.2}$ = Yield strength. ε =
Elongation. Rp = Polarization resistance.

The experimental alloy does respond to an age-hardening treatment; i.
e. after simulating the heating cycle of the baking of porcelain, followed by an additional age-hardening, at 700°C for 15 minutes, the
yield strength rises to 530 MPa, the hardness to 280 HVN, and the
elongation decreases to 18%. The alloy might therefore be considered
for orthopaedic applications, provided its fatigue and corrosion resistance are acceptable.

To be successfully used as an alternative to the dental gold alloys,
a non-precious alloy should meet the tough requirement of a strong
bond with a veneering porcelain. Since the color of non-precious alloys is not cosmetically acceptable, it is necessary to apply a porcelain veneer. The poor bond strength between the porcelain veneer
and the present day Ni-Cr alloys represents one of the problems. To
achieve a firm bond between alloy and porcelain, the coefficients of
thermal expansion of both materials should be almost identical and
the growth of the oxide layer, formed at the surface of the alloy,

should be capable of strict control during all the stages of porcelain veneering. A practical way to evaluate the strength of the bond is to measure the stress needed for breaking it. The design of specimen selected in this study was the proposed A.D.A. specification (ANSI/ADA 1980, Asgar and Giday 1978). A disk of opaque and gingival porcelain is baked around an alloy rod, using spacers for constant thickness. The test bar is then waxed and embedded in dental stone. After 7 days of setting, a load is applied to the upper metal rod, which induces a shear stress at the interface between the porcelain disk and the alloy rod. A sharp decrease in the recorded stress indicates the breaking strength of the bond. The values obtained with the 68Ni 13V 17Cr 2Nb alloy are reported in Fig. 5.

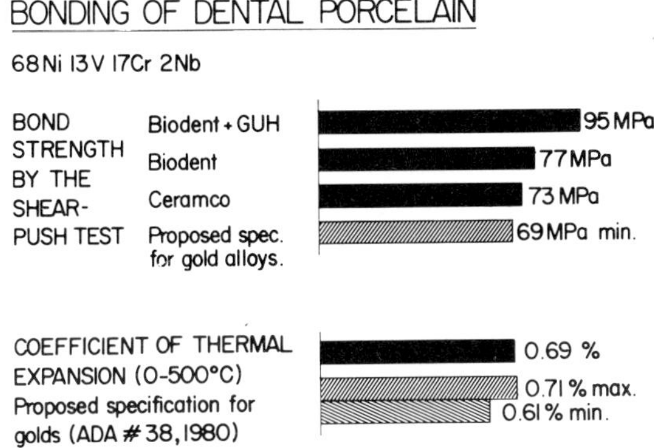

Fig. 5. Porcelain bond strength and coefficient of thermal expansion of the 68Ni 13V 17Cr 2Nb alloy, compared to the reference values in the proposed ADA specification for gold alloy-porcelain systems. All data are means of six specimens.

The use of a special bonding agent, GUH[1], with the Biodent[1] porcelain, leads to a bond strength value which exceeds that usually obtained with gold alloys. Without this bonding agent, or with another brand of porcelain (Ceramco[2]), the bond strength remains slightly above the minimum value required in the proposed specification. The linear thermal expansion (increase of the nominal length between 20 and 500° C) of the same alloy is also reported in Fig. 5. It fits well whithin the range of the proposed specification. The proposed values for dental porcelains are 0.70 % (max.) and 0.52 % (min.).

---

[1] De Trey GmbH, Wiesbaden, Germany

[2] Ceramco, Johnson & Johnson, East Windsor, N.J.

A preliminary in vivo testing of tissue tolerance, using cylinders of the studied alloys implanted subcutaneously in mice for up to 9 weeks (Geret et al; 1979), has indicated that the Ni-V-Cr and Ni-V-Cr-Nb alloys behave similarly to a dental gold alloy of the same usage.

ACKNOWLEDGEMENTS

This study has been supported by the Grant No. 3.820.076 from the Swiss National Science Foundation and by a research grant from the Swiss Society for Odontostomatology.

REFERENCES

Asgar, K., and Giday Z., 1978. Refinements on testing of porcelain to metal bond. Intern. Assoc. Dent. Res., 57th Gen. Session, Washington D.C., abstr. 870, in: J.Dent.Res., 57 (A), 292.

Barraud, R., Meyer, J.M., Susz, C.P., and Nally, J.N., 1978. Properties of nickel-vanadium-chromium alloys. Intern. Assoc. Dent. Res., 56th Gen. Session, Washington D.C., abstr. 719, in: J.D.Res., 57(A), 254.

Barraud, R., Meyer, J.M., Susz, C.P., and Nally, J.N., 1979. Properties of Ni-V-Cr-X alloys. Intern. Assoc. Dent. Res., Continental Europ. Div. 16th Annual Meeting, Athens. To appear in: J.Dent.Res.

Barraud, R., Susz, C.P., Meyer, J.M., and Nally, J.N., 1977. Effects of additions on the mechanical properties of V-Ni alloys. Intern. Ass. Dent. Res., Continental Europ. Div., 14th Annual Meeting, Rome, abstr. 14, in: J.Dent.Res., 56 (D), D-137.

Geret, V., Rahn, B.A., Mathys, R., Straumann, F., and Perren, S.M., 1979. Methode zur quantitativen Auswertung der Gewebsverträglichkeit bei verminderter Relativbewegung zwischen Implantat und Gewebe. Helvetica Chirurgica Acta, 46, 189-193.

Mansfeld, F., 1973. Simultaneous determination of instantaneous corrosion rate and Tafel slopes from polarisation resistance measurements. J. Electrochem. Soc., 120: 515-518.

Meyer, J.M., Barraud, R., Susz, C.P., and Nally, J.N., 1977. Electrochemical properties of V-Ni and V-Ni-X alloys. Intern. Assoc. Dent. Res., Continental Europ. Div., 14th Annual Meeting, Rome, abstr. 11, in: J.Dent.Res., 59 (D), D-136.

Proposed ANSI/ADA Specification No. 38 for porcelain-gold alloy systems, January 28, 1980.

Süry, P., and Semlitsch, M., 1979. Corrosion behavior of cast and forged cobalt-based alloys for double-alloy joint endoprostheses. J. Biomed. Mat. Res., 12 (5): 723-741.

Susz, C.P., Meyer, J.M., and Nally, J.N., 1977. Ni-V alloys as a possible dental casting alloy system. Intern. Assoc. Dent. Res. 55th Gen. Meeting, Copenhagen, abstr. 35, in: J.Dent.Res., 56 (A), A51.

Biomaterials 1980
Edited by G. D. Winter, D. F. Gibbons, and H. Plenk, Jr.
© 1982 John Wiley and Sons Ltd.

TANTALUM AND NIOBIUM AS POTENTIAL PROSTHETIC MATERIALS

S. Schider and H. Bildstein

Metallwerke Plansee A.G., Reutte/Tirol, Austria

SUMMARY

The pure metals tantalum and niobium are introduced as materials for the manufacture of heavy load-bearing prosthetic devices. They combine excellent corrosion resistance and bioinertness with good ductility and workability. Using powder metallurigal techniques such as pressing, sintering and cold working in combination with dispersion hardening, the mechanical properties of tantalum and niobium can be adapted over a wide range to particular implant applications, for example, cerclage wires, intramedullary nails and surface structured stems of joint endoprostheses for cementless implantation.

In this paper, the first mechanical test results are presented which show that cold-worked tantalum achieves a fatigue strength comparable to the best cobalt-based alloys despite the fact that it exhibits only about half the ultimate strength at the same elongation. These values were the same in distilled water and in Ringer's solution. Similarly good results have been obtained so far with niobium. Due to their greater ductility and very low tendency to stress-corrosion, tantalum and niobium can be regarded as an alternative to the ultra high strength alloys at present in use and under development for highly stressed implants.

INTRODUCTION

Metals constitute one of the most suitable materials for load-bearing implants: they are extremely hard and strong, but exhibit good ductility and can also be easily worked. The stainless steels and cobalt-based alloys that have hitherto been used for load-bearing implants exhibit the necessary strength and good biocompatibility as long as a smooth shape in a metallurgically perfect state is obtained. However, failure to achieve an optimal metal structure and the machining of the implant to obtain porous or surface structured shapes for mechanical interlocking with skeletal tissue can have a detrimental effect on the corrosion resistance and biocompatibility of the metal and even result in material failure. A decisive improvement in biocompatibility has been brought about by the introduction of titanium as an implant material, but the hexagonal crystal structure of this metal makes it liable to cracks and fractures: this has already been established, for example, with dental implants (Branemark et al, 1977).

In view of these limitations to the metallic implant materials at present in use, this paper now presents the metals tantalum and niobium which in the view of the authors exhibit excellent biocompatibility coupled with the necessary mechanical properties. Up until now the biocompatibility and ductility of tantalum have only been used for the manufacture of surgical nets and wires, vascular and other clips, pacemaker electrodes, etc. (Contzen et al, 1967, Frank & Zitter, 1971, Johnson et al, 1977). Tantalum has also been found suitable for dental implants (Scialom, 1962, Heinrich, 1971) for which long-term osseous anchorage has been demonstrated (Grundschober et al, in these Proceedings)..

The chemical and mechanical properties of niobium are similar to those of tantalum, and the present paper reports on the results obtained so far in improving the mechanical properties of both metals, which can now be used for the manufacture of load-bearing devices for orthopaedic and traumatic surgery.

MATERIALS AND METHODS

Chemical and physical properties: Tantalum and niobium belong to the 5th group of the periodic system of elements and are thus highly reactive, refractory metals (Kieffer & Braun, 1963, Frank & Zitter, 1971). For this reason they are spontaneously covered by an oxide layer. Their crystals are body-centred cubic, resulting in the excellent ductility of the pure metal due to the six possible slip planes. The most important physical properties of the two pure metals are listed in Table 1.

TABLE 1: Physical properties of tantalum and niobium

Physical properties	Tantalum	Niobium
Melting point	2996 °C	2445 °C
Density	16.6 g/cm^3	8.66 g/cm^3
Vickers hardness	500–1800 MPa	500–1800 MPa
Tensile strength	300–1000 MPa	350–1000 MPa
Elongation	10–40%	10–40%
Young's modulus	1.9×10^5 MPa	1.15×10^5 MPa
Specific electrical resistance	12.5 $\mu\Omega$cm	14.2 $\mu\Omega$cm
Coefficient of linear expansion	6.5×10^{-6}	6.9×10^{-6}

Corrosion properties and biocompatibility: The layer of oxide which forms spontaneously on tantalum and niobium makes these metals so resistant to corrosion that they will resist the attack of most chemical agents, with the exception of a few fluorinated and hot acidic mixtures and corrosive molten salts. For this reason they are used in the chemical industry, high-temperature processes, electronics and the aerospace industry. Stimulating electrodes of tantalum have also exhibited excellent corrosion resistance both in vitro and in vivo (Johnson et al, 1977). At the same time, this chemically stable oxide layer results in an inertness which in the opinion of the authors accounts for the good tissue compatibility of this base metal, whereas a noble metal such as gold, though resistant to corrosion, is not sufficiently biocompatible due to its catalytic metallic surface (Contzen et al, 1967).

Metallurgical techniques and workability: Tantalum and niobium are refractory metals and therefore unsuitable for casting (see Table 1). The pure metal is obtained in powder form chiefly by electrolysis and worked using powder metallurgical techniques such as pressing, sintering or arc melting under high vacuum conditions and cold working. Powder metallurgical techniques make it possible to obtain increased strength by dispersion hardening (for example, by mixing the powder with a hard phase powder or by heat treatment in a low pressure gas atmosphere).

Several types of implants and test specimens were manufactured from pure tantalum and niobium powders using these techniques.
a)   The porous material for bone ingrowth tests was pressed (1.5-3 t/cm2) together with 5% PMMA spheres ($\emptyset$ 100 - 300 μ m) which were burned out at 350° C under vacuum conditions. The specimens were then sintered for 30 minutes by indirect heating at 2050° C and 10^{-5} Torr. This method resulted in a porosity of 30-40% with pore sizes between 100 and 300 μ m (mean 190 μ m) (Figure 1a). The shafts of a hinged tantalum knee joint prosthesis (Figure 1b) were also given a porous coating using this method.
b)   The dense material for the intramedullary stems of these artificial knee and hip joint prostheses in animals, for smooth and grooved test specimens (Weiss et al, 1979) and for cerclage wire was pressed (2-4 t/cm2) and sintered by direct current heating (duration > 10 hours, temperature 0.8-0.9 of the melting temperature in K° at 10^{-5} Torr). The test specimens and cerclage wire were then cold forged and drawn, while the prosthetic stems were cold forged and drop forged to different shapes (Figure 2a-c). The conical grooves in the surface ($\emptyset$ 300 and 900 μ m, Figure 2b) were produced on the test specimens and on the stems of the hip joint endoprostheses by cold working. Some of the hip joint endoprostheses were sand-blasted to obtain a micro roughness (Figure 2b).
c)   Intramedullary nails for human patients were manufactured by isostatic pressing (1000-3000 bar), indirect sintering (duration > 10 hours, temperature 0.8-0.9 of the melting temperature in K° at 10^{-5} Torr), extrusion, forging and drawing. The special non-rotating shape (Otte et al, 1980) was obtained by rolling and drawing (Figure 3).

Mechanical properties and test procedures: The mechanical properties of tantalum and niobium as found in literature (Kieffer & Braun, 1963, Frank & Zitter, 1971) and as determined in our own tests are shown in Table 1. Tensile tests were performed on standard test specimens,   on cerclage wires (1-1.5 mm diameter, made of differently processed tantalum and niobium and of 316 L stainless steel (Synthes, Switzerland)), and on intramedullary nails (12 mm diameter) made of tantalum, niobium and 316 L stainless steel (Küntscher nail, Synthes, Switzerland),   using a computer-aided Instron machine. Yield strength, ultimate strength and elongation were determined. Bending tests were also performed on the intramedullary nails with a distance of 350 mm between the supports and loads of 800 N.

The alternating fatigue strength was determined by an ultrasonic resonance load test (Weiss et al, 1979) at different load levels (200-400 N) and at 20 kHz and at least 10^7 loading cycles were applied. The tests were performed on smooth and grooved test specimens in distilled water and in Ringer's solution; the values presented in this report are only preliminary and were calculated for a 50% probability of failure.

MECHANICAL TEST RESULTS

The tensile strength of tantalum and niobium test specimens depends on manufacturing parameters, such as sintering conditions and type and degree of cold working. The range of ultimate strengths and corresponding elongations is given in Table 1. The effects of cold working and dispersion hardening on the mechanical properties of tantalum and niobium cerclage wire can be compared with the values for stainless steel in Table 2.

TABLE 2: Tensile strengths of cerclage wire $\emptyset$ 1-1.5 mm

	Yield strength σS (MPa)	Ultimate strength σB (MPa)	Elongation ε B %
Stainless steel (316L)	365	730	48.7
Tantalum:	243	330	40.3
Cold worked	533	578	4.4
Dispersion hardened	490-540	520-590	17-22
Niobium:	316	390	17-20
Cold worked	550	590	1.4
Dispersion hardened	837	920	7.9

Pure and annealed tantalum and niobium are soft and ductile. Cold working and/or dispersion hardening will considerably increase their strength, but are accompanied by a reduction in ductility. The results of the tensile tests with intramedullary nails are presented in Table 3. In this type of implant, too, tantalum and niobium exhibited a considerably lower strength than stainless steel at comparable elongations. In the bending tests up to a load of 400 N both metals showed an elastic deformation comparable to that of stainless steel, but at higher loads a much more pronounced plastic deformation was observed (Figure 4).

TABLE 3: Tensile strengths of intramedullary nails ($\emptyset$ 12 mm)

	Yield strength σS (MPa)	Ultimate strength σB (MPa)	Elongation $\varepsilon B \%$
Stainless steel (316L)	692	764	11.1
Tantalum	444	471	6.5
Niobium	468	509	7.5

The preliminary test results for the fatigue strength of cold-worked tantalum
and niobium are presented in Table 4: these values were the same in distilled
water and in Ringer's solution.

TABLE 4: Ultimate and fatigue strengths and elongation of cold-
worked tantalum and niobium test specimens.

	Ultimate strength σB (MPa)	Fatigue strength σW (MPa)	Elongation $\varepsilon B \%$
Tantalum	520	383	26
Niobium	306	227	30

DISCUSSION AND CONCLUSIONS

Both tantalum and niobium were expected to have a good biocompatibility, and
this has been demonstrated both in a cell culture (Contzen et al, 1967) and in
soft tissue (Laing et al, 1967). Comparative studies with human fibroblast
cultures and implants in the jawbones of dogs (Zetner et al, in press) have
demonstrated that neither tantalum nor titanium inhibit the growth of cells
and that both are tightly enveloped by osseous tissue, whereas dental gold and
a cobalt-based alloy inhibited cell growth and caused bone resorption. Our own
animal experiments with porous and grooved cylindrical implants of tantalum
and niobium demonstrated the growth of osseous tissue right up to the
implants and into the pores (Pflüger et al, (a), in these Proceedings). The same
positive effect has been demonstrated under loaded conditions for porous
surfaced tantalum knee joint prostheses in rabbits and grooved hip joint
prosthesis shafts in beagle dogs (Pflüger et al, (b), in these Proceedings). This
mechanical interlocking with bone tissue under so-called "unloaded" conditions, and even under heavy loading, points to the excellent biocompatibility of
both tantalum and niobium. In addition, tantalum, and in particular niobium
have a modulus of elasticity closer to that of bone than other high strength
metals and alloys: this fact may have contributed to the favourable bone
reaction.

It must be emphasised that the mechanical properties of tantalum and niobium
can be adapted to particular circumstances over a wide range simply by the
manner in which they are worked. This does not result in a reduction of

corrosion resistance and thus of tissue compatibility, as is the case when, for example, stainless steel is cold worked (Schuster, 1975).

The example of the "Otte-Plansee" intramedullary nail provided with a non-rotating profile (see Figure 3) also demonstrates that a high degree of bending strength can be obtained by a suitable shape, although the tensile strength of tantalum and niobium is considerably less that that of stainless steel. The bending behaviour of both metals does not appear to be a disadvantage with regard to the mode of insertion of intramedullary nails and their adaptation to the bone. In comparison with the specifications for the high grade prosthesis material Protasul 10® (Süry & Semlitsch, 1978), cold-worked tantalum only achieves about half the ultimate strength at the same extension, but with a comparable fatigue strength (see Figure 5). It should be mentioned that the fatigue strength of tantalum is about 50% of its ultimate strength, whereas the wrought cobalt-based alloy reaches only about 40% of its ultimate strength. It is the fatigue strength coupled with biocompatibility that is the most important criterion for materials suitable for the manufacture of long-term load-bearing implants. The results of these mechanical and animal experimental investigations indicate that tantalum is a promising material for this purpose. Similarly good results have also been obtained so far with niobium, which offers further advantages due to its lower modulus of elasticity, lower specific weight and better availability. With respect to their material characteristics, both metals can therefore be regarded as an alternative solution in the search for alloys of even greater tensile strength.

ACKNOWLEDGEMENTS

These studies were supported in part by the Austrian "Forschungsförderungs-fonds der Gewerblichen Wirtschaft" grant no. 3/1851-1/P. The authors are indebted to Dr. H. Plenk Jr. for substantial help in the preparation of this manuscript and to Drs. G. Pflüger, F. Grundschober, N. Böhler, W.D. Otte, B. Weiss and R. Stickler for their cooperation in the experimental, clinical and mechanical trials reported on in this study.

REFERENCES

Branemark, P.I., Hansson, B.O., Adell, R., Breine, U., Lindström, J., Hallen, O. & Öhman, A. (1977) Osseointegrated implants in the Treatment of the Edentulous Jaw-Experiences from a 10-year period pp 7-132. Almquist & Wiksell International, Stockholm.
Contzen, H., Strauman, F., Paschke, E. & Geißendörfer, R. (1967) Grundlagen der Alloplastik mit Metallen und Kunststoffen, pp 1-179. G. Thieme, Stuttgart.
Frank, E. & Zitter, H. (1971) Metallische Implantate in der Knochenchirurgie (Werkstoff-Verarbeitung-Operationseinsatz), pp 1-160. Springer, Wien-New York.
Grundschober, F., Kellner, G., Eschberger, J. & Plenk H.Jr. (in press) Long term osseous anchorage of endosseous dental implants made of tantalum and titanium. In Proceedings of the First World Biomaterials Congress, (Eds. G.D. Winter, D.F. Gibbons & H. Plenk Jr.). J. Wiley, Chichester.
Heinrich, B. (1971) Schrauben-Implantate. Quintessenz, 22/9, 1-5.

Johnson, P.F., Bernstein, J.J., Hunter, G., Dawson, W.W. & Hench, L.L. (1977) In vitro and in vivo analysis of anodized tantalum capacitive electrodes: corrosion response, physiology and histology. J. Biomed. Mater. Res., 11, 637-656.

Kieffer, R. & Braun, H. (1963) Vanadin-Niob-Tantal. Die Metallurgie der reinen Metalle und ihrer Legierungen, pp 1-347. Springer, Berlin-Göttingen-Heidelberg.

Laing, P.G., Ferguson, A.B.Jr. & Hodge, E.S. (1967) Tissue reaction in rabbit muscle exposed to metallic implants. J. Biomed. Mater. Res. 1, 135-149.

Otte, W.D., Schider, S. & Weisner, O. (1980) Knochenmarknagel und Verfahren zu seiner Herstellung. Patent No. 0008758, European Patent Office, 19-03-1980.

Pflüger, G., Plenk, H.Jr., Böhler, N., Grundschober, F. & Schider, S. (a) (in press) Bone reaction to porous and grooved stainless steel, tantalum and niobium implants. In Proceedings of the First World Biomaterials Congress, (Eds. G.D. Winter, D.F. Gibbons & H. Plenk Jr.). J. Wiley, Chichester.

Pflüger, G., Böhler, N., Grundschober, F., Plenk, H.Jr. & Schider, S. (b) (in press) Experimental studies on total knee and total hip joint endoprostheses made of tantalum. In Proceedings of the First World Biomaterials Congress, (Eds. G.D. Winter, D.F. Gibbons & H. Plenk Jr.). J. Wiley, Chichester.

Schuster, J. (1975) Die Metallose. In Praktische Chirurgie, (Ed. G. Maurer), Vol. 90, 1-110.

Scialom, J. (1962) Immediate needle implants. Inform. Dent. 44, 1606-1611.

Süry, P. & Semlitsch, M. (1978) Corrosion behaviour of cast and forged cobalt-based alloys for double-alloy joint endoprostheses. J. Biomed. Mater. Res. 12, 723-742.

Weiss, B., Stickler, R., Femböck, J. & Pfaffinger, K. (1979) High cycle fatigue and threshold behaviour of powder metallurgical Mo and Mo-alloys. Fatigue of Engineering Materials and Structures 2, 73-84.

Zetner, K, Plenk, H.Jr. & Strassl, H. (in press) Tissue and cell reactions in vivo and in vitro to different metals for dental implants. In Dental Implants, Materials and Systems, (Ed. G. Heimke). Hanser, Munich.

FIGURES

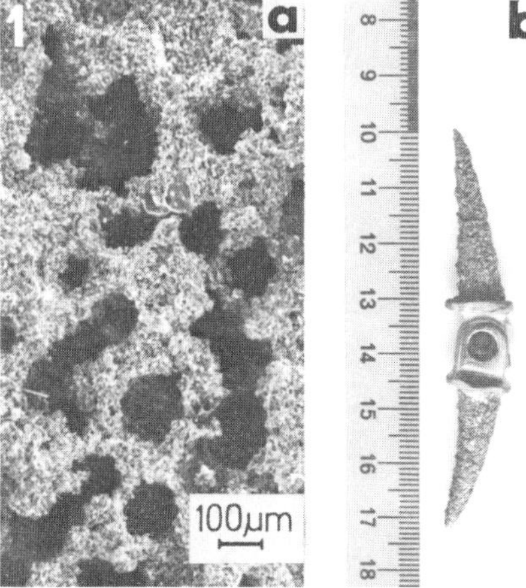

Figure 1: a) SEM picture of a porous sintered tantalum implant: b) Porous coated hinged tantalum knee joint endoprosthesis for the rabbit.

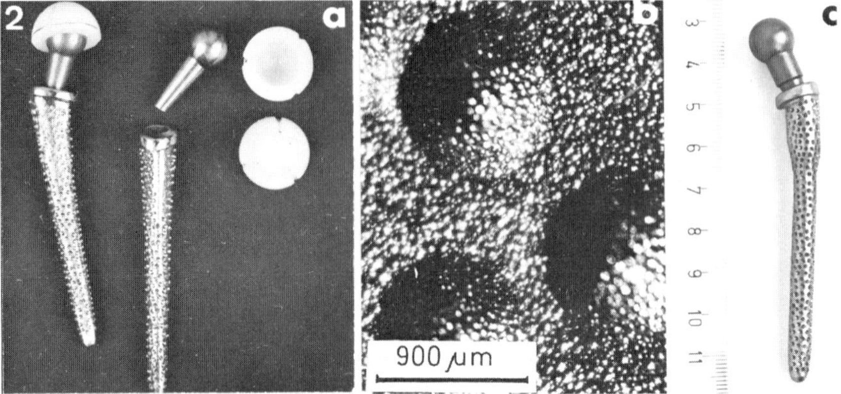

Figure 2: a) total hip joint endoprosthesis for the beagle dog, consisting of tantalum grooved stems and ball heads and polyethylene sockets; b) enlarged detail of the conical surface grooves of a tantalum stem after sand blasting; c) Niobium grooved stem and ball head for the same endoprosthesis.

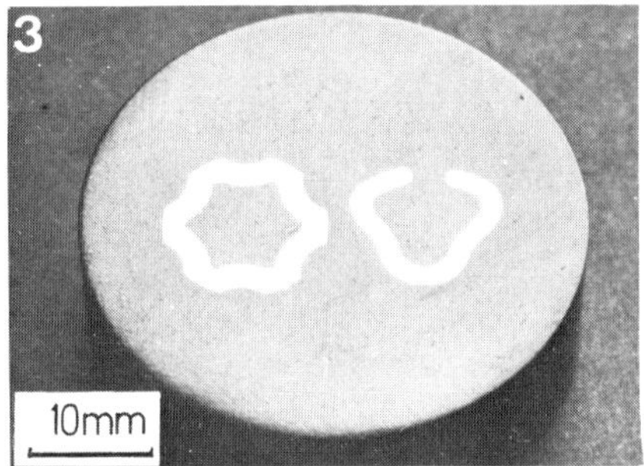

Figure 3: Surface polished cross sections of an "Otte-Plansee" intramedullary nail made of tantalum (left) and a stainless steel Küntscher nail (right).

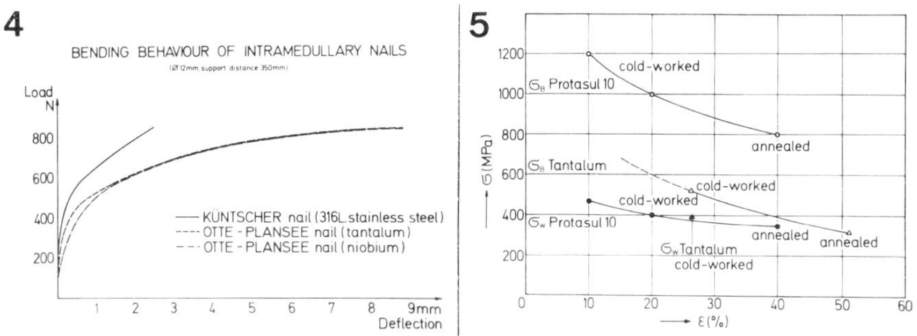

Figure 4: Bending behaviour of intramedullary nails ($\varnothing$ 12 mm) made of tantalum, niobium and 316 L stainless steel.

Figure 5: Relationship between strength (σ) and elongation (ε) for differently processed tantalum (Δ) in comparison to the data for Protasul 10® (o) as given by Süry and Semlitsch (1978).

Biomaterials 1980
Edited by G. D. Winter, D. F. Gibbons, and H. Plenk, Jr.
© 1982 John Wiley and Sons Ltd.

METAL FIBRE REINFORCED BIOGLASS COMPOSITES

P. Ducheyne and L.L. Hench

K.U. Leuven, Leuven, Belgium and University of Florida,
Gainesville, Florida

SUMMARY

The reinforcement of bioglass by ductile metal wires is an effective
means to prevent crack nucleation and propagation of the glass matrix. It has a major effect on the decrease of number of critical
crack length flaws, the formation of residual compressive stresses in
the glass and the crack blunting of the glass by suitable second
phase particles. The data show a strengthening effect by a factor 7
to 8 over the strength of the parent-glass. In addition, the ductility of the composites is large, since all bent test specimens are reproducibly bent over an angle greater than 90°. A major design advantage for implant applications of these bioglass composites is the
ability to be subjected to tensile stressing.

INTRODUCTION

Several new methods to attach permanent load bearing implants to the
skeleton have been proposed. Chemical bonding as a result of a sequence of reactions at the surface of a bioreactive implant material, such as bioglass, is one of the new methods developed
(Blencke et al., 1978, Clark et al., 1976, Ducheyne et al., 1979,
Hench et al., 1972, Pernot et al., 1979). Bioglasses however, have
limited mechanical strength and poor ductility.

Several approaches are possible to improve the mechanical properties
of bioglasses and make them suitable for practical implant purposes.
These include :
1) Apply bioglass as a coating on a suitable metal or ceramic substrate,
2) Crystalize the glass : it may reduce flaw size by the presence of
second phase crystals,
3) Reinforce the glass with a ductile second phase, which ideally
impedes crack formation and propagation.
These possibilities are the basis for a design rationale using ceramics in structural applications. Either the glass does not serve as
a structural component as is the case with bioglass coatings, or
strength and toughness can be increased by preventing crack initiation and propagation. To reach these goals, 1) the critical flaws in
the glass must be decreased, and/or 2) residual compressive stresses
in the glass must be achieved, and/or 3) cracks can be blunted by
adding second phase particles in the glass.

In this paper we report on the reinforcement of bioglass with ductile metal fibres. We also discuss the effectiveness of this reinforcement on strength and toughness and show that the increase of mechanical properties is mainly due to the mechanisms outlined above.

METHODS AND MATERIALS

Glass composites were made by dipping prepared metal fibre compacts into a molten glass batch. Stainless steel AISI 316 L fibres with a diameter of 50, 100 or 200 μm were moulded to different densities, typically between 40 and 60 volume %, yielding a metal to glass volume ratio of between 4/6 to 6/4. Stainless steel was chosen because of its appropriate thermal expansion coefficient which approaches that of bioglass. Bioglass type 45 S 5 with a composition (in weight %) 45 % SiO_2, 24.5 % Na_2O, 24.5 % CaO and 6 % P_2O_5 was used.

Flat specimens with a gauge length of 42 mm and a thickness of 2 mm were used. After dipping, the specimens were consecutively sand blasted and ground with a series of grits in order to remove the excess glass surrounding the composite. Tensile testing was performed in air with an initial cross-head speed of 0.2 mm/min. At 0.2 % yield stress the specimen was unloaded to clearly observe plasticity. Subsequently it was loaded till fracture at a cross-head speed which would yield fracture in about 15 minutes, i.e. 0.5 mm/min. An extensometer with span 10 mm and range 10 % was used throughout. Specimens were tested in three point bending with 3 cm span between supports and a cross-head speed of 0.5 mm/min.

Prior to testing some specimens were randomly selected for microstructural assessment. After testing, selected specimens were used for fractographic analysis, consisting of reflected light microscopy and scanning electron microscopy.

RESULTS AND DISCUSSION

Microscopic examination of untested specimens showed that initial cracks, if any, were present only in the outside rim of glass formed during the removal of the impregnated specimen from the melt. At no instance was cracking observed in the composite structure.

Energy dispersive X-ray analysis (EDXA) and electron microprobe analysis (EMP) revealed the presence of an interfacial oxide layer between the fibres and the glass. The transition from the stainless steel fibre to the bulk glass occurs through 1) a Fe-depleted and Cr-enriched oxide layer; 2) a layer with Fe in an amount comparable to the bulk composition, but with limited Cr; and 3) a glass layer displaying a gradual increase of Si-content. With a graded interface corresponding to chemical adhesion, stress transfer from the glass matrix to the reinforcing metal fibres may be expected to be much more effective than through purely frictional interaction at the interface.

In order to clearly see the onset of plastic deformation of the glass composite during tensile testing, the specimens were unloaded and reloaded. Fig. 1 shows a graph from a specimen with 60 vol % fibres of 100 μm diameter. Plastic deformation of up to 10 % elongation was reproducibly observed among the different types of composites.

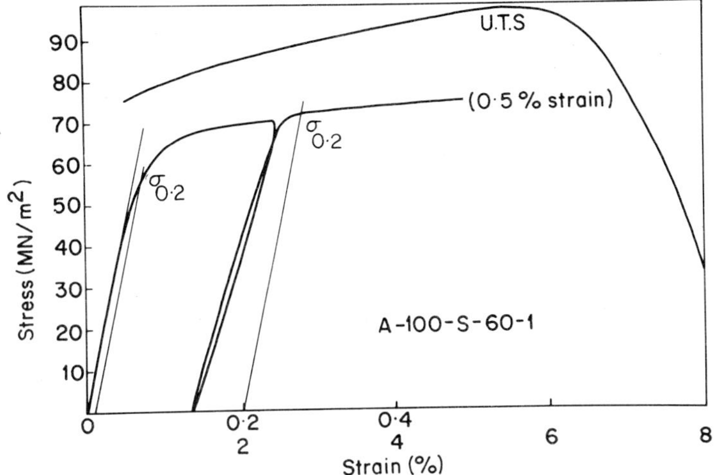

Fig. 1. Tensile graph of a composite with 60 vol % fibres of 100 μm diameter. Note the plastic deformation.

The mean strength values of these two types of bioglass fibre composites are represented in table 1. Results for the yield strength and ultimate tensile strength were obtained for a set of 20 specimens (tension) and 10 specimens (3-point bending).

TABLE 1. Mean strength values (0.01 % and 0.2 % yield strength and ultimate tensile strength) and standard deviation (s) of two types of composites, identified by fibre diameter and fibre content, as measured by tensile and three point bend testing.

	$\sigma_{0.01}$ (MPa)	s	$\sigma_{0.2}$ (MPa)	s	UTS (MPa)	s
50 μm, 45 vol %						
tension	61.9	11.8	78.3	11.2	91.9	15.2
bending			167.6	38.4	290.4	42.4
100 μm, 60 vol %						
tension	57.0	8.6	73.3	7.1	97.9	12.8
bending			162.9	31.4	339.9	71.9

The difference between strength as measured in tension and in three point bending, is however, striking. Three point bending produces a mean yield strength which is twice the value measured in tension and an ultimate strength three times the one obtained in tension. These differences are attributed to the nature of the tests and the distribution of microstructural flaws in the glass. In tensile testing,

the specimens fail in the weakest section since stresses are uniform
along the length of the specimens. In three-point bending the highest
stresses are generated under the load, which is not necessarily the
weakest section. In addition bend tests generally yield higher tensile strengths than tensile tests, depending upon the value of the
Weibull modulus, which describes the distribution of cracks (Lange,
1974). Flaws were located at the centre of the specimen due to en-
trapped air during dipping. These flaws will not markedly influence
strength in bending since normal stresses increase from nil at the
neutral axis to a maximum at the surface. Such flaws, however, will
influence the strength in tensile testing since the cross sectional
stress is uniform.

The data in table 1 provide substantial evidence for a large strengthening effect of bioglass by metal fibres. The ultimate tensile
strength previsouly measured in diametral compression was 42 MPa
(Housefield, 1972). The results obtained here show a strengthening by
a factor of at least 2 (tensile testing) and reaching as much as 8
(3-point bending). This result is markedly superior to any previously
reported strengthening of brittle matrix composites which was a
factor of 5.5 (Donald and McMillan, 1976).

The ductility of the composites is large. All specimens of both types
of composites were bent more than 90°, the maximum possible angle
with the set-up used (Fig. 2). Thus in addition to adding considerable
strength, the fibres transform a brittle glass into a plastically de-
formable glass composite.

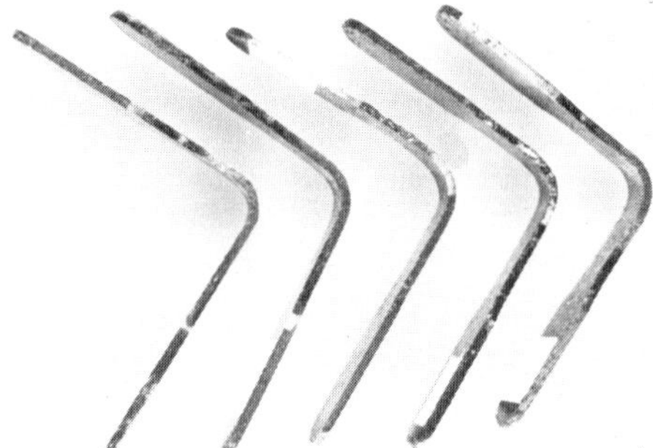

Fig. 2. Specimens (60 % fibres, 100 µm diameter) tested in
bending : a bend angle greater than 90° is obtained for
these brittle matrix composites.

Considering the tensile graph of fig. 1, one observes that strain
hardening is associated with the plastic deformation of the composite.
After reaching the maximum load the specimen continues to deform.
Specimens tested in tension up to 0.1 % plastic deformation did not
show any microstructural damage in the glass. Thus the onset of plastic deformation of the composite is probably due to plastic deformation of the metal fibres.
Microscopic analysis of fractured specimens, tested in tension, indicated that both at the fracture surface and remote from it cracks in

the glass were oriented perpendicular to the tensile direction.
Crack fronts were blunted at the metal fibre (fig. 3). Multiple
cracking in the glass at the fracture surface indicated that the
fibre-glass bonding remained good and there was effective stress
transfer between fibre and glass until final fracture. Scanning electron microscopy revealed that the extensive elongation at the fracture surface was almost exclusively due to the stretching and pull-
out of the fibres from the glassy matrix (fig. 4). These observations suggest a five step failure pattern for the composite :
1) failure is initiated by cracking of the glass perpendicular to the
tensile stressing direction; 2) the cracks are blunted by the presence of the fibres; 3) The fibres undergo plastic deformation followed by 4) debonding of fibres and glass; and 5) rupture of the metal fibres.
Since these failure steps are additive, a large increase in both
failure stress and strain to failure occurs for the composite.

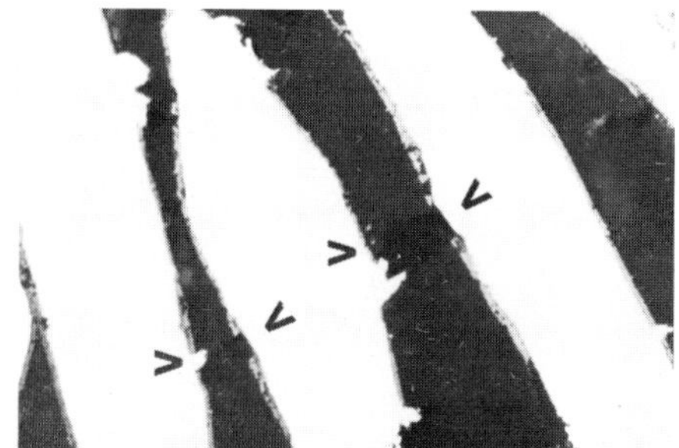

Fig. 3. Cross section of a tensile tested composite (45 %
fibres, 100 µm diameter) : the fibres blunt propagating
cracks.

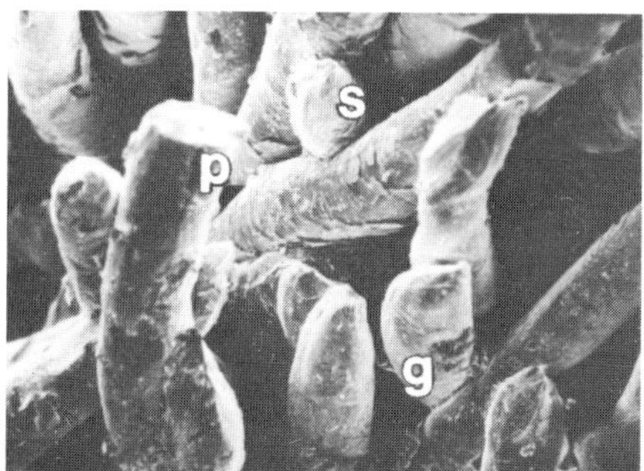

Fig. 4. Fracture surface of a tensile tested composite :
stretching and pull-out of the fibres and glass remnants are
indicated by S, P & G respectively.

CONCLUSIONS

Metal fibre reinforcement is an effective method for transforming bioglass into a structurally reliable material. Strength and toughness are markedly superior to the properties of the parent bioglass.

A major design advantage for implant applications of bioglass composites is the fact that they can be subjected to tensile stressing. Potential implant applications are coatings on permanent orthopaedic implants, bone plates and maxillofacial and dental implants. Additional work is directed towards the optimization of material properties through improvement of the fabrication technology, the study of composite laminates, in vitro corrosion testing, fatigue reliability and implantation.

ACKNOWLEDGEMENTS

The authors gratefully acknowledge the partial financial assistance of NATO Research Grant 1582 and the laboratory assistance of William Lacefield.

REFERENCES

Blencke, B.A., Broemer, H. & Deutscher, K.K. (1978) Compatibility and long term stability of glass-ceramic implants. J. Biomed. Mater. Res., 12, 307-316.

Clark, A.E. Jr., Hench, L.L. & Paschall, H.A. (1976) The influence of surface chemistry in implant interface histology : a theoretical basis for implant materials selection. J. Biomed. Mater. Res., 10, 161-174.

Donald, I.W. & McMillan, P.W. (1976) Ceramic-matrix composites. J. Mat. Sci., 11, 949-972.

Ducheyne, P., Hench, L.L., Kagan, A., II, Martens, M. & Mulier, J.C. (1979) Short term bonding behaviour of bioglass coatings on metal substrate. Archiv. Orthop. Traum. Surg., 94, 155-160.

Hench, L.L., Splinter, R.J., Allen, W.C. & Greenlee, T.K. Jr. (1972) Bonding mechanism at the interface of ceramic prosthetic materials. J. Biomed. Mater. Res. Symp., 2, 117-143.

Housefield, L.G. (1972) Mechanical property control of a bioglass-ceramic system. M. Sc. Thesis, U. Florida.

Lange, F.F. (1974) Strong, high-temperature ceramics, in Annual review of mater. sci. (Eds. Huggins, R.A., Bube, R.H., Roberts, R.W.) Annual Reviews Inc., 365-390, Palo Alto (California).

Pernot, F., Zarzycki, J., Bonnel, F., Rabischong, P. & Baldet, P. (1979) New glass-ceramic materials for prosthetic applications. J. Mat. Sci., 14, 1694-1706.

Biomaterials 1980
Edited by G. D. Winter, D. F. Gibbons, and H. Plenk, Jr.
© 1982 John Wiley and Sons Ltd.

NEW CARBON MATERIALS FOR JOINT PROSTHESES

H. Brückmann, H.-J. Mäurer, K. J. Hüttinger*,
H. Rettig**, U. Weber**

Schunk & Ebe GmbH, 6300 Gießen, FRG
* Institut für Chemische Technik der Universität Karlsruhe,
7500 Karlsruhe, FRG
** Orthopädische Klinik der Justus-Liebig-Universität,
6300 Gießen, FRG

SUMMARY

Three different carbon materials were developed for the use in endoprosthetics.
Their mechanical properties and tribological properties are described in comparison with other commonly used biomaterials and sliding combinations. The biocompatibility of the three carbon materials was tested by implanting powder
and bulk materials in rats, hares and dogs.

INTRODUCTION

In the early 1960 a solution to the problem of artificial joints seemed to be
found in the use of bone cement, special metal alloys and HDPE (Charnley,
1965). Satisfaction with the success of the first years soon changed to a con-
viction, that only by eliminating bone cement and replacing metal and HDPE
by more bioinert and wear resistant materials could long term stability and
function of artificial joints be obtained.

Carbon, known for its sliding capability under severe conditions (Savage and
Schäfer; 1956, Bowden and Tabor, 1964; Midgley and Teer, 1963) has excellent biocompatibility (Bokros, 1977; Weber, 1980). By varying the fabrication processes it is possible to manufacture carbon materials covering a wide
range of mechanical and tribological requirements (Brückmann and Hüttinger,
1980).

MATERIALS

For potential use as joint replacements, three materials were developed (Brückmann, 1979), two of which have good wear resistance, the third one being
capable of bearing high loads, as required for anchoring parts of endoprostheses.

27

(1) High strength isotropic carbon
    This material, having a glassy-carbon like, porous structure, is hard and
    highly wear resistant. In contrast to glassy carbon it is available in dimen-
    sions required for joint replacements. It is produced by pyrolysis of a
    semi-coke.

(2) Silicon-carbide/carbon composite (SiC/C)
    The manufacturing process includes the impregnation of a basic carbon grade
    with liquid silicon at a temperature of about 2.000 ^{o}C. In this process the
    silicon is completely transformed to silicon carbide. The resultant composite
    consists of two phases, SiC and C.

(3) Carbon-fibre reinforced carbon (CFRC)
    Most of the commonly known processes for manufacturing CFRC do not fit
    economic demands. A process has been developed, being capable of economi-
    cally manufacturing CFRC using pitch as a matrix precursor.

MECHANICAL PROPERTIES

Table 1 gives data on some characteristic properties of the three materials which
were evaluated.

TABLE 1. Mechanical properties of carbon based materials

		Isotropic C	SiC/C	CFRC
bulk density	(g/cm^3)	1,8	2,6	1,7
flexural strength	(N/mm^2)	140	220	800
Young's modulus	(kN/mm^2)	25	100	140
porosity	(%)	10	0	7

The Young's modulus of the isotropic carbon is nearly identical to that of
cortical bone. Considering that stress in artificial joints is not static, tests of
material behaviour under dynamic load are important. The most convenient
method was a bending test with a sinusoidaly varying load. Results from such
tests indicate, that isotropic C as well as SiC/C accept sinusoidal loading to
about 80 % of the level of static load to rupture. No significant difference
was found between experiments in air and Ringer's solution.

Figure 1 shows the fatigue strength and Young's moduli of all three carbon
materials in comparison with bone and two other commonly used biomaterials,
namely a CoCrMo alloy and alumina. This representation demonstrates possible
advantages of the carbon materials, especially if one compares the ratio of
fatigue strength and Young's modulus with that of femoral bone. The CFRC

material with its high fatigue strength may preferentially applied for shafts, whereas the isotropic carbon and the SiC/C materials are obviously suitable for sliding parts like ball and socket.

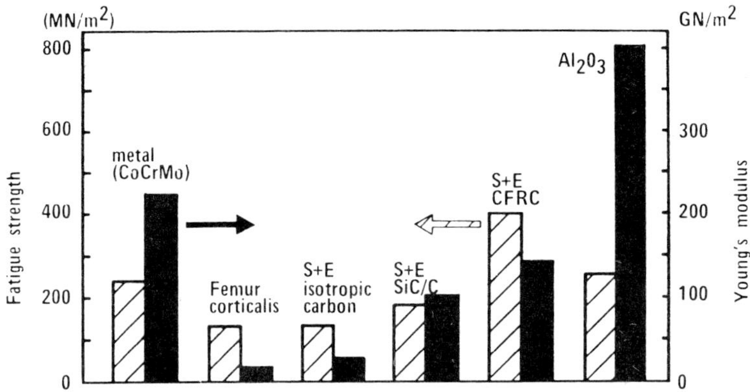

Fig. 1. Fatigue strength and Young's modulus of selected biomaterials (S+E = products developed by Schunk & Ebe GmbH)

TRIBOLOGICAL PROPERTIES

An extended program for testing friction and wear using ring-on-disk- and ball-in-socket have been used. In each case, the combinations SiC/C - isotropic C as well as SiC/C - SiC/C were found to give the best results. The ring-on-disk-test was carried out under specific pressures of 10 - 30 MN/m^2 and a relative speed of 0,05 m/sec. The ring is oscillating ± 30 degree.

The penetration depth of the ring in the disk was about 2 - 2,5 /um at 100 km sliding distance (specific pressure 20 MN/m^2). The coefficients of friction were clearly below 0,1 in the whole testing range. Due to the open porosity of the carbon surfaces, dry friction is not to be expected. The lubricant is always available close to the point of highest load.

Figure 2 shows a comparative study of different prostheses in the ball-in-socket-test. The in vitro data of the sliding combinations Al$_2$O$_3$ - HDPE respectively CoCrMo - HDPE are in agreement with clinical experiences, i. e. the combination with a femoral cup of alumina shows a better performance than with a CoCrMo-cup. The SiC/C - isotropic C-combination however represents the sliding pair with the absolutely lowest wear.

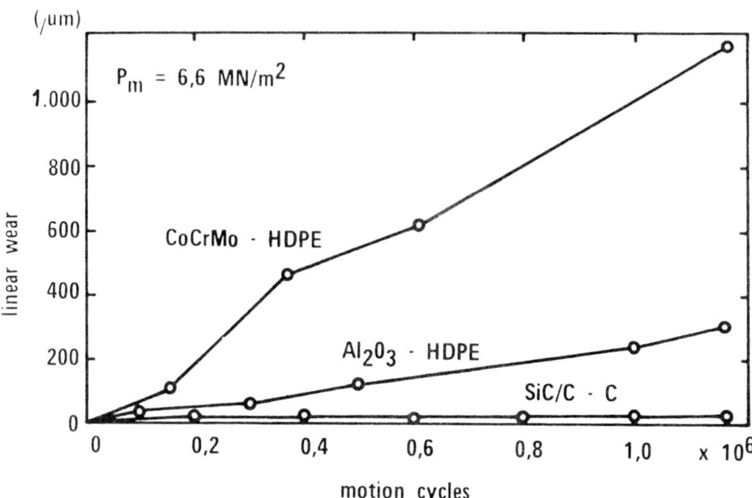

Fig. 2. Wear of different cups versus motion cycles, mean pressure of all prostheses 6,6 MN/m^2 (ball-in-socket-test).

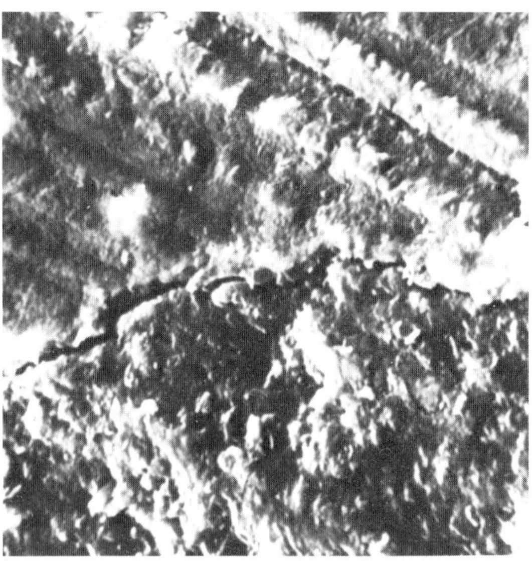

Fig. 3. Scanning picture of a carbon-bone interface of carbon implants in dog-femurs (20 weeks), top: bone, bottom: carbon

BIOCOMPATIBILITY

Biocompatibility of C, SiC and elemental Si was tested by implanting powders of different grain sizes as well as bulk materials in rats, hares and dogs. All three materials were found to be biocompatible. Bone was found to grow into contact with the material without gathering a layer of connective tissue (Fig. 3). Push out tests of non loaded implants in the femoral condyles of dogs show a complete ingrowth of bone into the thread of a carbon screw (lentgh 9 mm, thickness 7 mm, screw pitch 2 mm, thread depth 1 mm) (Fig. 4).

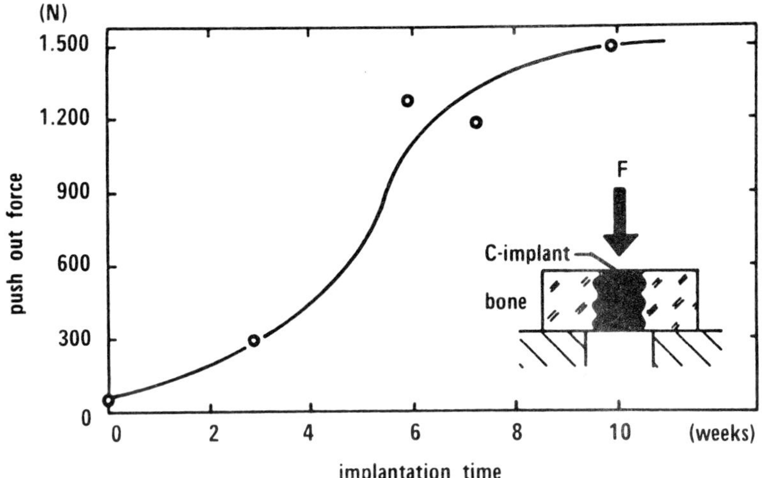

Fig. 4. Strength of osseous bone/implant interface (dog experiments)

CONCLUSIONS

The three fabricated carbon materials meet the requirements for joint replacement materials. The mechanical as well as tribological properties seem to show some advantages over other prosthetic materials. The biocompatibility gives hope, that cementless anchoring of joint prostheses might be possible.

REFERENCES

Bokros, J. C. (1977) Carbon 15, 355
Bowden, F. B. & Tabor, D. (1964) The friction and lubrication of solids II, Oxford University Press
Brückmann, H. & Hüttinger, K. J. (1980) Biomaterials 2, in press
Brückmann, H. (1979) Doctor thesis, University Gießen
Charnley, J. (1965) J. Bone Jt. Surg., 47 B, 354
Midgley, J. W. & Teer, D. G. (1963) Transact. of ASME, 12, 488
Savage, R. H. & Schäfer, D. L., (1956) J. Appl. Phys. 27, 136
Weber, U. (1980) Thesis submitted for the certificate of habilitation, Uni Gießen

Biomaterials 1980
Edited by G. D. Winter, D. F. Gibbons, and H. Plenk, Jr.
© 1982 John Wiley and Sons Ltd.

INVESTIGATION OF MECHANICAL BEHAVIOUR OF FIBRE-REINFORCED MATERIALS FOR ENDOPROSTHETIC DEVICES

U. Soltész, H. Richter

Fraunhofer-Institut für Werkstoffmechanik, Freiburg, GFR

SUMMARY

Seven carbon and glass fibre reinforced plastics are investigated.
Their quasistatic material properties are characterized by Young's
and bending moduli and by tensile and flexural strengths. The time
dependent properties are studied in creep and fatigue tests under
normal laboratory as well as simulated physiological conditions. In
addition the water absorption is also determined. With regard to
structural differences, the suitability of these composites for the
femoral stem component is discussed.

INTRODUCTION

Fibre-reinforced materials, because of their properties and behaviour, can offer a new approach to the development of improved implants and endoprostheses. Compared with isotropic materials they offer a greater possibility for matching the mechanical properties of
a structure to the problem to be solved; for example, to transfer
the load to bone in a physiological acceptable manner.

Most of the composites which are successfully used in engineering applications cannot be considered biocompatible because of purity or
composition. This paper deals with various fibre-reinforced plastics
which can be considered for medical applications since they are composed of materials proved to be biocompatible or of materials for
which no incompatibility is anticipated. These composites have been
developed by several companies as a bone replacement material, but
they are still in the developmental stage.

In this paper, only the mechanical behaviour of these materials is
described; the biological characterization is presented by Ehard et
al. (1980). The main purpose of the investigation was a screening,
using simple specimen geometries and test arrangements, in order to
determine the range of mechanical properties and evaluate the suitability of these composites for different endoprosthetic devices. However, a final assessment of the suitability can only be achieved by
testing the final device.

MATERIALS AND METHODS

The materials investigated consist of Polyethylene (PE), Polymethylmethacrylate (PMMA), Epoxy (EP), or a Cyanate (CY) resin as the ma-

TABLE 1. Characterization of materials

| MATERIAL CODE | FIBRES | | | | MATRIX | | STRUCTURE |
	MATERIAL	TRADE NAME	ORIEN-TATION	VOL %	MATERIAL	TRADE NAME	
GF-PE-X	E GLASS	GEVETEX	BIDIR. 0°,90°	40	POLYETHYLENE HMW	LUPOLEN 5261 Z	LINEN WEAVE
GF-PE-I	E GLASS	GEVETEX	MOSTLY UNIDIR. 0°	40	POLYETHYLENE HMW	LUPOLEN 5261 Z	LINEN WEAVE 840:100
CF-PMMA-I	CARBON HIGH TENSILE	SIGRAFIL A	UNIDIR. 0°	35-40	POLYMETHYL-METACRYLATE	PLEXIGLAS	ROVINGS
CF-EP-I	CARBON HIGH TENSILE	TORAYCA T 500	UNIDIR. 0°	65-70	EPOXY	ARALDITE EPN 1139 +HT 976	ROVINGS
CF-EP-II	CARBON HIGH MODULUS	TORAYCA M 40	UNIDIR. 0°	65-70	EPOXY	ARALDITE EPN 1139 +HT 976	ROVINGS
CF-CY-IV	CARBON HIGH MODULUS	MODMOR I + GRAFIL HM-S	UNIDIR. 0° FLEECE	40	CYANATE RESIN	TRIAZIN A	SANDWICH: ROVINGS +FLEECE
CF-CY-IV-PE	CARBON HIGH MODULUS	MODMOR I + GRAFIL HM-S	UNIDIR. 0° FLEECE	40	CYANATE RESIN	TRIAZIN A	SAME AS CF-CY-IV +PE-COATING

trix component and either carbon (CF) or glass (GF) fibres as reinforcing material. They are described in more detail in Table 1.

The composites differ with respect to structural features. Most of
the composites utilize unidirectional fibres; however in one case,
the glass-fibre reinforced PE, the fibres are oriented bidirectionally, and in another, the cyanate resin based materials, an even more
complicated structure is used. In the latter case, layers with long
unidirectional oriented fibres alternate with layers containing
short fibre fleeces. Because of these structural differences the measured properties must be compared with caution.

Because of the pronounced anisotropy of these composites it was necessary to characterize the influence of the matrix by performing
different tests such as uniaxial tension and bending with various
specimen lengths. The dimensions of the specimens and the support
conditions are listed in Table 2. In addition to the quasistatic properties the time dependent properties were also studied. Creep tests
were performed in a loading range which was expected to simulate the
actual physiological conditions. The fatigue strength was determined
under cyclic loading with a frequency of 10 Hz, a minimum load of
10 % of the quasistatic strength and up to $2 \cdot 10^7$ cycles. In addition
to testing under normal laboratory conditions (LAB) the tests were
also performed in a Ringer-solution at 37°C to simulate the physiological environment (PHYS).

The water absorption of the composite materials was determined by
storing square plate specimens in Ringer's solution (see Table 2).

RESULTS

Quasistatic conditions. The measured Young's Moduli and strengths
are depicted in Fig. 1 where the results obtained from different
test configurations are marked by different hatchings (cf. Table 2).
The highest moduli are measured in the tensile tests, in bending

they are lower and decrease with decreasing specimen length. This observation can be explained in terms of increasing nonuniformity of
the stress field, which accentuates the influence of the matrix on
the elastic behaviour. All CF-materials display a linear stress-
strain dependence whereas the GF-materials show various nonlineari-
ties due to the organization of the fibres in the linen weave. Comparison of the materials shows that the moduli vary over more than one
order of magnitude.

The strength measurements with continously increasing load exhibit a
similar influence of the test configuration and range of values.

Creep behaviour. To describe the creep behaviour a normalized deflec-
tion, which is equal to the reciprocal bending modulus, is plotted
versus the loading time in Fig. 2. For the EP based materials the
creep rate can be regarded as negligible and is most pronounced for
GF-PE. All materials show an increased creep rate under simulated
physiological conditions when compared with those under the normal

TABLE 2. Test methods,
specimen configurations
and conditions

TESTS	SPECIMENS	SYMBOL
UNIAXIAL TENSION	200×15×1-2 mm³	
3-POINT BENDING		
LONG BEAMS 16:1	100×10×5 mm³	
SHORT BEAMS 8:1	60×10×5 mm³	
ABSORPTION	50×50×5 mm³	

CONDITIONS		
ENVIRONMENTS	AIR, ROOM TEMP.	LAB
	RINGER SOLUTION, 37°C	PHYS
FATIGUE	PULSATING, 10Hz	

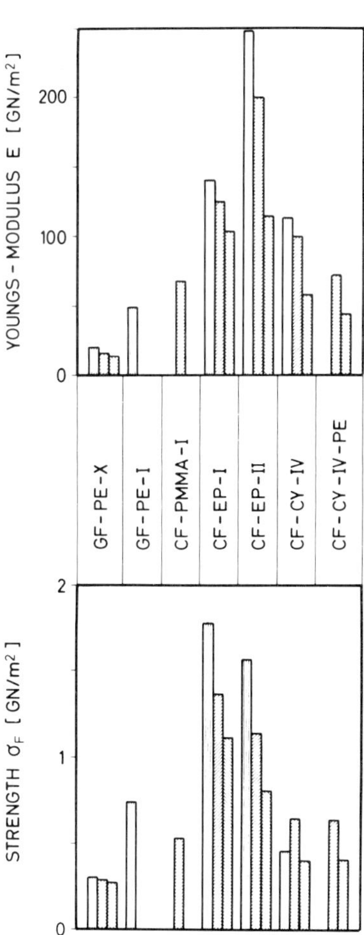

Fig. 1. Youngs-modulus and
strength for quasistatic
loading conditions

                  U. Soltész and H. Richter

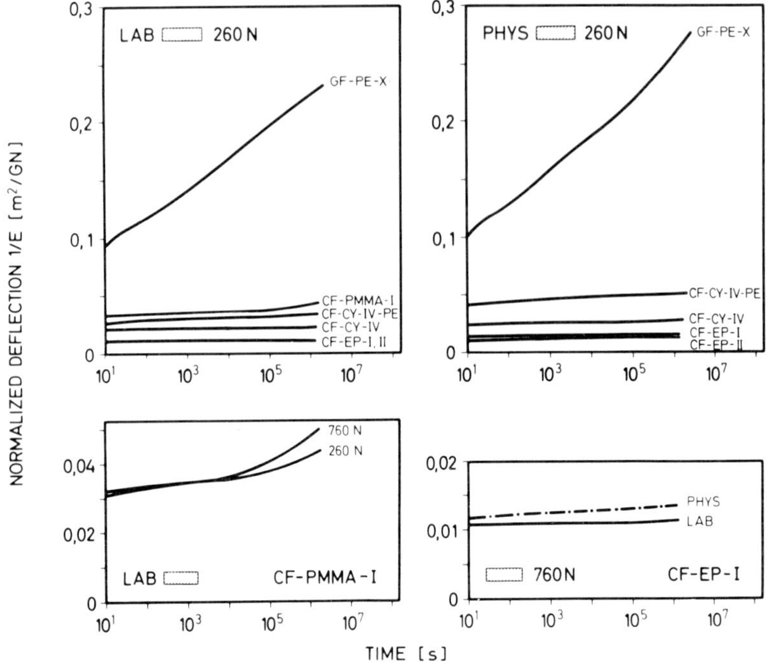

Fig. 2. Creep behaviour

environment. This influence is illustrated in more detail for CF-
EP-I in Fig. 2. An influence of load level can be observed for CF-
PMMA (Fig. 2) and even more pronounced for GF-PE.

Fatigue behaviour. The results of the fatigue tests are presented in
Fig. 3 as Wöhler-diagrams with the data fitted to straight lines.
For all materials the fatigue strength decreases markedly as the required number of cycles to failure increases. For some materials,
the strength decreases to about 30 % of the quasistatic strength
within the range of cycles investigated. Furthermore, they show an
additional decrease under simulated physiological test conditions
compared with their behaviour under laboratory conditions. This is
illustrated in more detail for CF-EP-II in Fig. 3. The test configuration also influences the fatigue strength in a way similar to quasistatic loading (Fig. 3).

Water absorption. The water absorption is depicted in Fig. 4. Within
the time investigated it amounts to about 0.5 - 1 % for the CF-materials but it is negligible for the GF-PE.

DISCUSSION

The data reported in this paper must be interpreted with caution
when applying them to actual clinical cases. This is because the measurements were partially performed utilizing specimens containing

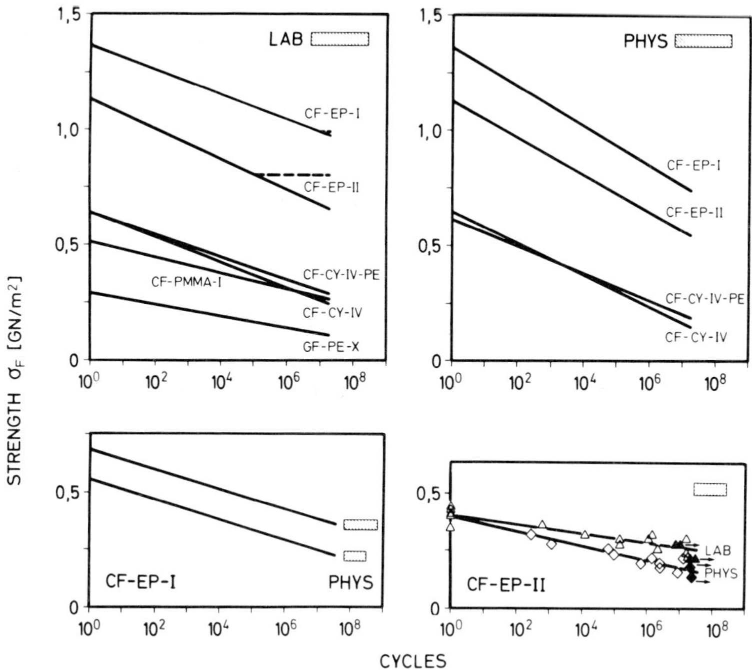

Fig. 3.: Fatigue behaviour

unidirectionally arranged fibres, whereas in real structures such fibre arrangements will generally not be acceptable. Therefore, in particular, the measured strength values are higher than the strengths of real structures. On the other hand, measurements performed on bidirectionally reinforced or fleece containing specimens simulate clinical conditions more closely.

Nevertheless, an attempt is made in Fig.5 to estimate the suitability of the materials investigated for application to the highly loaded femoral component of a hip-joint. The flexural fatigue strength for $2 \cdot 10^7$ cycles, represented by the bars, is compared with the range of maximum possible stresses in a conventionally designed stem which is indicated by the curves. Röhrle and Scholten (1978) found that in stems of identical shape the stresses increase with increasing stiffness. Therefore, the comparison is made using the

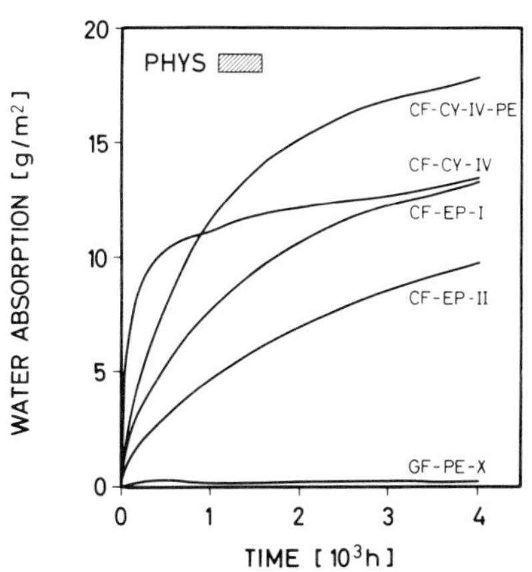

Fig. 4. Water absorption

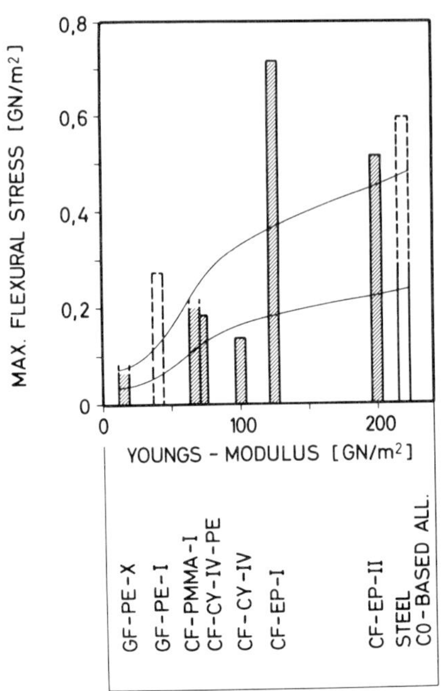

Fig. 5. Comparison of material strength (bars) with calculated stress levels (curves) in the femoral stem component for normal and extreme loading during walking

bending modulus. For evaluating the range of the maximum stresses different body weights (750 N up to 900 N) and increased loading due to inertial effects produced during normal or fast walking have also been considered.

It is to be seen that, even taking into account reduced values for the unidirectional tested materials, all materials would sustain the lower loads without failure, but that only the CF-EP-I would have a sufficient strength for the higher loads (Fig. 5). On the other hand, it seems possible that the stresses in the stem could be reduced by a suitable change in design and that the materials can be further improved. In any case, a final assessment of these materials has to be made on the basis of an actual clinical application.

REFERENCES

Ehard, H.; Köster-Lösche, K.; Kubicek, J. (1980) Tierexperimentelle und pathomorphologische Untersuchungen zur Reaktion des primären Knochenlagers nach Implantation verschiedener neu entwickelter Biomaterialien - CaP-Keramiken, CaP-Keramik-Polymere und Faserverbundwerkstoffe. 2. Münchner Symp. f. Exp. Orthopädie
Röhrle, H.; Scholten, R. (1978) Private communication, unpublished

This work is sponsored by the German Ministry for Research and Technology (BMFT) and several companies. The CF-EP materials were supplied by MAN-NT, München.

Tissue reaction to hard tissue implant materials

Biomaterials 1980
Edited by G. D. Winter, D. F. Gibbons, and H. Plenk, Jr.
© 1982 John Wiley and Sons Ltd.

CULTURED CELLS CONTACTING IMPLANT MATERIAL OF DIFFERENT SURFACE TREATMENT.

B. A. Rahn *, H.W. Gerber *, J. Simpson **,
F. Straumann **, and S. M. Perren *

* Laboratory for Experimental Surgery,
Swiss Research Institute,
Davos, Switzerland

** Straumann Institute,
Waldenburg, Switzerland

SUMMARY

The surface of titanium disks had been treated to result in a
different degree of roughness. Chondrocytes were cultured on these
disks. Cells presented a more flat shape on smooth surfaces and a
more rounded shape on rougher surfaces. An intimate contact
between cells and substratum seems to be advantageous to minimize
mechanical irritation, to prevent spreading of bacteria and to
reduce the accumulation of corrosion products.

INTRODUCTION

A given implant material may be provided with a variety of
different surface structures. Smooth surfaces have the least
surface area and therefore a low area-dependent corrosion rate and
possible stress concentrations caused by micronotches are avoided.
For these reasons most orthopedic implants are smooth. On the
other hand bone ingrowth into porous implants is a common finding
and rough implants are advocated for better anchorage. In this
paper we describe the morphology of cells after their exposure in
tissue culture to titanium surface structures of different
roughness.

MATERIALS AND METHODS

Commercially pure titanium disks (SNV 056 507, diameter 10.8mm, thickness 1.3mm) were provided with six different surfaces. 1.Mechanically polished with Al_2O_3 (grain size $1\mu m$). 2.chemically polished(20% HF, 20% HNO_3, 60% formic acid for 1 minute). 3.chemically etched(10% HNO_3, 1% HF for 1 minute at 40-50 ^{o}C) and anodically oxidized (80% H_3PO_4, 10% H_2SO_4, 70V, resulting in an oxyde layer of approximately 60nm). 4.chemically etched and anodically oxydized (120V, resulting in an oxyde layer of approximately 100nm). 5.sandblasted. 6.coated with plasma sprayed titanium.

The disks were defatted in Xylene, washed in ethanol, in distilled water and then steam sterilized. Chondrocytes from young adult rat sterna were enzymatically isolated (Hyaluronidase 3 minutes, Trypsin 30 minutes, Collagenase 90 minutes), and washed in F12 growth medium (Ham). A drop of the suspension (ca.7500 cells) was placed on the center of the specimen surfaces and also on glass coverslips. They were cultivated in F12 growth medium until there was a coherent cell layer in the center of the control coverslips as shown by phase contrast microscopy. Then all specimen were rinsed in Gey's balanced salt solution, fixed in 1.5% glutaraldehyde in a Na-cacodylate buffer, critical point dried and gold sputtered (ca.20nm). The examination was performed using reflected light Nomarski interference phase contrast and scanning electron microscopy (SEM).

RESULTS

The treatment of the titanium disks resulted in surfaces of different roughness. Sandblasting and plasma coating produced differences in altitude of up to one to two tenths of a mm between the deepest indentation and the highest elevation. The edges of the plasma coating were rounded, sandblasting produced sharp edges. The other finishing techniques provided smoother surfaces with differences in altitude smaller than a few micrometers. The multilayer arrangement of cells in the centre of the disks tapered towards the border to a monolayer, coherent groups and finally single cells. Depending on the degree of roughness of the substratum, two main patterns of cell contact morphology could be observed.

On <u>smooth</u> surfaces (mechanically polished, chemically polished, anodically oxidized) the cells were flat, adhering over a large area to the metal. On the mechanically polished disks the cells were flat and had relatively few and short processes. Chemically polished surfaces were covered with ´superflat´ cells (Fig.1) having short flat processes. On the anodically oxidized (ca.60nm) specimens there were flat or slightly raising cells comparable to the ones found on glass coverslips. On the ca.100nm oxide layer, a low cell density was observed, the cells being very flat and having short processes.

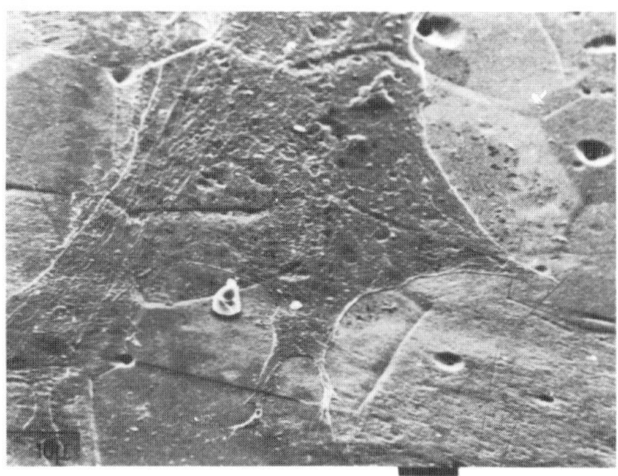

Fig.1 "Superflat" cell on a smooth (chemically polished) titanium surface. The cell plasma is widely spread and not influenced by the grain boundaries of the substratum. The cells reach a diameter of almost a tenth of a mm.

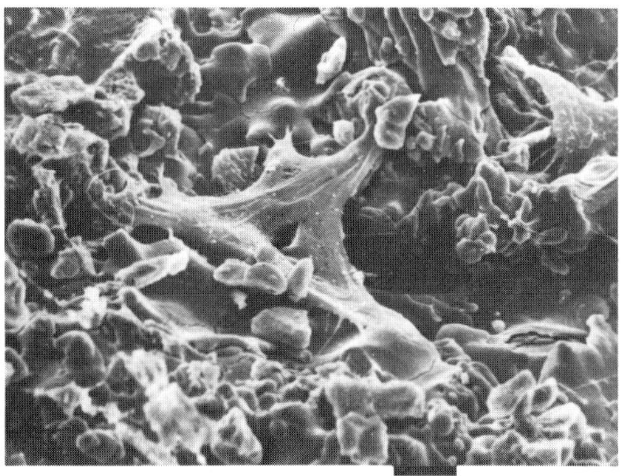

Fig.2 Thicker cell body in a valley of a rough (plasma coated) titanium surface. The cell processes are anchored on protruding edges of the substratum. There is a space between the cell body and the substratum.

On **rough** surfaces (sandblasted, plasma coated) the cells were thicker. They were mainly located within valleys and their processes were anchored on protruding edges. These cells covered five to ten times less area than the cells on smooth substrates. Sandblasted specimens were densely covered with thick cells having many fine processes with widely distributed anchoring points. On plasma coated disks (Fig.2) the cells had fewer processes and a larger contact area to the substratum than those on sandblasted disks but they clearly had more processes than those on the mechanically polished disks.

<u>DISCUSSION</u>

In testing the behavior of cultured cells grown on different surface structures the use of the same metal kept the variations of the chemical surroundings at a minimum. Reflected light Nomarski microscopy at relatively low magnification (80x) was useful in detecting the areas of cell growth and in determining the general arrangement of cells. The gold coated surface provided good contrast. In the low magnification range this technique was superior to the SEM in particular while observing smooth surfaces. At higher magnification (200x) the SEM is preferred to observe single cell shapes and their relationship to the microstructure of the substratum.

We found that cell morphology depends on the structure of the surface and this is supported by histologic observations. Tissues in contact with sandblasted metal cylinders (Geret et al., 1980) showed several layers of relatively large cells with a high number of nuclei per unit length of contact zone. On the other hand tissues in contact with smooth surfaces exhibited a layer of one to two cells thickness with few nuclei and capillaries were found in close vicinity to the implant.

Adaptation of cells to their surrounding is to be expected. Curtis and Büültjens(1973) suggest ´that cells can ´sense´ mechanical strains acting on them and suitably adjust their motile processes to compensate for changes in cell adhesion´. It seems probable that the same laws which control cell to cell contact (Weiss, 1970 a, b) are also valid for cell to substratum contact.

For initial cell spreading and adhesion such surface properties
as wettability and surface energy are important (Baier, 1970).
Long term adhesion is provided by a substance deposited by cells.
According to Taylor (1970) the composition of this substance is
independant of the substratum. With increasing contact area one
would therefore expect stronger adhesion. The strength of
attachment of flat normal fibroblasts was higher than that of
rounded tumor cells (Vasiliev and Gelfand, 1973). A firm
attachment of cells is desirable to avoid mechanical irritation
at the cell-implant interface. The intimate contact between cells
and substratum without intervening fluid spaces may prevent
spreading of bacteria potentially introduced at the time of
implantation. Because continuous removal of soluble corrosion
products keeps their tissue concentration low, there should be a
minimal barrier between the implant surface and blood vessels.
Therefore a contact area with minimal mechanical irritation and
minimal connective tissue elements based on good adhesion would
seem to be desirable. Minimal irritation would seem to be advantageous in relation to carcinogenesis. In this respect it is interesting to note that according to Andrews et al.(1979) the
physical rather than the chemical structure of the material surface seems to be important.

Although biological and metallurgical considerations speak in
favour of smooth surfaces there are clinical experiences which
would advocate rough surfaces (Schroeder et al., 1978, Mühlemann,
1975). Meeneghan et al. (1979) have found a more favourable tissue
reaction around glow-discharge treated implants, independent of
the surface microstructure.

In our studies using tissue culture and one type of cell,
comparing rough and smooth surfaces, a marked difference in the
morphology of the cell contact was found. We conclude that a
smooth surface, which leads to an intimate contact of finely
spread cells may be preferable to the point contact wich occurs
with rough surfaces. However which is more advantageous in
clinical practice is still undecided.

<u>ACKNOWLEDGEMENT</u>

The authors thank Miss R.Grunder for her excellent tissue culture
work. This study was supported by the "Swiss National Science
Foundation", credit 3.976.078

REFERENCES

Andrews, E.J., Todd, P.W. & Kukulinski, N.E. (1979) Surface charge in foreign body carcinogenesis. J.Biomed.Mater.Res.13,173-187.

Baier, R.E. (1970) Surface properties influencing biological adhesion. in Adhesion in biological systems. (Ed. R.S. Manly), pp15-48. Academic Press, New York.

Curtis, A.S.G. & Büültjens, T.E.J. (1973). Cell adhesion and locomotion. in Ciba Foundation Symposum 14, Locomation of tissue cells, pp 171-186. Elsevier, Amsterdam.

Geret, V., Rahn, B.A., Mathys, R., Straumann, F. & Perren, S.M. (1980) In vivo testing of tissue tolerance of implant materials: Improved quantitative evaluation through reduction of relative motion at the tissue implant interface. in Current concepts in internal fixation of fractures. (Ed. H.K.Uhthoff), pp 160-164. Springer, Berlin.

Meenaghan, M.A., Natiella, J.R., Movesi, J.L., Flynn, H.E., Wirth, J.E. & Baier, R.E. (1979) Tissue response to surface treated tantalum implants: Preliminary observations in primates. J.Biomed.Mater.Res.13, 631-643.

Mühlemann, H.R. (1975). Zur Mikrostruktur der Implantatoberfläche. Schweiz. Mschr. Zahnheilk. 85, 97-112.

Schroeder, A., Stich, H., Straumann, F. & Sutter, F. (1978) Ueber die Anlagerung von Osteozement an einen belasteten Implantatkörper Schweiz. Mschr. Zahnheilk. 88, 1051-1058.

Taylor, A.C. (1970) Adhesion of cells to surfaces. in Adhesion in biological systems.(Ed.R.S.Manly),pp 51-71.Academic Press,New York

Vasiliev, J.M. & Gelfand, I.M. (1973) Interactions of normal and neoplastic fibroblasts with the substratum. in Ciba Foundation Symposum 14, Locomation of tissue cellts, pp 311-331. Elsevier, Amsterdam.

Weiss, L. (1970a) Cell contact phenomena. in Advances in Tissue culture (Ed. C.Waymouth), pp 48-78. Williams & Wilkins, Baltimore. Weiss, L. (1970b) A biophysical consideration of cell contact phenomena. in Adhesion in biological systems. (Ed. R.S. Manly), pp 1-14. Academic Press, New York.

Biomaterials 1980
Edited by G. D. Winter, D. F. Gibbons, and H. Plenk, Jr.
© 1982 John Wiley and Sons Ltd.

BONE REACTION TO POROUS AND GROOVED STAINLESS STEEL, TANTALUM AND NIOBIUM IMPLANTS

G. Pflüger[1], H. Plenk Jr.[2], N. Böhler[1,4], F. Grundschober[2] and S. Schider[3]

1) Orthopaedic University Clinic
2) Bone Research Lab., Histological & Embryological Institute of the University of Vienna
3) Metallwerke Plansee A.G., Reutte
4) Research Institute for Traumatology of AUVA, Vienna, Austria

SUMMARY

The aim of this experimental study was on the one hand to test bone reaction to the pure metals tantalum and niobium in comparison to stainless steel, and on the other to study the osseous anchorage of porous and grooved implants. Porous and grooved cylinders of these metals (pore size: 40, 150 and 300 μm, conical grooves: $\emptyset$ 300 μm, size: 3 mm $\emptyset$ x 5 - 6 mm) were implanted under "non-loaded conditions" into holes drilled in the distal tibiae of rabbits. Sequential fluorochrome labelling was performed and the animals were sacrificed 3 and 6 weeks, 3 and 6 months postoperatively. Undecalcified ground sections were evaluated using fluorescence and polarized light microscopy and radiomicrographs.

After three weeks a vigorous growth of new bone was observed in the medullary cavity and in the periosteum with all three materials. The osseous tissue had grown right up to the grooved surface and into pores of the cylinder with a diameter of 100 μm or more. As early as 6 weeks after implantation there was a reduction in the formation of new bone and at the end of the period of observation there was only functional support of the implant. Whereas the structured cylinders were closely surrounded by osseous tissue, osseous tissue had grown into the porous cylinders mainly at the base and in continuation of the cortex.

These results led us to conclude that both tantalum and niobium were just as biocompatible as stainless steel. However, as tantalum and niobium are much more resistant to corrosion, it is possible to manufacture porous or grooved implants which can be anchored over an extended period of time by the osseous tissue itself.

INTRODUCTION

The pure metals tantalum and niobium are chemically extremely inert. They have proved very compatible with soft tissue (Laing et al, 1967) and have already been used with success in surgery. However, due to their low mechanical strength these metals have not so far been considered for heavily loaded orthopaedic implants. Schider (in these Proceedings) has now been able to demonstrate that tantalum and niobium can indeed achieve strengths comparable with those of stainless steel and even cobalt-based alloys. What is more, they are more resistant to corrosion than these alloys, and the surface area can therefore easily be increased by pores or structures which make possible the durable anchorage of joint endoprostheses by the mechanical interlocking of osseous tissue. This paper reports on the reaction of osseous tissue to unloaded tantalum and niobium implants compared to stainless steel implants. The results with loaded tantalum joint prostheses are reported on in another paper (Pflüger et al, in these Proceedings).

MATERIALS AND METHODS

The implants were cylinders (size: 3 mm $\emptyset$ x 5 - 6 mm), some of which were fitted with an extraction hook. They were either porous or had a finely grooved surface and were manufactured of the following materials:

a) Stainless steel powder (316 L - coldstream) was pressed at 2 - 2.5 t/cm^2 and sintered for 1 hour at 1100° C in an H_2 atmosphere to produce an open porosity of 20 - 30% (max. pore size 40 μm) or 30 - 40% (pore size 100-150 μm) after addition of burn-out PMMA spheres ($\emptyset$ 50-120 μm).

b) Pure tantalum and niobium powders were either pressed with PMMA spheres ($\emptyset$ 100-300 μm) and sintered (30 min. at 2050° C and 10^{-5} Torr) to produce a open porosity of 30 - 40% (pore size 150-300 μm) or processed by powder metallurgical methods (pressed and sintered by direct current heating at 1800-2700° C and cold worked) and machined to produce a grooved surface (conical grooves, $\emptyset$ 300 μm).

These cylinders were implanted under general anaesthetic and sterile conditions into two drill holes ($\emptyset$ 3.2 mm) 1 cm apart in the distal tibiae of rabbits, one in the metaphysis and 1 in the diaphysis on either side.

Material	Form of Cylinders	Number	Number of animals	Observation periods
Stainless steel	small pores ($\emptyset$ 40 μm)	20	5	3 & 6 weeks
	large pores ($\emptyset$ 150 μm)	56	14	3 & 6 weeks
Tantalum	large pores ($\emptyset$ 300 μm)	40	10	3 & 6 weeks and
	dense, grooved	36	9	3 & 6 months
Niobium	large pores ($\emptyset$ 300 μm)	8	2	3 & 6 weeks and
	dense, grooved	12	3	3 & 6 months

Table 1: Experimental schedule of stainless steel, tantalum and niobium implants in rabbits.

The operated limbs were not immobilised postoperatively. Sequential fluoro-chrome labelling was carried out two weeks after implantation and one week before sacrifice. The implants were excised together with the surrounding bone, embedded in methylmethacrylate and cut and ground into sections 80 to 100 μm thick. The sections were evaluated using fluorescence and polarized light microscopy and radiomicrographs were prepared from selected sections.

Pull-out tests were only performed with the stainless steel cylinders and the results have been published elsewhere (Pflüger et al, 1979).

RESULTS

Three weeks after implantation, all types of implant were surrounded by a vigourous new growth of intramedullary and periosteal woven bone. The former was more pronounced in the metaphysial than in the diaphysial site of implantation. The osseous tissue had grown into the larger pores, mostly around the base of the implant and in continuation of the drilled cortex (Fig. 1 and 2). On the other hand, the growth of osseous tissue into the pores of the stainless steel cylinders with a smaller pore size extended only as far as the surface of the implant. The same observation was made with the grooved cylinders of tantalum and niobium (Fig. 3).

Six weeks after implantation the reaction of the osseous tissue was already somewhat less marked, but all the implants were tightly enveloped by newly formed osseous tissue. Bone ingrowth and osteon-like bone formation were found in all the larger pored implants. In the case of the stainless steel cylinders with larger pores, osseous tissue was found only in the pores at the base of the implant and in the area of the hole into the cortex.

Three and six months after implantation, only the tantalum and niobium cylinders were examined, and these, too, showed a reduction in the surrounding osseous tissue. Bone ingrowth into the pores was still found in the same areas as described above, and the bone tissue within the pores and of the supporting structures at the base showed a lamellar character (Fig. 4 and 5). The surrounding fat marrow was separated from the implants without cell reaction by a thin layer of connective tissue.

DISCUSSION

The results of these experiments with stainless steel cylinders point to the importance of a porous structure in bone reaction. As stated by Hulbert et al (1973) a minimum pore diameter of 100 μm is required for fibrous trabeculae to grow into the implant. The small pored steel cylinders were thus only anchored in the same way as the grooved tantalum and niobium implants. On the other hand, bone ingrowth was found in the larger pored steel cylinders, but the osseous tissue did not continue to fill all the pores. On the contrary, the formation of new bone was reduced to the areas that seemed necessary for the stable support of the implant. This "functional incorporation" points out the effects of loading, which appears to play a part even under so-called "non-loaded conditions" in the bone.

These observations are apparently in contrast with the findings of Nilles and Lapitsky (1973), who reported that bone ingrowth completely filled the porous stainless steel implants by 12 weeks. There is no doubt that the pore size used in Nilles' study was considerably greater than that used in our study, and we are unable to say anything about the interconnected pore size. However, the implants of Nilles and Lapitsky (1973) were only as thick as the cortical bone, and we too could observe the durable formation of bone mainly in continuation of the cortex. In addition, the fact that the pores of our implants were sufficiently interconnected was demonstrated not physically but biologically and biomechanically by the occurrence of osteon-like lamellar bone formation in this area.

On the other hand, the tissue compatibility of the implant materials could have had an effect on the ingrowth of bone into the pores. During an observation period of six weeks, the corrosion of the porous stainless steel may have caused the reduction in bone formation. A similar reduction in bone formation did occur somewhat later with the porous and grooved tantalum and niobium implants, which were of course more resistant to corrosion and more compatible with tissue. On the contrary, no such reduction has been reported from similar porous implants made of an equally good cobalt-based alloy (Welsh et al, 1971) or of titanium (Galante et al, 1971). However, as mentioned above, there are many variables affecting the mechanism of bone ingrowth into porous materials, and this method of approach alone is not suitable for the evaluation of differences in the tissue compatibility of these materials.

On the basis of the present results it may be concluded that the pure metals tantalum and niobium exhibit a tissue compatibility every bit as good as that of stainless steel. Whereas the manufacture of porous sintered elements of suitable porosity and pore size and with adequate mechanical strength is always problematical, the manufacture of cold worked grooved implants is a more practical proposition. The mechanical strength and the means of anchorage by mechanical interlocking offered by tantalum and niobium make it possible to make the shafts of joint endoprostheses of either metal. Initial trials with a tantalum hip-joint prosthesis are reported on by Pflüger et al (in these Proceedings).

ACKNOWLEDGEMENT

These studies were supported by the Austrian "Forschungsförderungsfonds der Gewerblichen Wirtschaft" Grant No. 3/1851-1/P and by Metallwerke Plansee AG, Reutte, Austria.

REFERENCES

Galante, J., Rostoker, W., Leuck, R. & Ray, R. (1971) Sintered fiber metal composites as a basis for attachment of implants to bone. J. Bone & Jt. Surg. 53A, 101-114.
Hulbert, S.F., Cooke, F.W., Klawitter, J.J., Leonard, R.B., Sauer, B.W., Moyle, D.D. & Skinner, H.B. (1973) Attachment of prostheses to the musculo-skeletal system by tissue ingrowth and mechanical interlocking. J. Biomed. Mater. Res. 7, 1-23.

Laing, P.G., Ferguson, A.B.Jr. & Hodge, E.S. (1967) Tissue reaction in rabbit muscle exposed to metallic implants. J. Biomed. Mater. Res. 1, 135-149.
Pflüger, G., Bösch, P., Grundschober, F., Kristen, H., Plenk, H.Jr. & Schider, S. (1979). Untersuchungen über das Einwachsen von Knochengewebe in poröse Metallimplantate. Wien. klin. Wschr. 91, 482-487.
Pflüger, G., Böhler, N., Grundschober, F., Plenk, H.Jr. & Schider, S. (in press). Experimental studies on total knee and total hip joint endoprostheses made of tantalum, in Proceedings of the First World Biomaterials Congress (Eds. G.D. Winter, D.F. Gibbons & H. Plenk Jr.). John Wiley, Chichester.
Schider, S. (in press) Tantalum and niobium as potential prosthetic materials, in Proceedings of the First World Biomaterials Congress (Eds. G.D. Winter, D.F. Gibbons & H. Plenk Jr.). John Wiley, Chichester.
Welsh, R.P., Pilliar, R.M. & Macnab, I. (1971). Surgical implants - the role of surface porosity in fixation to bone and acrylic. J. Bone & Jt. Surg. 53A, 963-977.

FIGURES

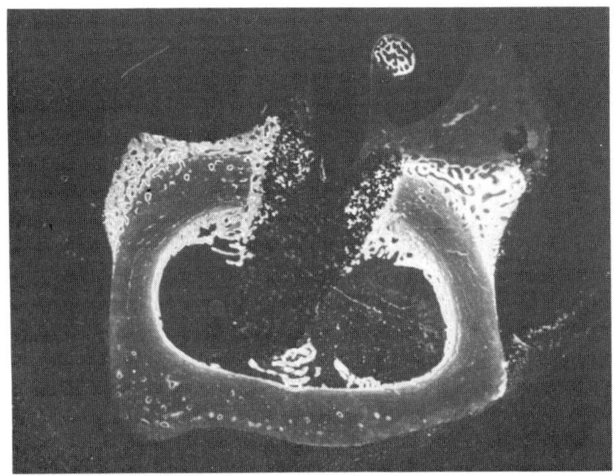

Figure 1: Porous ($\emptyset$ 150 µm) stainless steel cylinder in the diaphysis 3 weeks postoperatively (magn. 7 x). Fluorochrome labelled bone has grown into the open pores.

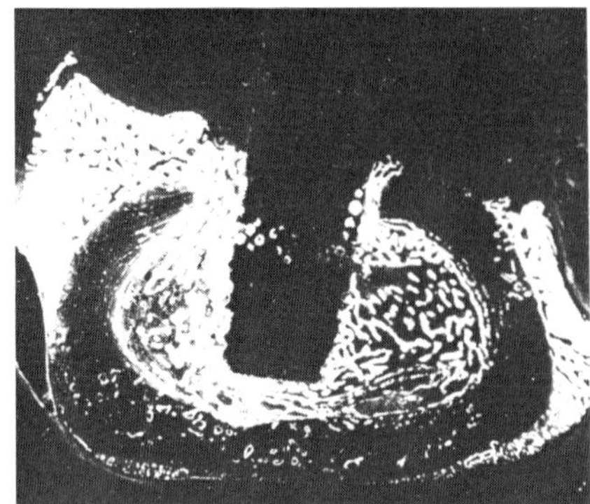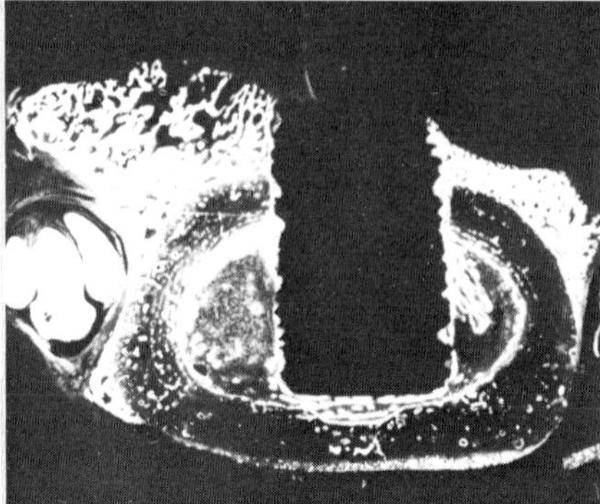

Figure 2   Figure 3

Figure 2: Porous ($\emptyset$ 300 μm) tantalum cylinder in the diaphysis 3 weeks postoperatively (magn. 5 x). Vigorous endosteal bone formation around the implant and within the open pores.

Figure 3: Grooved tantalum cylinder in the diaphysis 3 weeks postoperatively (magn. 5 x). Endosteal and periosteal bone formation has tightly enveloped the implant.

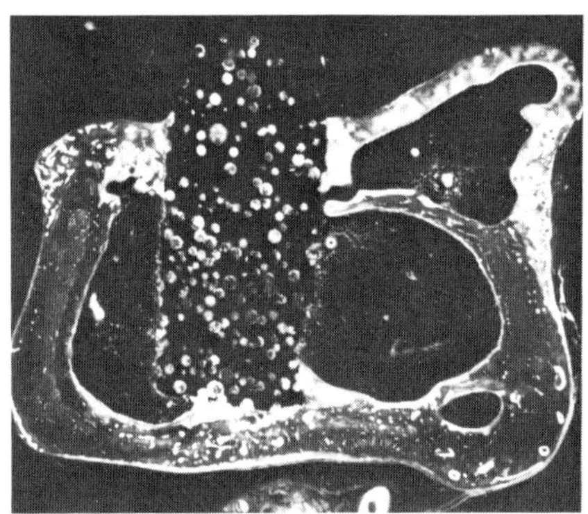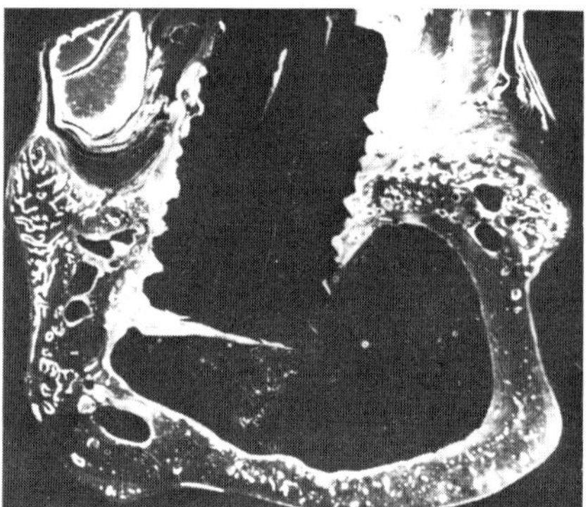

Figure 4   Figure 5

Figure 4: Porous ($\emptyset$ 300 μm) tantalum cylinder in the diaphysis 6 months postoperatively (magn. 6 x). The bone reaction is now restricted to supporting structures, but bone ingrowth is again found mainly in the continuation of the cortex.

Figure 5: Grooved niobium cylinder in the diaphysis 6 months postoperatively (magn. 6 x). Abutment by lamellar bone structures from endosteal and periosteal sides.

Biomaterials 1980
Edited by G. D. Winter, D. F. Gibbons, and H. Plenk, Jr.
© 1982 John Wiley and Sons Ltd.

BONDING OSTEOGENESIS INDUCED BY CALCIUM PHOSPHATE CERAMIC IMPLANTS

J. F. Osborn* and H. Newesely**

* North-West-German Clinic for Maxillo-Facial
  Surgery, University Hospitals, D-2000 Hamburg 20
** Free University of Berlin, Department for
  Materials Science FB 7, WE 5, D-1000 Berlin 33,
  West Germany

SUMMARY

The way in which intra-osseous implants interact with living tissues is examined. In the case of the most metals defense reactions are induced by the corrosion products. Metallic implants and bone tissue become separated by an intervening fibrous layer, a process called 'distance osteogenesis'.
Ceramics composed of low solubility calcium phosphates show bioactive interface reactions. A hydroxyapatite material causes a particularly osteotropic effect in new-forming bone near the implant site characterised by a centripetal mode of growth within open pores.
Calcium and phosphate ions liberated from the bioactive material diffuse into the surrounding tissues and participate in the physiological turnover. Exchange processes starting from the interface region induce 'bonding osteogenesis' and connect the ceramic implant with bone. Our experimental results show borderless confluence of synthetic hydroxyapatite material and bone apatite. We believe there is epitaxy between bone crystals and the crystal phase of the ceramic and between protein molecules and the ceramic apatite.

INTRODUCTION

The clinical success of an intraosseous implant depends on, among other things, the type of bond which develops between implant and bone. A survey of the materials suitable for intraosseous implantation makes it clear that there is a certain antagonism between the mechanical qualities and the biological properties. The metals form the optimal end to the continuum with regard to the technical aspects of material and manufacture, but the highest degree of biocompatibility is provided by hydroxyapatite ceramic, which is identical with the bone mineral in terms of crystal chemistry (Newesely and Osborn, 1978)(Table 1).

In terms of their interaction with living bone, materials can be classified as biotolerant, bioinert and bioactive

(Osborn and Weiss, 1978)

TABLE 1. Mechanical and biological properties of biomaterials

<u>Mechanical properties</u>

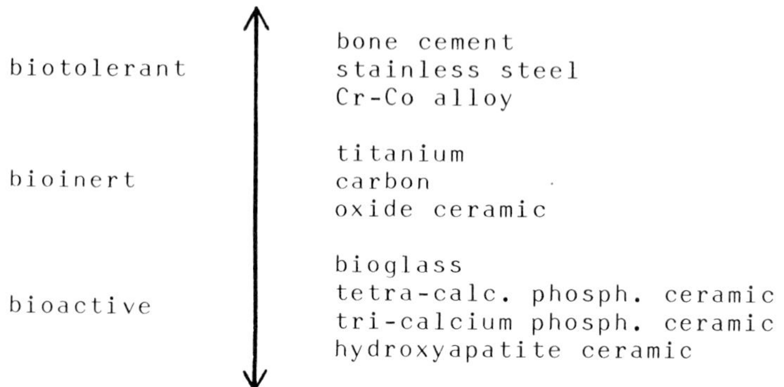

<u>Biological properties</u>

Every type of material evokes a group specific reaction. Most metals are incorporated in bone by osteogenesis at a distance, bioinert materials by contact osteogenesis, and bioactive implants by bonding osteogenesis (Table 2).

TABLE 2. The different patterns of osteogenesis

material	reaction of implant bed	biodynamics
1. bone cement metals	distance osteogenesis	biotolerant
2. alumina carbon materials	contact osteogenesis	bioinert
3. bioglass Ca-phosphate ceramic hydroxyapatite ceramic	bonding osteogenesis	bioactive

The foreign body response of the living bone to metallic implants, called 'metallosis', is induced by the corrosion products and enhanced by premature loading resulting in relative implant-tissue motion. Metallosis is character- ised by the formation of a fibrous membrane at the bone- implant interface (Escalas et al., 1975). The connective tissue layer adjacent to the implant is specific to the

material (Griss et al., 1978) and does not depend exclusively on the functional stress to which the implant is
subjected.
In contrast to metals which release toxic ions, hydroxyapatite ceramics liberate physiologically acceptable
calcium and phosphate ions (Köster et al., 1977a; Osborn
and Newesely, 1979).

If the meaning of biocompatibility is broadened in the
sense that implant materials must not only resist the
solvent attack of the biological environment, but should
also stimulate bone growth, then according to our studies
(Osborn and Newesely, 1979; Osborn et al., 1980) the chemical and physicochemical nature of the implant material
must simulate bone mineral which comprises up to 70% fine
crystalline hydroxyapatite (Termine and Posner, 1966).
Of the calcium phosphate materials, only hydroxyapatite
ceramic has the same Ca/P ratio of 1.67 as bone mineral
and the same structure type as shown by X-ray diffraction
analysis (Osborn and Weiss, 1978; Osborn and Newesely,
1980). The mean diameter of the macropores of our porous
hydroxyapatite ceramic is estimated to be about 150 to
200 um corresponding almost exactly to those of the in-
tertrabecular spaces in cancellous bone (Osborn and Newesely, 1980). Cancellous bone exhibits a network of inter-
trabecular spaces opening on to each other and our porous
materials also have a system of interconnecting pores.
The three-dimensional uninterrupted connection between
the macropores is of major importance to bony incorporation and anchorage of the implant (Osborn, 1979).

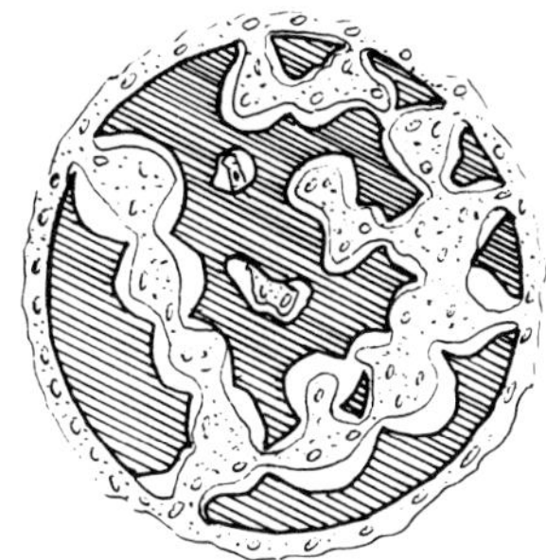
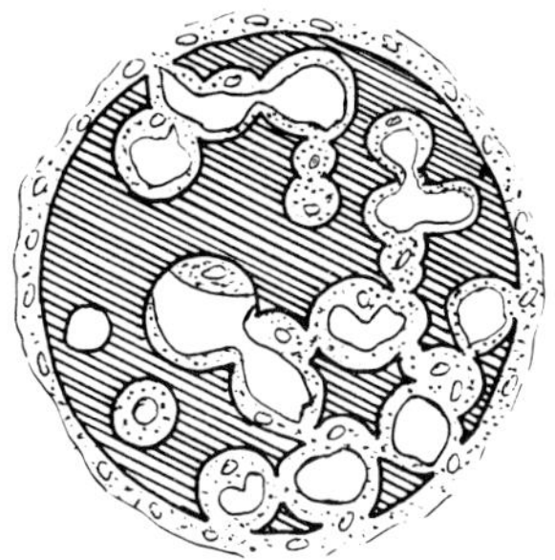

Osteogenesis within porous ceramic implants
(diagramatic)

Fig. 1. Osteogenesis within porous ceramic implants

Figure 1 explains the different principles of bone ingrowth into porous materials. In the case of bioinert
oxide ceramics (Köster et al., 1977b) osteogenesis takes
place in a centrifugal manner and there is initially a
layer of connective tissue between the new bone and the
ceramic. A long time elapses before the intervening
fibrous layer is reduced and the bone comes into direct
contact with the implant.
With bioactive materials, such as hydroxyapatite ceramic,
osteogenesis begins directly on the surface of the implant
without connective tissue intervention and proceeds in a
centripetal direction towards the centre of the pores
(Osborn and Weiss, 1978; Osborn, 1979; Osborn et al.,
1980). This centripetal bone growth is the characteristic
feature of bioactive materials.

MATERIALS AND METHODS

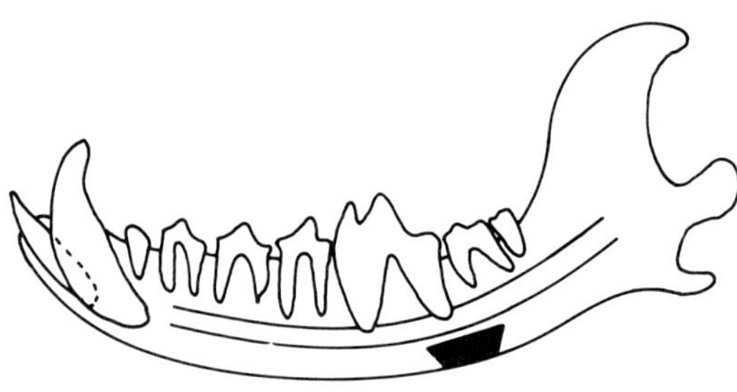

For animal experi-
ments we used the
hydroxyapatite ce-
ramic described in
our previous papers
(Osborn and Weiss,
1978; Osborn and Ne-
wesely, 1980).
Porous and dense
specimens of this
hydroxyapatite ce-
ramic were implanted
into the mandibular
bone of three Alsa-
tian dogs (Fig. 2).

Fig. 2. Location of implants
in the mandibula of dogs

This location was
selected because at this point of the lower jaw an implant is loaded exclusively by compression forces. Healing
of the implants was uneventful in all animals.

RESULTS

Eight weeks after implantation, the ceramic specimens
were so firmly embedded that separation of bone and implant by mechanical means was impossible. Histological
evaluation was carried out with the light and scanning
electron microscope (SEM).
The centripetal pattern of bone growth within the pores
of hydroxyapatite ceramic is shown in figure 3. Osteogenesis took place in direct contact with the surface of the
implant. Depositing new bone, a row of osteoblasts mi-
grates to the center of the pores.
The interlocking growth of the calcifying tissue at the
bone-ceramic interface is illustrated in figure 4.

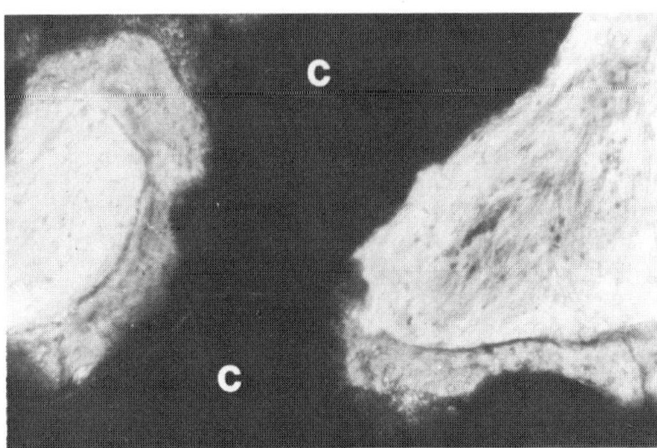

Fig. 3. Osteoblasts deposit
bone initially on the ce-
ramic lining the pores.
These cells gradually mi-
grate to the centre, filling the pores with bone.

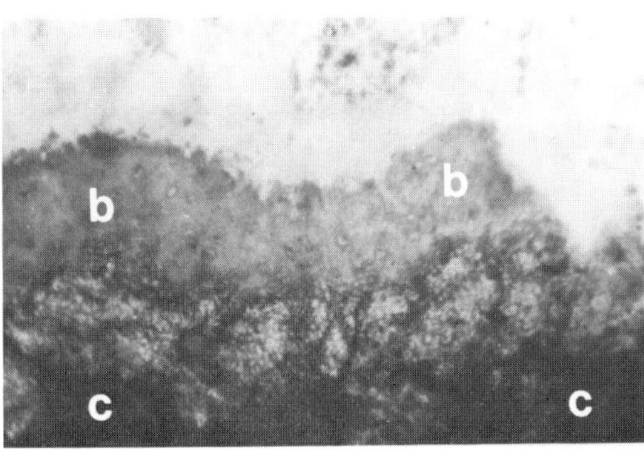

Fig. 4. Interlocking growth
of the calcifying tissue (b)
at the bone-ceramic interface; C = ceramic (light
microscopy, x 100).

The regular rhythm
of physiological bone
growth within a po-
rous hydroxyapatite
ceramic implant be-
comes evident by fig-
ure 5 and by the mon-
tage of images ob-
tained by scanning
electron microscope
(Fig. 6). Osteogene-
sis, originating from
the primary cortical
bone on the right mar-
gin of the picture,
proceeds continuously
through the system of
the interconnecting
pores. The X-ray dis-
tribution scan for
calcium shows varying
degrees of mineral-
isation corresponding
to the maturity of
bone tissue. The in-
timate association
between the hydroxy-
apatite implant and
the bone tissue leads
to strong bonding at
the bone-ceramic in-
terface.
As critical point
drying procedures
were not performed
during the prepara-
tion of the samples
for SEM analysis, the
bone-ceramic inter-
faces were subjected
to a variety of
stresses. These re-
sulted from cutting
operations, dehydra-
tion procedures and the heat associated with the preparation of the surface coating. Scanning electron microscopy
showed that some cracks occurred, but the bone-ceramic
interface always remained intact.
Even at x 2400 magnifications (Fig. 7) it is still difficult to make a distinction between the hydroxyapatite of
the ceramic and the mineral of bone. In general, the biological apatite obtained from the octacalcium precursor
transformation exhibits a more finely dispersed texture
than our synthetic equivalent.

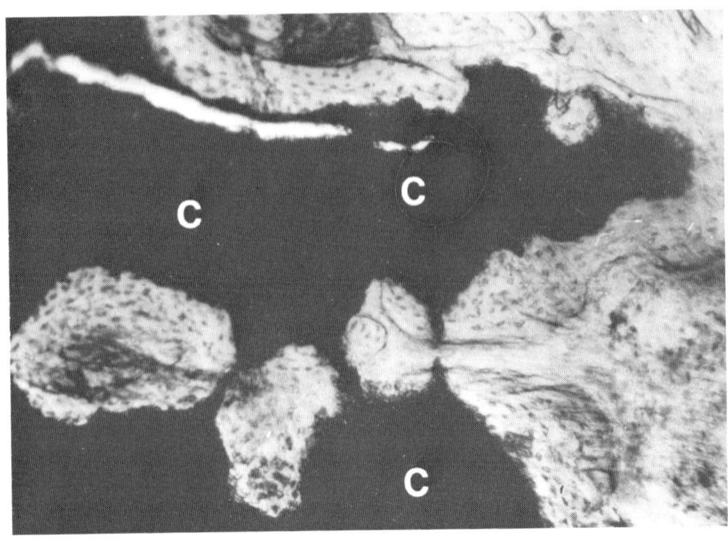

Fig. 5. The interconnection of the pores of the ceramic is of decisive importance to the continuous proceeding of osteogenesis; C = ceramic (light microscopy, x 82).

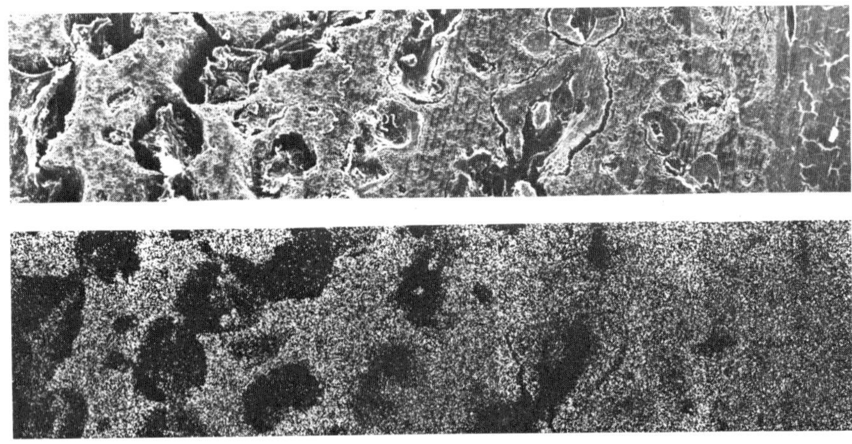

Fig. 6. Montage of scanning electron micrographs (x 50).
top: Gradation of bone growth in porous hydroxyapatite, 8 weeks after implantation.
bottom: X-ray distribution picture of calcium in the specimen shown above.

DISCUSSION

This interdigitation of the two phases of minerals with
their almost identical chemistry and crystal structure,
supports our hypothesis (Osborn and Newesely, 1979) of
the epitaxy concept featuring the strong bonding between hydroxyapatite in ceramic and bone in terms of physico-chemical interaction. The physico-chemical intergrowth of similar types of crystals happens if certain
atomic spaces in the ultrastructure be-tween the two partners are about the same size or are identical, in other
words when the structure of the host mineral and the

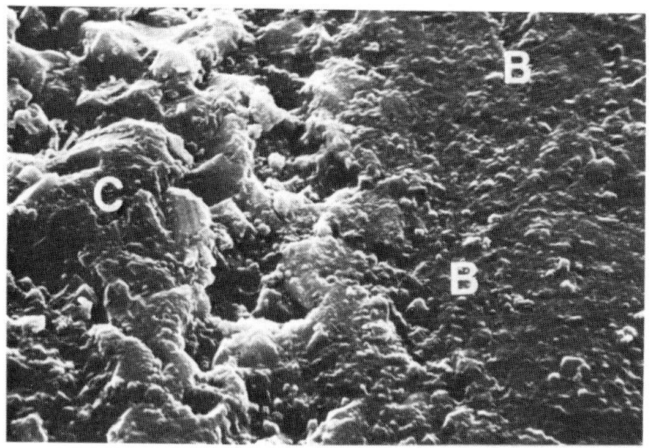

Fig. 7. Interdigitation of
the ceramic (C) and the hydroxyapatite mineral (B)
of bone (SEM, x 2400).

guest mineral show a high degree of similarity. Epitaxy
is sometimes also possible in inorganic/organic systems,
e.g. epitaxy of ß-keratine and apatite (Newesely, 1969).
Epitaxy, or in a wider sense mineral impregnation, can
also occur between partners with different and more differentiated bond systems, e.g. between the fibrillar texture of collagen and hydroxyapatite, as long as the organic partner exhibits spatial quantities with which the
hydroxyapatite can interact (Newesely et al., 1980).

The interaction model in the case of hydroxyapatite ceramic and bone involves both mechanisms: epitaxy between
the bone crystals and the crystal phase of the ceramic as
well as intergrowth between the protein molecules and the
ceramic apatite. Both processes govern the dynamics of
of the intraosseous incorporation. Their order of magnitude is in the range of the individual protein molecules,
and thus 100 times lower in the metric scale than the
dimensions of the textured elements adjacent to the ceramics visible in the scanning electron micrograph at
10,000 magnification.

We are of the opinion that for the implant's maintenance
in the continually remodelling bone the implant substance
itself must be integrated into the basic processes of
bone physiology. By virtue of its chemical and structural
likeness to bone, hydroxyapatite ceramic will ably fulfill the requirements of an implant material.

REFERENCES

Escalas, F., Galante, J., Rostocker, W. & Coogan, P.S. (1975) $MP_{35}N$: A corrosion resistant, high strength alloy for orthopaedic surgical implants: Bio-assay results. J. Biomed. Mater. Res., 9, 303-313

Griss, P., Werner, E. & Heimke, G. (1978) Alumina Ceramic, Bioglass and Silicon Nitride: a comparative biocompatibility study. In Advances in Biomaterials, Vol. 2, (Eds., Hastings & Williams) John Wiley, Chichester, in press

Köster, K., Heide, H. & König, R. (1977a) Resorbierbare Calciumphosphatkeramik im Tierexperiment unter Belastung. Langenbecks Arch. Chir., 343, 173-181

Köster, K., Heide, H. & König, R. (1977b) Histologische Untersuchungen an der Grenzfläche zwischen Knochengewebe und Calciumphosphat-, Calciumaluminat- und Aluminiumoxid-keramik. Z. Orthop., 115, 693-699

Newesely, H. (1969) Chemische Affinitäts- und Strukturbeziehungen zwischen organischen und Proteinkomponenten biogener Mineralisationen. Dtsch. zahnärztl. Z., 24, 473-483

Newesely, H. & Osborn, J.F. (1978) Structural and textural implications of calcium phosphates in ceramics. In Advances in Biomaterials, Vol. 2, (Eds., Hastings & Williams), John Wiley, Chichester, in press.

Newesely, H., Hosemann, R. & Uther, B. (1980) Kollagen-Einschlußverbindungen. Z. Naturforsch., 35c, 177-187

Osborn, J.F. & Weiss, T. (1978) Hydroxylapatitkeramik - ein knochenähnlicher Biowerkstoff. Schw. Mschr. Zahnheilkd., 88, 1166-1172

Osborn, J.F. (1979) Biowerkstoffe und ihre Anwendung bei Implantaten. Schw. Mschr. Zahnheilkd., 89, 1138-1139

Osborn, J.F. & Newesely, H. (1979) Dynamic aspects of the implant-bone interface. In Dental Implants - Materials and Systems (Ed., Heimke, G.) Carl Hanser, München, in press.

Osborn, J.F. & Newesely, H. (1980) The material science of calcium phosphate ceramics. Biomaterials, 1, 108-111

Osborn, J.F., Kovacs, E. & Kallenberger, A. (1980) Hydroxylapatitkeramik - Entwicklung eines neuen Biowerkstoffes und erste tierexperimentelle Ergebnisse. Dtsch. zahnärztl. Z., 35, 54-56

Termin, J.D. & Posner, A.S. (1966) Infrared analysis of rat bone: age dependency of amorphous and crystalline mineral fractions. Science, 153, 1523-1525

Biomaterials 1980
Edited by G. D. Winter, D. F. Gibbons, and H. Plenk, Jr.
© 1982 John Wiley and Sons Ltd.

EPITHELIAL ATTACHMENT AND BONE TISSUE FORMATION ON THE SURFACE OF HYDROXYAPATITE CERAMICS DENTAL IMPLANTS

M. Ogiso, H. Kaneda, J. Arasaki and T. Tabata

Dept. Prosthodontics II, School of Dentistry,
Tokyo Medical and Dental Univ.

SUMMARY

An histological study was made of the biocompatibility of
hydroxyapatite ceramics for dental implant material.
Apatite implants in the jaw bone of adult dogs, ranging in duration
from 5 days to 6 months without functional load, were carried out in
order to observe epithelial attachment and bone formation on the
surface of apatite implants.
Epithelial attachment: 6 months after implantation the gingival sulcus
around apatite implants was shallow. The epithelial cell layer in
contact with the apatite under the sulcus became thinner depending on
its depth. TEM examination indicated that there was an internal
basement lamina between the epithelial cell membrane and the apatite,
and hemidesmosomes along the membrane.
Bone formation: The first contact of new bone with the apatite was
found 5 days after implantation. 10 days after implantation, the area
of bone formation on the apatite was enlarged, and the entire surface
of some specimens was covered by new bone. At the same time, the
calcification of new bone on and near the surface of the apatite had
begun. 60 days after implantation, bone tissue and bone crystallization on the apatite were almost the same as those of normal bone.

INTRODUCTION

Dental implant materials must have a high biocompatibility with bone
and soft tissue. The authors have observed that a tooth adheres to
bone when it is replanted or transplanted (Ogiso, 1977). However, the
absorption of the tooth takes place concurrently. We took the view
that this absorption is caused by an immunologic response to organic
bodies in the dentine. We argued that if inorganic bodies in dentine
or any other similar inorganic materials are used as the implant
materials, constant bone adhesion without such an absorption could be
obtained (Ogiso, 1977). As a preliminary experiment, ceramics of
apatite from tooth or bone, and those of synthetic apatite, were
implanted in bone. Both materials showed very high biocompatibility
with bone tissue, particularly when the relative density was high, in
which case almost all the surface of the ceramic was covered with new
bone tissue.

M. Ogiso et al.

In this paper, a summary of the results from our studies on the biocompatibility of synthetic apatite ceramics is reported, and particular emphasis is placed on bone tissue formation on apatite ceramics
and the relation between apatite ceramics and oral epithelium.

MATERIALS and METHODS

The experimental method of observing the response of jaw bone to the
apatite ($Ca_{10}(PO_4)_6(OH)_2$) consisted in drilling a 5.5 mm in diameter
socket in an adult dog mandible 3 months after tooth extraction,
inserting a cylinder-shaped apatite (the relative density was from 56%
to 99%) 5.0 mm in diameter and 12 mm in length into the socket, and
then crosing the gingival tissue over the implant using mucosal
sutures. The dog was placed under systematic anesthesia.
An histological examination of the specimens was made 3 days to 6
months after implantation.
The experimental method of observing the response of epithelial cell
to the apatite consisted of drilling a socket 5.5 mm in diameter and
12 mm in depth, into an adult dog mandible 3 months after tooth
extaction, implanting a cylinder-shaped apatite (the relative density
was more than 99%) 5.0 mm in diameter and 18.0 mm in length, into the
socket so that the apatite extended 6 mm above the bone surface, and
then suturing gingival tissue around the apatite after cutting away
the gingival tissue from where the apatite protruded. Immediately
after implantation, the apatite was splinted to the proxymal teeth.
One month after implantation, the splint apparatus was removed, and an
histological examination was made 5 months later of the specimens
which had not undergone decalcification.

RESULT

Figure A shows the initial stage of bone growth 5 days after
implantation. There are osteoblasts near the apatite and a number of
collagen fibers between cells. This represents the early stage in the
formation of an osteoid. The density of collagen fibers is
particularly low near the apatite in comparison with other areas.
Figure B shows the initial stage of calcification of the osteoid and a
region of delayed calcification 10 days after implantation. There are
crystal deposits in the osteoid on the apatite surface which are shown
at higher magnification in Figure C.
In this region (Figure C) are discrete crystal deposits, matrix-
vesicles among the collagen fibers and direct crystal deposits on the
apatite surface. Collagen fibers have been formed near the apatite,
but have not yet reached the surface (Figure D), although crystal
deposits were beginning to be formed directly on the apatite surface.
Evidently, once calcification of osteoid begins, crystal deposition
takes place independently of collagen formation on the apatite surface.
Figure E shows the condition on 10 days after implantation in an area
of more advanced calcification than that shown in Figure C.
Independent crystal deposits have fused together as a result of the
expansion of crystal deposits along the collagen fibers surrounding
them. The crystal deposits expanding in this way are incorporated into

the crystal layer on the apatite surface where the crystals were deposited without relation to collagen fibers. Figure F shows the bone growth 10 days after implantation with the area of calcification already advanced. The calcified region of bone which grew into the apatite surface has been largely extended. Figure G is a magnification of Figure F. The bone crystals observed are thinner and shorter on the whole than those of mature bones. 60 days after implantation, the bone tissues are almost the same as those of normal bones, as shown in Figure H. The bone matured 120 days after implantation. Bone cavities and bone canaliculae can be observed and bone crystallization is normal (Figure I,J).
About 50 apatite teeth were used to study the response of the epithelial tissue to the apatite. There were no cases of implant loss or movement during the six-month experimental period.
Figure K shows the relation between the apatite and gingiva. The gingival sulcus is extremely shallow, and the downward growth of epithelial cell is minimal. The gingival connective tissue reveals a low-grade type of inflammation, similar to that in healthy gingival tissue around natural teeth. The inner epithelial cell layer has become narrow in width, including the apical displacement of the cell layer (Figure L).
Epithelial cells are firmly connected with each other by intercellular bridges (Figure M). The junction of epithelial cells and the apatite was observed in the transmission electron microscope (figure N). The cellular membrane of the epithelial cells adheres to the apatite by an internal basement lamina (500Å − 700Å). There are well-developed hemidesmosome along the epithelial cellular membrane. Also present are numerous filaments, mitochondria, free ribosomes, pynocytotic vesicles and other cellular components, indicating that the epithelial cells which were closely adapted to the apatite were functioning normally.

DISCUSSION

The gingival sulsus around apatite implants is extremely shallow and the downward growth of epithelial cells was minimal. Moreover, there was adhesion between the implants and the epithelial cells.
Our next experiment will be to observe the details of the growth process of epithelial attachment and the gingival sulcus themselves.We found that the formation of bone tissue around and on the apatite occured simultaneously. Also, the formation of calcified crystal deposits occured simultaneously within osteoid tissue around and on the surface of the apatite.
These developments signify the high level of biocompatibility between the bone and epithelial tissue, and the apatite. The apatite is therefore an ideal substance for the construction of dental implant materials.

REFERENCE

Ogiso, M. (1977) Histological changes in the mandibular tissue by implantation of apatite ceramics. J. Stomatol. Soc., Jpn., 45, 170-221.

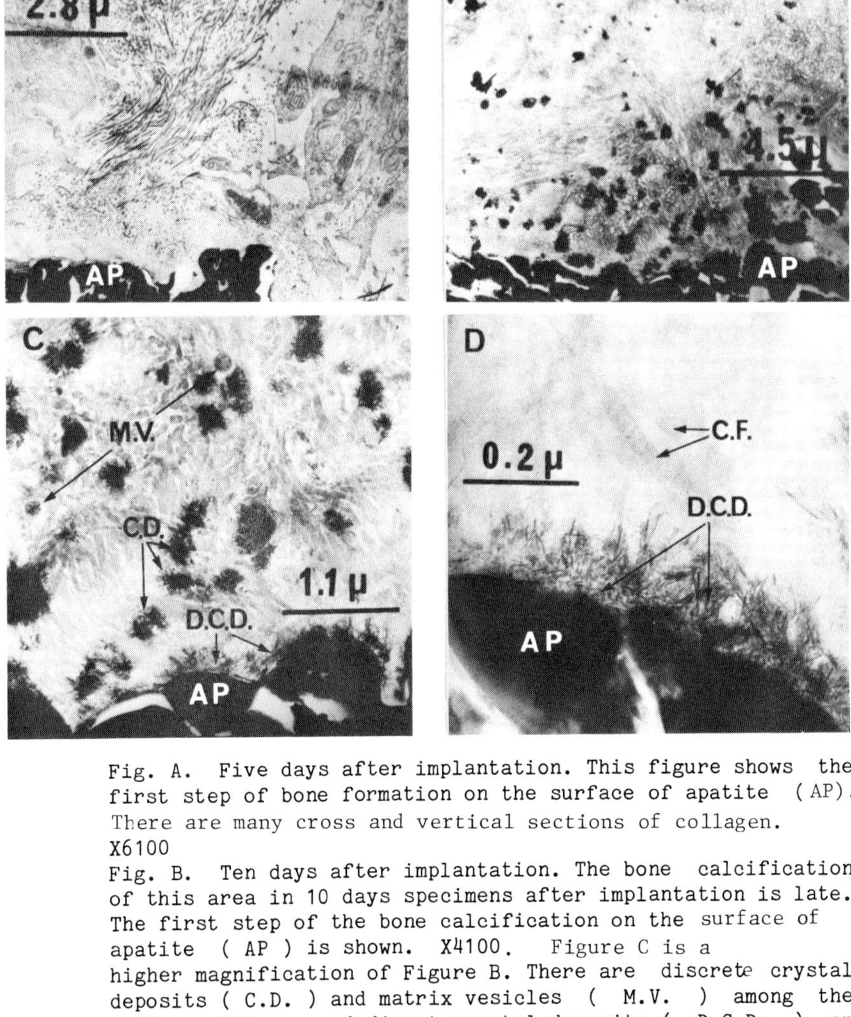

Fig. A. Five days after implantation. This figure shows the
first step of bone formation on the surface of apatite (AP).
There are many cross and vertical sections of collagen.
X6100
Fig. B. Ten days after implantation. The bone calcification
of this area in 10 days specimens after implantation is late.
The first step of the bone calcification on the surface of
apatite (AP) is shown. X4100.   Figure C is a
higher magnification of Figure B. There are discrete crystal
deposits (C.D.) and matrix vesicles (M.V.) among the
collagen fibers, and direct crystal deposits (D.C.D.) on
the surface of apatite.   X14600
Fig. D. Figure D is higher magnification of Figure C. Direct
crystal deposits (D.C.D.) on the surface of apatite (AP)
takes place independently of collagen fibers (C.F.)
formation on the apatite surface.   X81200

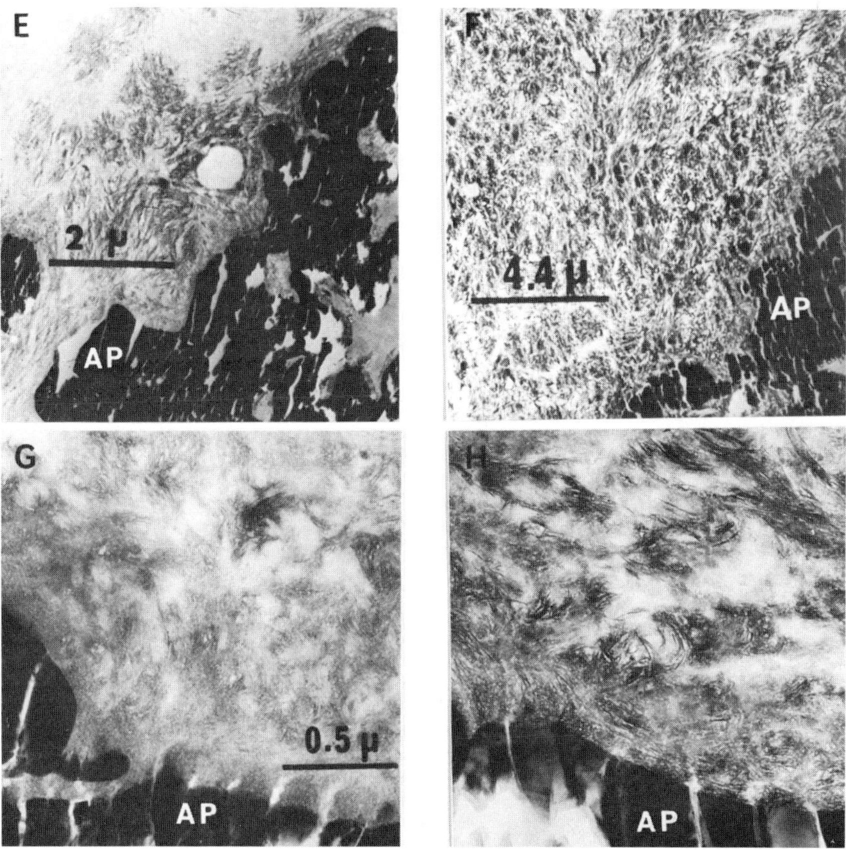

Fig. E. Ten days after implantation. The bone calcification
of this area in 10 days specimens is more advanced than
Figure B. X8700
Fig. F. Ten days after implantation. The bone calcification
of this area is most advanced in 10 days specimens. X4400
Fig. G. Figure G is higher magnification of Figure F. Bone
crystal is rougher, shorter and thinner than that of normal
bone. X31500
Fig. H. Sixty days after implantation. Bone tissue are
almost the same as those of normal bones. X40000

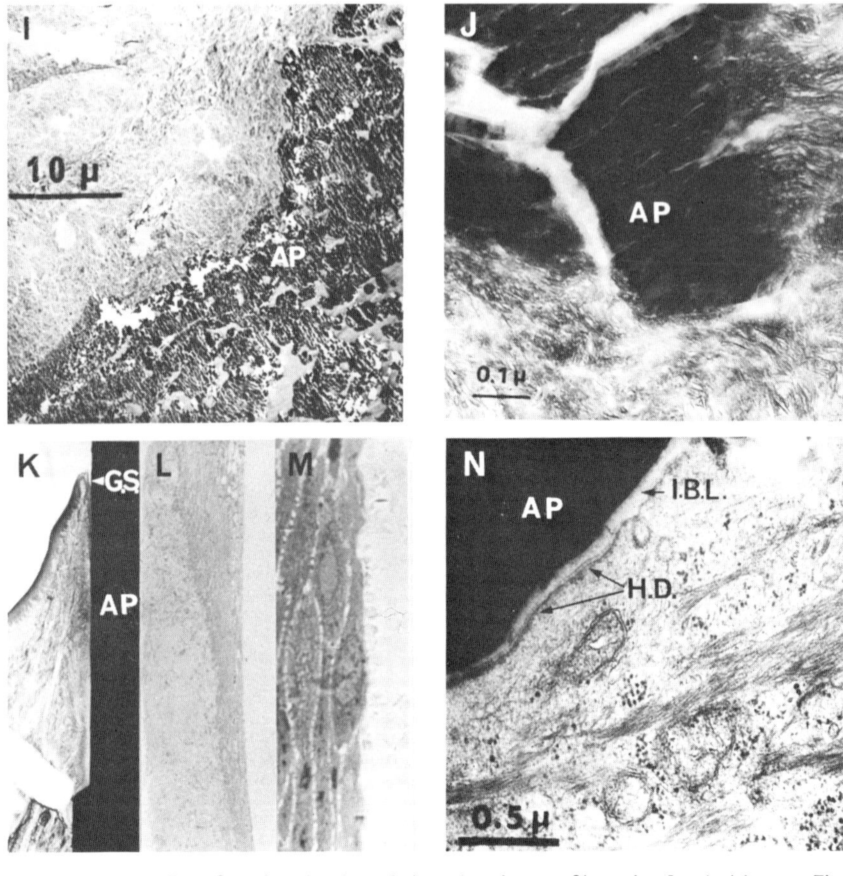

Fig. I.   One hundred and twenty days after implantation.   The
are bone canaliculae and bone cavities in the bone tissue   on
the apatite surface.   X1600
Fig. J.   This figure is higher magnification of Figure I.
Bone crystal on the surface of apatite are the same as those
of normal bone.   X81600
Fig. K.   The relation of gingival tissue and apatite (AP)
is shown. Gingival sulcus (G.S.) is extremely shallow.   The
gingival tissue presents a low grade type of inflammation.
Fig. L.   Up side is sulcus side. The epithelial cell layer
has became narrow in width with the apical displacement.
Fig. M.   Higher magnification of Figure L   shows that
epithelial cells are firmly connected with each other by
intercellular bridges and adhering to apatite crystals.
Fig. N.   The epithelial cell membrane is electron
microscopically adhering to apatite (AP) through internal
basement lamina (I.B.L.) The well-developed hemidesmosomes
(H.D.) are shown along the cell membrane.   X27800

Biomaterials 1980
Edited by G. D. Winter, D. F. Gibbons, and H. Plenk, Jr.
© 1982 John Wiley and Sons Ltd.

EXPERIMENTAL STUDIES ON THE IMPLANTATION OF HYDROXYAPATITE IN THE MEDULLARY CANAL OF RABBITS

S. Niwa, K. Sawai, S. Takahashi, H. Tagai*, M. Ono** and Y. Fukuda**

Aichi Medical University, Aichi-ken, Japan
*Chiba Institute of Technology, Chiba-ken, Japan.
**Mitsubishi Mining and Cement Co., Ltd., Japan.

SUMMARY

This report concerns the histological investigation of bone following the introduction of synthetic hydroxyapatite in the medullary canal of rabbits. Two holes were made in the proximal femoral shaft of rabbits and a composite of synthetic hydroxyapatite powder and physiological saline was implanted into the medullary canal. The animals were killed one week to six months after implantation and the specimens were observed by decalcifying and undecalcifying methods. By seven days after implantation, half of the hydroxyapatite granules were already tightly covered with newly formed bone which had active osteoblasts on its surface. The rest of the granules were filled with connective tissue, in which no appreciable foreign body reaction was observed. By 21 days the whole implanted granules were embedded in the new bone, which formed new cancellous bone in the femoral canal. By six months this cancellous bone became porotic by the bone resorption except in the area of the drilled holes. These porotic changes could be regarded as the result of the proper function of the rabbits marrow. These results suggest the clinical application of the synthetic hydroxyapatite.

INTRODUCTION

The recent development of biomaterials in the orthopaedic field, especially of ceramics including alumina, has been remarkable but reports on the clinical application of these materials have been limited mostly to replacement arthroplasty. We have taken an interest in the induction of bone by these ceramics and have investigated this phenomenon by an original method, described in this paper.

The purpose of this paper is to present our observations that a synthetic hydroxyapatite, which closely resembles bone mineral, possesses high osteogenic capacity and excellent potential as a bonegraft material.

MATERIALS AND METHODS

In the conventional methods, biomaterials in the hard tissue are studied either by inserting the material into the bone through a gap, or by fixing screw-shaped materials into bone. These methods, however, have the shortcomings that the bone reaction caused by the operation itself or by mechanical stress affects the results. We have developed a new technique which avoids these problems as much as possible and the interface between the materials and the tissue is made maximum.

65

                                           S. Niwa et al

Under intravenous anaesthesia two small holes were made by drilling in the proximal femoral shaft of adult rabbits and bone marrow was washed out by injecting physiological saline into the hole with a syringe. Four kinds of material were injected into the spaces between the two holes in the bone:

1. Synthetic hydroxyapatite $Ca_{10}(PO_4)_6(OH)_2$ powder with the calcium phosphorous ratio of 1.67.

2. Tricalcium-phosphate, $3Cao.P_2O_5$ powder which was reported to have high osteogenic capacity for bone graft (Koster, 1979).

3. 99.9% high density alumina powder.

4. Polymethylmethacrylate (Simplex C bone cement).

Each of the powders was mixed with physiological saline (Fig. 1). The animals were killed from one to six months after implantation and the specimens were observed by the decalcifying and undecalcifying methods.

RESULTS

Hydroxyapatite injected group: By seven days after the implantation half of the apatite was buried in the connective tissue, in which no appreciable foreign body reaction was observed. The rest of the granules were already tightly covered with newly formed bone or osteoid, the surface of which showed active osteoblasts. Some of the surrounding cells, which resembled fibroblasts, were turning to osteoblasts and were forming new bone (Fig. 2). The newly formed bone produced a variety of cancellous bone by joining with other new bone, made by intramembranous ossification. In the decalcified specimens, some osteocyts were seen to adhere directly to the granules (Fig. 3). Radiomicrographs showed growth of newly formed bone of low density (Fig. 4). The fluorescence micrographs at this stage showed increase of new bone formation within the marrow cavity.

This active bone formation around the granules continued until four weeks after implantation, when all of the granules were embedded in the new bone, which then formed the new cancellous bone in the femoral canal. Radiographically, the density of the trabeculae in the new cancellous bone was still lower than in the cortical bone, but the lacunae within the trabeculae were arrayed in regular order (Fig. 5). After four weeks no vigorous bone formation was observed and the trabeculae appeared to be fully mineralized. By six months this cancellous bone became porotic as a result of bone resorption. However, the drilled part in the bone, which had been filled with lamellar bone composed of hydroxy-apatite, remained nonporotic.

Tricalcium phosphate injected group: By fourteen days after implantation little new bone formation could be seen. By four weeks nearly one third of the granules formed new bone by connecting with one another, though the other two thirds did not produce any new bone. Some multinucleated giant cells were detected between the granules (Fig. 6).

Alumina injected group: By two weeks after the operation there was almost no bone formation, and the alumina particles were simply encapsulated in fibrous connective tissue. By four weeks, a few new bone trabeculae were formed between the granules, some of which connected directly with alumina, and the others across the membrane (Fig. 7).

Polymethyl methacrylate powder injected group: The mass of all the cement granules was covered with fibrous membrane which separated it from the normal tissue. Numerous foreign body giant cells were found within the mass, while no bone formation was observed.

DISCUSSION

Synthetic hydroxyapatite injected into the marrow cavity of the rabbit's femoral shaft induced new bone formation by one week. In the undecalcifying specimen, many osteblasts adhered to the apatite granules and formed osteoid and new bone. Microradiographically there was no cleavage plane between the bone and the hydroxyapatite. By four weeks apatite granules served as the nuclei to form new lamellar cancellous bone. Subsequently, the density of bone continued to increase. However, at six months, the new bone became porotic as the result of resorption. This porotic change could be regarded as a reversion to the normal from and function of the rabbit's marrow. Tricalcium phosphate granules also produced new bone, although the time required was longer than for hydroxyapatite and the amount of bone produced was less. Alumina granules did not produce new bone, neither did bone cement. Until now, synthetic hydroxyapatite has been studied mainly in the dental field, and its high capacity for bone induction and bone-bonding was reported by Aoki et al. (1977), Onchi et al. (1977) and others. But mechanisms of bone formation by hydroxyapatite is not well understood. However, the results of the above experiment indicates that in the marrow cavity the hydroxyapatite stimulates osteogenesis and induces bone formation (Takahashi et al., 1979). In the case of the transplantation of bone, it has been long a matter in question whether the organic matrix or the inorganic salts of the implanted bone plays an advancing part, though Wells (1911) observes that calcium salts make connective tissue cells active and cause metaplasia not only into osteoblasts but even into marrow cells with hematogenic function. As substitute materials for bone tissue with good biocompatibility, Al_2O_3, TCP, Carbon and Bioglass (Hench, 1971) which is thought to be connected with bone directly and chemically are studied and developed, and partly in use, but these materials are different from human bone tissues and continue to be foreign bodies forever. On the other hand, synthetic hydroxyapatite is very similar to bone component, and if the possibility of the clinical use of this hydroxyapatite in the orthopedic field is to be considered, it is an ideal material for bone-grafting because of its good histocompatibility and high osteogenic capacity, and also because its supply is inexhaustible and its application easy.

REFERENCES

AOKI, H., KATO, K., OGISO, M. and TABATA, T. (1977). Hydroxyapatite for new Dental Implant Materials. Dental Outlook, 49, 567–575.

HENCH, L. L., SPLINTER, R. J., ALLEN, W. C. and GREENLEE, T. K. (1971). Bonding Mechanisms at the Interface of Ceramic Prosthetic Materials. J. Biomed. Mater. Res. Symposium, 2, 117–141.

KOSTER, K., EHARD, H., KUBICEK, J. and HEIDE, H. (1979). Experimentelle Anwendung von Kalziumphosphatgranulat zur Substitution von Konventionellen Knochentransplantaten. Z. Orthop., 118, 398–403.

ONCHI, T., HURUYA, M., IIDA, M. and AOKI, H. (1977). Hydroxyapatite for new Biomaterials. J. Jap. Orthop. Ass., 51, 1039–1040.

TAKAHASHI, S., NIWA, S., SAWAI, K., TAGAI, H., ONO, M. and FUKUDA, Y. (1979). Experimental Studies on the Implantation of synthetic Hydroxyapatite. Cent. Jap. Orthop. Traumat., in press.
WELLS, H. G. (1911). Calcification and Ossification. Arch. Int. Med. 7, 721–753.

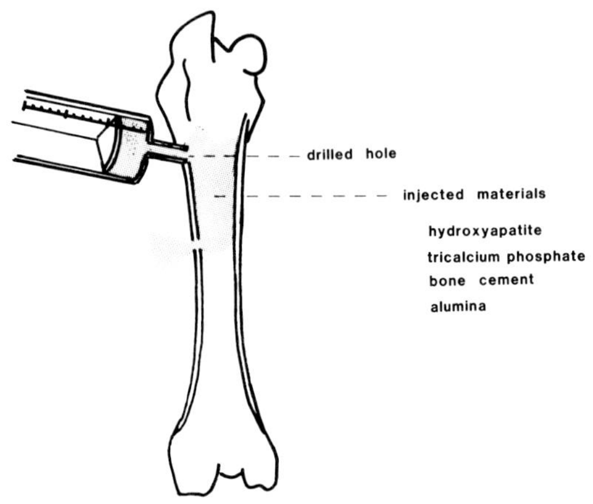

Fig. 1

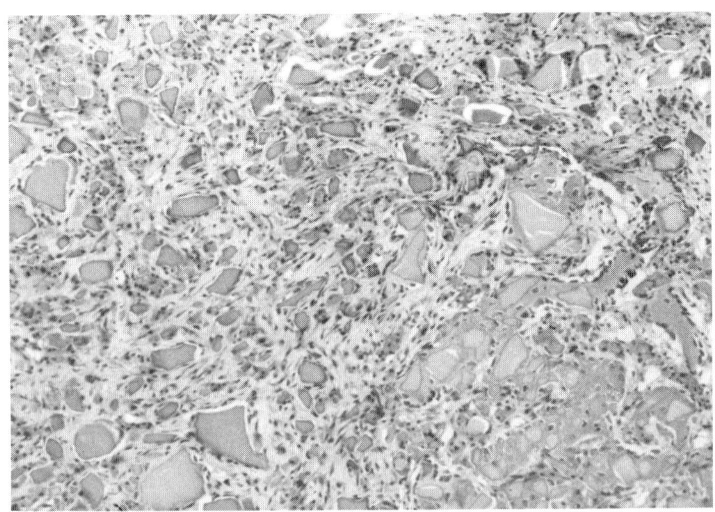

Fig. 2

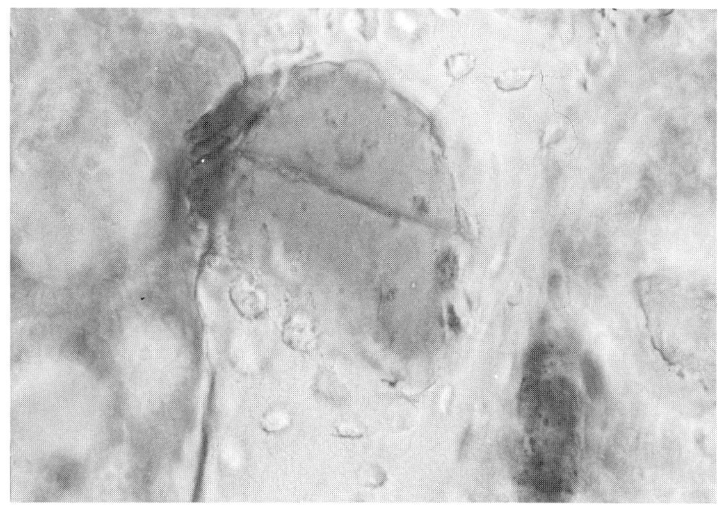

Fig. 3

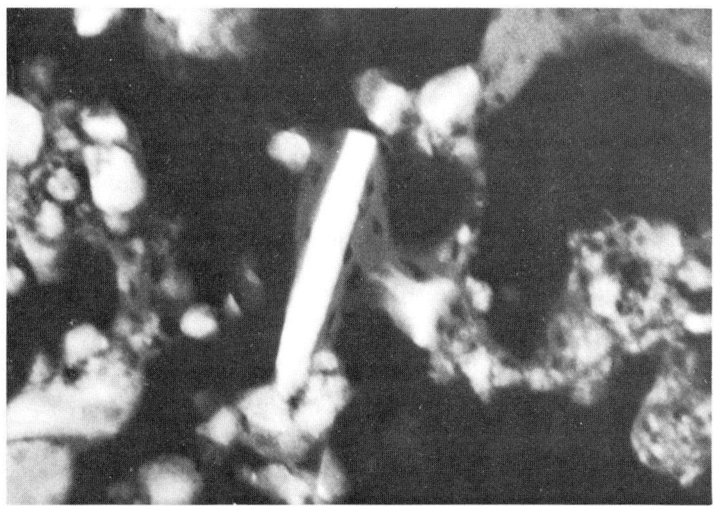

Fig. 4

S. Niwa et al

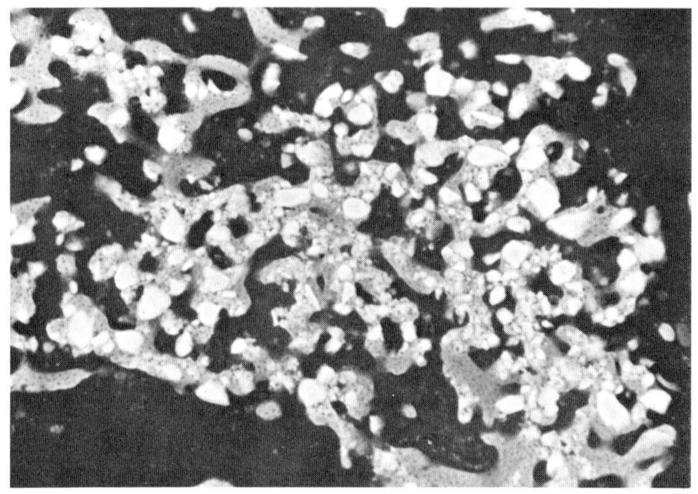

Fig. 5

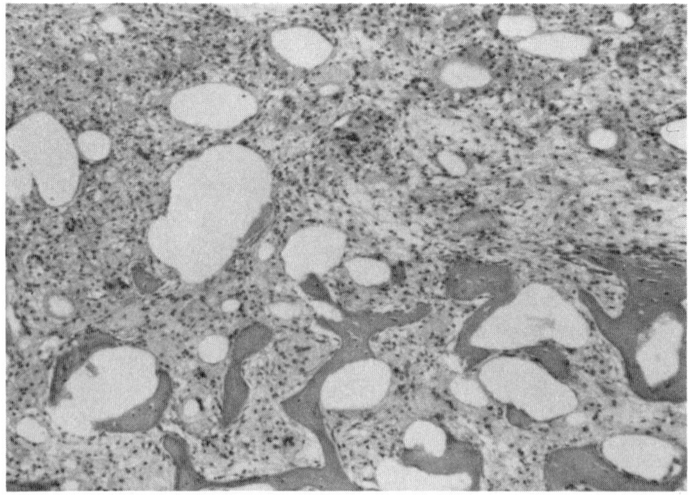

Fig, 6

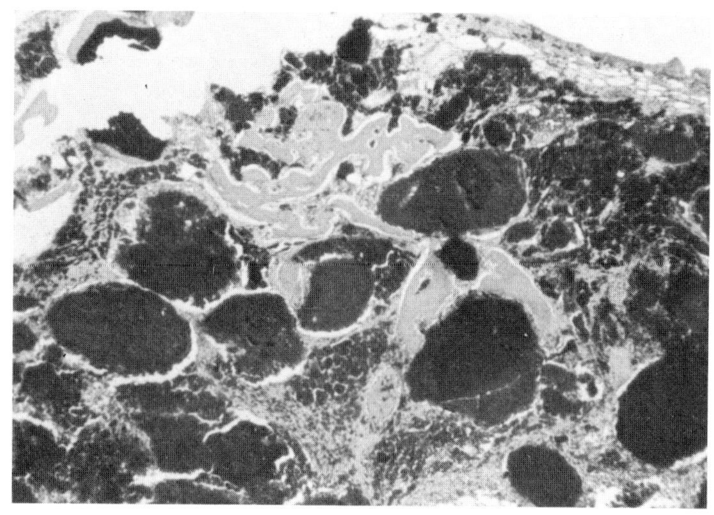

Fig. 7

Biomaterials 1980
Edited by G. D. Winter, D. F. Gibbons, and H. Plenk, Jr.
© 1982 John Wiley and Sons Ltd.

STUDY OF BONE INGROWTH IN POROUS CALCIUM
ALUMINO-PHOSPHATE GLASS CERAMICS

P.Baldet,[*] F.Pernot,[**] J.Zarzycki,[**]
F.Bonnel, and P. Rabischong.[***]

[*] Laboratoire d'Anatomie Pathologique, Hopital
Gui de Chauliac, 34059 Montpellier, France.
[**] Laboratoire des Verres du CNRS et Laboratoire
de Science des Matériaux, Université Montpellier II,
34060 Montpellier Cedex, France.
[***] Unité de Recherches Biomécaniques U. 103, INSERM,
Avenue des Moulins, 34000 Montpellier, France.

SUMMARY

Porous glass-ceramics prepared by controlled crystallization of a
calcium alumino-phosphate "foam" glass were implanted in rabbits'
bones and the resulting bone ingrowth studied by histological methods.
It is shown that the growth process is conditionned by the texture of
the material : satisfactory results were obtained with an average
interconnection diameter between the pores greater than 25 microns.
The ingrowth then presents general characteristics of intramembranous
ossification : condensation of collagen fibers around capillaries,
embedding of connective cells, followed by deposition of calcium salts.
Trabeculae of primary woven bone were totally formed from the 2nd
month. The transformation in lamellar bone with specialization of
osteoblasts took place between the 2nd and 3rd months. Development of
hematopoietic marrow began after 6 months. The degree of bone
ingrowth could reach more than 40%. When the average interconnection
diameter was less than 25 microns only an ingrowth of fibrous tissue
was observed.

INTRODUCTION

Metal bone prostheses have long been used in orthopaedic surgery but
as they have a much greater strength than the surrounding bone, the
living organism reacts unfavourably towards both the metallic implant
and the cement used for fixation. This led to the consideration of the
particular advantages offered by ceramics and to the synthesis of
materials which would promote a direct bond between the bone tissue
and prostheses.

One solution consists in replacing the metal by a vitreous or glass-
ceramic material which reacts chemically with the bone. This
technique was proposed in the U.S.A. (Hench et al., 1971 ; Beckham et
al., 1971 ; Hench & Paschall, 1973) and in Western Germany (Brömer et
al., 1975 ; Strunz et al., 1977 ; Bunte et al., 1977).

P. Baldet et al.

Another solution is to use porous materials with interconnected pores. Such structures with optimal morphological characteristics permit tissue ingrowth and thus ensure a perfect anchoring with the surrounding bone. Interesting results were obtained with the Replamine® form process which consists of replicating the structure of corals in metals, ceramics or organic polymers (Weber & White, 1973 ; Chiroff et al., 1975). Other attempts were made to use porous alumina or calcium aluminates (Klawitter & Hulbert, 1971 ; Lyng et al. 1973 ; Benum et al., 1976 ; Benum et al., 1977). These ceramics were well tolerated and showed successful bone ingrowth but their mechanical strength was rather low. This led to the investigation of the possibility of using glass-ceramics which are extremely fine grained ceramics obtained by controlled crystallization of suitable glasses and which may be tailored to possess excellent mechanical properties. Such a material was previously synthesized (Pernot et al., 1979), and the present paper describes the biological results obtained with this new material.

MATERIALS AND METHODS

To obtain a porous glass-ceramic, porosity is introduced into the base glass by the classical method of making a "foam" glass (Schulz, 1954). A foaming agent (in this case $CaCO_3$) is added to a suitable glass (previously ground) and the mixture heat-treated above the transformation temperature T_g of the glass. This thermal treatment allows the sintering of the glass particles imprisoning the $CaCO_3$ particles, then at the same temperature the foaming agent reacts, gives off gas within the low viscosity glass mass and produces the foaming effect. Finally, after the onset of foaming, ceramization occurs. Crystallization has a twofold function, it arrests foaming when the pores have reached a suitable size and brings about a general increase in the mechanical strength of the material resulting from the convertion of glass into a microcrystalline phase.

In practice the method requires a careful choice of base-glass, foaming agent and heat-treatment temperature. This was achieved using differential thermal analysis techniques (Pernot et al., 1979). Moreover the glass should be well accepted by the living organism. All these criteria led to the choice of calcium alumino-phosphate glass ($80\%Ca(PO_3)_2-20\%\ AlPO_4$). Such a glass with the appropriate heat-treatment temperature allows sintering and foaming to be obtained prior to crystallization. By controlling these different steps, selecting the granulometry of the powdered base glass and by adding different quantities of $CaCO_3$ it is possible to prepare samples with various textural and mechanical properties.

To study the texture, the following characteristics were measured : bulk density (picnometric method); apparent density, open porosity (Archimedes' method) ; total porosity from apparent volume and, by mercury porosimetry, interconnection pore size distribution which is obtained from a plot of the incremental volume of the mercury intruded versus diameter (Klawitter & Hulbert, 1971) ; an average diameter can be defined where half of the pore volume is filled with

mercury. To evaluate the mechanical properties, samples of
approximate dimensions 40x5x3 mm were subjected to a bending test
in a four point loading mode on a Instron machine with a cross-head
speed of 0,2 mm/mn^{-1}.

The general tolerance of materials was tested by implanting powders
with various granulometry (50-80 microns) into rats' peritoneum
(0,50 per animal). A histological study was realized on animals
killed after uniform periods (3 months). To study the bone ingrowth ,
samples of various porosity and interconnection pore size
distribution were implanted under the tibial plate or in the
diaphysal and medullary bone of New Zealand white rabbits. The
animals were killed after periods ranging from 1 to 15 months.
Immediately after sacrifice the operated bone was removed and fixed
in 0,2 M sodium cacodylate-buffered, 3% glutaraldehyde for 4 days.
The specimen was dehydrated by soaking for 10 days in 80 percent
alcohol and finally embedded in "BIOPLASTIC" . Sections of about
1 mm thick were cut and then ground down to about 50 µm thickness.
The samples were stained with Villanueva's osteochrome, Masson's or
Goldner's trichrome and observed by ordinary or polarized light
optical microscopy. Some specimens were prepared for scanning
electron microscopy. Morphometric studies were made from photographs
with an automatic analyser.

RESULTS

Total porosity of the samples ranges from 40% to 70% (Fig.1). This
porosity is almost entirely an open one ; as may be seen from Table 1
the difference between the open and total porosity does not exceed 4%.
The interconnection between the pores may be easily observed on
scanning electron micrographs (Fig.2). Fig.3 shows the interconnection
pore size distribution for each sample studied, the average diameter
varies between 14 and 55 microns (Table 1).

TABLE 1. Properties of the materials

Materials	Apparent density g/cm3	Porosities Open (%)	Total (%)	Average interconnection diameter (m)	Fracture bending stress $(10^7 Nm^{-2})$	Young's modulus $(10^7 Nm^{-2})$
A	0.90	66	70	55	1.0	750
B	1.33	53	55	43	2.0	1200
C	1.40	46	50	26	2.4	1500
D	1.67	36	40	14	4.0	2400
Bone	–	–	–	–	12.0	1800 to 2000

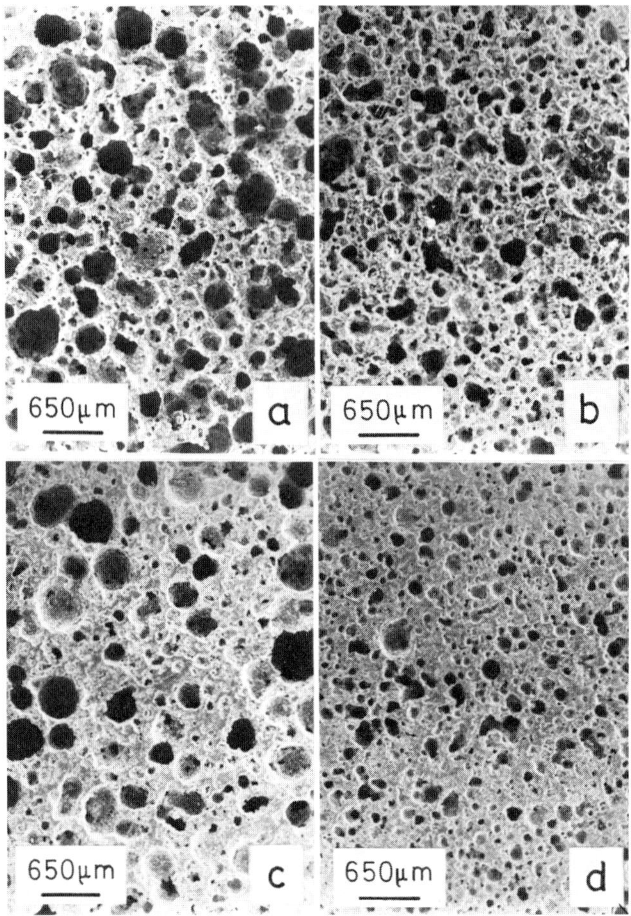

Fig.1. Scanning electron micrographs of some porous
glass-ceramics; porosity of the materials:
(a) 70% ; (b) 55% ; (c) 50% ; (d) 40%.

The stress/strain curves are given in Figure 4. The fracture bending
stress which is about 4.10^7 Nm^{-2} for the material with 40% porosity
falls to $1\ 10^{-7} Nm^{-2}$ for the 70% porosity (Table 1). Young's modulus
was calculated from the linear portion of the curves : it is
situated between 750 and $2400\ 10^7 Nm^{-2}$ (Table 1) and depends directly
on porosity. While the fracture bending stress is always rather low
compared with that of bone $(12.10^7 Nm^{-2})$, Young's modulus of C and D
materials appears rather similar to the bone's modulus (1800 to 2000
$10^7 Nm^{-2}$).

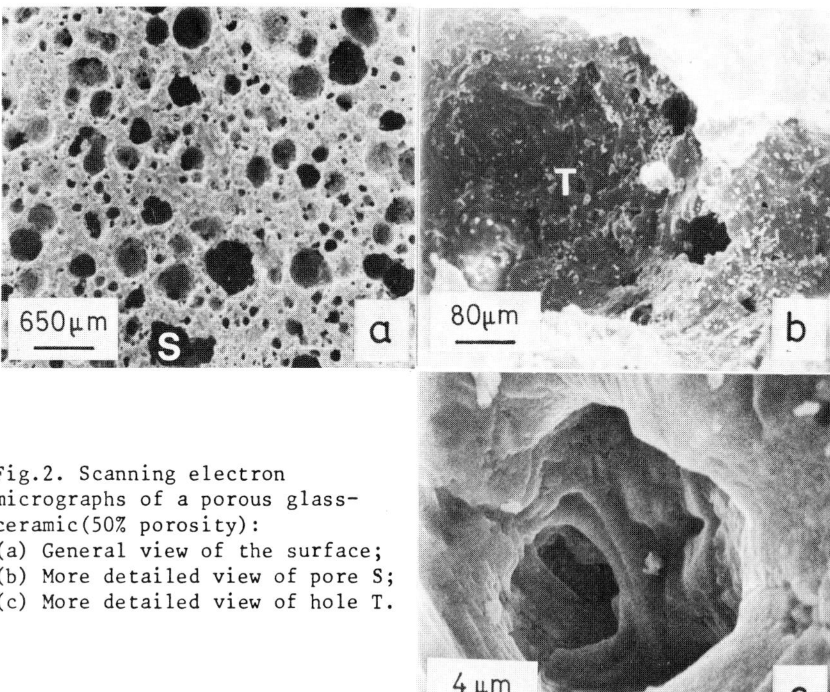

Fig.2. Scanning electron
micrographs of a porous glass-
ceramic(50% porosity):
(a) General view of the surface;
(b) More detailed view of pore S;
(c) More detailed view of hole T.

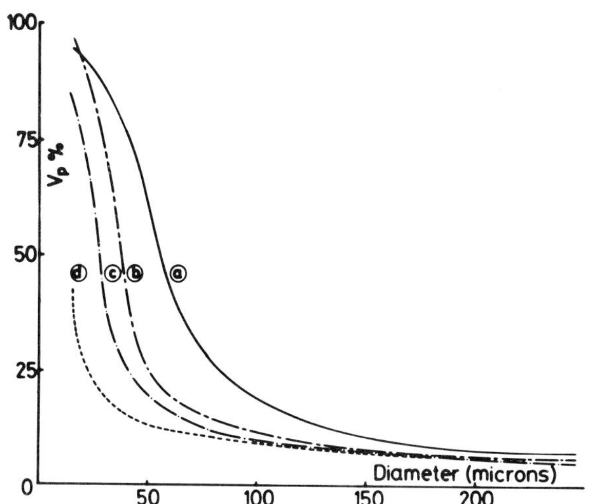

Fig.3. Interconnection pore size distribution curves.
Porosities of glass-ceramics studied :
(a) 70%; (b) 55%; (c) 50% ; (d) 40%.

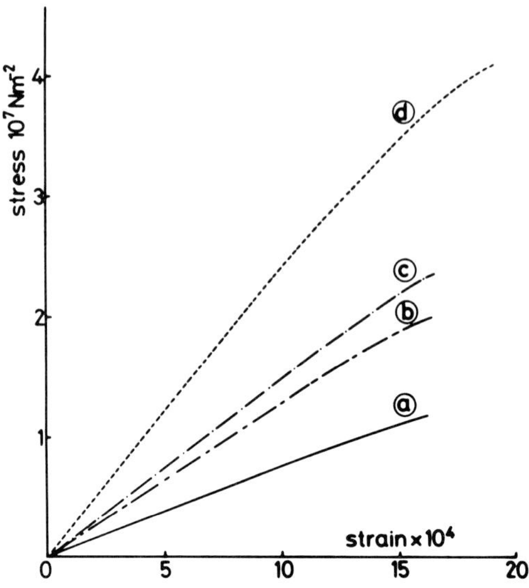

Fig.4. Stress/Stain curves for some porous materials.

The optimal porosity for bone ingrowth was evaluated after three to
six months implantation by qualitative study of bone ingrowth in
samples with various textural characteristics (Bonnel, et al. 1979)
Satisfactory ingrowth required an average interconnection diameter
between the pores greater than 25 microns, the open porosity being
more than 45%. For materials with lower porosity (36%) and average
interconnection diameter less than 15 microns, only vascular fibrous
tissue with scanty woven bone was observed.

The study of bone ingrowth was realized on samples with open porosity
ranging from 45 to 66% for periods of 1 to 15 months.

After one month, a fibroblastic reaction with resorptive giant cell
(Fig.5a) and a beginning of embedding by a woven bone tissue was
observed around the implants. The hematopoietic marrow was not
modified which was felt to be indicative that an adverse tissue
reaction had not taken place. The implantation hole was totally
filled by reparative compact bone.

The pores of the implant were completely invaded by a highly
vascularized, loose fibroblastic tissue (Fig.5b), which condensed
close to the periphery of the pores, embedding connective cells and
preforming bone trabeculae. Calcium salt deposition occured, but at
this time no oesteoblasts were observed. However, some surface pores
already contained trabeculae of primary woven bone.

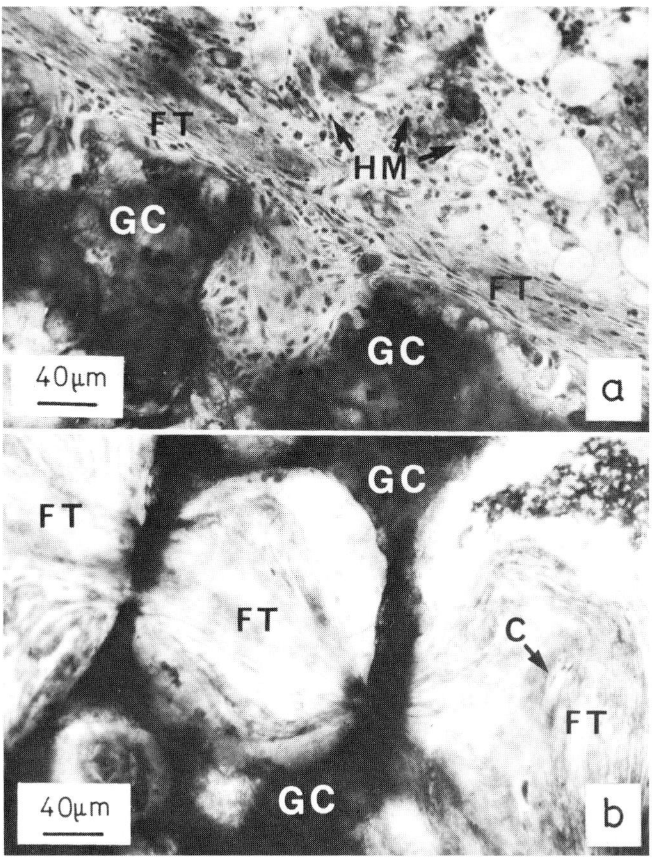

Fig.5. Aspect of bone ingrowth after 1 month :
a) Fibroblastic reaction FT and hematopoietic marrow HM
at the periphery of the glass ceramic implant GC.
b) Highly vascularized (C: capillaries) fibrous tissue FT
enters the pores .; H:haemorrhage.

After two months, the implant was totally embedded by bone tissue
but the ceramic was separated from the bone by a thin layer of
connective tissue of 10 to 15 μm thickness in which persisted
resorptive giant cells.

In the pores of the implant, perivascular condensation of fibrous
tissue appeared very distinctly and the amount of primary woven bone
was considerable (Fig.6a). The first lamellar bone trabeculae with
parallel orientation of collagen fibers (Fig.6b) and lining
osteoblasts (Fig.6c) were differentiated.

 P. Baldet et al.

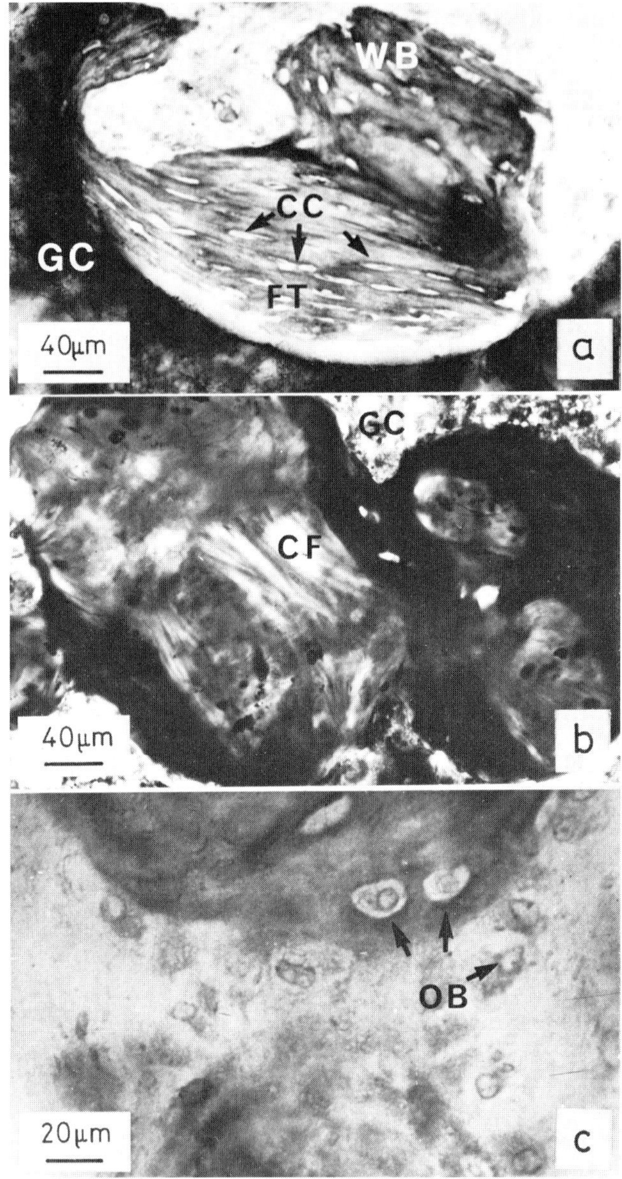

Fig . 6. Aspect of bone ingrowth after 2 months :
a) Close to the periphery of a pore, condensation of fibrous tissue FT
embedding connective cells CC and formation of woven bone WB.
b) Formation of lamellar bone ; parallel orientation of collagen
fibers CF (polarized light)
c) Differentiation of lamellar bone LB with lining osteoblasts OB.

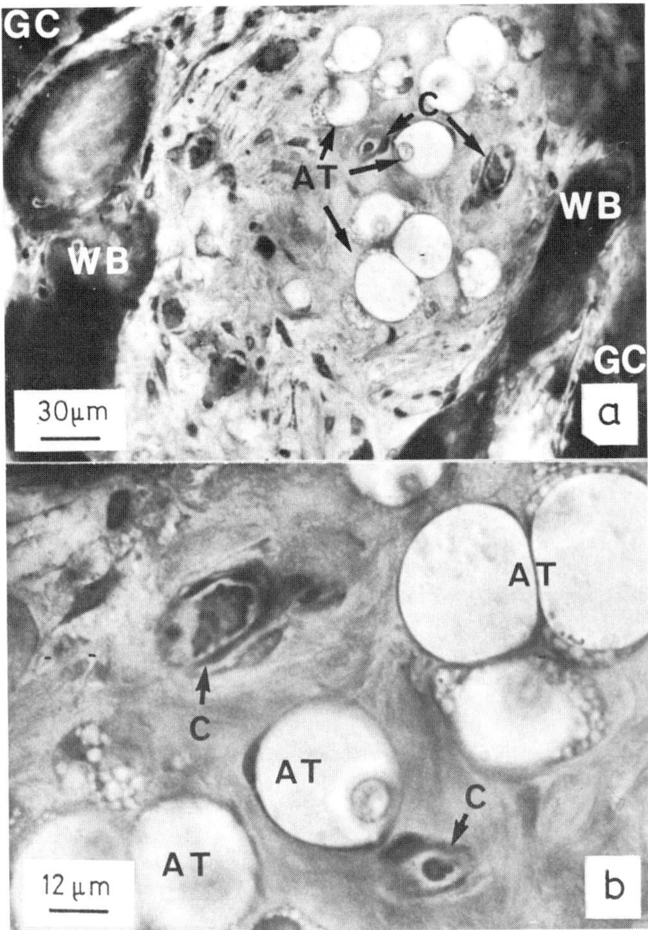

Fig. 7. Aspect of bone ingrowth after 3 months :
a) In a pore, woven bone trabeculae WB with adipose tissue AT
   and capillaries C.
b) More detailed view of adipose tissue AT
   with capillaries C.

After three months, bone ingrowth was nearly complete. Immature bone
trabeculae were seen to mould the walls of all the pores (Fig.7a)
a capillary network was well developed and adipose tissue without
hematopoietic cells appeared (Figs. 7a and 7b).

After six months, differentiation of lamellar bone was almost
complete (Fig.8) and the first hematopoietic cells were observed in
adipose tissue. Peripheral embedding reaction was very intense as is
shown by scanning electron microscopy (Fig.9).

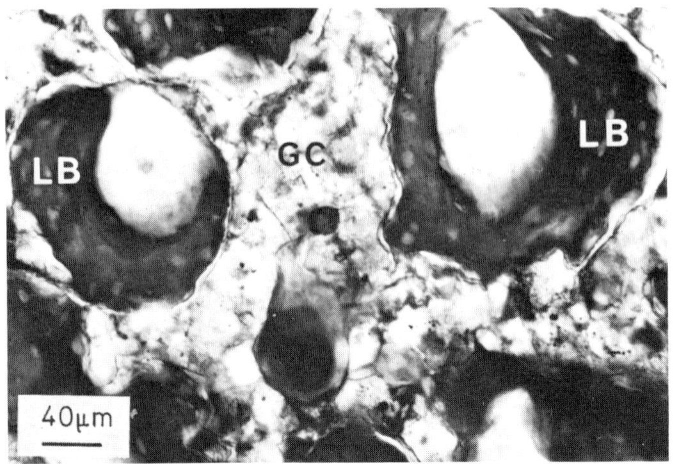

Fig. 8. Aspect of bone ingrowth after 6 months.
LB : lamellar bone ; GC : glass-ceramic.

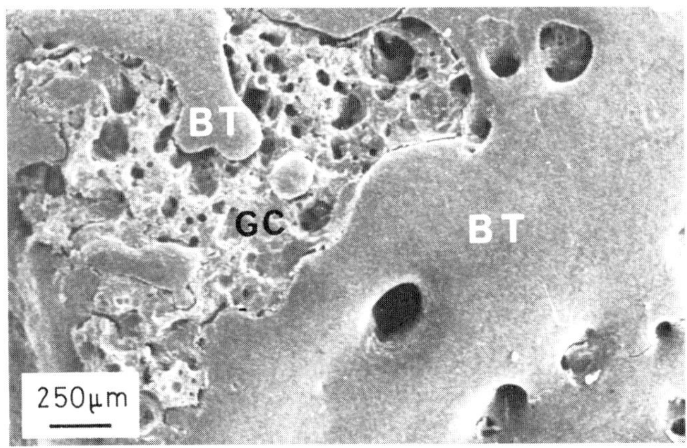

Fig. 9. Scanning electron micrograph of embedding
by bone tissue after 6 months.
BT : bone tissue ; GC : glass-ceramic.

From the 9th to 15th month, histological aspects showed no great
change. Lamellar bone was still not mature but was lined by
osteoblasts and osteoclastic cells. Hemotopoietic cells were
completely differentiated. Microfractionning of material without
breaking, with a histiocytic resorptive reaction, was observed after
fifteen months. The evolution of this has not yet been studied, but
the phenomenon could be due to a beginning of biodegradation.

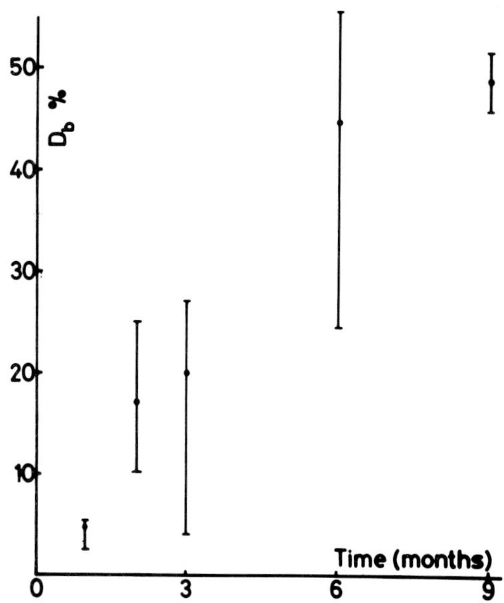

Fig. 10.   Degree of bone ingrowth (%) versus time (months)

A quantitative study of bone ingrowth was made by comparing, for a given material, the respective volume fraction V_p and V_b of pores and bone ; the degree of bone ingrowth was defined by the ratio :

$$D_b = \frac{V_b}{V_p} \times 100$$

and a plot of D_b versus time (Fig. 10.) showed an important increase in D_b from the 1st to the 9th month when it reached about 50%.

DISCUSSION

The study of general tolerance reported in a previous paper (Bonnel et al., 1977) already suggested that there was a good tolerance of the material ; the histological tests showed a limited giant-cell resorptive reaction with fibrous tissue and an absence of extensive inflammation.

The results of this experimental study of bone ingrowth seem to prove that, in all cases, calcium aluminophosphate glass-ceramics were well accepted by the bone tissue. The quality of bone ingrowth depends on the texture of the samples studied. When the average interconnection diameter between the pores was lower than 25 microns, only an ingrowth of vascular fibrous tissue was observed. The development of bone tissue was rather low, only some primary woven bone trabeculae were obtained (Fig. 11.). The degree of bone ingrowth was not higher than 10%. In more porous implants with larger average interconnection

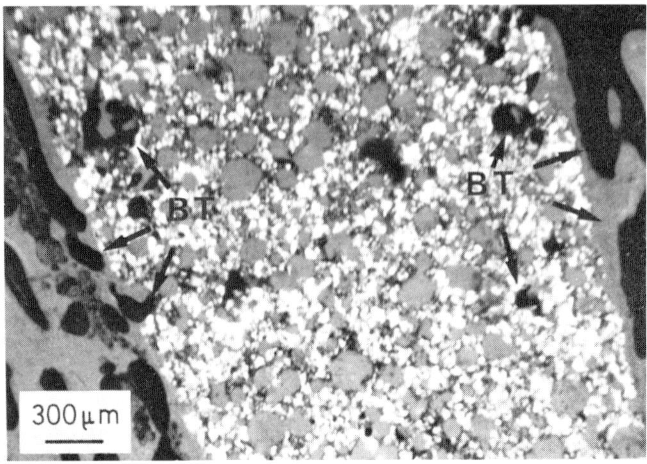

Fig. 11. Aspect of bone ingrowth for a material with low
porosity (6 months implantation).
BT : bone tissue ; GC : glass-ceramic.

diameters, differentiation of bone trabeculae took place in various
steps which be compared with "intramembranous ossification" phenomena:
condensation of collagen fibers around capillaries, embedding
connective cells, followed by deposition of calcium salts.

Trabeculae of primary woven bone were totally formed from the second
month. The transformation in lamellar bone with specialization of
osteoblasts took place between the 2nd and 3rd months.

Development of hematopoietic marrow occurred later, beginning after
6 months, and seem to be additional proof of the good tolerance of
the material. From the 9th month, the histological appearance of the
bone trabeculae did not change but further increase of calcium salt
deposition could take place during this period. This will be the
object of a microradiographic study. The degree of bone ingrowth
could reach more than 40%.

The mechanical properties of the implants were rather low compared
with those of ordinary bone. Therefore it seems necessary to improve
these properties, for example, by preparing a transition between a
porous and a dense material. Once this is achieved, these products
might be used in orthopaedics for both bone prostheses and bone
tissue replacement.

REFERENCES

Beckham, C.A., Greenlee, T.K. & Crebo, A.R. (1971) Bone formation at
a ceramic implant interface. Calc. Tiss. Res., 8, 165-171.

Benum, P., Lyng, S., Bø, O., Rafn, I. & Haffner, J.F.W. (1976)
Porous ceramics as bone substitute in the medial condyle of the tibia.
An experimental study in sheep. Acta orthop. scand., 47, 158-166.

Benum, P., Lyng, S., Alm, T. & Johannessen, N. (1977) Porous ceramics as bone substitute in the medial condyle of the tibia. An experimental study in sheep. Long-term observations. Acta orthop. scand., 48, 150-157.

Bonnel, F., Rabischong, P., Baldet, P., Pernot, F. & Zarzycki, J. (1977) Tolérance et pénétration osseuse des alumines et vitrocéramiques poreuses. Journées d'études internationales sur les matériaux et implants artificiels en chirurgie osteoarticulaire, Nancy - Vandoeuvre, pp 63-78.

Bonnel, F., Pernot, F., Baldet, P., Rabischong, P. & Zarzycki, J. (1979) Bases anatomiques de la colonisation osseuse des vitrocéramiques poreuses. Anatomia clinica, 2, 89-91

Brömer, M., Kaes, M.M. & Pfeil, E. Ernst Leitz G.m.b.H., Wetzlar, Germany (1975) Process of making biocompatible glass-ceramic U.S. patent n°3.922.155.

Bunte, M., Strunz, V., Gross, U.M., Kühl, K., Brömer, H. & Deutscher, K. (1977) Kiefer-Augmentation mit Glaskeramik im Tierversuch. Implantate. Dtsch. zahnärztl. Z., 32, 323-325.

Chiroff, R.T., White, E.W., Weber, J.N. & Roy, D.M. (1975) Tissue ingrowth of Replamineform implants. J. biomed. mater. res. Symposium 6, 29-45.

Hench, L.L., Splinter, R.J., Allen, W.C. & Greenlee, T.K. (1971) Bonding mechanism at the interface of ceramic prosthetic materials. J. biomed. mater. res. Symposium, 2, (part 1), 117-141.

Hench, L.L. & Paschall, H.A. (1973) Direct chemical bond of bioactive glass-ceramic material to bone and muscle. J. biomed. mater. res. Symposium, 4 , 25-42.

Klawitter, J.J. & Hulbert, S.F. (1971) Application of porous ceramics for the attachement of load bearing internal orthopedic applications. J. biomed. mater. res. Symposium, 2, (part 1) 161-229

Lyng, S., Sudmann, E., Hulbert, S.F. & Sauer, B.W. (1973) Fixation of permanent orthopaedic prosthesis use of ceramics in the tibial plateau. Acta orthop. scand., 44, 694-701.

Pernot, F., Zarzycki, J., Bonnel, F., Rabischong, P. & Baldet, P. (1979) New glass-ceramic materials for prosthetic applications. J. mater. sci., 14, 1694-1706.

Schulz, E.O. (1954) Schaumglas, Teil II : Zur verfahrenstechnik bei der Herstellung von Schaumglas. Silikattechnik, 5, 343-346

Strunz, V., Bunte, M., Stellmach, R., Gross, U.M., Kühl, K., Brömer, H. & Deutscher, K. (1977) Bioaktive Glaskeramik als Implantat-material in der Kieferchirurgie. Implantate. Dtsch. zahnärztl. Z., 32, 287-290.

Weber, J.N. & White, E.W. (1973) Carbonate minerals as precursors of new ceramic, metal and polymer materials for biomedical applications. Miner. sci. engng., 5, 151-165.

Biomaterials 1980
Edited by G. D. Winter, D. F. Gibbons, and H. Plenk, Jr.
© 1982 John Wiley and Sons Ltd.

TISSUE TOLERANCE OF CARBON MATERIALS

P. Christel[*], B. Buttazzoni[**], J.L. Leray[*], C. Morin[*]

[*] : I.N.S.E.R.M., Pavillon Ollier, Hôpital Cochin,
75674 Paris, France.

[**]: S.E.P., Bordeaux, France.

SUMMARY

Carbon-carbon composite materials are considered good candidates for orthopaedic implants because of their excellent tissue compatibility and versatile mechanical properties. The three materials selected for investigation of tissue tolerance were a carbon matrix prepared by chemical vapor decomposition and reinforced with carbon fabric, either pure or with 22% SiC, and pyrolysed pitch reinforced by a carbon felt. Subcutaneous implantations in rats (up to 90 days) and osteosynthesis plates in sheep (up to one year) showed that inflammatory reaction was strongly dependent upon the concentration of released particles. A pyrolytic coating slowed down the migration of particles from implants without fully preventing it. The pyrolyzed pitch was found to be inadequate for orthopaedic application because of rapid disintegration. SiC addition enhanced the stability of the material structure without causing adverse tissue reaction. However, extreme care must be taken to avoid any damage to the coating with ancillary tools during surgery.

INTRODUCTION

It is commonly accepted that metals and alloys used for prostheses and osteosynthesis devices are subject to corrosion, wear and subsequent loosening. Their comparatively high Young's modulus with respect to the skeletal tissue greatly disturbs bone remodeling (Moyen et al., 1978) and may lead to excessive bone atrophy and pathological fractures. Among the new materials recently developed for space technology, carbon-carbon composites have raised some hopes for orthopaedic applications on the basis of their excellent blood compatibility and of the broad range of their mechanical characteristics related to the versatility of their manufacturing process (Bokros, 1977). For orthopaedic implants requiring high ultimate tensile strength, a carbon fibre reinforced carbon matrix prepared by chemical vapor decomposition (CVD) was selected. This reports the investigations of the tissue tolerance of this and two other candidate carbon materials for orthopaedic applications.

MATERIALS

Three carbon composites with different matrix and reinforcing structures were tested:

a) The first one called <u>pyrolytic CRFC</u>, is manufactured by stacking several plies of high strength carbon fabric and embedding them in a pyrolytic carbon matrix prepared by chemical vapor decomposition – CDV process. The fibres of the carbon fabrics are prepared by pyrolysis of a poly-acrylonitrile precursor (PAN). After heat treatment, the final product has a specific weight of 1.73 g/cm^3 associated with 10% open porosity and a purity higher than 99%. The pore size ranges from 10 to 500 microns. Its mechanical characteristics (ultimate bending strength 300 MN/m^2, Young's modulus 70 GN/m^2) make this material suitable for building the inner core of a femoral stem in a total hip prosthesis.

b) The reinforcement of the second material, called SiC/CFRC, is made of a stack of graphitized carbon fabric plates embedded in a matrix of pyrolytic carbon and silicon carbide, deposited consecutively by CVD (Christin et al., 1979). The carbon fabric is prepared by pyrolysis of staple PAN fibre strands. The final product has a specific weight of 1.9 g/cm^3 associated with 14% open porosity, 64% v/v carbon and 22% v/v SiC. The pores are smaller than in the pyrolytic CFRC and by raising the compressive strength to 500 MN/m^2 and improving hardness, addition of SiC makes this material suitable for sliding surfaces in artificial joints.

c) The third material, called Pitch-CFRC, is made of a rayon precusor carbon felt impregnated with petroleum pitch and pyrolysed under high pressure (7 MN/m^2) at high final temperature (1600°C). The final product has a density close to 1.7 g/cm^3 associated with less than 6% closed porosity and carbon purity higher than 99%. Its mechanical properties are similar to those of polycrystalline graphite (ultimate bending strength 60 MN/m^2).

METHODS

Tissue reaction to these materials was studied using subcutaneous implants in rats and bone plates implanted in sheep.

Rat experimentation involved 90 animals with subcutaneous implants in the interscapular region. Each material was tested with three implant shapes : squares (5 x 5 x 2mm) coated with dense pyrolytic carbon, bare grooved cylinders (diameter and length were 4 x 7mm) and carbon dust collected during machining of the cylinders.

Under general anesthesia, the implants were slipped subcutaneously through a small lumbar-sacral skin incision into the interscapular region.

After 8, 30 and 60 days, the implants with surrounding tissues and

adjacent lymph nodes were retrieved for histological examination and
embedded in methylmethacrylate. Except for carbon powder, because of
the high hardness of carbon material, the histological sections were
200 μm thick and were stained by floating them on the surface of
Giemsa or Paragon solutions.

Eight 2-hole carbon plates were implanted with anodized titanium
screws on the tibias of two sheep without osteotomy. The plates were
made of pyrolytic CFRC material and four of them were coated with
dense pyrolytic carbon. In each animal two uncoated plates were implanted on one tibia and two coated ones on the contralateral bone.

RESULTS

<u>Subcutaneous implantations in rats</u>: At eight days post-op the com-
pact implants were surrounded by a fibrous tissue layer, whereas the
dust was encapsulated and invaded with fibrous tissue. There was a
mild inflammatory reaction associated with every material tested.
Increased porosity was already evident on every uncoated material
whilst coating prevented CVD materials from disintegration.
Migration of carbon particles was confined to the immediate vicinity
of the implant within the fibrous layer (Fig. 1). The larger fragments were found extracellular and embedded in fibrous tissue, the
smaller ones within macrophages and giant cells. Regional lymph nodes
were slightly swollen.

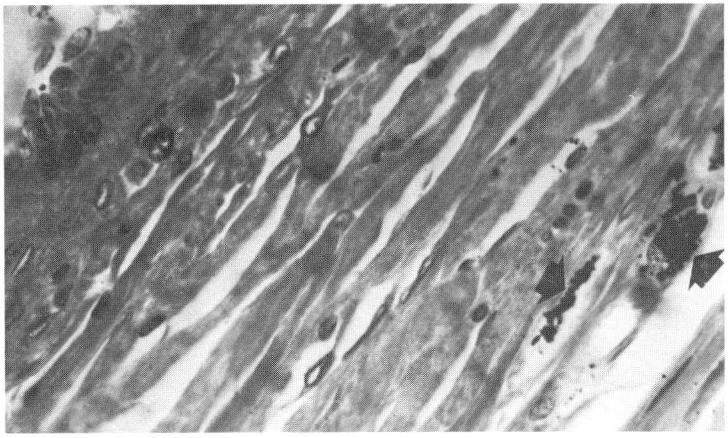

Fig. 1. Fibrous tissue layer surrounding an implant of pyro-
lytic/CFRC at 8 days (subcutaneous implantation in rat).
Arrows : carbon particles (x 400, trichrome).

At 30 days post-op, the inflammatory reaction had receded as the thickness of the fibrous layer reached 50 to 200 μm. This fibrous layer
was well vascularized, showed histiocytes in some areas and embedded
carbon particles.

Few carbon particles had migrated from the coated implants of pyrolytic
CFRC and SiC/CFRC. On the contrary the coating of the pitch-CFRC
material was disrupted from the pyrolyzed pitch matrix, the implants
had deteriorated extensively and the released carbon particles had induced a secondary foreign body reaction. The loss of carbon was even
larger from those materials which were not coated. The powder
material (Fig. 2) was well encapsulated whatever the size of the particles ranging from less than 1 μm to 200 μm.

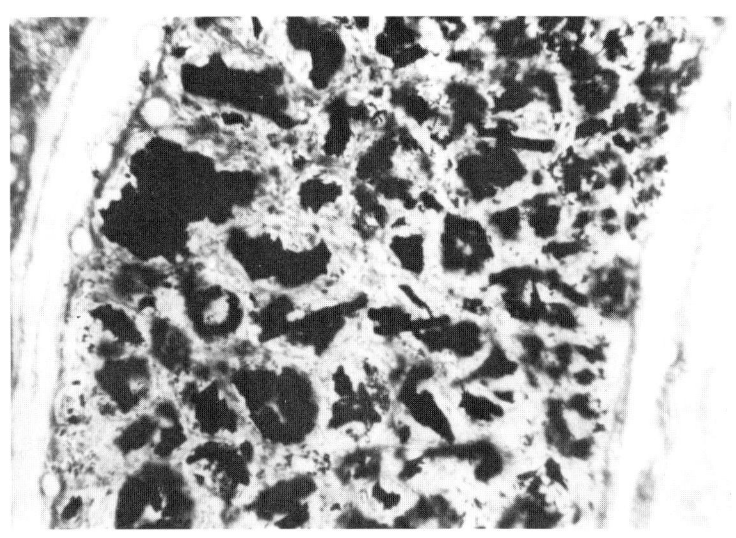

Fig. 2. Thin fibrous encapsulation of carbon powder from
pitch/CFRC implanted subcutaneously in a rat for one month.
Paragon stain (x 100).

The increased density of carbon particles released around the implants
induced increased vascularization and oedema of lymph nodes. Sinus
areas increased at the expense of follicles areas (Fig. 3). Plasmocytes and young lymphoblasts were found within the follicles and
mesenchymal cells in the sinus.

Activation of the regional lymph nodes increased from coated to bare
materials and was maximum with powder. No carbon particles were detected in the lymph nodes with the light microscope.

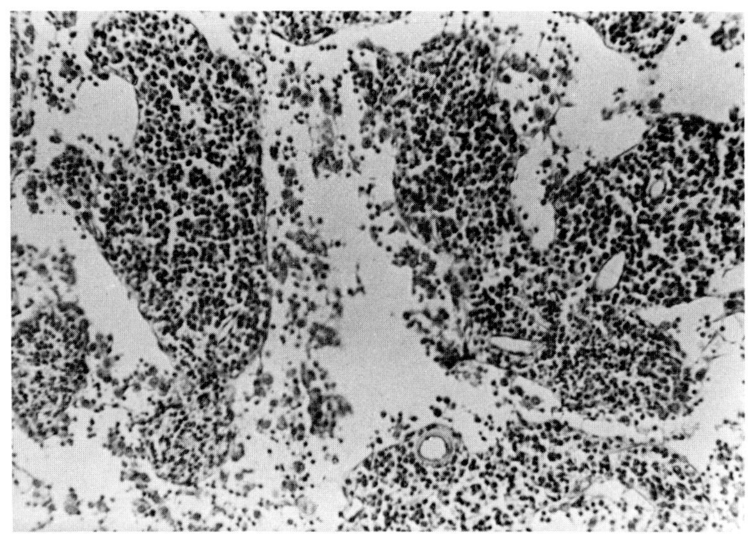

Fig. 3. Axillary lymph nodes in rats after one month implantation of carbon powder (pitch-CFRC) in the intercapsul-
ar region : oedema, vascularization and increased sinus areas
(x 100, Hematoxylin-Eosin).

At 60 days the fibrous capsule was stable without any histiocytic
clusters. Inflammatory areas, when present, corresponded to recent
coating disruption. At this stage, giant cells were observed around
grains of pyrolytic powder with fragmentation of the larger lumps.
Carbon particles were observed within the fibrous tissue layer around
every implant, whether coated or bare. The porosity had increased in
all implants except the SiC-CFRC. Pitch-CFRC was extensively degraded
and invaded by connective tissue (Fig. 4). The lymph nodes were
normal and no carbon particles were observed within them at highest
magnification of light microscope.

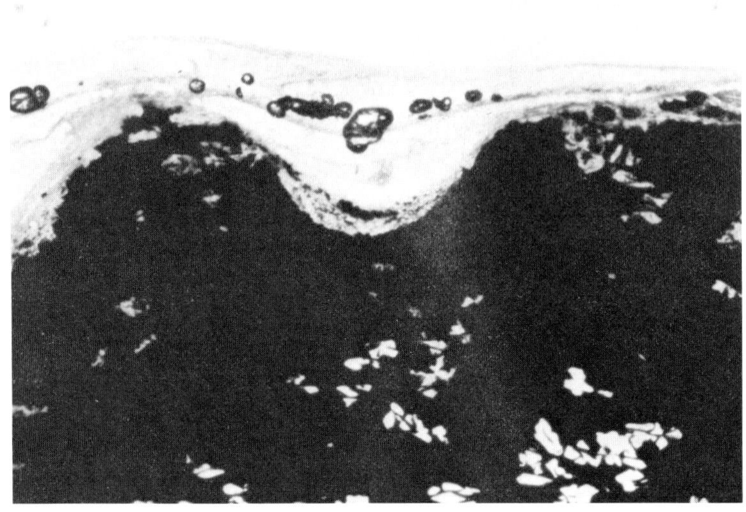

Fig. 4a.

Fig. 4 a & b. Grooved cylinders of uncoated pitch/CFRC subcutaneously implanted in rat (x 25, Paragon).
a)   one month implantation time.
b)   two months implantation time.
Cohesion of the material was poor and the material was extensively degraded after two months.

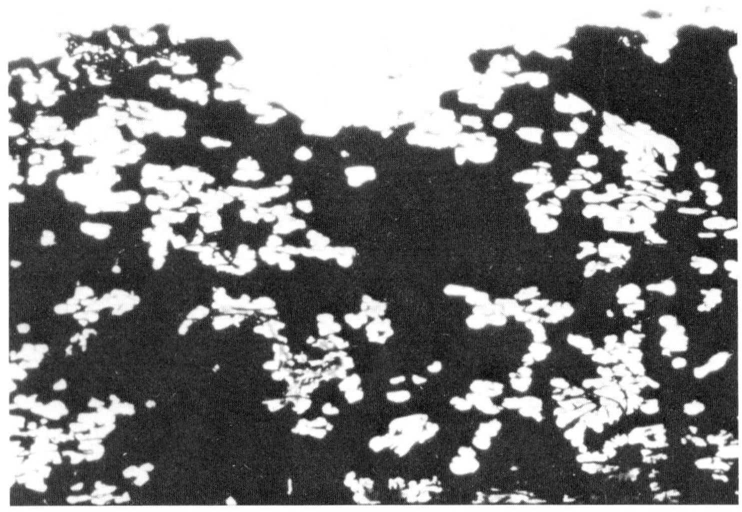

Fig. 4b.

<u>Sheep experimentation</u>. The first animal was killed 60 days post-op-
eratively because of an intriguing inflammatory reaction around the
bone plates (Fig. 5). This reaction without fistulae or abcess had
the macroscopic appearance of a malignant bone tumor. Histology
showed an intense foreign body reaction with a fibrous capsule invaded with inflammatory granuloma containing fibroblasts, lymphocytes,
monocytes and a dense vascularization.

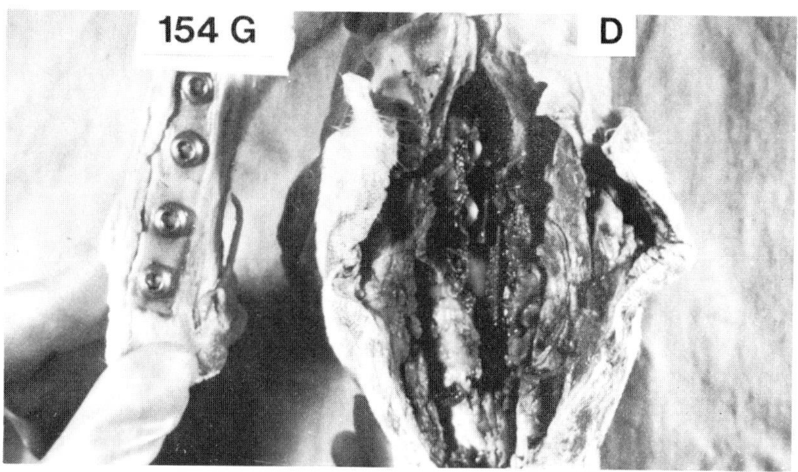

Fig. 5. Macroscopic views of the tissue reaction around
bone plates at 60 days on sheep tibias. Plates were made
of Pyrolytic/CFRC.
154 G : Material coated with pyrolytic carbon, thin
         fibrous layer surrounding the plates.
    D : Bare material ; intense foreign body reaction.

A very high number of carbon particles had been released into the soft
tissues and many of them were intracellular. The medullary cavity
exhibited the same features. Necrotic areas were located around screws,
plate and endosteal bone. Histological examination did not reveal the
presence of any malignant cell. The lymph nodes were swollen with
dense sinus reticular hyperplasia invested by macrophages, plasmocytes
and young cells within connective trabeculae without any sign of infection. Histological examination of the contralateral side with
coated plates revealed a normal fibrous tissue layer with few carbon
particles, present also within the medullary cavity.

The second animal carried its four plates for twelve months. A normal
fibrous tissue layer formed around each plate. Carbon particles
migrated from the coated and bare plates, more extensively however in
the case of bare plates (Fig. 6). Both types of plate exhibited
cracks but there were more in the plates that were not coated. Bone
remodeling beneath the plates was minimal (Fig. 7). The cracks were
invaded by primary bone. Carbon particles were also found perivascular

in the medullary cavity. The lumbar-inguinal lymph nodes did not exhibit any abnormal features and no carbon particles could be detected
within them.

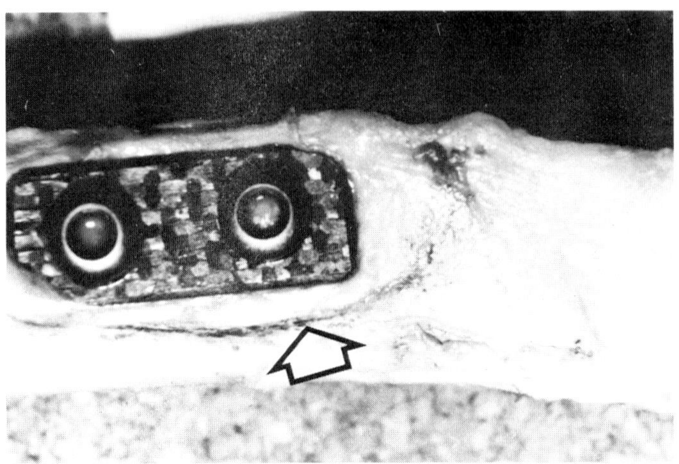

Fig. 6. Macroscopic view of the tissue reaction around a bone
plate (coated pyrolytic-CFRC) after one year implantation on
sheep tibia. Note a black halo (single arrow) made of carbon
particles surrounding the upper side despite the coating.

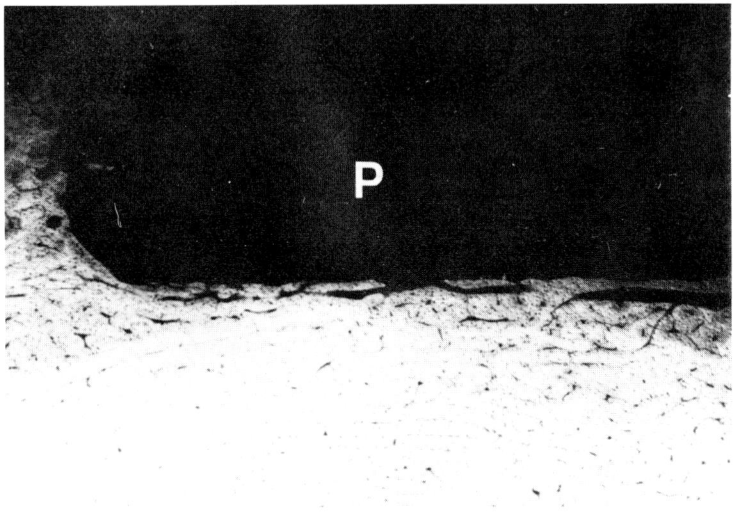

Fig. 7. Radiomicrograph of cortical bone beneath the upper
left plate shown in Fig. 6. Minimal bone remodeling under
plate (P).

DISCUSSION

The investigations of Wolter et al. (Wolter et al., 1978) indicated
migration of carbon particles within the lymph nodes following intra-
articular and intra-peritoneal injection of carbon powder material in
rats. Such particles could be found by optical microscopy, in rats or
sheep, where ever lymph nodes were activated. We did not find any
carbon in the lymph nodes in our experiments. This could be related
to the site of implantation. After subcutaneous implantation and for
bone plates, the fibrous encapsulation might prevent or slow down the
migration of particles. After increasing implantation time, particles
were found far from the implantation site. In agreement with others
(Wolter et al., 1978) we found that depending upon their size, the
smallest particles were intracellular and the largest ones extracellular. Macrophages and giant cells with phagocytosed carbon particles
did not exhibit any sign of damage, using optical microscopy and conventional histological staining techniques. This should be further
investigated with electron microscopy.

The intensity of the tissue reaction appeared to be strongly dependent
upon the amount of released particles. This is relevant to the use of
carbon-carbon composites for anchoring parts of articular prostheses.
The foreign body reaction induced by the released particles would lead
undoubtedly to prosthesis loosening (Willert and Semlitsch, 1976). The
pyrolytic coating significantly lowered the release rate but did not
fully stop it, probably because of local breakage of the pyrolytic
carbon layer. Cohesion of the implant material is an important factor.
The Pitch-CFRC material having poor cohesion showed fast disintegration.
even when coated. In this study it appears that addition of silicon
carbide to carbon did not bring about any local tissue toxicity, but
further investigations need to be carried out to evaluate tissue compatibility of wear debris from carbon-SiC materials.

In the first sheep a very intense foreign body reaction to carbon particles was diagnosed around the bare plates. It must have been initiated by an excessive release of carbon particles in the absence of coating
and also by abrasion of the plate at the time of initial surgery, because the drill and tap damaged the plates. In the second animal,
special care was taken to avoid damage of the uncoated plates, nevertheless, the presence of carbon particles within the medullary cavity
indicates some damage to the carbon matrix during the initial surgical
procedure. Their location one year after surgery implies a very slow
migration.

In summary, after subcutaneous implantations in rats, an early formed
fibrous tissue layer was regularly observed. The inflammatory reaction
was strongly dependent upon the density of released particles. Activation of lymph nodes was maximum at 30 days and related to the intensity of the carbon particles release. No carbon particles visible with
the light microscope were found within the lymph nodes.

The pyrolyzed coating slowed down the particle migration from compact
material but did not fully prevent it. The pyrolyzed pitch reinforced
with carbon felt disintegrated rapidly, even when coated, and was

found to be unsatisfactory for orthopaedic application. The silicon
carbide addition strongly enhanced the stability of the material
structure.

For tibia plates on sheep the coating did not fully prevent carbon
particle release but slowed it down in such a way that after one year
the tissue reaction remained slight. A pyrolytic coating is apparently required to avoid excessive particle release. When implanting
these materials, extreme care is needed to avoid damaging the coating
with ancillary tools.

It is concluded that carbon materials are well accepted by connective
tissue provided that intrinsic cohesion is adequate to avoid excessive
production of particles.

ACKNOWLEDGEMENTS:

The authors thank Mrs Hott for her very active co-operation at surgery
and histology and Mrs Henry-Amar for typing the manuscript.

REFERENCES

Bokros, J.C. (1977) Carbon medical devices. Carbon, 15, 355-371.
Christin, F., Naslain, R., & Bernard, D. (1979) A thermodynamic
and experimental approach of silicon carbide-CVD application to
the CVD-infiltration of porous carbon-carbon composites.
Proceedings of 7th International Conference on chemical vapor deposition 14-19th October - Los Angeles (Ed. Thomas O. Sedgwick),
499-507. (Electrochemical Soc. Inc., Princeton, N.J.)
Moyen, B.J.L., Lahey, P.J.Jr., Zeinberg, E.H. & Harris, W.H. (1978)
Effects on intact femora of dogs of the application and removal of
metal plates. Journal Bone Joint Surgery, 60A, 940-947.
Willert, H.C. & Semlitsch, M. (1976) Reactions of the articular
capsule of artificial joints prostheses, in Williams, D., Biocompati-
bility of implant materials, London, Sector Publ. Ltd., 39-48.
Wolter, D., Burri, C., Helbing, G., Mohr, W. & Rüter, A. (1978)
Die Reaktion des Körpers auf implantierte Kohlenstoffmikropartikel.
Arch. Orth. Traum. Surg., 91, 19-29.

Biomaterials 1980
Edited by G. D. Winter, D. F. Gibbons, and H. Plenk, Jr.
© 1982 John Wiley and Sons Ltd.

PRELIMINARY FINDINGS USING WOOD AS AN IMPLANT MATERIAL

H. Bednar[1], H. Kristen[2], P. Bösch[2], H. Plenk Jr.[3] and G. Punzet[4]

1) Institute of Wood Research, University of Agriculture
2) Orthopaedic University Clinic
3) Bone Research Lab., Histological–Embryological Institute,
University of Vienna
4) Surgical Department, University of Veterinary Medicine,
Vienna, Austria.

SUMMARY

Wood is a natural fibre-composite material with a porous structure which has mechanical and elastic properties similar to those of bone. In this study the suitablility of wood as a skeletal implant material was investigated.

Biocompatibility testing in bone was concentrated primarily on birch and ash using small cylinders which were implanted in the distal tibiae of rabbits. Despite a foreign body reaction, new bone formation was observed on the surface and in the larger vessels of the wood. A similar bone reaction was observed after implantation into the calcaneus of rabbits under dynamic loading conditions.

Wood implants were also inserted to bridge diaphyseal defects of the humerus and the ulna in human patients following the resection of tumour metastases. No bony anchorage was observed after different periods of implantation. However, full function and painless use of the limb were achieved. Experiments with a spacer application in the femur of dogs point to the limitations imposed by the mechanical properties of the woods tested. The tropical timber green-heart, now under test, appears to have many advantages.

INTRODUCTION

The first reports on the implantation of wood in the human body date back to the days of the Aztecs in Central America (Gall, 1940). The resin content of pine twigs was believed to improve wound healing, and they were used to treat fractures of the upper extremities that were slow to heal. However, wood also has many properties in common with bone tissue; there are species of wood with the same modulus of elasticy as bone and similar strength characteristics. Apart from these mechanical properties, many morphological features, such as the porosity of wood vessels, are also of importance in the selection of wood as a skeletal implant material. The purpose of our experiments was to investigate the bone reaction to wood implants under different loading conditions and to test a possible clinical application.

MATERIALS AND METHODS

The experiments were started with the two indigenous species birch and ash. Due to its greater strength, tropical greenheart was later included. Fig. 1 shows the modulus of elasticity of these species with a moisture content of 12% compared to bone. See Kristen et al (1977, and in press) for more detailed information on the mechanical properties of the species tested.

Birch (Betula verrucosa Ehrh.) is a typically diffuse-porous species (Fig. 2a). The vessels are narrow, the tangential diameter ranges from 20 to 130 µm (mean value 90 µm). Ash (Fraxinus excelsior L.) is a ring porous species. The springwood vessels are solitary or in pairs with a diameter of 250 to 350 µm, forming a zone of one to four rows. Late wood vessels are much narrower, averaging 50 µm (Fig. 2b). Greenheart (Ocotea rodiaei (Schomb.) Mez) is a diffuse-porous species, the vessels are solitary or in pairs with a diameter ranging from 95 to 170 µm (mean value 145 µm).

Animal experiments: The two series of experiments with wood implants in bone are shown schematically in Fig. 3. Test 1: Ethanol extracted and steam sterilized cylinders (size 5 x 5 mm) of ash (n = 21) and birch (n = 7) were implanted under "unloaded" conditions on one or both sides into the distal tibiae of 13 rabbits (two animals received 2 implants on one side). The implants together with the surrounding tissues were removed after 3, 5, 14 and 32 weeks. Test 2: The dorsal parts of the calcanei of rabbits were resected and replaced with rod-shaped implants of ash. The Achilles tendon was then reinserted into the projecting part of the implant so as to subject the latter to the dynamic loads imposed by use of the limb. The implants were removed from 10 animals after 5 weeks and from 5 animals after 14 weeks. Details of the histological techniques used for the investigation of the tissue reaction are published elsewhere (Kristen et al, 1977, 1979).

To test this material under high stress conditions, a diaphyseal defect of 4 cm in the femur of 8 German shepherd-dogs was bridged by ash spacers. The intramedullary taps on both sides had randomly distributed predrilled transverse holes (∅ 2 mm). In 4 animals additional fixation was provided by means of a 6 hole bone plate. The implant area was controlled radiologically and after different observation periods (see results) these implants were also investigated histologically.

Clinical applications: In 5 patients (3 female, 2 male) with tumour metastases and imminent or painful pathological fractures of the upper extremity, alcohol extracted and steam sterilized ash wood implants were adapted intraoperatively to the necessary shape and were inserted to bridge large diaphyseal defects (8 to 10 cm) of the humerus or ulna after resection of the tumour metastases. In two cases the implants were also fixed by a bone plate. The observation periods until the death of the patients from their initial diseases ranged from 19 days to 9 months. Further clinical details are presented in Kristen et al (in press).

RESULTS

<u>Experimental findings</u>: Under "unloaded" conditions, the bone implants of all 3 wood species were covered by a granulation tissue in which abundant multi-nucleated giant cells developed and persisted during the whole observation period. After 3 weeks, bone ingrowth was found in the larger pores, and after 5 weeks, osteon-like structures were formed in these larger pores, whereas radiodense deposits were found in the smaller vessels (Fig. 4).

Under dynamic loading conditions, no breakage or loosening of the calcaneal implants was observed, and there was again bone formation in contact with the wood surface. The intramedullary stem was closely surrounded by new bone formation which was also evident in the larger pores (Fig. 5). The fork-shaped end of the implant, however, showed no contact with the periosteal exostoses, but fibrocartilage had formed on the wood and joint-like spaces had developed.

Under high-stress conditions, the ash spacers in the canine femoral diaphysis showed breakage of the proximal intramedullary taps after 4 to 7 weeks. In the second group of dogs (Fig. 6a), breakage of the wood implants and of the bone plates occurred (Fig. 6b), but 10 to 20 weeks after operation. However, histological examination showed that bone ingrowth into larger pores and the predrilled holes (Fig. 6c) had taken place in both the proximal and distal intramedullary taps.

<u>Clinical observations</u>: In the human patients, breakage of both intramedullary taps occurred only in one case after 6 and 20 weeks respectively. None of the wood implants were anchored by bone ingrowth, but they were clinically stable at least at one end. The operated limbs functioned well and painlessly in every case until the death of the patients (Kristen et al, in press).

DISCUSSION

A pronounced foreign body reaction around wood implants was oberved in hard tissues (Kristen et al, 1977, 1979) and in soft tissues (Bösch et al, 1979). This may be related to the constituents of the wood species under test and may be one of the reasons for the tissue reactions after traumatical insertion of wood into the body. As far as can be concluded from light microscopical observations, no structural changes of the wood occurred in the biological environment. However, this adverse cell reaction did not seem not to have hindered the new bone formation which was observed in close contact with the wood surface and resulted in the anchorage of these porous implants. The findings with the calcaneus implants in the rabbit showed that this anchorage occurred also under dynamic loading conditions. They demonstrate the favourable isoelastic proper-ties of the material, as bone ingrowth was also found at the distal end of the rod, where in more rigid implant materials the greatest movement would occur and bone ingrowth would therefore be most unlikely.

The experiments under high stress conditions, however, showed the limits imposed by the material and by the experimental model using a spacer. It seems obvious that a thin intramedullary rod cannot exhibit the same bending strength as a hollow cylinder of the surrounding long bone, despite similar elastic and mechanical properties. In addition, the fibre orientation and the porous structure of the wood cannot be compared to the structure of bone. However, the use of wood with a considerably greater strength would again result in a mechanical mismatch such as occurs with other high-strength materials.

Nevertheless, the clinical trials justified the application of this material: the size and the shape of the implant could easily be adapted during operation to the individual patient after resection of the bone tumour. Despite the lack of bony anchorage, functional restoration and painless utilization of the limb were obtained for a more or less short time until the death of the patient. The abovementioned tests using wood as an implant material in bone have shown that this natural, fibre-reinforced and porous composite offers favourable conditions for bone ingrowth despite adverse cell reactions due to leachable constituents. Further investigation of mechanically more suitable wood species, e.g. the tropical timber greenheart, will show whether this natural material has similar advantages to artificially produced fibre composite materials.

REFERENCES

Bösch, P., Kristen, H., Braun, F. & Kovac, W. (1979) Das Verhalten des Bindegewebes und der quergestreiften Muskulatur gegenüber implantiertem Eschenholz. Wien. Med. Wschr., 15, 419-423.
Dempster, W.T., & Liddicoat, R.T. (1952) Compact bone as a nonisotropic material, Amer. J. Anat. 9, 331-362.
Gall, A., Freiherr von (1940) Medizinische Bücher (tici-amatl) der alten Azteken aus der ersten Zeit der Conquista, in Quellen und Studien zur Geschichte der Naturwissenschaften und der Medizin, vol. VII, no. 4 and 5. Springer, Berlin.
Kristen, H., Bösch, P., Bednar, H. & Plenk, H. Jr. (1977) Verträglichkeitsuntersuchungen von Holz im Knochengewebe. Arch. orthop. Unfall-Chir., 89, 1-14.
Kristen, H., Bösch, P., Bednar, H. & Plenk, H. Jr. (1979) The Effects of Dynamic Loading on Intracalcaneal Wood Implants and on the Tissue Surrounding them, Arch. Orthop. Traumat. Surg., 93, 287-292.
Kristen, H., Bösch, P., Bednar, H. & Plenk, H. Jr. (1980) Eschenholz zur Überbrückung diaphysärer Defekte nach Tumorresektionen an der oberen Extremität, Acta chir. Austr. Suppl. (in press).

FIGURES

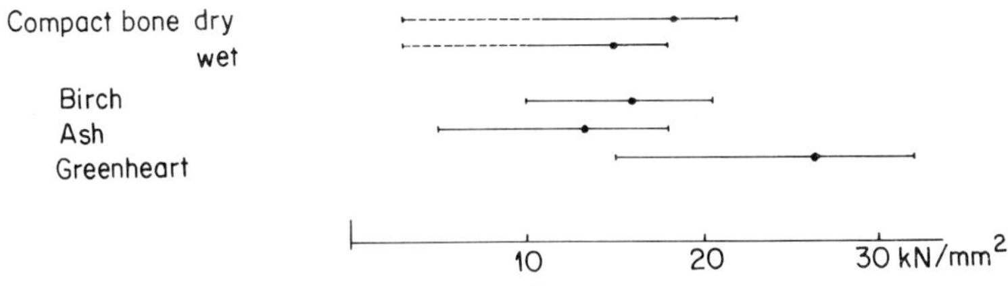

Fig. 1: Moduli of elasticity (mean $\pm$ range) of different wood species compared to compact bone (after Dempster & Liddicoat, 1952).

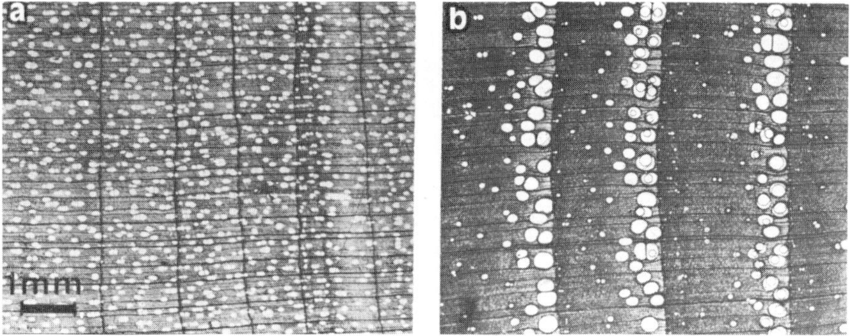

Fig. 2: Transverse microtome sections of a) birch and b) ash
(Hematoxylin-eosin-stain, magn. 9x).

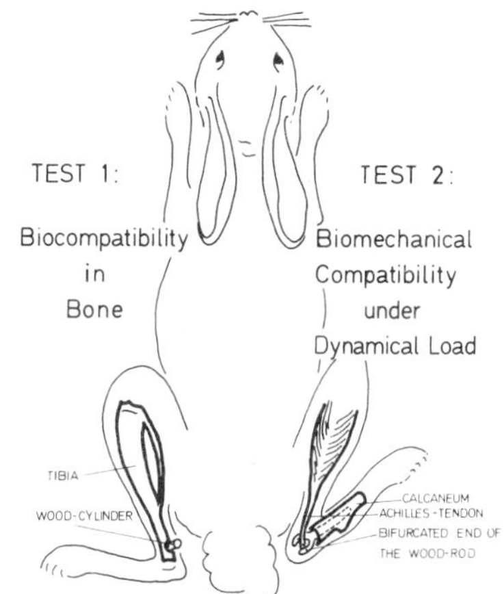

Fig. 3: Schematic drawing of biocompatibility test and dynamic loading experiment in the rabbit.

Fig. 4: Radiomicrograph of a longitudinal ground section of an ash cylinder in the rabbit tibia, 5 weeks after implantation (magn. 25x). Osteon-like bone formation in the larger spring-wood vessels (arrows right) and mineral deposits in the smaller vessels (arrows left). CB = cortical bone.

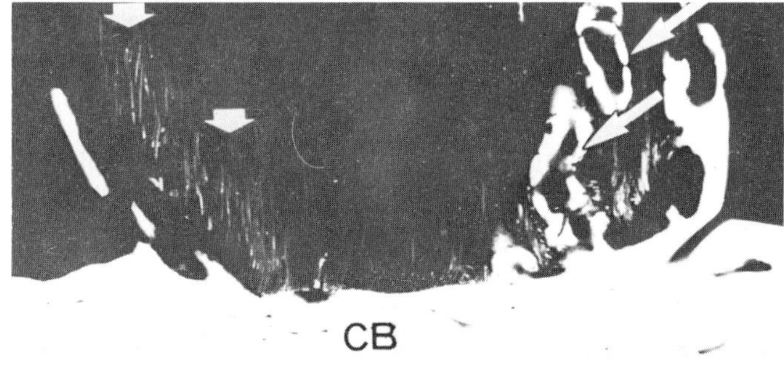

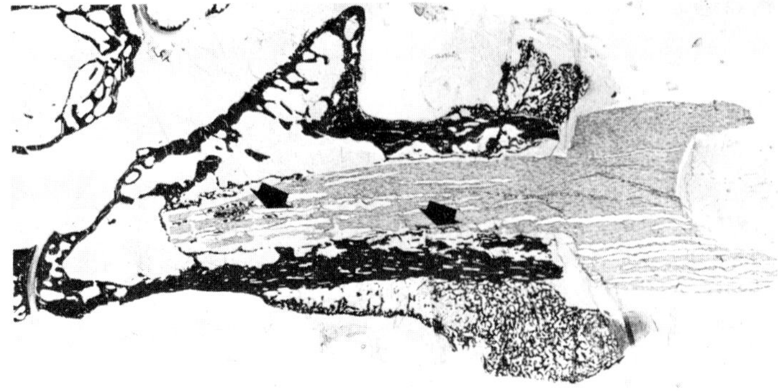

Fig. 5: Longitudinal microtome section of an ash implant in the rabbit calcaneus (modified Kossa stain, methylgreen–pyronin, magn. 5x). The intramedullary part of the implant is closely surrounded by new bone which has also grown into the larger pores (arrows).

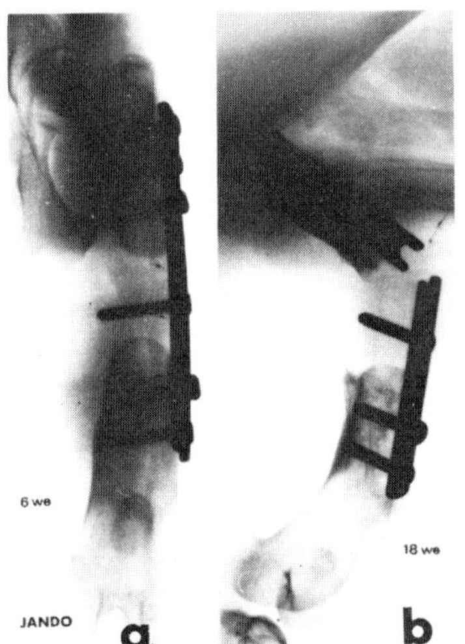

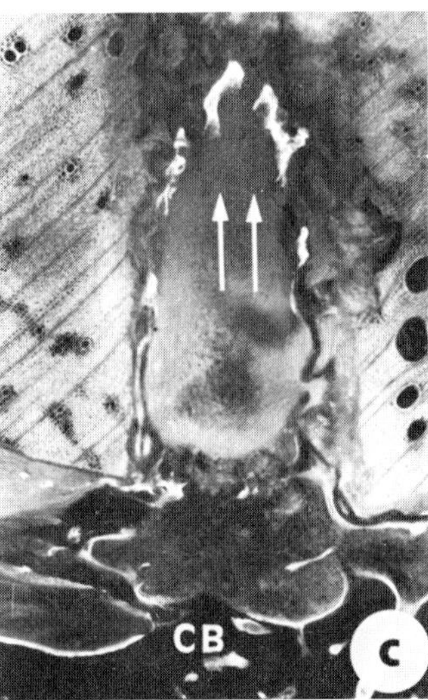

Fig. 6: a–b) Radiograph of an ash spacer fixed with a bone plate in the canine femur, a) six weeks after implantation, b) after breakage of both implants 18 weeks after implantation.
c) Detail of a ground section from the proximal intramedullary tap of this ash spacer (magn. 25x). Formation of fluorochrome labelled bone spiculae (arrows) in the connective tissue in a predrilled hole. (CB = cortical bone).

Joint replacement

Biomaterials 1980
Edited by G. D. Winter, D. F. Gibbons, and H. Plenk, Jr.
© 1982 John Wiley and Sons Ltd.

COMPUTER ANALYSIS OF THE BENDING STIFFNESS OF A SEGMENT OF THE LOWER LEG

I.A. JANSONS and H.A. JANSONS

Department of Biomechanics and
Biomaterials

Riga Scientific Research Institute of
Traumatology and Orthopaedics, USSR

SUMMARY

The bending stiffness of the extremity section varies
greatly with the condition of the soft tissue. Taking
into consideration the real properties of biomaterials
when straining the muscles, the stiffness may increase
several times. The behaviour of the soft tissue should
be taken into account when designing fixation devices
and endoprosthesis and when implanting them.

INTRODUCTION

The complicated surgical and biomechanical problems encountered in the rehabilitation of limbs when endoprostheses are used to repair serious bone defects can be
partly solved by computer modelling of biomechanical
systems.
We report here on theoretical analyses of the bending
stiffness of an extremity section model. The first task
was to determine the properties and biomechanical functions of biomaterials constituting the extremity section.

DEFINITIONS

Bending stiffness is the product of the modulus of material elasticity (E modulus) and the inertia moment of
the bending element cross-section. The extremity section
consist of bony and various soft tissues. Therefore the
geometrical characteristics of muscles are multiplied
by E modulus ratio of muscles and bony tissue. The modulus of elasticity of compact bone depends on the zone
of cross-section and ranges within 17000-21000 MPa
(Jansons H. 1975). We assumed that E modulus of strained muscles might increase to 1000 MPa (Rabischong 1965,
Fung 1970).

                    I.Jansons and H.Jansons

METHODS

The extremity section is regarded as a curved, nonhomogenous rod consisting of different biomaterials - compact and spongiose bony tissue, muscular tissue, tendons, ligaments and fascia. The extremity section is conventionally divided into separate parts along its entire length. The tissue geometrical parameters and deformation properties are assumed to have constant values within the limits of each part. All the transverse cross-section components are approximated by polygons (Fig. 1). The material of bone is regarded as transversaly isotropic. The inhomogeneity of deformation properties along said zones are taken into account. The muscles are substituted by idealized material with longitudinal deformation, equivalent to real muscle. The muscle deformation properties conventionally are described by their modulus of elasticity, which varies with muscle stress and the modulus of elasticity of fascia surrounding the muscle. The bending stiffness of the model's cross-section was calculated using a special computer program "PIVEX-I" for computer model EC-1022 (Jansons I. 1979).

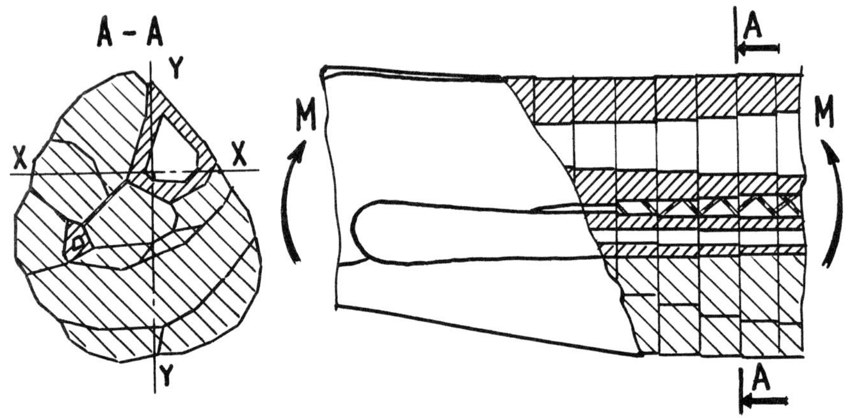

Fig. 1. Model of extremity section.

RESULTS

Maps of stiffness for two extreme cases ($K_B = K_M = 0$ and $K_B = K_M = 1$) are drawn in polar coordinates (Fig. 2). Fig. 1 shows the bending stiffness of the model relative to axis X-X with respect to the bond coefficients and the elasticity of muscles.

<u>DISCUSSION</u>

The bending stiffness of the tibia relative to X-X axis was 1.52 kNm^2 , of the fibula - 0.08 kNm^2 (Fig. 2). The total stiffness of the bones varied from 1.6 to 3.7 kNm^2, depending on the degree of bonding between them. The reduced stiffness of the model was increased to 10-12 kNm^2, i.e. four times, because of existing bonds between muscles. The effect of soft tissue and the bonds between the constituent elements of the model varies with the direction of bending.

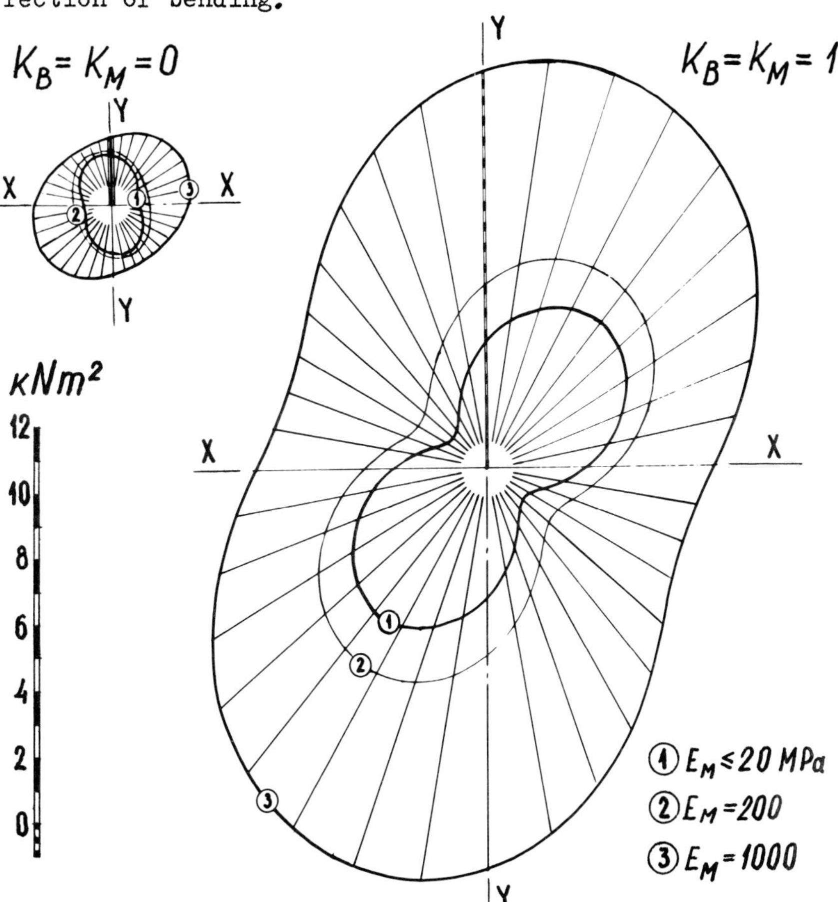

Fig. 2. Relationship of stiffness to bending in different directions.
K_B= the bond coefficient between tibia and fibula.
K_M= the bond coefficient between the muscles and between the muscles and the bone surface.
E_M= modulus of elasticity of muscles.

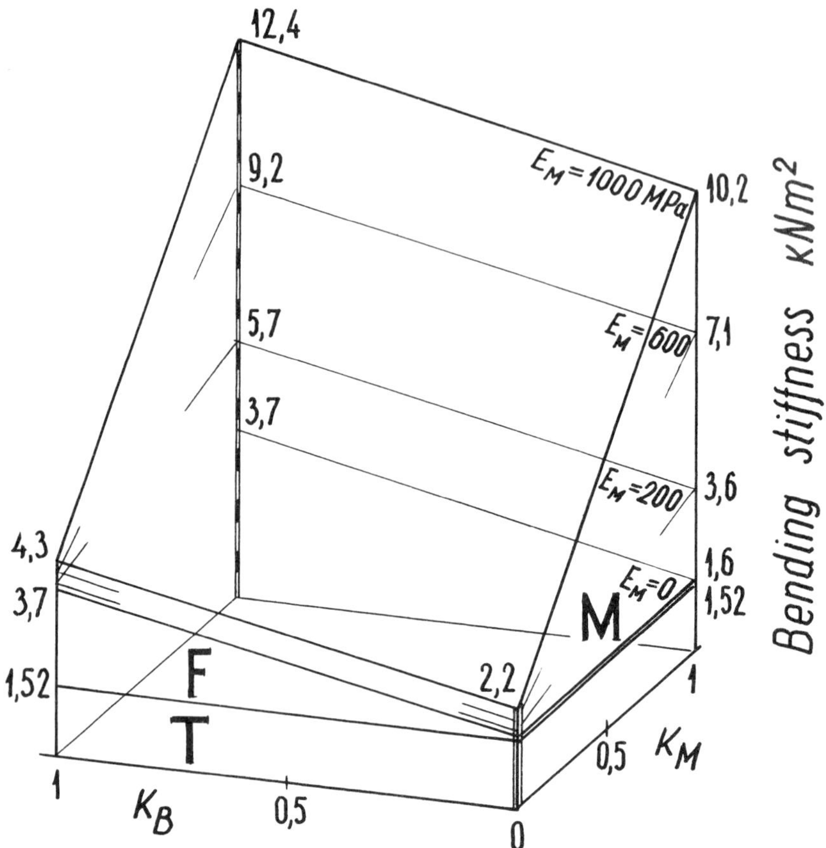

Fig. 3. Bending stiffness relative to axis X-X
with respect to bond coefficients K_B and K_M
(see Fig. 2) and modulus of elasticity of muscles (E_M).
T = tibia. F = fibula. M = muscles.

<u>REFERENCES</u>

Fung Y.Ch. (1970) Mathematical representation of the mechanical properties of the heart muscle. <u>J.Biomechanics</u>,
<u>3</u>, 381-404. Jansons H.A. (1975) Biomechanics of the Hu-
man Leg. Riga, "Zinatne", pp 59-112 (in Russian). Jansons I.A., Kirpichnikow V.S., Jansons H.A.& Kuzmina N.D.
(1979) The metod of determination of geometrical characteristics of total complex constituent sections of any
shape, in <u>Proceedings of the Second Allunion Conference</u>
<u>on Problems of Biomechanics, 4</u>, Riga, "Zinatne", pp18-22
(in Russian). Rabischong P.& Avril J. (1965) Rôle bio-
mecanique des poutres composites os-muscles. <u>Rev. chir.</u>
<u>orthop.</u>, <u>51</u>, 437-458.

Biomaterials 1980
Edited by G. D. Winter, D. F. Gibbons, and H. Plenk, Jr.
© 1982 John Wiley and Sons Ltd.

Optimum Design of Biomaterials For A
Bone Bridge Prosthesis

H. A. Jansons

Department of Biomechanics and Biomaterials
Riga Scientific Research Institute of
Traumatology and Orthopaedics, USSR

SUMMARY

Biomechanical studies have determined that the rheological mechanisms
responsible for the adaptation of human long bones to large loads depends upon anisotropy, inhomogeneity and yielding of the bone. These
data suggest that a composite constructed from hybrid elements could
be used for the design of a tubular bone endoprosthesis. We therefore have used as the basis for our design a simple spirally wound
element which resembles the natural osteon. This basic element is
repeated as a series of parallel interconnected spirally wound cylinders. Such a structure allows the individual elements to relax
in a periodic manner.

INTRODUCTION

Biomechanical theories based upon studies of the structure and function of the human system have led to the development of a new approach to the design of implants and endoprostheses (R. Huiskes,
1979; V.K. Kalnberz et al, 1979; H.A. Jansons, 1979). Several successful designs of shoulder, hip and knee joint endoprostheses have
been based on studies of live biomechanical systems. However, these
designs imitate only the external or kinematic features of joints,
without taking into account the properties of the natural bone or the
materials from which they are constructed. Recent studies on the biomechanics of the living human leg have provided a new understanding of
the structure and function of these tissues and in particular the significance of the internal three-dimensional structure of its components. The results of more than 10,000 measurements on the strength,
deformation and ultrasonic measurements of bones, together with the
biomechanics of the human system, lead to the following conclusions:
1. The hybrid construction of the human extremity allows the internal stresses to be redistributed under increasing external load.
2. The structure of the right and left load bearing elements of tubular bone elements have a corresponding left or right handed symmetry. These elements cannot be interchanged. The elements must be
fabricated with anisotropic materials and be of inhomogeneous construction.

3. The contribution of muscle to the total load bearing ability of
the segment increases considerably as the load is increased.
4. The natural protective mechanism of the bone is effective only if
there is adequate yielding.

METHODS AND DESIGN

The complex structure and function of the natural biomechanical system places the designer of a human tubular bone endoprosthesis in a
predicament. Live bone must be regarded as an active component of
this precisely defined and complex biomechanical system. The results of both experiment and theoretical studies show that tubular
bone must be considered as an optimumly designed, composite biomaterial, created by nature. A complex computer-based method for the
optimum design of composite materials was suggested by W. Prager and
Y. Taylor (1968). It is necessary, however, to discuss some possible methods to optimumize the construction of the artificial bone.
Optimumization of design and construction of implants has been described as an ideal approach (D.F. Williams and R. Roaf, 1973).
The optimum selection of material and design of the endoprosthesis
requires:
1. The definition of the basic criteria for design optimumization.
2. The development of a computer program to calculate the spacial
orientation and volume ratio of the reinforcing elements as well as
the necessary geometrical shape and size of the prosthesis.
3. The development of the technology necessary to produce the optimum reinforced composite.
Isotropic and homogeneous materials - metals, polymers and ceramics -
fail to satisfy the requirements for optimum materials. A possible
design for a bone segment replacement prosthesis in the diaphysis of
the human tibia, which is developed by means of a composite approach,
is presented in Fig. 1.
The shape of the natural bone proved to be the most favorable outer
shape of the endoprosthesis. The matrix method of press-molding does
not cause any special technical difficulties for the fabrication of
such a composite (V.K. Kalnberz et al, 1979). The selection and manufacturing of a mechanism for the fixation of the prosthesis is an
independent and complex problem not dealt with in the present paper.
The simplicity of the outer shape of the prosthesis conceals the
complex multistage reinforcing of the internal structure. Areas for
muscle and fascia fixation are envisaged along the external sheath
of the prosthesis.
The elements of the multistage constuction which are located under
the outer sheath (Fig. 2) are spirally wound composites consisting
of three load-bearing elements located around a central reinforcing
rod. The right or left handed spirals, spiral angle, packing density
and diameter of the load bearing elements at each level and in each
segment of the endoprosthesis was established by the computer program
for optimal design. The space between the spiral members is filled

with spirals, rods or sheets of spirally wound reinforced material.
The outer sheath is made of the same reinforcing material, which
adds to the rigidity of construction. The fourth stage composite
resembles the model of a tibia based on measurements of its spacial variation of stiffness (H.A. Jansons, 1975).
The design of the third stage reinforcing element - bearing element -
was based on a partial solution to the problem. This element could
be given the shape of a spirally-wound tube with a smooth or checker-
ed surface, a triple helix rope or a rope twisted in a spiral; the
choice is dependent upon the rigidity required at each cross-sectional
region of the prosthesis. The internal design of the element is relatively complex (Fig. 3).
Rope, with a right or left handed twist to the second stage reinforcement, is packed between the layers of the initial mesh reinforcement
and forms a velvet-like material. Spirally wound components of different diameters were made of metal and polymer in accordance with the
requirements of the designer. Alternation of the diameter of the second stage element, and/or increasing the number of right and left
handed spiral ropes, produced a wide range of anisotropy and properties of the composite, i.e., to create the right or left handed spiral
type material analogous to the right or left handed spiral material of
the human compact bone tissue. The third stage reinforcement remotely
resembles the structure of the tissue osteon.
Judged on a basis of their design and manufacturing technology, the
second stage reinforcement elements are relatively simple (Fig. 4).
The direction of reinforcement was easily alternated and depends upon
the angle of the mesh twisting along the spiral of the right or left
handed spiral. Each layer of the element consisted of two first stage
reinforcement nets. The design of this stage of reinforcement resembles the mulitlayer construction of an osteon. The first stage reinforcement components were made from fine meshes of high strength alloys
with an effective low modulus of elasticity. An alternative reinforcing net was made with strong polymeric filaments. Both types of nets
were aligned at an angle of 10-20º in parallel planes. Reinforcement
at this stage resembles collagen structures observed in human tissues.

DISCUSSION

It is quite obvious that the method suggested for the design of a human tubular bone endoprosthesis is relatively complex. However, the
principle is simple - the same type of spiral structure is repeated at
each level with a higher degree of reinforcement.
The approach cannot be regarded as a simple replacement for a defective
bone segment, but it does simulate the biomechanical functions of the
injured system, with an effective protection from mechanical overloads
by an adaptive mechanism.
The method of optimum design of the composite and implant enabled us to
achieve the essential properties of bone tissue and biomechanical system, namely a uniform stress distribution at all levels of the endo-

prosthesis and on all types of the surrounding tissue. More and more
new elements take up and redistribute increasing stresses, and the
total system functions only under extreme conditions. Under normal
stress conditions several elements are relaxed and unloaded. We assume that the application of this concept, with the suggested technical construction, will provide long-term functionality of an implant
and stability of the rehabilitated biomechanical system in the whole.

REFERENCES

Huiskes, R. (1979) Some fundamental aspects of human joint replacement.
Analyses of Stress and Heat Conduction in Bone-prosthesis Structures,
Eindhoven, 208.
Kalnberz, F.D., Jansons, H.A., Knets, I.V. and Saulgozis, J.Zh. (1979)
Material for making bone endoprosthesis and endoprosthesis of said
material. Patent GBr. No 1549328 fil.16.09.1976.
Jansons, H.A. (1979) Biomechanics and endoprosthesis materials design.
Abstracts of VII-th Internat. Congress of Biomechanics, Warszawa, 10-
11.
Jansons, H.A. (1975) Biomechanics of the Human Leg, Riga, "Zinatne",
324.
Prager, W. and Taylor, Y. (1968) Problems of optimal structure design.
J. Appl. Mech., 35, 102-106.
Williams, D.F. and Roaf, R. (1973) Implants in Surgery. W.B. Saunder
Co., Ltd., London.

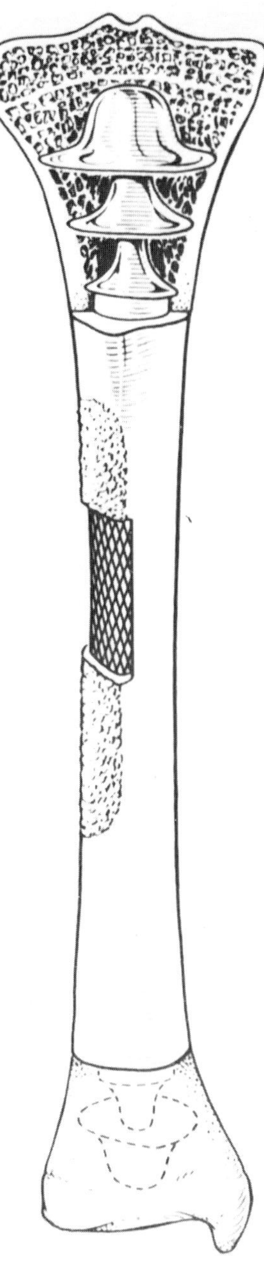

Fig. 1. Endoprosthesis of human tibia

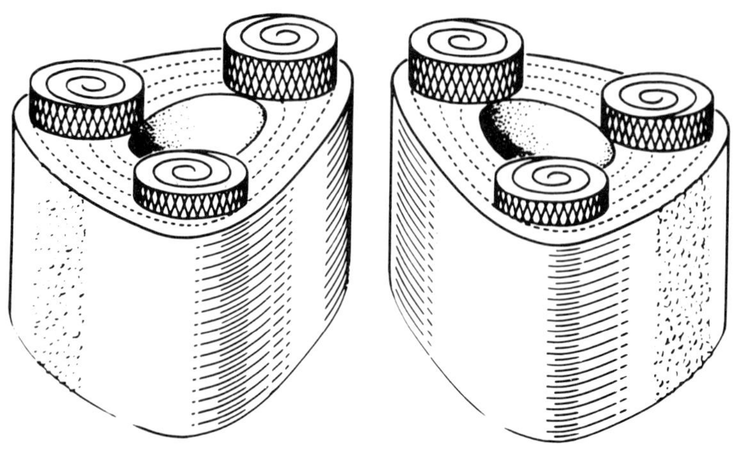

Fig. 2. Internal structure of endoprosthesis
(fourth stage level of construction)

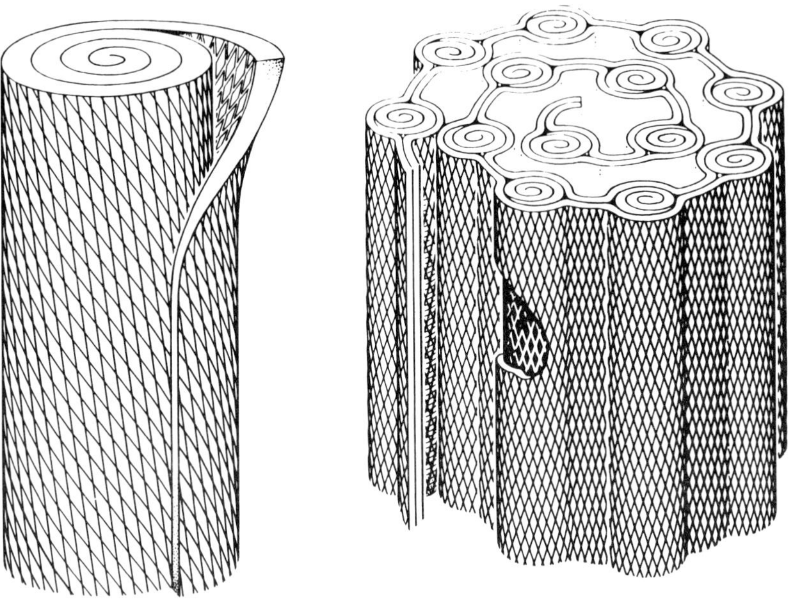

Fig. 3. Third stage level of
the construction.

Fig. 4. Spirally wound
second stage element.

Biomaterials 1980
Edited by G. D. Winter, D. F. Gibbons, and H. Plenk, Jr.
© 1982 John Wiley and Sons Ltd.

SYSTEMATIC APPROACH TO THE EXPERIMENTAL AND THEORETICAL
STUDY OF HIP PROSTHESIS COUPLINGS

P.M. Calderale, M.M. Gola and A. Gugliotta

Politecnico di Torino, Torino, Italy

SUMMARY

The present work describes the experimental techniques used in the
Authors' Department for the stress analysis of the stem-femur coupling.
After a general discussion of the problems encountered in the mechanical evaluation of the coupling, the tests that were performed with
two special transducer stems on two human femurs, one dry and one
embalmed, are described.

INTRODUCTION

The study of the coupling conditions between prosthesis' stem and
femoral bone can be accomplished, in principle, either theoretically
or experimentally. This problem happens to be a many faced one; if
just the mechanical problems are singled out, the following areas of
interest can be considered:
a) coupling conditions, as to flexural phenomena,
b) coupling conditions, as to axial phenomena,
c) coupling conditions, as to torsional phenomena.
The following two lines of approach can be followed:
1) optimization of both length and distribution of stiffness of the
   stem,
2) optimization of only the length, since the other dimensions must
   closely match the medullary channel's dimensions.
Both approaches 1) and 2) can include all areas a), b), c), or a part
of them.
The choice between approach 1) or 2) depends on which is considered
to be the governing phenomenon in the long term duration of the
implant; if, for instance, a relatively thin layer of cement is
considered mandatory, or if cement-less insertions are sought for,
approach 2) must be followed. In this case, the optimization of
cross-sectional shapes is used only in order to relieve stress
concentration peaks, without of course forgetting torsional coupling
problems.
Theoretical work on the mechanical coupling can be tentatively
classified according to the areas of interest. The flexural-only
phenomena have been studied in (Gola et al., 1979a), (Huiskes et al.,
1979a), (Huiskes, 1979b); coupled flexural and axial phenomena are
the object of most two-dimensional analyses, such as in (McNiece et
al., 1976), (Wood, 1975), (Svensson et al., 1977), or in other works

discussed in (Huiskes, 1979b).
The axial phenomena have been treated in (Huiskes, 1979b) but this
analysis depends upon the assumptions regarding the nature of the
stem-cement coupling, which is considered to fully and continuosly
transmit tangential stresses.
Complete analyses, including torsional phenomena, have been treated
by (Röhrle et al., 1979), (Crowninshield et al., 1979), (Tarr et al.,
1979).
A comparison of these studies leads to the conclusion that even if
the complete, i.e. axial-flexural-torsional, analysis is considered
with the finite element approach, it is possible to split the study
in two parts: torsional and axial-flexural.
The efforts of the authors have been concentrated in the axial-
flexural area; after a first attempt to examine only the flexural
area (Gola et al., 1979), they have become convinced that both the
geometry and the nature of the constraints require simultaneous axial-
flexural analysis (Calderale et al., 1979a,b,c, and d).
They have also become increasingly convinced that experimental
analysis is an unavoidable complement to the theoretical analysis,
because the mathematical model itself has to be shaped on those facts
which emerge as relevant.
This can be appreciated by discussing the following crucial problems:
i) the role of creep in fresh or embalmed bones: this does not seem
to be a governing phenomenon, at least in the conditions referred in
(Huiskes, 1979b), where an embalmed femur subjected to physiological
loads and instrumented with strain-gages reached the definitive
strains in about 3 minutes, and manteined them constants for at
least 72 hours thereafter (Huiskes et al., 1977); this is confirmed
by data gathered by the authors, who measured asymptotic variations
of less than 3% on a stem inserted in an embalmed femur under
physiological loads and after 8 minutes (Calderale et al., 1980);
therefore, studies in the elastic range should be adequate.
ii) the problem of shear at the stem's surface: this has always been
taken into account, either by implicitily assuming the existence of
a no-slip contact (which is easier for finite element or composite
beam formulations), or by assuming the existence of no tension
(Gola et al., 1979), (Calderale et al., 1979a,b,c, and d) or by
simulating both conditions and discussing the differences (Huiskes,
1979b), (Svensson et al., 1977); the conclusions are that normal
stresses at the interfaces and flexural stresses in bone and stem
are not altered of a relevant amount, apart from local peaks;
considering that the elastic energy content of such local regions is
small and considering that the stem-cement contact is not adhesive,
it seems nearer to reality the adoption of a no-tension model; the
accuracy of a model based on an energy approach is anyway impaired
by the presence of frictional phenomena at the interfaces, as it is
suggested by experimental findings (Calderale et al., 1980).
iii) the origin of forces that sustain the axial load: this is a
very difficult subject to evaluate, since axial load can be
contemporaneously sustained through friction, stem's taper, non-
uniform curvature of stem's axis, support of the shoulder on the
calcar. The non-adhesive nature of the contact between cement and
stem, and, in general, the difficulty of taking into account the
contribution of friction which would depend on the system's time

history, led us to exclude it from the model; the contribution of
the calcar support is perhaps questionable (Jacob et al., 1979), and
it depends on the ability of stem's taper and non-uniform curvature
to share the load, but it can be easily included both in a three-
dimensional or in a two-dimensional model.
iv) <u>the importance of three-dimensionality for the axial and
    flexural phenomena</u>: it has been shown on a simplified model that,
apart from the stress state in cement, stem and bone behave very
closely to a slender beam in bending (Huiskes, 1979b), except in the
proximal zone of the bone; this was confirmed also in a more realistic model (Röhrle et al., 1979); this indicates the feasibility
of a two-dimensional model for the study of the overall axial-
flexural behaviour, apart from local effects.
In conclusion, the authors believe that a two-dimensional model of
the stem-femur coupling can supply all the relevant informations on
the mechanics of the coupling; a more refined analysis is not
necessarily more realistic because of uncertainties in the physical
parameters.
Such a simplified model, which nevertheless takes into account the
principal equilibrium and compatibility conditions, leads itself to
a fast parametric analysis and allows guidelines for the interpretation of experimental results to be formulated. Experimental data can
be obtained either by strain-gaging the stem or the femur or both
(Huiskes, 1979b), (Svensson et al., 1977), (Huiskes et al., 1977),
(Jacob et al., 1979), (Weightman, 1976), (Markolf et al., 1976),
(Breyer et al., 1979), or by using a special re-usable instrumented
stem which we have developed (Calderale et al., 1979a,b,c, and d) and
used in a first series of experiments on dry and embalmed bones
(Calderale et al., 1980).

THEORETICAL ANALYSIS

The theoretical analysis follows substantially a Rayleigh-Ritz procedure for a two-dimensional model, and is based on a polynomial
description of the kinematics of stem and bone. The assumptions of
the model are:
i)   the axis of the bone is considered approximately straight,
ii) the axis of the stem has a curvature,
iii) the stem has a taper,
iv) the position of the stem relative to the bone can be rotated
     and shifted compatibly with the dimension of medullary channel.
This theoretical procedure is described at length in (Calderale et
al., 1979a,b and c).
Unfortunately the theoretical results do not match well with the
experimental ones; probably this is due to the fact that the contact
at the interface stem-cement and cement-bone play a very relevant
role in the coupling as the experimental results (Calderale et al.,
1980) show. On this grounds we are now developing an improved
mathematical model which can take into account the contact at the
stem-cement interface.

     P.M. Calderale, M.M. Gola and A. Gugliotta

EXPERIMENTAL ANALYSIS

In order to better clarify the effect of the variables, e.g.
distribution of cement and/or contact, rate of loading, relative
position of stem and bone, etc...., the authors endeavoured a
systematic approach to the experimental analysis, by developing a
reusable instrumented stem.
As an initial approach to the problem a first set of experiments in
pure bending was performed. The stems used in the experiments are
both medium length (120 mm), straight (code P3) and curved (code P4);
these have been calibrated and then implanted in femurs, two dry and
two embalmed. Care was taken that the quantity of cement would be
sufficient to surround the whole length of the stem after it was
implanted; visual inspection at the end of the loading test, with
destruction of the bone confirmed the regular distribution of cement
in all the cases (figure 1).

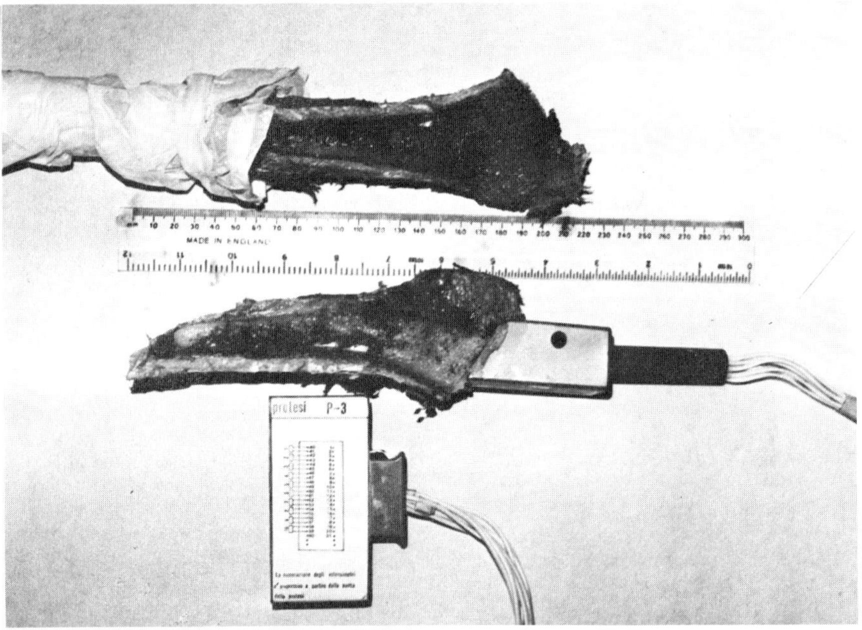

Figure 1

All the loading tests were performed by using an Instron machine and
the signals from the strain-gages were collected via a manual
switching and measuring system (Hottinger Baldwin MTK and UMK 50).
Figure 2 shows the time history of the two loading cycles for the
case P4-dry bone. Figures 3 and 4 summarize the results in terms of
bending moments, in two of the four cases examined (P4-dry bone and
P3-embalmed bone). The full lines represent the loading cycle and
the dotted lines the unloading cycle.

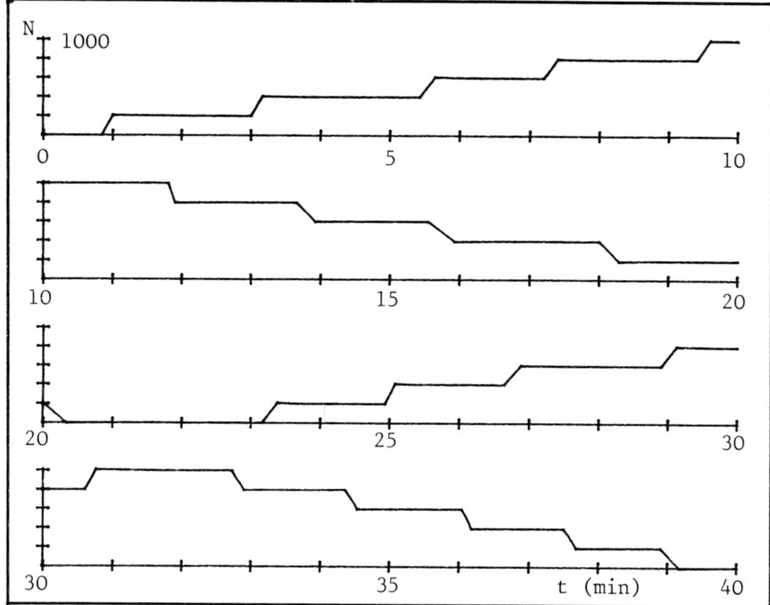

Figure 2: Time history of the two loading cycles for the case P4-dry bone

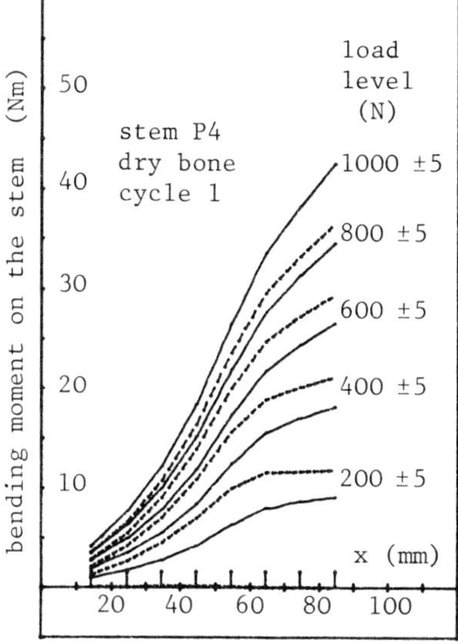

Figure 3: Experimental results for the case P4-dry bone (x is the abscissa from the stem's tip)

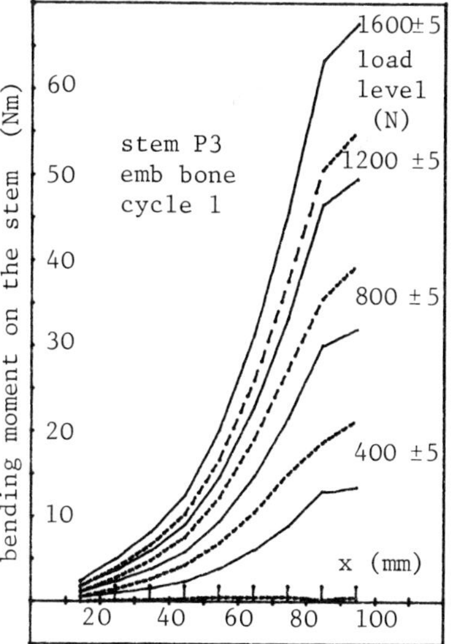

Figure 4: Experimental results for the case P3-embalmed bone (x is the abscissa from the stem's tip)

The difference between loading and unloading is not understood.
Dry-friction effects, suggested by the rather constant differences
between the loading and unloading values, do not account for the
return to the initial values as the load returns to zero.

REFERENCES

Breyer, H.G., Enes-Gaiao, F., Kühn, H.J. (1979) Biegebeanspruchung
desFemurkopfprothesenschaftes bei pertrochanterer Osteotomie.
Pauwels Symposium, Freie Univ. Berlin.

Calderale, P.M., Gola, M.M., Gugliotta, A. (1979a) New theoretical
and experimental developments in the mechanical design of implant
stems. Pauwels Symposium, Freie Univ. Berlin.

Calderale, P.M., Gola, M.M., Gugliotta A. (1979b) Analisi teorica
e sperimentale dello stato di tensione in steli protesici. VII Con
vegno Naz. AIAS, Cagliari.

Calderale,P.M., Gola, M.M., Gugliotta, A. (1979c) Theoretical and
experimental analysis of stem-femur coupling: new improved procedure.
II E.S.B. Meeting, Strasbourg.

Calderale, P.M., Gola, M.M., Gugliotta, A. (1979d) Mechanical stress
distribution in stem of implants. Biomechanics VII, Warsaw.

Calderale, P.M., Gola, M.M., Gugliotta, A. (1980) Experimental
results for stem-femur couplings loaded in bending. II Nat. Symposium
of Experimental Stress Analysis, Cluj Napoca, Romania.

Crowninshield, R.D., Brand, R.A., Johnston, R.C. (1979) An analysis
of femoral stem design in total hip arthroplasty. 25th Ann. Meet.
Orthop. Res. Soc., San Francisco.

Gola, M.M., Gugliotta, A. (1979) Analytical estimate of stresses in
bones and prosthesis stems. Journal of Strain Analysis, vol. 14, n. 1.

Huiskes, R. et al. (1977) Strain-gauge measurements on loaded femur,
intact as well as provided with orthopaedic implants. Poster Session,
Biomechanics VI, Copenhagen.

Huiskes, R., Sloof, T.J. (1979a) Experimentelle und rechnerische
Spannungsanalyse der Hüftgelenkverankerung. Pauwels Symposium, Freie
Univ. Berlin.

Huiskes, R. (1979b) Some fundamental aspects of human joint replacement. Proefschrift Doc. Techn. Wet., Techn. Hoge. Eindhoven.

Jacob, H.A.C., Huggler, A.H. (1979) Spannungsanalysen an Kunststoff-
modellen des menschlichen Beckens sowie des proximalen Femurendes mit
und ohne Prothese. Pauwels Symposium, Freie Univ. Berlin.

Markolf, K.L., Amstutz, H.C. (1976) A comparative experimental study
of stresses in femoral total hip replacement components: the effects
of prostheses orientation and acrilic fixation. Journal Biomech.,
vol. 9, 73-79.

McNiece, G.M., Amstutz, H.C. (1976) Finite element studies in hip
reconstruction.Biomechanics V, P. Komi ed., Univ. Park Press,
Baltimore.

Röhrle, H., Scholten, R., Sollbach, W. (1979) Der Kraftfluss bei neuartigen Hüftendoprothesen, Pauwels Symposium, Freie Univ.Berlin.

Svensson, N.L., Valliappan, S., Wood, R.D. (1977) Stress analysis of human femur with implanted Charnley prosthesis. Journal Biomech., vol. 10.

Tarr, R.R., Lewis, J.L. et al. (1979) Effects of materials, stem geometry and collar-calcar contact on stress distribution in the proximal femur with a total hip. 25th Ann. Meet. Arthop. Soc., San Francisco.

Weightman, B. (1976) The stress in total hip prosthesis femoral stems: comparative experimental study. Artif. hip knee technol., Springer.

Wood, R.D. (1975) Stress analysis of the femur. Thesis, Univ. of New South Wales, Australia.

Biomaterials 1980
Edited by G. D. Winter, D. F. Gibbons, and H. Plenk, Jr.
© 1982 John Wiley and Sons Ltd.

UNCONSTRAINED TOTAL ANKLE PROSTHESIS:
REPORT OF FOUR YEARS EXPERIENCE

Paul K. Odland, M.D.,

Mercy Hospital,
Janesville, Wisconsin, U.S.A.

SUMMARY

Total ankle arthroplasty, as an alternative to arthrodesis of the
ankle, is a fairly new concept. Available prostheses are semi-
constrained, constrained, or unconstrained. The device here
presented is unconstrained, congruous and anatomically designed.

The prosthesis design rationale, development and usage in 45 cases
over 4 years are presented. This paper is prepared to present the
design criteria, the clinical indications and contraindications
developed to date.

PROSTHESIS DESIGN

This unconstrained anatomical total ankle system was developed based
on the anatomy, physiology and biomechanics of the ankle joint, and
the properties of the prosthetic materials utilized. The design is
intended to minimize the amount of bone resection necessary for
installation. It is unique in that it allows mediolateral laxity,
which is important in prevention of loosening and restoring near-
normal function. An extensive study of ankle models, specimens, and
roentgenograms was made to obtain data for the specifications of
this unconstrained total ankle.

Anatomical considerations. The ankle joint has three sets of articular
surfaces; the tibiotalar joint bears most of the body weight and
joint forces. The articular surfaces conform. The talar surface is
trapezoidal, tapering posteriorly with an anterior/posterior width
ratio of 1.4 to 1.

This trapeziodal configuration exerts a wedging effect on the malleoli
as the foot dorsiflexes. The malleoli grip the talus, and full
stability occurs in full dorsiflexion.

Measurements of the tibiotalar joint surfaces were grouped into three
categories; a small joint, 8.3 cm^2 (1.3 sq.in.); a medium joint,
10.5 cm^2 (1.6 sq.in.); and a large joint, 12.9 cm^2 (2 sq.in.).

<u>Biomechanical considerations</u>. Force plate studies have shown that
peak loads in a normal subject may be five times the body weight.
The large contact area of the tibiotalar joint minimizes stresses
in the ankle joint.

<u>Design considerations</u>. Therefore, the ideal ankle prosthesis should
have the following features:

1. It should replace the tibiotalar joint
2. It should be trapezoidal in shape
3. It should restore the natural radius of the joint
4. The potential range of motion should be 45 degrees
5. It should allow some mediolateral movement.

There are a number of advantages for replacing the tibiotalar joint
only. The ankle joint stabilizes quickly in dorsiflexion, thus an
impact load may arise. By retaining the natural malleoli, the
potential for prosthetic loosening due to this impact should be
minimized. Since the ankle joint also sustains injuries such as
sprains and strains, leaving the malleoli structures intact would be
helpful in minimizing prosthetic loosening due to ankle injury postoperatively. In the event that fusion may become necessary, the
malleoli structures can also provide the height needed to maintain
leg-length equality.

The trapezoidal contact surface is advantageous, since the ankle joint
is in dorsiflexion most of the time during the walking cycle. Thus,
the prosthetic components will have a maximum contact area which is
expected to minimize the stresses transmitted to the prosthetic
materials.

If the natural radius of dorsiflexion and plantar flexion is not
restored, the ligaments may be placed under undue strain. The
stresses developed in the ligaments may also affect the motion of
the prosthesis and the fixation mechanism. The natural radius can
be restored, and near normal function postoperatively can be
achieved, using the range of available sizes.

By providing a maximum potential range of motion, the malleoli
structures, rather than the prosthesis, will stabilize the joint at
extreme dorsiflexion. Again, the stresses on the prosthesis
fixation mechanisms will be minimized.

By allowing some mediolateral motion in the prosthesis, the stresses
exerted on the ligaments in the joint can be minimized. To allow
such motion, the width of the tibial component is made slightly
wider than the talar component. This also helps provide a safety
margin to the surgeon in the installation of the device.

Observation shows that the talus shifts gradually from lateral in
plantar flexion to medial in dorsiflexion, thereby mandating slight
medial to lateral motion in the prosthesis design.

Motion of the ankle occurs primarily in the sagittal plane in a
hinge action (Inman, 1969). To determine the location of this axis,
220 unselected lateral ankle roentgenograms were measured and the
profile of the talus and distal tibia were observed and the radii
recorded.

The data grouped into three ranges. The most common was 23 mm to
25 mm (41%). Next was 20 to 22 mm (31%), and last, 26 to 28 mm
(16%). Twelve percent of the cases fell outside these ranges.

From the same films, the potential range of ankle motion was
determined by subtracting the arc subtended by the talus from
that of the tibia. The potential range of motion was 45 degrees.

The load surfaces of the ankle joint are the dome of the talus and
the distal tibia. The lateral facets of the ankle joint provide
side to side stability only (Lambert, 1971).

Motion through the ankle joint can be approximated by rotating
around a simple axis (Inman, 1969). Only the mid 35 degrees of
ankle motion is used during normal walking (Sammarco, 1975). The
possible separation of the malleoli that can occur in the ankle is
very small, 0.13 - 1.8 mm (Williams, 1976).

During the walking phase, the ankle joint does not internally or
externally rotate, but simply rotates from dorsiflexion to plantar
flexion (Morris, 1977). The study of Morris shows that during one
walking cycle the ankle joint is plantar flexed 30% of the cycle,
and dorsiflexed 70% of the cycle. The subtalar joint is inverted
45% and everted 55% of the cycle (Inman, 1969).

The maximum peak load in the joint occurs at 85% of the walking cycle
and has been reported to be 5.3 times the body weight in normal
subjects (Stauffer, 1969).

SPECIFICATIONS AND MATERIALS

The dimensions and size of the unconstrained total ankle were based
on the previous studies. Three sizes were developed to allow the
surgeon to restore the radius of the ankle joint to within 1 mm of
the natural configuration. The combined thickness of the tibial and
talar components is 15 mm and only 6 mm of bone must be removed from
the talus.

To minimize wear, the articular surfaces of the plastic tibial
component and the metal talar component have a surface roughness of
less than 20 and 2 millionths of an inch respectively.

The talar component of this prosthesis is made from cast Cobalt-
Chromium-Molybdenum alloy. The tibial component is made from ultra
high molecular weight polyethylene. Both of these materials have
been widely used and well studied (Figure 1).

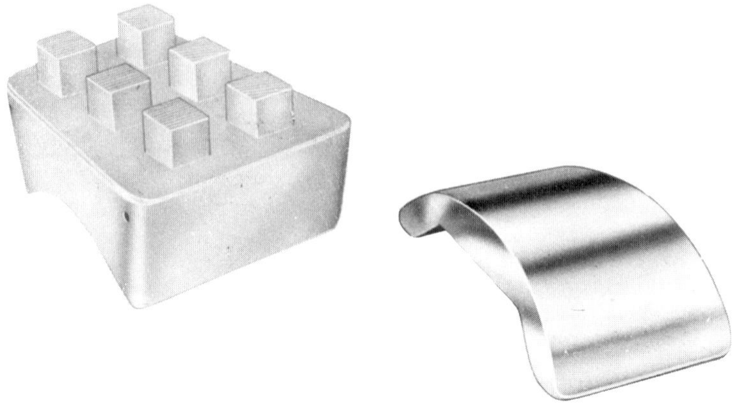

Figure 1.   Perspective and laterial views
of the prosthesis

For this total ankle system the relative curvature of the prosthetic
components for the three sizes are above the 12 mm threshold
curvature and the final contact stresses are below 8.7 MPa. Trent
and Walker have suggested that if the relative curvature of the
prosthetic components is above 12 mm and the final contact stress
below 8.7 MPa the wear rate of the prosthesis is not expected to
be excessive (Trent & Walker, 1976).

INDICATIONS AND CONTRAINDICATIONS

Generally, patients with a painful and disabling ankle joint may
elect to undergo total ankle replacement. The patient ideally
should have normal motor power, normal stability of the ankle,
absence of severe deformity, good circulation, good sensation, skin
coverage and condition. Subtalar, talonavicular or calcaneocuboid
arthritis is not a contraindication for total ankle replacement.
By restoring good ankle motion, those arthritic syndromes may be
alleviated. This should be explained preoperatively to patients
when such syndromes are observed in the roentgenograms.

Indications

1. Painful and disabling ankle joint arthritis, such as rheumatoid,
degenerative or post-traumatic arthritis.
2. Painful, stabilized, partial aseptic necrosis of the talus.
3. Failed previous ankle arthroplasty or fusion in which the medial
and lateral malleoli were maintained.

Contraindications

1. Unexplained fever or laboratory tests suggesting infection.
(elevated sedimentation rate, elevated WBC, or more marked shift
in differential count)
2. Severe angular deformity of the ankle that exceeds 20 degrees
of valgus or varus.

3. Marked instability of the ankle joint, such as a Charcot joint.
4. Inadequate circulation.
5. Inadequate sensation.
6. Abnormal or reduced motor power.
7. Inadequate soft tissue and skin coverage.

RESULTS

From January 1976 to February 1980, forty-five total ankle replacements have been done. Of these procedures, thirty-three cases (73%) have been followed longer than 12 months. Eighteen have been followed longer than two years. The follow-ups have ranged from two to fifty-one months with an average of twenty-three months. There were 22 females and 23 males, with an age range from 22 to 72 years, an average age of 46 (Figure 2).

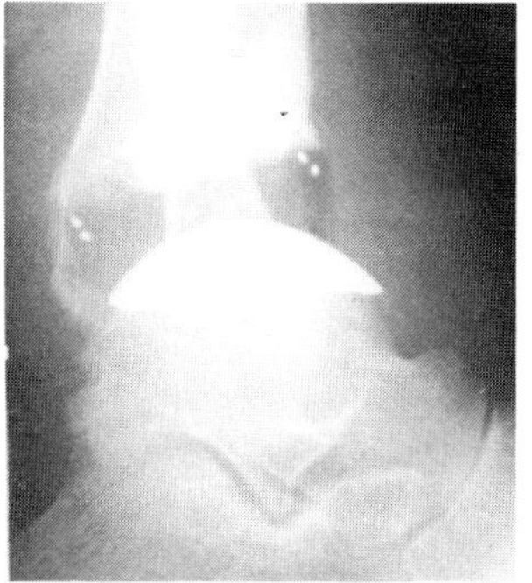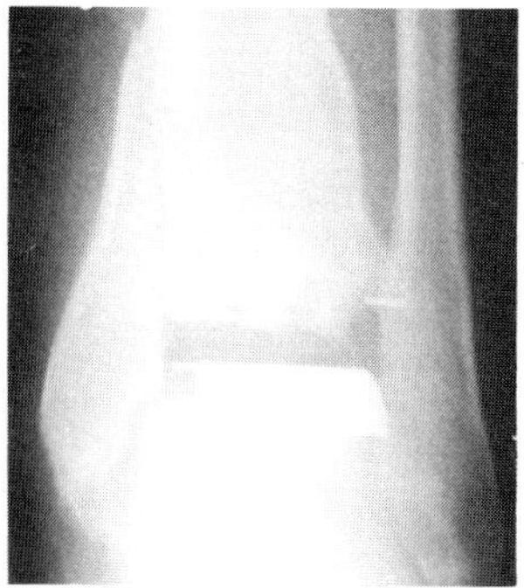

Figure 2. Four years post-operative X-rays of working auto-assembly factory man

Preoperative diagnoses	Cases
Post-traumatic arthritis	28
Degenerative joint disease	8
Rheumatoid arthritis	2
Failed total ankle arthroplasty	3
Failed ankle fusion	2
Aseptic necrosis	1
Absent talus	1

Postoperative results

Rating		Pain		Swelling	
Excellent	30	None	34	None	34
Good	5	Slight	9	Slight	10
Fair	8	Moderate	1	Severe	none

The average range of motion achieved was 25 degrees. The patients
who also had Achilles tendon lengthening averaged 29 degrees of
motion. The overall improvement of the patients' symptoms, motion,
and discomfort in this series was 78% as adjudged by available
criteria of pain, motion, swelling and lack of support. As judged
by the patients themselves, there was an 82% improvement. One
ankle was later arthrodesed. Two prostheses loosened (4.4%) and
were re-done.

CONCLUSION

The chief benefit from this prosthetic replacement has been the
relief of pain, and, secondly, the improvement in ankle motion.
Excluding the ankle fusion, all patients have maintained their
activity as before the operation and have a greater walking tolerance,
less pain and swelling, and better motion than they averaged before
the operation.

RECOMMENDATION

Total ankle replacement should be considered as an alternative to
arthrodesis. When carefully applied with meticulous surgical
detail and selection of patients, this unconstrained prosthesis is
expected to function well in a high percentage (77% - 82%) of
patients.

REFERENCES

Inman, V.T. (1969) UC-BL dual axis ankle control system and UC-BL
shoe insert, biomechanical considerations. Bulletin of Prosthetic
Research, Spring, 10-11.
Inman, V.T. (1976) The joints of the ankle. Williams and Wilkins Co.,
Waverly Press, Baltimore, MD., 24-25, 92-93.
Lambert, K.L. (1971) The weight-bearing function of the fibula: A
strain-gauge study. J.Bone & Joint Surg., 53A, 507-513.
Morris, J. (1977) Biomechanics of the foot and ankle. Clin. Orth.
Rel. Res., 122, 10-17.
Sammarco, G.J., Burstein, A.H., Frankel, V.H., (1973) Biomechanics
of the ankle; a kinematic study. Orth. Clin. N.America, Jan. 75-96.
Stauffer, R.N. (1976) Total ankle joint replacement as an alternative
to arthrodesis. Geriatrics, 31, 79-82.
Trent, P.S. and Walker, P.S. (1976) Wear and conformity in total
knee replacement. Wear, 36, 175-187.

Biomaterials 1980
Edited by G. D. Winter, D. F. Gibbons, and H. Plenk, Jr.
© 1982 John Wiley and Sons Ltd.

BIOMECHANICAL MEASUREMENTS OF STRESS-DISTRIBUTION AFTER CUP-PROSTHESIS IMPLANTATION IN THE TRABECULAR BONE OF THE FEMORAL NECK

Gerngross, H., Burri, C., Claes, L., Rüter, A.

Department of Traumatology (Prof. Dr. C. Burri), University of Ulm, Steinhövelstraße 9, 7900 Ulm, West-Germany

SUMMARY

The biomechanical considerations of Wagner (1979) and Freeman (1979) emphasize the need for a precise 20°-valgus-cup-position and a need to avoid damage to the cortex of the femoral neck. After cup-prosthesis implantation femoral neck fractures occurred. Strain and stress under different loading conditions in the femoral neck were measured by using strain gauges. We found that the reaming of the femoral head and the implantation of the cup reduces the strength of the femoral neck: varus orientation significantly more than valgus orientation. The results of our experimental investigation confirm the requirements of Wagner and Freeman.

INTRODUCTION

In patients whose femoral head had been resurfaced by a cup prosthesis several femoral neck fractures occurred in the absence of any trauma. Further investigation proved that the reduction of blood-flow or osteoporosis under the cup (induced by stress-protection) could not account for the fractures (Hipp, 1979). Therefore we have examined the changes in the stress distribution in the femoral neck after reaming of the head and implanting the cup prosthesis.

MATERIAL AND METHODS

Six fresh human femora were prepared for testing. To measure the strains in the tension-band region of the femoral neck, five strain gauges were glued to the lateral cortex of the neck. To measure the strains in the compression region a hole 1.5 cm diameter was drilled into the femoral neck near the Adams´-arch and a rosette-strain-gauge glued to the specially prepared spongy bone.

The strain gauges were compensated for changes of temperature. In a mechanical testing machine with a jig capable
of changing the orientation of the load relative to the
axis of the femur, all relevant loading conditions of the
femoral head could be simulated: We chose to apply the
load at angles 16°, 0° and -12° relative to the vertical
axis of the femur with a constantly increasing load with
a deformation rate of 2 mm/min up to 1 kN. The applied
load and the response from the strain gauges were simultaneously plotted as a function of time. Therefore, direct
comparison of load and strain was possible. All femora
were tested first without cup (= no cup), then after
reaming and implantation of the cup first in a valgus-
and then in a varus position.

RESULTS

After reaming, the stress distribution in the proximal end
of the femur changes even without load. Figure 1 shows the
main tension strains (stresses) after both slight and extensive reaming.

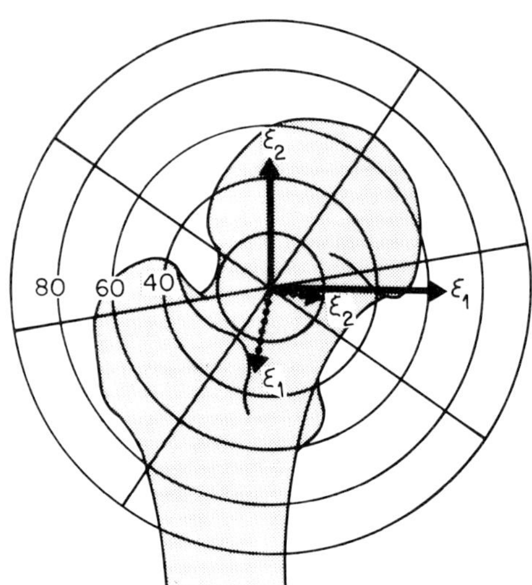

Fig. 1. Strain-distribution after reaming:
·······▶ slight reaming
——▶ extensive reaming
$\varepsilon_1, \varepsilon_2$ main tension strains (μm/m), with no applied
load.

The more extensively the head is reamed, the greater the
strain (stress) weakening in the femoral neck; the orientation of the principal tensile stresses also markedly
changes.

After cup implantation no significant change in the
strains in the lateral cortex was found for the 16° load
orientation, either for valgus or varus positioning of
the cup (Fig. 2, left). For the 0° load orientation valgus
positioning of the cup does not differ from the unreamed
femoral head, however varus positioning of the cup decreases the strain (Fig. 2, middle). The -12° load orientation reduces the strain for both varus and valgus
orientations of the cup (Fig. 2, right).

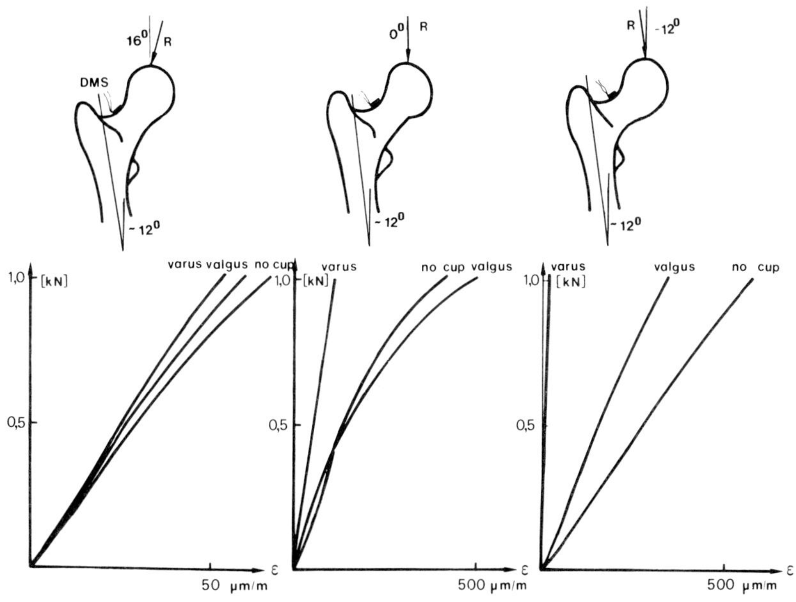

Fig. 2. Strains after cup-implantation with different load angles.

Under normal conditions (no cup) both the strains in the
lateral cortex and the shear stress in the compression
region increase when the orientation of the load on the
femoral head is changed from 16° to -12° (Fig. 3). If the
cup is implanted in the valgus orientation the increase
in shear stress (s) is significantly lower than when it
is implanted in the varus orientation.

DISCUSSION

Weakening of the femoral neck and increase of shear
stress in the compression region could be the cause for
the observed femoral neck fractures in the absence of
trauma. While the one-leg-stand phase in normal gait,
with a static maximum load, does not appear to be dangerous because of the direction of the resultant-force

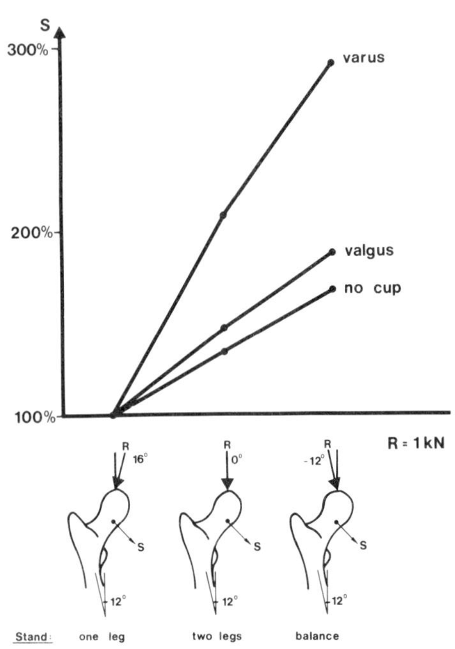

Fig. 3. Shear stress after cup-implantation with
different load angles. For the one leg stand
(R = 1 kN, 16°) similar shear stress occurred for
no cup, valgus or varus orientation of the cup,
and was set 100 %.

R (16°). All the other phases of gait (stand and balance)
approximated by resultant forces at angles (0°, -12°)
could excessively stress the femoral neck after cup-implantation. We are of the opinion, that the increased
shear in the compression region, after partially cutting
the tension band region by reaming, could be the origin
of the observed femoral neck fractures, after cup-implantation, in the absence of trauma.

REFERENCES

Freeman, M.A.R. (1978) "Some anatomical and mechanical
considerations relevant to the surface-replacement of the
femoral head". Clin. Orthop., 134, 19-24.
Hipp, E. (1979) Blood supply of the femoral head in
Symposium on Orthopedic Surgery: the Hip, Conference
Digest, 14, München 1979
Wagner, H. (1979) "Die Schalenprothese des Hüftgelenks -
Oberflächenersatz als Gelenkerhaltung". Orthopädie, 8,
276-295

Biomaterials 1980
Edited by G. D. Winter, D. F. Gibbons, and H. Plenk, Jr.
© 1982 John Wiley and Sons Ltd.

CUP ENDOPROSTHESIS OF THE HIP.
EXPERIMENTAL STUDIES IN RABBITS.

W. Pforringer, R. Bassermann and B. Rosemeyer

Orthopadische Klinik und Poliklinik der Universitat
Munchen.
Pathologisches Institut der Universitat Munchen.

SUMMARY

Cup arthroplasties of the hip joint have been performed in rabbits
to study the problems arising from this type of joint replacement as
far as the attachment of the cup and the vitality of the bone underneath the cup are concerned. It was found that the attachment of
the cup with the use of bone-cement gives no problems of loosening
as long as certain technical procedures are performed thoroughly.
The bone underneath the cup attaches itself to the inner layer of
bone-cement and this connection holds strong as long as there is no
avascular necrosis of the head or infection. The rest of the femoral
head stays vital as long as the vascular supply is not damaged
during the operation. There is still bone metabolism underneath the
cup which can be proved by tetracycline marking.

Connective tissue is found wherever the contact of bone and bone-
cement is insufficient. This happens in loose cups as well as in
centers where there has been insufficient contact between bone and
bone-cement from the moment of implantation.

INTRODUCTION

The cup arthroplasty of Wagner (1978) or the double cup of Freeman
(1978) are the latest link in the chain of prosthetic replacements of
the hip. In contrast to total hip replacement, cup arthroplasty
preserves most of the anatomical conditions of the hip joint. The
damaged head of femur is capped with a metal cup attached with bone-
cement. The acetabulum is replaced by plastic prostheses matching
the size of the metal cup. With this procedure there are more
retreatment possibilities than with the total hip.

Such failures as do occur are caused by loosening of the implanted
components of the hip joint prostheses and by infection, requiring
further intervention. Cup arthroplasty leaves more of the coxal end
of the femur untouched than does the stem of a total hip. This can
lead to two complications; firstly loosening of the cup at the line
of contact between bone-cement and cancellous bone and secondly
reduced vitality of the head of the femur underneath the cup.

MATERIALS AND METHODS

We tried to analyse these problems in an experimental study using
rabbits, over a period of one year. No similar studies are to be
found in the literature. We implanted cup endoprostheses in the
left hip joint of 25 rabbits. The cups were made of highly
polished, non-corrosive V4A steel which had been produced out of
steel balls of 10 mm diameter. A hole was drilled into the cup's
middle as is done in Wagner's original cups. The operation was
performed by dorsal approach to the hip and after luxation of the
joint the head of the femur was freed of cartilage with the use of a
special reamer, until the cancellous bone was exposed and bleeding.
Then the head was shaped until the cup could be attached and fixed
with bone-cement. The bone-cement was mixed and while still fluid
filled into the cup and the cup was then attached with high pressure
on to the reamed head of the femur. Superfluous cement came out of
the hole in the middle of the cup due to the high pressure during
attachment and only a thin layer of cement was left between cup and
femoral head.

We did not replace the natural acetabulum because this had no direct
connection or importance for our experiment. There was no external
fixation post-operatively for the affected limb, but it was observed
that the animals protected the operated hip from full weight bearing
for up to two weeks.

Having lost some rabbits due to post-operative infection, we started
to inject tetracycline post-operatively (once a week 1 mg/kg body
weight) for four weeks. It was used for bone marking by fluoroscopy
as well as protection from infection. By this procedure we did not
lose any more animals. The rabbits were killed 14 to 200 days postoperatively and the hip joints were X-rayed and then excised
(Fig. 4a & b).

We had, as complications, two cases of infection, two luxated hips
and one avascular necrosis of the neck of the femur, which led to a
fracture. In two cases, radiographs showed a complete loosening of
the cup combined with a complete luxation of the hip joint. After
exclusion of these cases 20 animals were left for evaluation. Of
these, 15 had their cup endoprostheses between 100 and 200 days, an
average time of observation of about five months. The hip joint
specimens, including the steel cup, were cut in half with a water
cooled diamond grinding disc and photographs were taken.
Histological specimens were then made. The surface of the rest of
the femoral head as well as the femoral neck were examined by high
magnification microscopy of unstained specimens as well as by fluoroscopy examination. Special attention was paid to the borderline of
bone and bone-cement.

RESULTS

30 days: Microscopic views showed that the cortical layer of bone
underneath the cement was of different strength and most of the

osseous laminae were free (Fig. 2). Only occasional osteoblasts were
seen covering the bone. At this early stage a reactive and reparative
inflammation was found within the marrow spaces. There was no
fibrous tissue between bone and cement and intraosseous necrosis was
not observed.
60 days: As at 30 days, there was cortical bone of variable
thickness underneath the cement. There was no longer any inflammation
and we did not find osteoporosis or osteonecrosis (Fig. 3).
90 days: The 90 day specimens are similar. Tetracycling labelling
is clearly visible within the femoral head and neck on fluoroscopic
examination. Directly underneath the metal cup and cement it is
absent. We believe that because the tetracycline was given only
during the four weeks post-operatively the absence of labelling is
due to this fact. Histologically it was clearly visible that the
bone was not dead. This proves that the bone underneath the cement
was formed later, which suggests normal osseous metabolism underneath
the cup endoprosthesis. The specimens from the 120th to the 200th
days are no different. Macroscopically they are without abnormalities
and microscopically there are no interpositions of connective tissue
at the borderline. Inflammation, necrosis and other signs of a
disturbed metabolism are not apparent.

<u>DISCUSSION</u>

Connective tissue was always found where the contact of bone and
cement was insufficient from the very beginning, i.e. in hips where
the bone-cement showed air bubbles which contacted with the surface
of free cancellous bone (Fig. 1a & 1b). Connective tissue was found
also where cups had loosened.
We want to add some clinical observations: Examining some of our
clinical cases where the cup had to be changed to a total replacement
due to loosening or infection, we always found a thick layer of strong
connective tissue on top of the rest of the femoral head when there
had been loosening of the cup. This was not seen in cases where there
was reintervention, for example, due to a fracture of the neck of the
femur. In addition, we found in our clinical cases a clear shrinking
of the rest of the head and neck of the femur as well as osteoporosis of a high degree.

Summarising, we found all examined coxal ends of the femur showed
primarily a varying tissue reaction to the surface replacement. The
main centre of this reaction was towards the middle of the femoral
head rather than at the border line to the bone-cement. The
reactions diminished with increasing temporal distance to the
operation. The border line bone-cement showed only morphological
changes during the time of observation. The trabeculae soon had
adapted themselves to the molding form of the inner layer of bone-
cement, fresh or old zones of necroses were not found. Furthermore,
at the border line a bone growth of varying degrees took place. We
gained the impression that this growth decreased proportional to the
timelag to the implantation of the cup. The hips which after excision
showed no macroscopic signs of loosening, also microscopically, did
not show any insufficiencies of the contact zone bone/bone-cement.

It can be concluded that the osseous structures of the femoral end
of the hip tolerates the bone-cement during the full time of
observation and that the trabeculae adapted themselves to the surface
irregularities of the cement layer. There was no observation of
changes in the structure of the trabeculae. Our clinical cases
induce the impression that intra-operatively it is necessary to
smooth the surface of the femoral head, where the cup is to be
attached, as much as possible. It is of special importance to
remove all cavities (induced by avascular necroses or degenerative
changes) which may have been opened by the reaming of the head. In
addition, it is a fact that pre-operatively damaged areas of the
femoral head or neck, i.e. in cases of an idiopathic or post-
traumatic avascular necrosis, have a reduced chance of survival to
the heat induced damage resulting from the hardening of the bone-
cement. In spite of the fact that the mechanics of the hip of the
rabbit differ clearly to those of man, these differences are of no
important relevance in the discussion of the problems arising at
the border line bone/cement during the implantation of a cup endoprosthesis. The vitality of the bone tissue in the whole coxal end
of the femur underneath a cup underlies the same conditions in man
as well as in animals.

The observations of Draenert and Hofmann (1979, that there is reinforcement of cancellous bone underneath the cup in cases of
surface replacement of the coxal end of the femur matches with our
results. Cserhati et al (1979) have drawn the conclusion that
there is always a layer of fibrous tissue between cement and
cancellous bone underneath a cup arthroplasty. This conclusion is
based on the fact that they checked only clinical cases where the
cup implantation had failed and the cup was loose. Hereby a
negative series was used to study the behaviour of bone underneath
a metal cup in positive cases and this fact had to lead to
conclusions into the wrong direction. The studies of Mendes et al
(1974) and Hedley et al (1979) are not, in our opinion, comparible
to our studies. They have used different techniques and a different
approach to the problem which is discussed in this paper. But they
are, without doubt, a valuable contribution as far as experimental
studies in animals for surface replacement of the hip are concerned.

<u>REFERENCES</u>

Cserhati, M.D., Oliveira, L.G., Jacob, H.A.C. & Schreiber, A. (1979)
Histomorphological investigations of coxa femoral ends following
double-cup arthroplasty according to Freeman. <u>Arch.Orth.Traumat.</u>
<u>Surg.</u>, <u>94</u>, 223-240.
Draenert, K.& Hofmann, H. (1979) The reinforcement of cancellous bone
under the cup. <u>The Hip</u>, Verlag Art. & Science, Munchen.
Mendes, D.G., Walker, P.S., Figarola, F. et al (1974) Total surface hip
replacement in the dog: a preliminary study of local tissue reaction.
<u>Clin. Orthop.</u>, <u>100</u>, 256-264.
Hedley, A.K., Moreland, J., Bloebaum, R.D., Coster, I. & Clarke, I.C.
(1979) Canine surface replacement model: press-fit, cemented and
bone ingrowth fixation. <u>Trans. 11th Internat.Biomat.Symp., Clemson,</u>
<u>Vol. 3. p 107</u>.

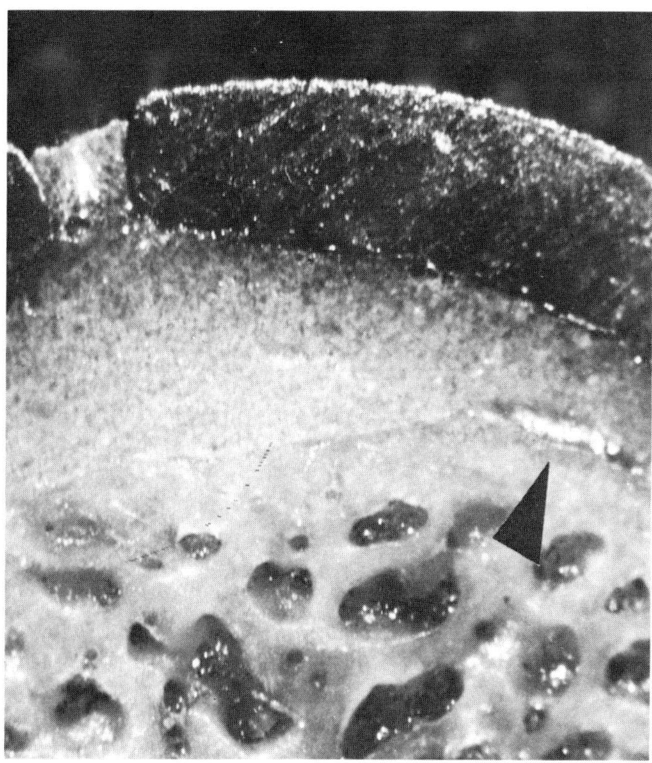

Fig. 1a. Macroscopic view (magnification x 16, unstained) cross section of femoral head, 54 days after implantation. Arrow marks insufficient contact between cement and bone surface (air bubble)

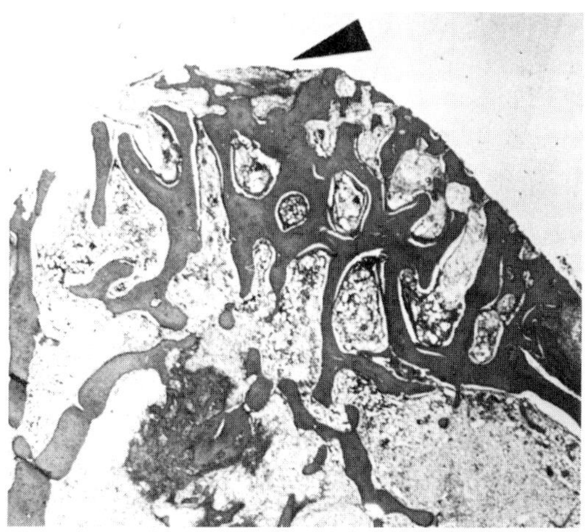

Fig. 1b.
Microscopic view of specimen of Fig. 1a. Arrow marks layer of fibrous tissue covering the area of insufficient contact of cement and bone surface. Regular structure of cancellous bone (magnification x 24, HE)

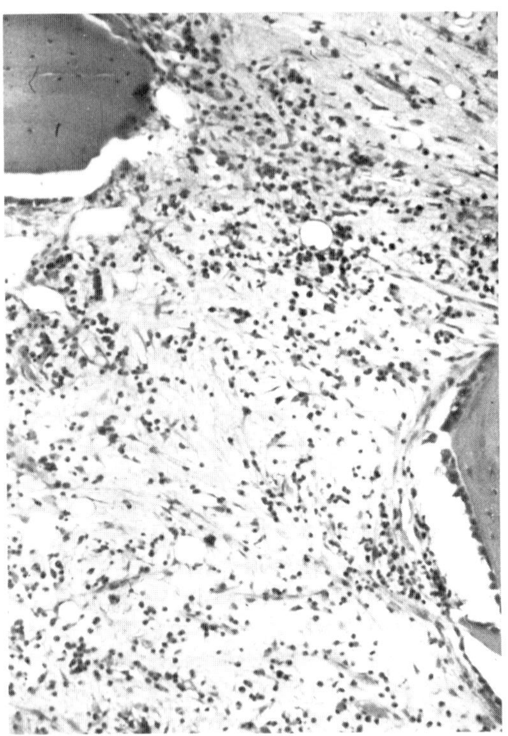

Fig. 2.
Cross section of center
of femoral head, 24 days
after implantation.
(magnification x 60, HE)
Moderate reactive and
reparative inflammation

Fig. 3
Cross section of specimen
60 days after cup
implantation (magnification
80, HE). Interposition of
fibrous tissue in the
cavities of the bone
marrow. Regular spongious
structure with significant
activity of osteoblasts
covering the trabecula

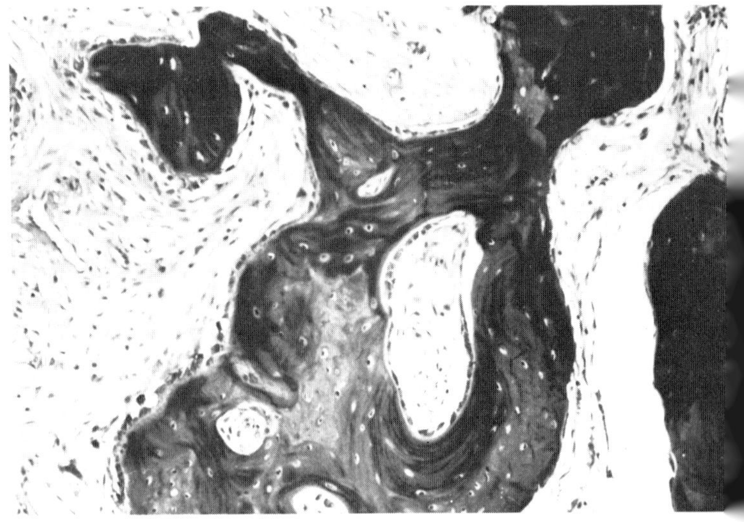

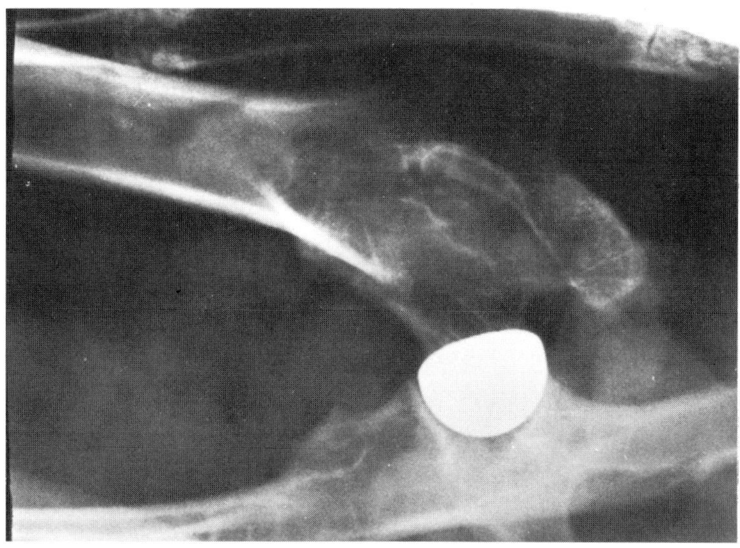

Fig. 4a. Roentgenogram of rabbit hip with surface replacement, 200 days after cup implantation

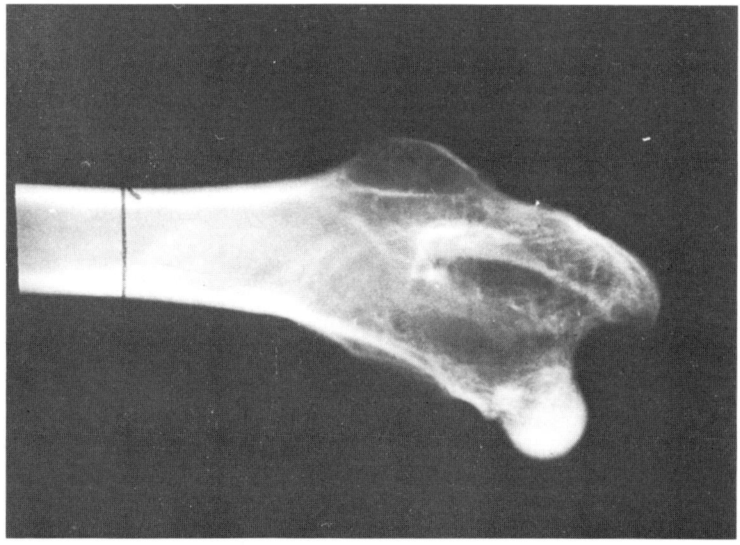

Fig. 4b. Same hip as in Fig. 4a after explantation at the day of X-ray control. The metal cup has been removed, the femoral head is still covered with cement

Biomaterials 1980
Edited by G. D. Winter, D. F. Gibbons, and H. Plenk, Jr.

CLINICAL AND HISTOLOGICAL OBSERVATIONS OF BIOCERAMIC DOUBLE–CUP HIP PROSTHESES INSERTED WITHOUT CEMENT

K. Knahr*, H. Plenk Jr.**, F. Grundschober** and M. Salzer*

* Orthopaedic Department of the Orthopaedic Hospital Wien-Gersthof, Vienna, Austria

** Bone Res. Lab., Histological and Embryological Institute of Vienna University, Schwarzspanierstrasse 17, Vienna, Austria

SUMMARY

Between 1976 to 1978 19 double-cup hip prostheses made of dense Al_2O_3 ceramic were implanted without using bone cement in 16 patients suffering from idiopathic coxarthrosis, ancylosing spondylitis, severe polyarthritis, idiopathic osteoarthrosis with confirmed allergy to metals and necrosis of the femoral head. Their ages ranged from 28 to 67 years.

The follow-up indicated a high complication rate of 68.4 % loosening of the femoral component, which occurred 1 to 45 months after surgery. Histologically, a lack of bony anchorage was established as the reason for failure. This was primarily because of a rotational instability of the implants and secondly because of the inferior quality of the femoral head and neck bone. In one case biomechanically incorrect implantation of the femoral cup caused the loosening.

There was no clinical evidence of loosening in the corresponding socket prosthesis, despite the fact that no ingrowth of bone into the ceramic grooves occurred.

INTRODUCTION

The search for alternatives to the traditional cemented stem endoprosthesis has led to the development of various types of prostheses which have replaced only the surface of the femoral head. These prostheses are usually fixed in place with the aid of bone cement (Amstutz, 1978, Freeman et al, 1978, Furuya et al, 1978, Trentani and Vaccarino, 1978, Wagner, 1978) but, starting in 1976, we implanted ceramic double-cup hip-joint endoprostheses without cement, hoping to avoid the complications of stem prostheses (Beckenbaugh and Ilstrup, 1978, Huggler and Schreiber, 1978, Bösch et al, 1980) as well as of bone cement (Hupfauer and Oest, 1975, Kellner, 1976). The results were unsatisfactory and the purpose of this paper is to analyse the reasons for failure.

MATERIAL AND METHODS

In the period from 1976 to 1978 19 double-cup hip prostheses made of dense
alumina ceramic were implanted in 16 patients. 6 male and 10 female patients
were operated (in 3 cases on both hips) at an average age of 53.5 years (range
from 28 to 67 years). The indications for operation were: idiopathic coxarthrosis
(10), severe polyarthritis in 2 female patients operated on both hips, ancylosing
spondylitis (2), 1 patient with an idiopathic osteoarthrosis with confirmed
allergy to metals who was operated on both hips and 1 patient with necrosis of
the femoral head.

The detailed operative procedure is described in a previous paper (Salzer et al,
1978). The femoral head and neck portion is reamed to a conical stump of
macroscopically healthy looking trabecular bone. In 14 of the 19 cases the
resected proximal portion of this stump was investigated histologically using
transverse undecalcified microtome sections. In typical cases, the volume
density of trabecular bone was determined morphometrically.

9 patients had revision surgery because of loosening of the femoral component.
Histological examination of the cup-supporting femoral neckbone was performed in all of these 9 cases and in one case (no. 13) where death occurred 5
weeks after operation due to septic complications related to cholecystitis.

CLINICAL RESULTS

Loosening of the femoral component has so far been detected in 13 operated
hips (Fig. 1). Autopsy (no. 13) revealed a rotational instability of the femoral
cup. In another case (no. 12), the loosening of the femoral cup occurred 4 weeks
after surgery as a result of a technical mistake during operation. In the other 11
cases clinical and radiological symptoms of loosening were found after observation periods of 3 to 34 months (Fig. 2). 8 of these patients have been
reoperated. 3 Patients (cases no. 1, 3, 8) have so far refused revision surgery,
because their complaints are minimal despite evident radiological loosening of
the femoral cup. Clinically and radiologically stable implants were found in 5
patients with 6 operated hips 27 to 49 months (average 39.8 months) after
surgery (Fig. 3).

HISTOLOGICAL FINDINGS

Condition of supporting bone structures at the time of implantation. In 10 of 13
loosened femoral cups the resected proximal portion of the femoral head could
be analysed. All cross sections revealed a network of cancellous bone except in
the cranial area where there was connective tissue, degenerative cysts and
cartilage remnants (Fig. 4a). Beyond the surfaces viable bone and active bone
remodelling was found.

The evaluation of 4 of the 6 cases with stable implants showed a more dense
structure of the bone trabeculae in nos. 14, 16 and 18. Case no. 14, for example,
exhibited 58.6 % volume density (Fig. 4b). In case no. 19, however, suffering
from ancylosing spondylitis, a more porotic bone structure was found (23.8 %

volume density, Fig. 4c). Generally, in all 4 cases the degenerative lesions seemed to be less pronounced then in the cases with loosened implants.

Condition of supporting bone structures at the time of reoperation. In 6 cases (nos. 2, 9, 10, 11, 12, 13) reoperated shortly after loosening became evident, longitudinal and cross sections of the femoral neck removed showed that the bone structure had not significantly altered. In contrast, a remarkable decrease in the diameter of the femoral neck was found in 2 cases (nos. 4 and 6) in which revision surgery was performed 5 and 10 months after the first clinical and radiological signs of loosening became evident.

In 2 cases (nos. 5 and 7) the histological evaluation was done on ground sections and corresponding radiomicrographs of the resected bone stump with the cup in situ. No bone ingrowth into the grooves of the ceramic head occurred, indicating rotational instablility and varus migration of the implants. As a counter-reaction, the density of the bone trabeculae had increased in the cranial region (Fig. 5).

X-ray examination showed that in all the corresponding 19 bioceramic sockets there was a radiolucent zone between prosthesis and bone. During revision surgery, the sockets were held in place by osteophytes and were clinically stable. After removal of these osteophytes the sockets could easily be extracted by a special instrument. In all cases a layer of soft connective tissue was found between ceramic and pelvic bone.

DISCUSSION

The concept of the double-cup hip joint endoprosthesis made of dense alumina-ceramic and inserted without using bone cement was adopted for two reasons: on the one hand, the low friction and wear properties of the ceramic material, and on the other its good biocompatibility, which promised a direct bony anchorage to avoid the well known disadvantages of bone cement fixation. Despite the good results in some cases, a loosening of the femoral cup was observed in 68.4 % of the implantations, making reoperation necessary. The radiological and histological analyses revealed three main reasons for failure of these cement-free bioceramic endoprostheses:

1. Biological inferiority of the bone of the femoral head and neck. If the femoral neck is transected and profuse bleeding occurs from the divided intraosseous vessels, a sufficient weight-bearing bone might be expected (Amstutz, 1978, Freeman, 1978). This bleeding was seen in all 19 operated hips.

Histological evaluation of the resected femoral parts demontrated that the bone was alive and well vascularized. The bone tissue beneath the loosened cups again showed no signs of devitalisation because of poor nutrition and seemed well able to react to mechanical impact.

The total amount of tissue degenerated because of the primary disease could not be estimated from these small sections. Nevertheless, analysis of similar material points to a higher incidence of loosening in cases where the cross sections of the femoral bone reveal more degenerative lesions.

2. Biomechanically incorrect implantation of the femoral cup. The correct positioning of the cup is essential for a stable and permanent fixation (Swanson & Mach, 1978). It is necessary, to insert the cup in a 20 degree valgus position to the axis of the femoral neck (Freeman, 1978).

Initial fixation is also a decisive factor for a stable and permanent anchorage. We attempted to achieve this by twisting the cup onto the conically reamed femoral neck. Unfortunately, this fixation did not last until biological stabilisation took place by bone tissue growing into the preformed grooves within the cup.

3. Unfavourable design due to the use of dense alumina ceramic. Encouraged by our favourable experiences with the cement-free extracortical attachment of bioceramic endoprostheses (Plenk et al, 1978) and the promising experimental results with cement-free bioceramic double-cup hip prostheses in dogs (Plenk et al, in press), the principle of conical sleeve fixation was applied to the femoral cup prostheses for human patients. The brittleness of the bioceramic material needed the construction of a thick-walled prosthesis, which required extensive resection of the femoral head and neck bone. Nevertheless, no femoral neck-fracture or break-down of the supporting bone structures was observed. The bone ingrowth into the preformed grooves of the inner surface of the cup, however, which we anticipated because of the good biocompatibility of the ceramic material, did not occur. In all the 13 cases of loosening a layer of connective tissue was found between bone and implanted prosthesis as a result of inadequate stabilisation of the femoral cup. This instability hindered the ingrowth of bone into the circular grooves of the inner surface of the cup.

In all the 6 stable cases, however, biomechanically correct implantation and possibly also bony anchorage of the cup can be assumed.

Our analyses lead us to suggest that a successful surface replacement using a cement-free femoral cup endoprosthesis requires the following: minimal preparation and resection of the supporting bone. The bone of the femoral head and neck should not be extensively damaged by primary disease. Initial fixation must be stable enough to prevent rotation. Only on this condition can permanent bony anchorage be expected.

REFERENCES

Amstutz H.C., Graff-Radford A., Gruen Th.A & Clarke I.C. (1978) Tharies Surface Replacements: A Review of the First 100 Cases. Clin. Orthop., 134, 87-101.
Beckenbaugh R.D., & Ilstrup D.M. 1978. Total Hip Arthroplasty.
J. Bone & Jt. Surg., 60-A, 306-313.
Bösch P., Kristen H. & Zweymüller K. (1980) An analysis of 119 loosenings in total hip endoprostheses. Arch. Orthop. Traumat. Surg., 96, 83-90.
Freeman M.A.R. (1978) Some Anatomical and Mechanical Considerations Relevant to the Replacement of the Femoral Head. Clin. Orthop., 134, 19-24.
Freeman M.A.R., Cameron H.U. & Brown G.C. (1978) Cemented Double Cup Arthroplasty of the Hip: A 5 Year Experience with the ICLH Prostheses. Clin. Orthop., 134, 45-52.

Furuya K., Tsuchiya M. & Kawachi S. (1978) Socket-Cup Arthroplasty. Clin. Orthop., 134, 41-44.

Huggler A.H. & Schreiber A. (1978) Alloarthroplastik des Hüftgelenkes. Thieme, Stuttgart.

Hupfauer W. & Oest O. (1975) Die spezielle Problematik der Anwendung der Knochenzemente im klinisch-operativen Bereich, in Die Knochenzemente, (Eds., Oest O., Müller H. & Hupfauer W.) Enke, Stuttgart.

Kellner G. (1976) Untersuchungen zur Eluierbarkeit von Knochenzement. Orthop. Praxis, 12, 624-629.

Plenk H. Jr., Salzer M., Locke H., Stärk N., Punzet G. & Zweymüller K. (1978) Extracortical Attachment of Bioceramic Endoprostheses to Long Bones without Bone Cement. Clin. Orthop., 132, 252-265.

Plenk H. Jr., Locke H., Punzet G., Salzer M. & Zweymüller K. (in press) Biomechanical aspects of bone reactions on total bioceramic hip-joint endoprostheses. J. Biomed. Mater. Res.

Salzer M., Knahr K., Locke H. & Stärk N. (1978) Cement-Free Bioceramic Double-Cup Endoprosthesis of the Hip Joint. Clin. Orthop., 134, 80-86.

Swanson S.A.V. & Mech M.I. (1978) Engineering Considerations in the Design of Double-Cup Hip Replacement Prostheses. Clin. Orthop., 134, 12-18.

Trentani C. & Vaccarino F. (1978) The Paltrinieri-Trentani Hip Joint Resurface Arthroplasty. Clin. Orthop., 134, 36-40.

Wagner H. (1978) Surface Replacement Arthroplasty of the Hip. Clin. Orthop., 134, 102-130.

FIGURES

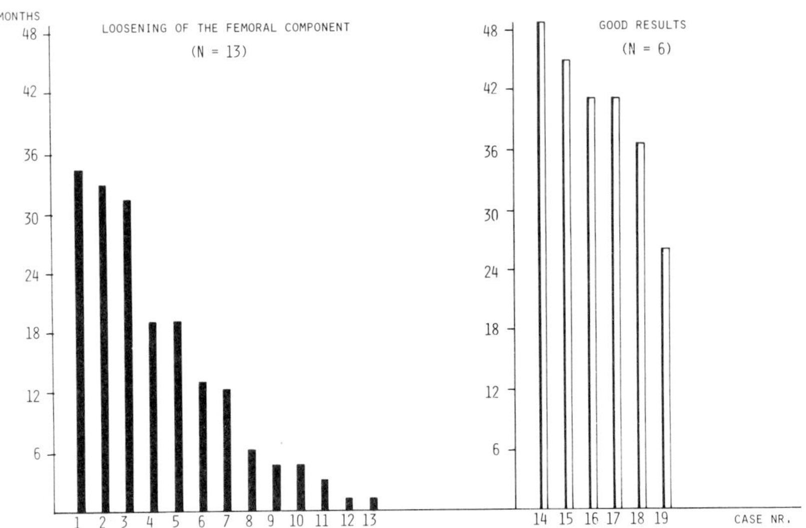

Fig. 1: Observation periods of loosened and stable bioceramic double-cup endoprostheses

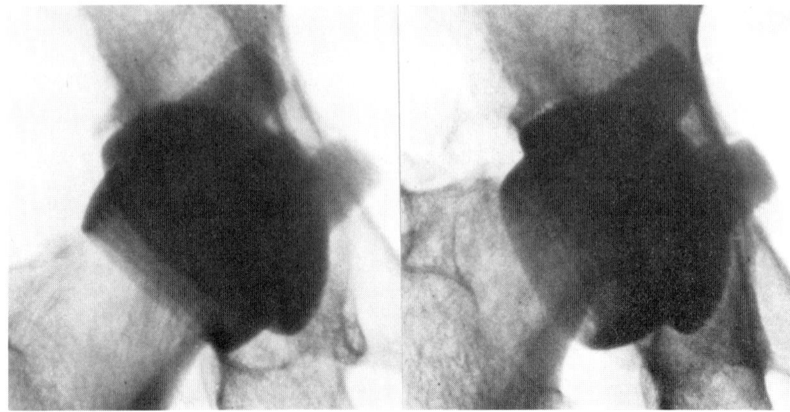

Fig. 2: H.F., 58a, male (case no. 9): idiopathic arthrosis of the right
hip
a) Postoperative radiograph. The femoral cup is in slight valgus
position.
b) The radiograph 5 month postoperatively shows a varus migration
of the femoral component and a thin radiolucent zone around the
socket.

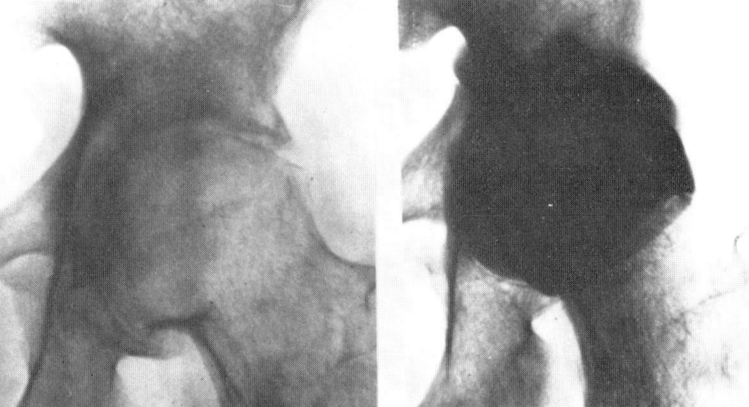

Fig. 3: T.B., 27a, male (case no.19): ancylosing spondylitis
a) Preoperative radiograph. Degenerated cartilage of the left hip
joint due to the primary lesion.
b) The radiograph 27 months postoperatively shows a stable anchorage of the endoprosthesis.

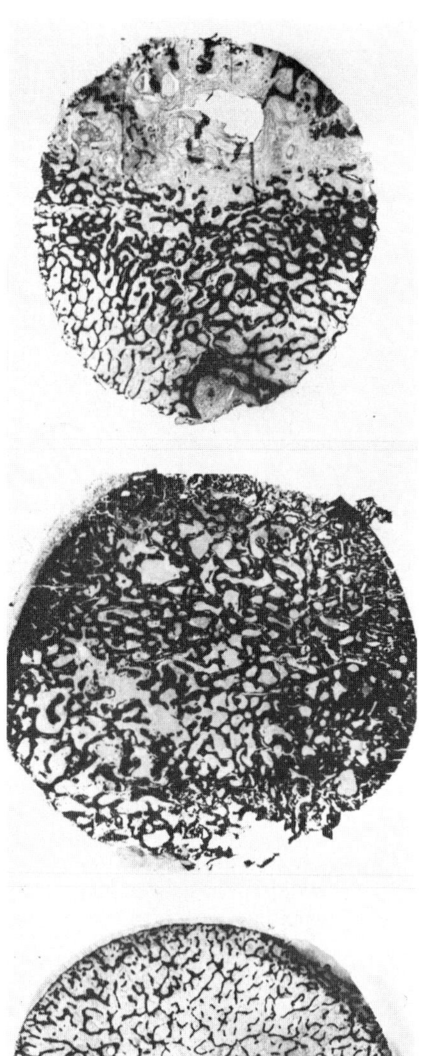

Fig. 4 (a-c): Cross sections of the resected femoral head and neck portion after reaming (Modified calcium-salt and methylgreen-pyronin staining, 3.5x).

a) H.F., 58a, male (no. 9): loosening 5 months postop. Degenerated cartilage, cysts and connective tissue have replaced the bone in the cranial portion (above).

b) S.Th., 65a, female (case no. 14): stable anchorage of the implant 49 months postop. The femoral neck consists of a very dense bone structure (58.6 % volume density).

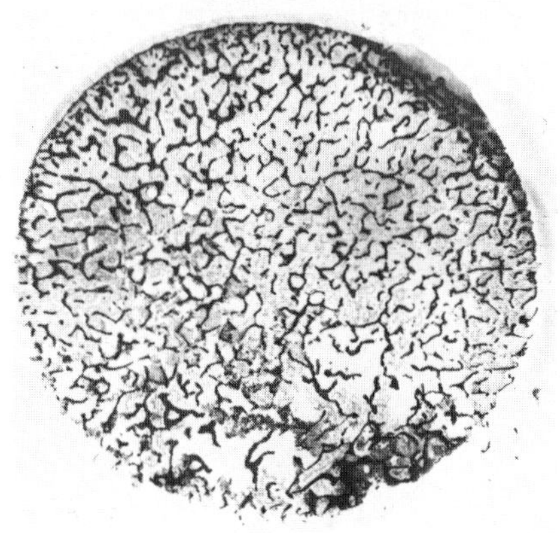

c) T.B., 27a, male (case no. 19) stable anchorage of the implant 27 months postop. A very delicate network of trabecular bone is found (23.8 % volume density).

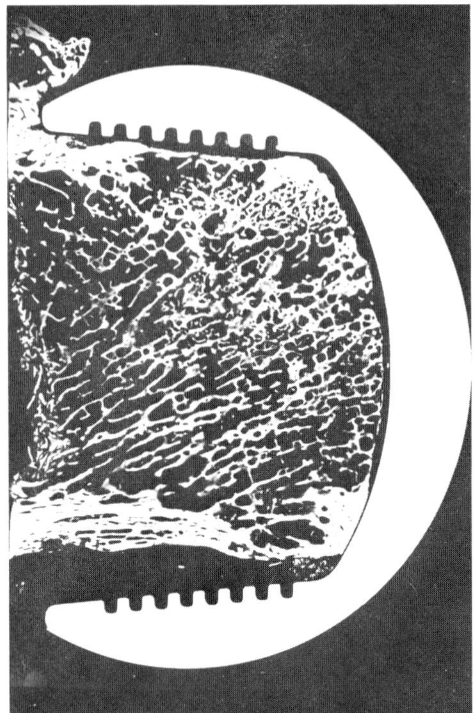

Fig. 5: Radiomicrograph (2.5x) of a frontal ground section through the loose ceramic-cup prosthesis and the femoral neck, resected at reoperation (20 months after implantation). The original trabecular pattern of the femoral neck is still visible, but a densening of bone can be seen in the cranial region. No bone ingrowth into the grooves of the ceramic cup.

Biomaterials 1980
Edited by G. D. Winter, D. F. Gibbons, and H. Plenk, Jr.
© 1982 John Wiley and Sons Ltd.

CEMENTLESS FIXATION OF THE ACETABULAR COMPONENT IN TOTAL HIP ARTHROPLASTY

E. Morscher, W. Dick and R. Bombelli

Orthopaedic University Clinic, Basle, Switzerland
Clinica Ortopedica, Busto Arsizio, Italy

SUMMARY

For a lasting cementless anchorage of an acetabular component it is required, that this component can be 'biomechanically incorporated' due to the absence of relative motion
between implant and bony pelvis, that the component is held
safely in place by proper fixing until the ingrowth of bone
is sufficient, and that no secondary loosening occurs.
In this aim 150 cementless fixed polyethylene sockets have
been implanted since 1976 in combination with conventional
cemented shaft prosthesis. Two deaths without relation to
the arthroplasty are reported. All other acetabular components have been performing successfully in patients for up
to 48 months with an average of 18 months. Up to now no
loosening has been observed.

INTRODUCTION

Aseptic mechanical loosening of the implant is by far the
most common cause for surgical revision after total hip arthroplasty. Although the annual number of primary operations
has not increased in Switzerland since 1973, secondary operations, necessary because of loosening, are increasing
from year to year.
Among the various factors known to cause loosening of the
prosthesis as technical errors, infection, microfractures
of the surrounding bone, stress protection, trauma, fractures of cement, excessive wear, biomechanical factors and
failures of the material, we have long been interested in
the difference between the mechanical behaviour of bone and
implant: As in fracture treatment, the use of a rigid implant in joint replacement surgery can result in stress-
protection of bone which leads to a local osteoporosis and
favour loosening of the prosthesis. Conditions are particularly unfavorable if movement occurs at the boundary bet-

ween bone and implant because the latter does not follow
the elastic deformation of the bone.
The boundary between the implant and bone is therefore a
weak point in the biological-implant combination. For this
reason, numerous attempts to improve the bone cement and
cementing methods have been reported (Oest et al, 1975;
Willert and Semlitsch, 1976; Huggler and Schreiber, 1978).
Our work has led us in another direction, namely the implantation of a so-called 'iso-elastic' prosthesis, i.e. a
prosthesis with same elastic properties as bone. It is
clear that perfect 'isoelasticity' is difficult to achieve
with a foreign material. Bone is anisotropic because of its
trabecular and lamellar structure whereas many foreign materials exhibit isotropic properties. In addition, bone
continually alters its structure and rigidity depending on
the mechanical situation. Moreover marked differences in
mechanical behaviour of bone occur with ageing and among
different individuals. Although anisotropic structure, remodeling and a mechanical behaviour specific to the individual can never be achieved (Morscher, 1979), we can at
least attempt to approach the optimum by choice of a suitable material, a suitable geometric structure and a proper
fixation of the implant. This should allow permanent incorporation of the implant into the bone without relative movement. Provided that there is a perfect fit between prosthesis and the surgically prepared site the use of bone cement, with its disadvantages as toxicity of the monomers,
heat, changes of volume, ageing, rigidity, allergy, would
no longer be necessary.

If we aim at permanent anchorage of the implant without
the use of a rigid cement, the following 5 conditions must
be fulfilled:
1. The artificial acetabulum must possess mechanical properties comparable to those of bone and in a suitable form so
that it can be biomechanically incorporated into the latter,
i.e. it should be 'isoelastic'.
2. It must be made of a material that is well tolerated by
tissue and thus allows close contact with the bone, that is
to say it should be 'osteocompatible'.
3. It must be sufficiently firmly anchored mechanically until it is incorporated into the bone.
4. There must be no secondary loosening after primary incorporation caused by intrusion of products of abrasion
between socket and bone, shearing forces or relative motion.
5. There must be a second line of defense which is as good
as the primary installation of a conventional acetabular
component.

DESIGN AND RESULTS

In 1973, we used an artificial acetabulum manufactured
from polyacetal resin (Morscher and Mathys, 1976). During
testing in vitro, the elastic values were similar to those
of bone and the gliding properties satisfactory. In vivo,
however, there was unexpectedly marked abrasive wear which
eliminated this material for use as a sliding surface and
thus for acetabular reconstruction.
In 1976, we introduced the high density polyethylene acetabular component to be fixed without cement. It is true
that this material has a lower modulus of elasticity than
polyacetal resin and bone, but, when used as an artificial
acetabulum, it becomes surrounded on all sides by bone and
is only under compressive stress. We are convinced that it
follows the deformation of the bony pelvis and loading so
that there is no motion at the bony interface and the cup
can be incorporated into the bone. Experimental work on
proving it is going on.

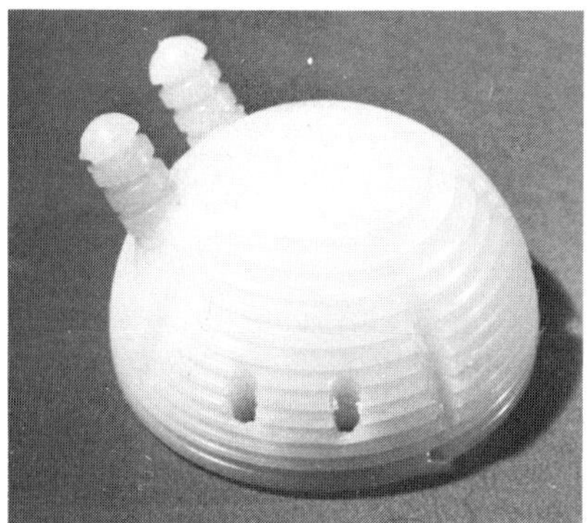

Fig. 1. Polyethylene socket for cementless
fixation in total hip arthroplasty.

Before implantation, the cartilage of the acetabulum is
removed and shaved off with the hemispherical rasp until
disseminated blood points appear in the cortex. The sclerotic layer should not be reamed away up to the free cancellous bone, it must remain intact to absorb pressure.
The exact fitting is facilitated since cup sizes in 2 mm
intervals are available. The implant has 2 studs cranially
to fit into corresponding holes in the acetabular roof
which are bored with a special centering device. This anchorage protects the artificial acetabulum from the action
of rotatory forces. In addition, holes for fixation screws

are present in the rim of the artificial acetabulum. It is,
however, primarily the tonicity of the hip muscles which
holds the acetabular component in place so that recently
we have taken to omitting the screws.

Immediately following correct reconstruction, the greater
part of the surface of the polyethylene cup is in direct
contact with the bone. As there is no mechanical motion,
the bone can grow into the grooves of the artificial acetabulum. In the first models from 1976 which had broader
grooves than today's version, the bone ingrowth is visible
radiologically:

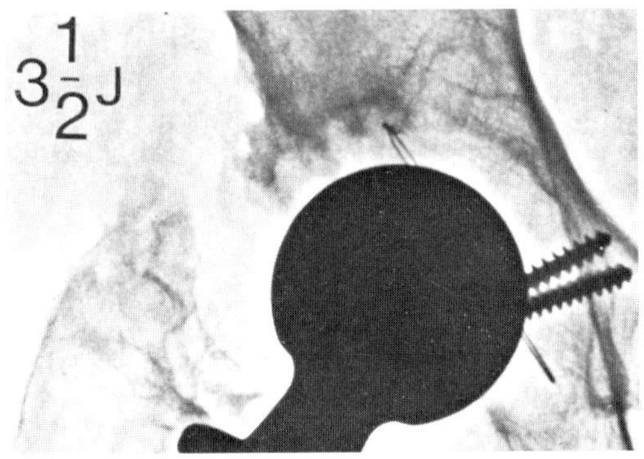

Fig. 2. Stable fixation of the socket by ingrowth
of bone in the grooves 42 months after operation.

We have only one histological sample: An 83 year old female
patient died 3 weeks after the operation of a ruptured
aortic aneurysm. At this time connective tissue filled the
grooves of the acetabular component.
It is noticeable that the formation of a radiolucent line
around the socket, to which we are accustomed with cement,
has not been observed in a single case. Sequential X-rays
show that the firm primary incorporation is stable and no
secondary loosening has occured up to the present time.
(Fig. 3).

Since 1976 we have implanted 150 polyethylene acetabular
components without cement in combination with the conventional cemented shaft prosthesis. These acetabular components have been performing successfully in patients for up
to 48 months, with an average of 18 months. Apart from the

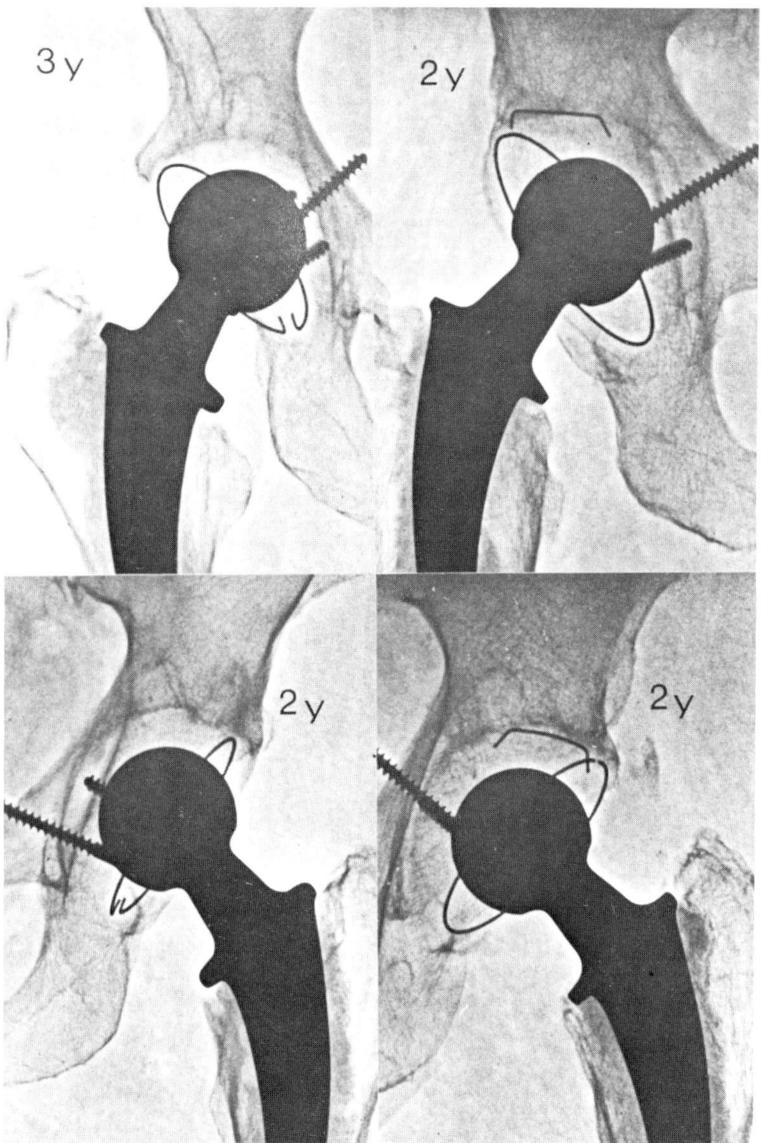

Fig. 3. Some examples of cementless fixed polyethylene sockets (today's model with small grooves).

case mentioned, one other patient died 1 year postoperatively. All the remaining patients have received continual
follow up. In one recent case we found early infection of
the stem with osteolysis. On surgical revision the stem
had to be changed but the socket was perfectly stable and
could be left in place. All patients are free of complaints
and all hips can fully be loaded. No other patient has been
reoperated and no radiological signs of loosening have been
observed in any patient.

In any kind of operation it is important to have a second
line of defense. This is particularly favorable for the
polyethylene acetabular component fixed without cement:
At reoperation for loosening, the situation of the acetabulum would hardly differ from that found at a primary operation, as practically no bone has been resected. Any normal artificial socket should be easy to fix with cement.
If the necessity occurs to remove a socket which is not
loose, the polyethylene socket can easily be cut and removed without damage to the bone. This is not possible with
metal or ceramic sockets.

The clinical results of 'isoelastic' cups implanted without
cement are so far good, however the maximum duration of implantation is only 4 years and no long term results are
available. The substantiation of the 'isoelastic' concept
will only be apparent in 10 years. We consider, however,
that the method is promising and propose to continue it
with caution.

REFERENCES

Huggler, A.H. & Schreiber, A. (1978) Alloarthroplastik des
Hüftgelenkes. Thieme, Stuttgart.
Morscher, E. & Mathys, R. (1976) First experiences with a
cementless isoelastic total prosthesis of the hip, in Total
hip prosthesis (Eds., Gschwend & Debrunner), pp. 289-297.
Huber, Bern Stuttgart Vienna.
Morscher, E. (1979) Isoelastische Prothesen. Langenbecks
Archiv für Chirurgie, 349, 321-326.
Oest, O., Müller, K. & Hupfauer, W. (1975) Die Knochenze-
mente. Enke, Stuttgart.
Willert, H.-G. & Semlitsch, M. (1976) Problems associated
with the cement anchorage of artificial joints, in Enginee-
ring in Medicine, 2, Advances in Artificial Hip and Knee
Joint Technology (Eds., Schaldach & Hohmann), pp. 325-346.
Springer, Berlin Heidelberg New York.

Biomaterials 1980
Edited by G. D. Winter, D. F. Gibbons, and H. Plenk, Jr.
© 1982 John Wiley and Sons Ltd.

POROUS POLYSULFONE COATED FEMORAL PROSTHESES
IN DOGS

M. Spector, J.T. Eldridge, S.L. Harmon and
A. Kreutner

Medical University of South Carolina
Charleston, South Carolina, U.S.A.

SUMMARY

Porous polysulfone coated cobalt-chromium femoral prostheses were implanted in dogs in order to investigate the cement-free fixation
achieved by bone ingrowth. Fourteen coated prostheses were evaluated
clinically and histologically for periods up to 3 years. Characteristic radiographic and scintigraphic features were demonstrated. Bone
ingrowth was found to some degree in all but 2 of the coated prostheses. One of these two prostheses was recovered 4 days after implantation and the second was loose after insertion due to overreaming.

INTRODUCTION

Recent studies demonstrate that porous coatings affixed to the intramedullary stems of femoral prostheses may be suitable for cement-free
fixation. The bone growth into the porous coating produces an interlocking bone with the surrounding bone which serves to anchor the
prosthesis in the femoral shaft. Previous investigations of several
different porous materials have shown that the shear strength of the
porous material-bone interface developed in minimally loaded intramedullary implants is more than adequate to support load-bearing prostheses (Galante et al., 1971; Corn et al., 1978; Spector et al., 1978).
Studies of canine femoral prostheses with porous metallic coatings
(Lembert et al., 1972) have demonstrated that bone can form and be
maintained in the porous coating of functioning, load-bearing prostheses.

The objective of this study was to evaluate the tissue response to
porous polysulfone (Spector et al., 1978) coated femoral prostheses
in dogs.

MATERIALS AND METHODS

Porous polysulfone (medical grade) coatings approximately 1mm thick
were fabricated by sintering particles of the material (Fig. 1).
Fourteen porous polysulfone coated cobalt-chromium canine femoral
prostheses were implanted in 12 dogs weighing from 25-40kg. Ten pros-

theses had porous coatings with an average pore size of about 125μm
and four had a 250μm pore size; all the coatings were approximately
33% porous. The coated prostheses were implanted with an interference fit in cavities prepared in the medullary canal. Ten dogs
received polyethylene acetabular cups implanted with bone cement.
Clinical evaluation included radiography and radionuclide bone
imaging. Bone images were made 2 hours after intravenous injection
of 8 mCi of Tc^{99m} methylene diphosphonate (MDP). Sacrifice times for
11 prostheses ranged from four days to over 1 year postoperatively.
Tissue specimens were allocated for conventional paraffin processing
and for embedment in plastic in preparation for microradiography,
ground section histology and electron microscopy.

<u>RESULTS</u>

Of the fourteen hip arthroplasties two were infected and four dis-
located. These complications came early in the study. Three of the
four dislocations were successfully reduced. Three prostheses still
functioning range in time from 1 1/2 to 3 years. One prosthesis
which was not placed with an interference fit due to overreaming was
found to be loose at postmortem examination.

Radiographic changes included 1) a transient periosteal reaction
along the femoral shaft surrounding the prosthetic stem from 2-8
weeks postoperatively, 2) a radiodense line at the porous poly-
sulfone-bone interface, 3) a radiodense zone distal to the tip of
the prosthesis, and 4) a radiolucent seam at the bone cement-bone
interface of the polyethylene acetabular cups (Fig. 2). The
prominence and time course of these radiographic features varied.
The loose prosthesis displayed radiographic evidence of periosteal
reaction and a radiodense zone distal to the tip of the stem.
However, no radiodense line was seen along the porous polysulfone-
bone interface of this implant.

Scintigraphic investigations were conducted to augment the radiographic evaluations by detecting areas of bone turnover. Bone
images recorded 2 hours after radionuclide injection revealed
differences in the pattern of uptake in operated and unoperated
limbs. Unoperated limbs typically displayed increased radionuclide
uptake in the femoral condyles and slight labeling in the femoral
head and trochanter regions. The operated limbs generally displayed
high uptake at the distal tip of the prosthesis and along the
femoral shaft surrounding the implant (Fig. 3). In order to obtain
a quantitative measure of the change in uptake with implantation
time the bone/soft tissue ratios at selected regions of interest
were computed. The uptake in comparable regions of the operated
femurs was divided by the uptake in the soft tissue adjacent to the
femur. One week after surgery significant activity (as indicated
by the bone/soft tissue ratio) could be seen in the operated femurs.

The uptake increased to a maximum intensity after about 4 weeks and
then decreased to a stable level after about 2 months postoperatively. Corresponding radiographs generally revealed
extensive periosteal reaction at the postoperative time periods just
after the bone images revealed maximal uptake. However, in a few
cases increased radionuclide uptake along the prosthesis could not
be correlated with periosteal reaction. In these cases scintigraphy
may be detecting bone ingrowth into the porous coating. In some
longer term implants radiographs revealed radiodense areas which,
on radionuclide imaging, showed little uptake suggesting that these
were areas of stable osseous structure.

Histological evaluation revealed bone ingrowth into the coatings of
all the prostheses except the one that was sacrificed 4 days postoperatively and the prosthesis that was loose at the time of
implantation. The relative amounts of osseous tissue, marrow, and
fibrous tissue in the pores of the prostheses varied. Six implants
in the time period of 2-5 months had bone and marrow in approximately
20-30% of the coating. Of three prostheses recovered after about
one year, 2 had bone in 60-70% of the coating and one implant had
osseous tissue (and marrow) in approximately 90% of the porosity
(Fig. 4). The balance of the porosity of these implants contained
fibrocollagenous material which varied from a loose, well
vascularized substance to dense scar-like material. No leukocytic
infiltrate and few to moderate numbers of foreign body giant cells
were found. No difference was noted in the tissue response to
prostheses having the 125 and 250µm pore size coatings.

Transmission electron microscopy of selected specimens occasionally
revealed an amorphous, granular substance on the surface of the
polysulfone particles. This substance appeared to be related to
cellular breakdown in the area and could be cellular debris (Fig. 5).
Fibrous tissue with normal ultrastructural appearance was adjacent
to these areas of cellular degeneration.

DISCUSSION

The present results evidence the bone ingrowth into functioning,
load-bearing porous polysulfone coatings on canine femoral
prostheses, and support the hypothesis that cement-free fixation can
be achieved by a bone ingrowth attachment vehicle.

Radionuclide bone imaging appears to be of greatest value when used
in conjunction with radiography to determine if radiodense features
represent stable osseous structures or areas of active bone turnover.
This can be of particular value in assessing the status of porous
coated prostheses since radiographic changes seen around loosened
cemented prostheses may have a different meaning when seen adjacent
to prostheses fixed by bone ingrowth.

The cause or importance of the layer of cellular debris occasionally
seen on the plastic particles within the porosity by the transmission
electron microscope is not yet clear. This feature may be an
artifact of tissue preparation or reflect deficiencies in the micro-
environment within internal pores for supporting cell viability.

ACKNOWLEDGEMENTS

The technical assistance of J.C. Lilga and W.B. Wigger is gratefully
acknowledged. The assistance of N.J. Ballintyn of Union Carbide
Corporation in fabricating the porous coatings is greatly appreciated.

REFERENCES

Corn, R., Berry, J., Black, J. and Greenwald, A. (1978) Mechanical
and microangiographic analysis of porous implant system. Trans. 4th
Ann. Mtg. of the Soc. for Biomat'l., San Antonio, Texas, p. 91.
Galante, J., Rostoker, W., Leuck, R. and Ray, R. (1971) Sintered
fiber metal composites as a basis for attachment of implants to bone.
J. Bone Jt. Surg., 53A, 101.
Lembert, E., Galante, J. and Rostoker, W. (1972) Fixation of skeletal
replacement by fiber metal composites. Clin. Orthop., 87, 303.
Spector, M., Michno, M., Smarook, W. and Kwiatkowski, G., (1978)
A high-modulus polymer for porous orthopedic implants: Biomechanical
compatibility of porous implants. J. Biomed. Mater. Res., 12, 665.

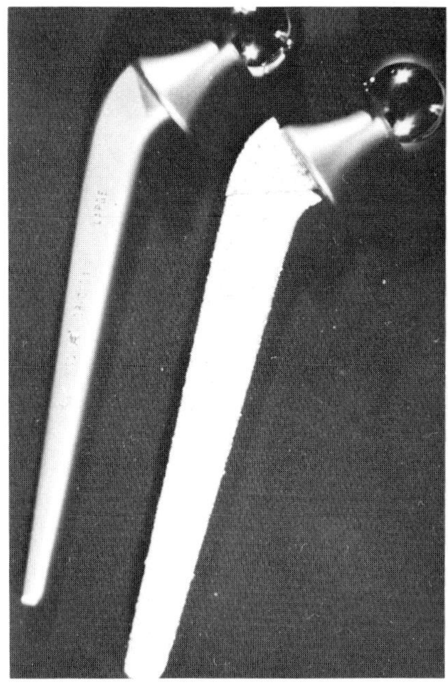

Fig. 1. Uncoated and coated
canine femoral prostheses.

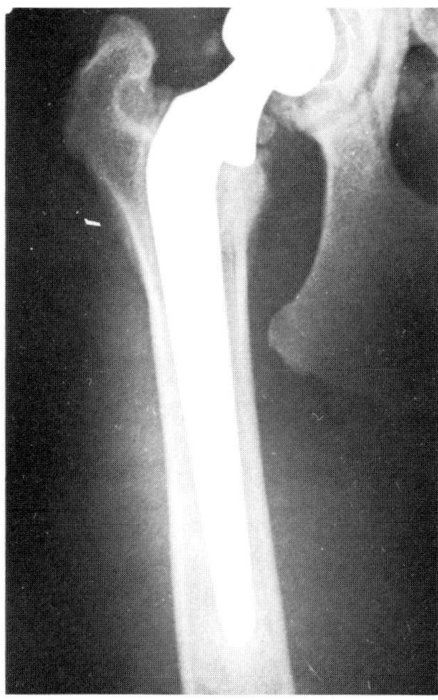

Fig. 2. Radiograph 1 year postoperatively showing radiodense zone distal
to tip of stem

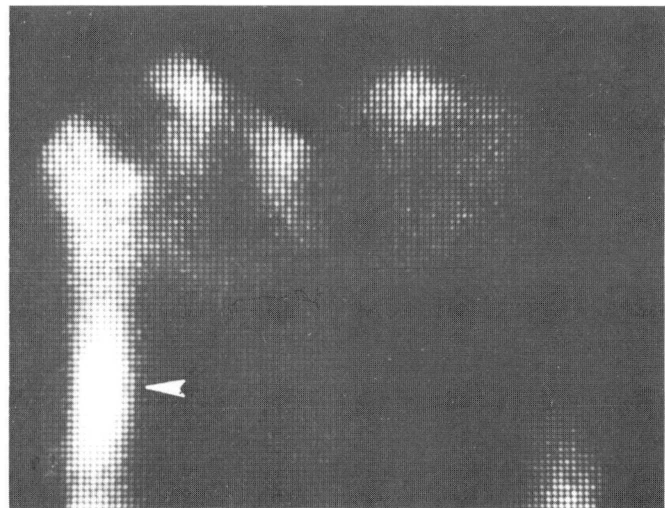

Fig. 3. Radionuclide bone image of operated (left) and unoperated (right) limbs in anteroposterior view. Arrow points
out uptake at distal tip of prosthesis.

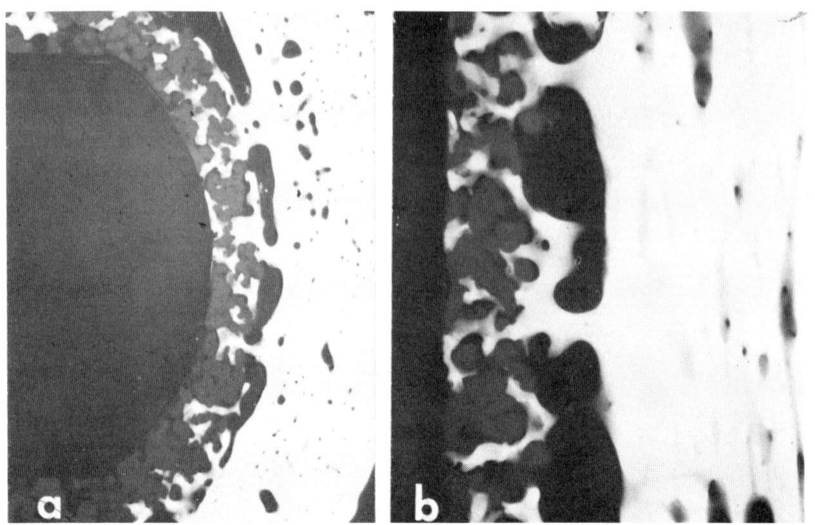

Fig. 4. Microradiographs of a) cross-section and b) longitudinal sections through a coating 1 year after implantation.

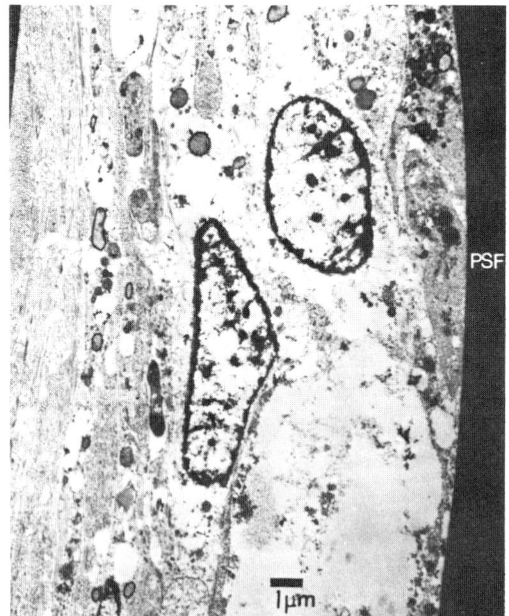

Fig. 5. Transmission electron micrograph of
cell debris on the surface of a polysulfone
particle in a coating 22 weeks after
implantation.

Biomaterials 1980
Edited by G. D. Winter, D. F. Gibbons, and H. Plenk, Jr.
© 1982 John Wiley and Sons Ltd.

EXPERIMENTAL STUDIES ON TOTAL KNEE AND HIP JOINT ENDOPROSTHESES MADE OF TANTALUM

G. Pflüger,[1] H. Plenk Jr.,[2] N. Böhler,[1,4]
F. Grundschober[2] and S. Schider[3]

1) Orthopaedic University Clinic
2) Bone Research Laboratory, Histological & Embryological Institute of the University of Vienna
3) Metallwerke Plansee A.G., Reutte
4) AUVA Research Institute for Traumatology, Vienna, Austria

SUMMARY

A cementless attachment for the intramedullary stems of artificial joint replacements was tested in two series of experiments using the highly biocompatible metal tantalum as a prosthetic material.

In the first series, the knee-joints of 20 rabbits were replaced by a hinged prosthesis, the femoral and tibial components of which were designed as tantalum stems adapted to the size and shape of the medullary cavities and coated with an open porous layer of tantalum. Great difficulties were encountered with incongruities of the stem dimensions, with the mechanical stability of the coating, and the postoperative fixation of the operated extremity. Due to primary instability of one or both components and post-operative infection, more than 60% of the prostheses were lost. In stable implants, tight bone-tantalum contact and attachment by bone ingrowth into the pores were demonstrated histologically. This process started 2 weeks after implantation and lasted at least another 8 weeks. After 11 and 12 months, however, after which 2 of the animals were more or less fully utilizing their operated extremities, the prostheses became loose and no bony anchorage could be found.

In the second series, total hip-joint endoprostheses for beagle dogs were developed using a grooved tantalum femoral stem for cementless implantation, a replaceable tantalum ball head and a cemented polyethylene socket. No postoperative fixation of the operated extremity was provided. So far, in 22 dogs only one case of loosening has occurred due to an incongruent stem size. There has been one case of luxation and one of the loosening of the ball head; both could be corrected operatively. Histologically, anchorage by intra-medullary bone formation was found after 6 weeks, leading to an abutment of the stem after 3 months. At 5 months the stem was nearly totally enveloped by new bone which showed tight contact with the implant surface, especially in the grooves of the surface. At 6 months after implantation there was no mechanical failure of the stems and no clinical or radiological signs of loosening were observed.

Whereas in the first series the experimental model proved unsuitable, the second series has so far shown very encouraging results. It has yet to be seen whether tantalum will withstand the heavy loads imposed on implants in humans, but its excellent biocompatility and corrosion resistance make it a very promising material for implants attached by mechanical interlocking with the skeletal tissue.

INTRODUCTION

In view of the problems involved in the implantation of artificial joints using bone cement, attempts have been made to obtain a durable anchorage at least for younger patients using the body's own tissue. One possibility is the mechanical interlocking of the bone with the enlarged surface of the implant. Metals and alloys particularly well suited for heavy load-bearing endoprostheses must exhibit not only the necessary mechanical strength, but must also be sufficiently biocompatible and corrosion resistant.
Tantalum exhibits good biocompatibiliy, ductility and workability, and has been used successfully in many areas of surgery (e.g., Hempel & Knothe 1977, Meyer et al., 1977). Thanks to its excellent resistance to corrosion, it has also been used for pacemaker electrodes (Johnson et al., 1977). However, as far as we know, tantalum has not so far been used for the manufacture of artificial joints because of its low mechanical strength. Nevertheless, its mechanical properties can be improved by suitable treatment (Schider & Bildstein, in these Proceedings), and previous experiments have shown that porous and grooved tantalum implants can be securely anchored in the bones of rabbits under so-called unloaded conditions (Pflüger et al., in these Proceedings). In this paper we report on our experiments with two artificial joints made from tantalum which were implanted in animals. The first was a hinged knee-joint with a porous coated, drop forged shaft which we implanted in rabbits, whilst the second was a total hip-joint prosthesis with a grooved stem which we implanted in dogs.

MATERIALS AND METHODS

Endoprostheses: The endoprostheses were manufactured from an extremely pure (capacitor grade) tantalum powder (Norton Comp., Newton, Mass., USA). The dense material for the intramedullary stems of the hinged knee-joint endoprostheses (Fig. 1a) and the hip-joint replacements (Fig. 1b) was pressed and sintered (for technical details see Schider & Bildstein in these Proceedings) and then cold forged and drop forged to form the different shapes of Xanthopren® moulds of each of the medullary cavities.
The porous coating of the knee-joint stems was created by pressing and sintering tantalum powder onto the stems (for technical details see Schider & Bildstein in these Proceedings). This resulted in an open porosity of 30 - 40% with pore sizes between 100 and 300 μm (mean 190 μm). The hinge pin was also made of tantalum and was screwed in place.
The femoral stems of the hip-joint endoprostheses received conical surface grooves (Ø 900 μm) by cold working, and some of the stems were sand blasted to obtain a micro-roughness. The ball heads were made of the same dense tantalum material and provided with different neck lengths and a self-locking cone or screw for fixation to the stem. The moving surface was polished and electrically oxidized. This femoral component was combined with a polyethylene socket for implantation with bone cement (Fig. 1b).

                163

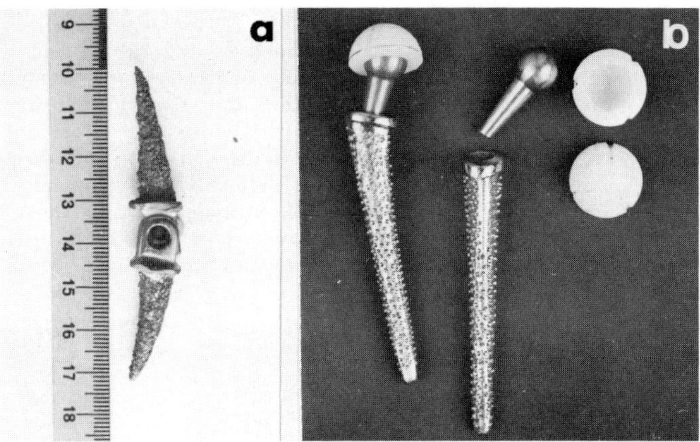

Figure 1: a) Porous coated, hinged tantalum knee-joint endoprosthesis for a rabbit. b) Total hip-joint endoprosthesis for a
beagle dog, consisting of grooved tantalum stems and ball heads
and polyethylene sockets.

<u>Experimental animals:</u> 20 chinchilla rabbits of either sex (Versuchstier-
zuchtanstalt WIGA, Sulzfeld, FRG) with a mean age of 1.5 years and a body
weight of 3.5 to 5 kg were used for the knee-joint experiments. In the hip-joint
experiments we employed 22 beagle dogs of either sex (Immuno AG., Vienna,
Austria) 1 to 1.5 years old and with a body weight of between 14 and 20 kg.

<u>Operative procedures and animal keeping:</u> Under general anaesthesia and
sterile conditions, the prostheses were implanted in the left knee-joints of the
rabbits and the left hip-joints of the dogs. The artificial joints were implanted
using the same surgical techniques as are used for human patients.
After implantation, the knee-joints of the rabbits were immobilised for
6 weeks using a pelvico-femoro-tibial plaster cast or an external fixation with
Kirschner wires. The rabbits were kept in solitary cages during the period of
observation. The dogs, on the other hand, were allowed to load their operated
extremities immediately and were transferred to an outer courtyard after
2 weeks.
X-ray controls and mobility checks of the operated extremities were carried
out monthly or when the sequential fluorochrome labelling was done (in the
case of the rabbits after 2 and 6 weeks and 1 week before sacrifice; in the
case of the dogs after 6 weeks, 6 months and 1 week before sacrifice).

<u>Histological examination:</u> After sacrifice, the joint regions were dissected, the
implants were removed together with surrounding tissue and embedded in
methylmethacrylate. Longitudinal and cross ground sections were prepared and
investigated microscopically using fluorescence and polarized-light microscopy
and radiomicrographs. The newly formed capsule of the joints was also
examined light- and electronmicroscopically.

RESULTS

Knee-joint experiment: Due to the brittle bone of the rabbit and to incongruities of the stem size with the medullary cavities, during implantation fracture of the femur and/or tibia occurred in 8 animals, and a stable implant was not achieved in 5 animals. Great difficulties were also experienced with postoperative fixation due to bone fractures at the drill holes and breakage or removal of the plaster casts by the animals themselves. Suppurative inflammation of the operated joint occurred in 14 animals. Due to these complications, loosening of at least one of the components was observed in 16 of the 20 rabbits, and most of the animals died or had to be sacrificed before the end of the scheduled observation periods.

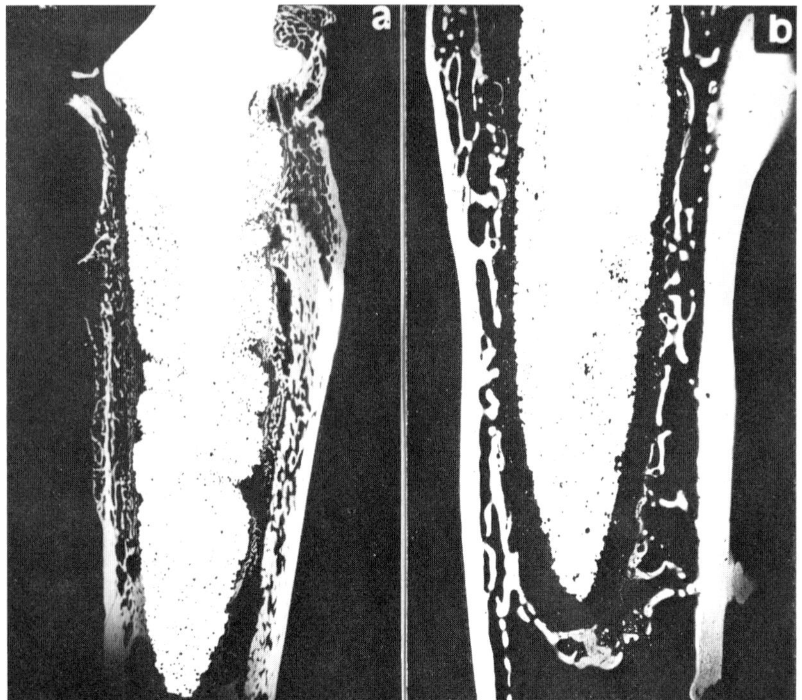

Figure 2: Radiomicrographs of longitudinal ground sections of the tibial components of porous coated, hinged tantalum knee-joint endoprostheses in rabbits.
a) Stable component, 8 weeks after implantation (magn. 3 x). The fractured tibia has healed and anchored the implant. Note the "spongification" of the cortex.
b) Loosened component, 12 months after implantation (magn. 5 x). Intramedullary bone formation has walled off, but not anchored the implant (the empty space contained a layer of fibrous connective tissue).

The first intramedullary bone reaction was observed in one animal after 2 weeks, when new bone trabeculae had reached the implant and were growing into the pores. In spite of inflammation, the tibial component was stable in one animal after 5 weeks and in another after 6 weeks, and new bone formation had enveloped and infiltrated the implants. Stable anchorage of the tibial component and tight bone contact at the collar were evident in a radiomicrograph of a longitudinal section taken after 8 weeks (Fig. 2a).
Stable attachment of both components was achieved in only two animals, after 7 and 10 weeks respectively, and this was confirmed microscopically. No postoperative complications occurred in two animals, which showed excellent mobility after removal of their plaster casts and were kept until 11 and 12 months after implantation. At sacrifice, the mobility of the operated joints was more or less restricted by contracture of the capsules and exostoses, the implants were all loosened, and there was no microscopic evidence of bony anchorage (Fig. 2b). In these cases, and also after shorter observation periods, particles of tantalum originating from wear of the hinge or the porous coating - which had come loose in some areas - were found in the connective tissue sheath and in macrophages surrounding the implants.

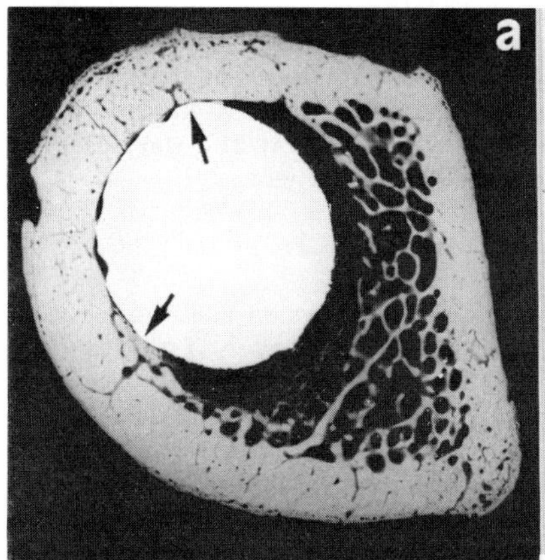
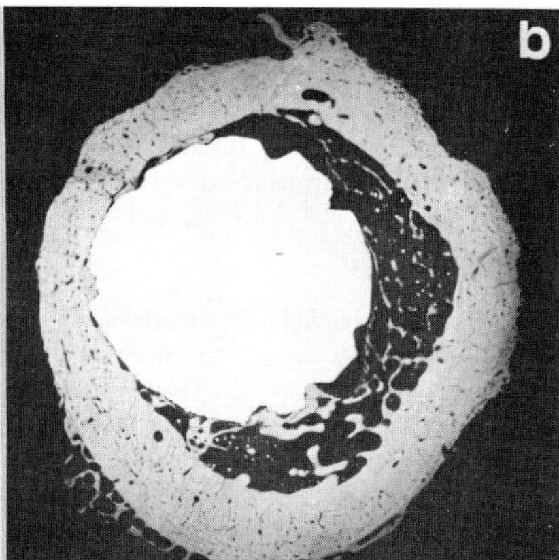
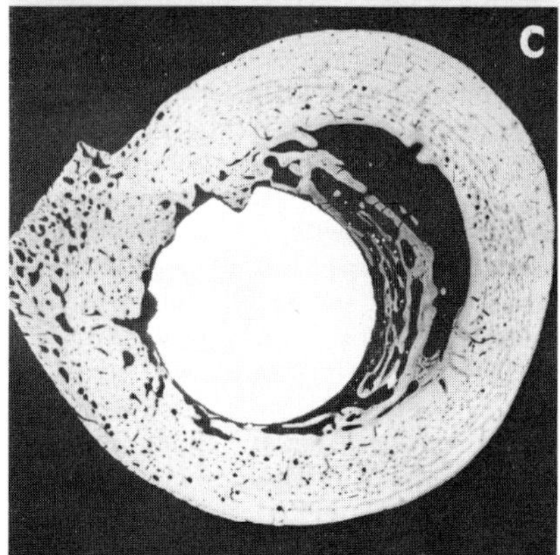

Figure 3: Radiomicrographs (magn. 8 x) of ground cross-sections of the grooved tantalum stems of hip-joint endoprostheses in the femoral diaphyses of beagle dogs.
a) 6 weeks after implantation: anchorage of the stem within the cortex is just beginning (arrows).
b) 3 months after implantation: anchorage of the stem in the cortex and by intramedullary bone formation.
c) 5 months after implantation: the stem is now enveloped by newly formed bone which shows tight contact with the surface.

<u>Hip-joint experiment</u>: So far there has only been one case of an endoprosthesis working loose in a dog. This was because the stem was too small for the dog. In one case, the ball head came loose and there was one case of luxation. The last two complications were eliminated operatively. Radiologically we have so far observed close contact of the stem in the area of the medial corticalis of the femur and the formation of a bony abutment at the tip of the stem. The prostheses did not subside into the medullary canal. 3 dogs have so far been subjected to histological examination. After 6 weeks there was evidence of intramedullary bone formation which, however, had only reached the implant in contact zones with the corticalis (Fig. 3a). The formation of an abutment at the tip of the stem was already clearly visible. After 3 months the formation of new bone was already in contact with the implant in several places (Fig. 3b), and the implant appeared to be well supported proximally. 5 months after implantation the entire stem was enveloped by newly formed osseous tissue (Fig. 3c) which was in close contact with the surface of the metal, particularly in the grooves. The medullary canal beneath the tip of the prosthesis was closed off by trabeculae which supported the tip.

Up until 6 months after implantation, all the animals exhibited good mobility clinically and there was no sign of any of the prostheses working loose. After an even longer period of observation we noticed an increase in the rate of wear of the tantalum in the artificial joint: this was evident macroscopically in the form of a black colouration of the surrounding connective tissue. Using both light and electron microscopy, we found evidence that the particles of tantalum were accumulating without reaction in macrophages.

DISCUSSION

The high failure rate in the knee-joint experiment was due on the one hand to infection caused by decubital ulcera in the thin soft tissue cover of the joint in the plaster cast or through the drill holes of the exteral fixation. On the other hand, the experimental animals varied too much in size, so that prostheses of the same size resulted either in the fracture of the diaphysis or in primary instability. It is certainly due to the material used that individual components were anchored in the bone in spite of infection. This anchorage appears to have withstood the load after confinement of the animals until at least 10 weeks after implantation. However, even with rabbits, the hinged knee-joint is not a satisfactory solution if the movement of the animals is unrestricted. As Ducheyne et al. (1977) have already emphasised, the bony anchorage of conventional designs of endoprostheses cannot to be expected even when compatible materials of sufficient porosity are used, and such anchorage will not stand load-bearing over a long period of time. Although this experimental model failed to provide evidence of the suitability of tantalum, the results so far with the grooved stems of the hip-joint endoprostheses are very promising. The stable bony anchorage observed in the so-called unloaded implants was also evident in the dynamically loaded endoprostheses. The grooves in the surface of the tantalum are simpler to manufacture and mechanically stronger than producing pores by sintering, and provided adequate stable anchorage by the ingrowth of osseous tissue. The prosthesis also withstood the loads imposed on it by the dogs, but did not meet the requirements of a wear resistant joint. We had made allowance for this deficiency, which enabled us to demonstrate the favourable tissue reaction of the tantalum particles produced by wear of the joint. Long term observation of this experiment will show whether the bony anchorage will withstand continuous loading and thus whether tantalum endoprostheses can also be considered for humans if sufficient mechanical strength can be ensured by metallurgical processing.

ACKNOWLEDGEMENT

These studies were supported by the Austrian "Forschungsförderungsfonds der Gewerblichen Wirtschaft" Grant No. 3/1851-1/P and by Metallwerke Plansee AG, Reutte, Austria.

REFERENCES

Ducheyne, P., De Meester, P., Aernoudt, E., Martens, M. & Mulier, J.C. (1977) Influence of a functional dynamic loading on bone ingrowth into surface pores of orthopaedic implants. J. Biomed. Mater. Res., 11, 811-838.

Hempel, D. & Knothe, C. (1977) Die Nakayama-Technik zur Shuntbildung für die chronische Hämodialyse. Chirurg, 48 (11), 713-718.

Johnson, P.F., Bernstein, J.J., Hunter, G., Dawson, W.W. & Hench, L.L. (1977) In vitro and in vivo analysis of anodized tantalum capacitive electrodes: corrosion response, physiology and histology. J. Biomed. Mater. Res., 11, 637-656.

Meyer, C., Alexiou, D., Calderolo, H. & Hollender, L.F. (1977) Les matériaux de synthése dans la cure des grandes éventrations abdominales. Enseignements à propos de 78 observations. Ann. Chir., 31, 221-228.

Pflüger, G., Plenk, H. Jr., Böhler, N., Grundschober, F. & Schider, S. (in press) Bone reaction to porous and grooved stainless steel, tantalum and niobium implants. In Proceedings of the First World Biomaterials Congress, (Eds. G.D. Winter, D.F. Gibbons & H. Plenk Jr.). J. Wiley, Chichester.

Schider, S. & Bildstein, H. (in press) Tantalum and niobium as potential prosthetic materials. In Proceedings of the First World Biomaterials Congress, (Eds. G.D. Winter, D.F. Gibbons & H. Plenk Jr.). J. Wiley, Chichester.

Tribology and safety of joint replacements

Biomaterials 1980
Edited by G. D. Winter, D. F. Gibbons, and H. Plenk, Jr.
© 1982 John Wiley and Sons Ltd.

THE POSSIBILITIES OF THE DYNAMIC TESTING
OF KNEE-JOINT ENDOPROSTHESES

M. Ungethüm and H. Stallforth

AESCULAP-Werke AG, D-7200 Tuttlingen

SUMMARY

The tribological behaviour of knee joint endoprostheses depends on
various wear mechanisms and therefore it cannot be studied but by a
large number of systematic experiments. For this purpose we developed a knee joint simulator and a model testing machine, the results
of which are thought to enable us to find out some of the characteristics leading to different wear rates. We have used the simulator
to study joint stresses in relation to different designs of knee
joint endoprostheses.

INTRODUCTION

The average failure rate of knee endoprostheses is approximately 15 to
20 per cent and is mainly due to complications caused by the biomechanics of the joint. The principal reasons for failure are fracture of
the articulating surfaces, breakdown of the fixation cement, loosening,
instability and wear of the sliding materials. Knee prostheses are subject to particularly high stresses and this must be taken into account
in their design. Before clinical evaluation it is therefore necessary
to carry out tests which determine the mechanical properties of the
prosthetic joint and confirm its suitability for long-life alloarthro-
plasty. Apart from static and dynamic design stability tests, machines
which simulate the specific biomechanical functions of the implant are
also required to obtain comparative results with various prosthesis
designs and so develop criteria for improved designs.

                    M. Ungethüm and H. Stallforth

KNEE JOINT SIMULATOR DESIGN

A simulator has been developed in which the movements of the knee
joint while walking on level ground are optimally simulated and tests
the fatigue strength and wear characteristics of the prosthesis. The
main consideration is the relative movement of the tibia with respect
to the femur under conditions of physiological load (Fig. 1). The type

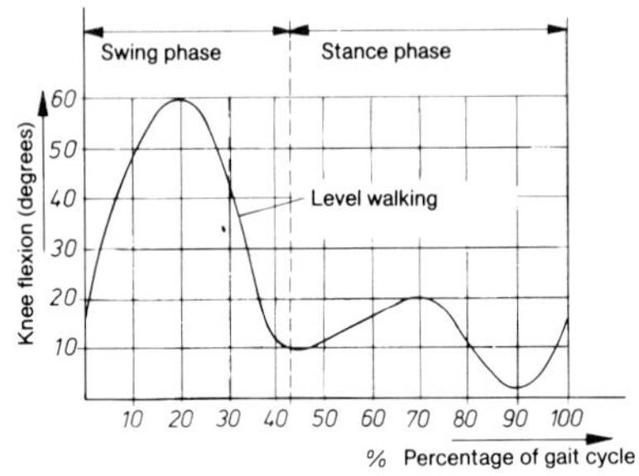

Fig.1: The relative bending movement of the tibia with respect to the femur

of motion depends on the design of the joint. In the natural knee joint
a rotation around the tibia axis is superimposed on the flexing action
in the sagittal plane. The factors responsible for the load are the
forces acting in the direction of the tibia axis (usually called the
normal force), the moment around the fronto-dorsal axis (M_x) and the
moment around the tibia axis (M_y) (Fig. 2). In the case of constrained
joints, i.e. hinge and ball prostheses, a bending moment takes place
around a fixed point of rotation. Unconstrained models, also known as
sliding prostheses, often have movements where the poles around which
the moment turns, form pole curves as in the case of the natural knee
joint. The normal walking cycle is characterised by two maxima in
flexion, the smaller of which is caused by the active absorption and
damping of the gravitational forces during the weight-bearing phase. In
addition, some designs of prosthesis provide for a physiological rotation around the tibial axis which is in the range of $\pm 6^0$. The normal
load on the joint is produced by the forces resulting from the ground-

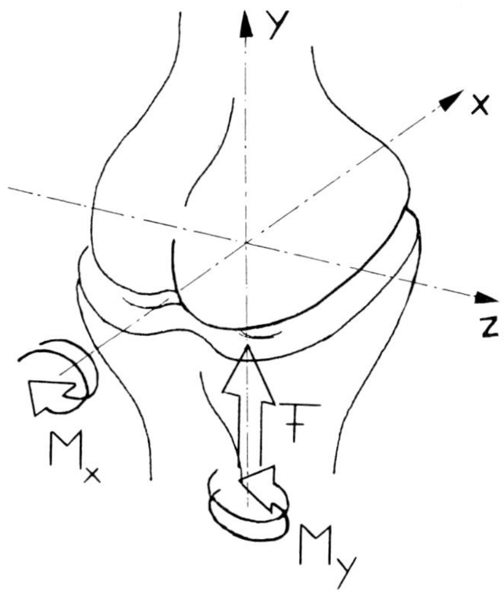

Fig. 2: The forces which have to be superimposed in order
to simulate the loading of the knee

foot contact, superimposed upon those of muscles and ligaments. This
load can only be calculated theoretically and as demonstrated in figure 3 considerable differences between the various measuring techniques are obtained, Seireg & Arvikar (1975); Morrison (1970). The curve

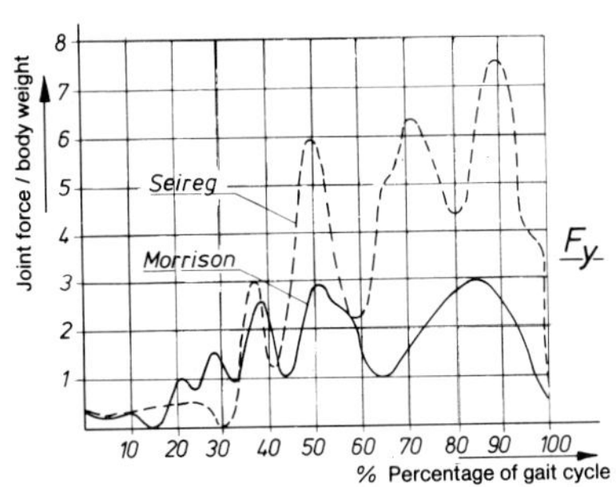

Fig. 3: The loading pattern of the knee joint found by
Morrison (1970) and Seireg (1975)

exhibits a number of maxima which may be explained by the activation
of the various muscule groups. In designing the test machine, we used
three times the body weight as the maximum normal force. One factor
which also is of major importance and influences the distribution of
load on the articulating surfaces is the moment around the fronto-
dorsal axis which lowers the force acting on the lateral parts of the
joint. The moment around the tibial axis is produced primarily as a
result of the contact between the foot and the ground. The knee-joint
simulator we have designed simulates the above functions of motion
and load as optimally as possible with relatively simple mechanical
system and at acceptable cost. Apart from minor deviations, the
bending angle is produced exactly as stated for the natural knee joint.
It should be remembered that the joint parameters of individuals may
vary greatly and that a number of factors, such as walking speed, will
influence the actual joint cycle. The load cycle had to be idealized
(Fig. 4) since such large force gradients could not be achieved and
would also have compromized the long-term behaviour of the machine;

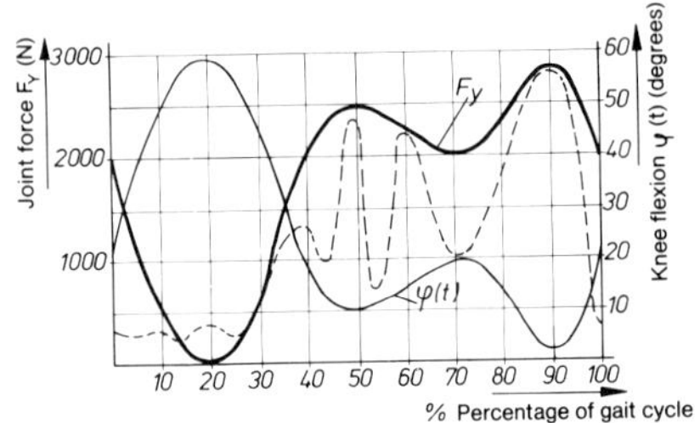

Fig. 4: The curves of knee flexion and axial loading realized
by the simulator

the same is true for the moments M_x and M_y, figure 2. The simulator is
designed such that all load functions are in inverse proportion to the
bending motion, (Fig. 4). Another criterion was that the machine would
test all known prosthesis models, with their various types of motion

and degrees of freedom. It is important therefore that no constraint
forces were produced which might lead to erroneous results. This requirement means that no additional centering devices are required to
place the prosthesis in the appropriate adapters. The test is carried
out in pseudo-synovial fluid whose temperature is kept constant at
37°C. The load reversal cycle is 0.85 Hz; this corresponds to a mean
walking speed of approximately 4.5 km per hour. On average, the number
of load cycles should be 1.5 to 2 x 10^6. In addition to the tribological behaviour of the prosthesis, the simulator may also be used to measure the strength of prosthesis fixation in the surrounding bone material when cement is used. For this purpose, the joint is inserted in
the usual way in a cadaver knee which later is then placed in modified
adapters. Our initial results on joint wear have shown that the simulator is capable of comparing individual prosthesis models; however, among
the prostheses now on the market there is so much variety in design regarding load transmission, active surface construction and fitting of
stabilizing elements that the simulator tests do not enable us to draw
any valid conclusions regarding the various factors which are responsible for wear. The main obstacle appears to be the variation in design
of the articulating surfaces; apart from different radii of curvature,
congruence of the femoral and tibial condyles also varies over a wide
range.

SPECIFIC DESIGN PARAMETER TESTING MACHINE

Because of the complications which accompany the knee simulator we have
developed a model test stand which enables us, on the basis of simple-
shaped test bodies, to assess how the tribological behaviour is affected
by different types of material combinations, varying congruence of the
sliding surfaces, varying sliding speeds and different contact pressures.
The test body which simulates the femoral condyle is a cylinder which is
moved, under load (Fig. 5), with respect to the tibia plateau (these also
have a constant radius of curvature). The most obvious material combinations to be tested are metal/polyethylene and ceramics/polyehtylene. The
sliding speed is varied in the experiment by using cylinders with diffe-

rent diameters, and the degree of congruence is adjusted by varying
the radius of curvature of the polyethylene plateaus. For each cylinder diameter, the ratio of the radii of curvature of the cylinder and

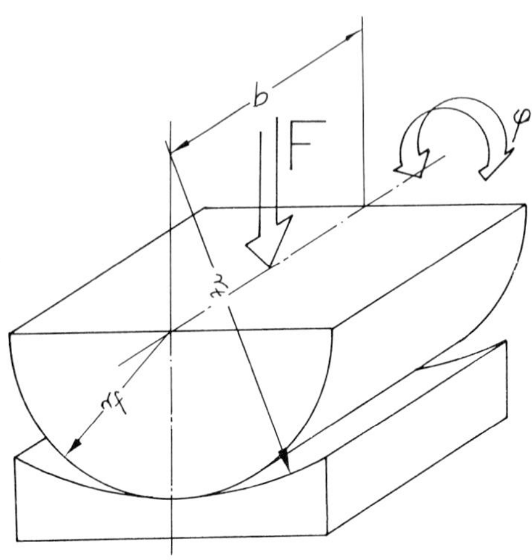

Fig. 5: The geometry of the test bodies

the plastic sliding surface is 1, 1.5, 2 and ∞. These values correspond to the ratios most frequently found knee-joint prostheses. The
value of the contact pressure is largely predetermined by the curvature
of the two sliding surfaces which are taken into account in calculating
Hertz's pressure, but may be modified by specifying a certain value for
the bearing surface. By placing a groove and ridge in the centre of the
samples, we obtain a geometry similar to that of the surfaces in the
knee joint. As a reference for measuring the specimens before and after
the test, comparative surfaces are fitted at one end of the plates. There
are two possibilities of subjecting the test bodies to loads. First, the
dynamic load can be synchronized with the cycle of movement so that it
reaches its maximum in the one reversal point of the movement while the
articular space is almost completely unloaded in the other (Fig. 6). In
this case, the load cycle is that of a sinoidal function. Second, the
oscillating motion of the cylinder can take place under static load. The
total rotation angle is 60° and a container with pseudo-synovial fluid at

37°C surrounds the specimens and the frequency is 2 Hz.

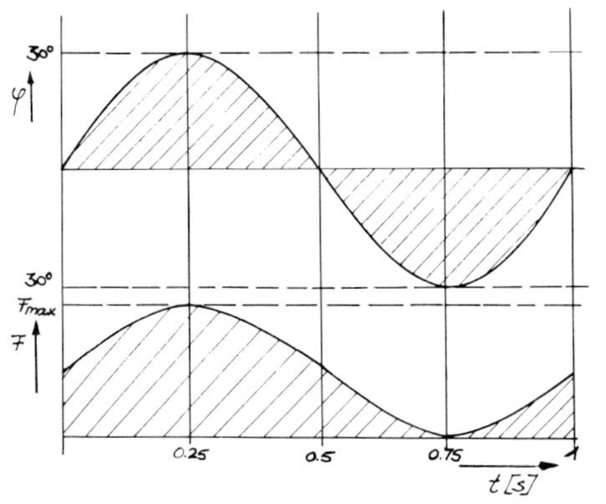

Fig. 6: The rotational movement and the load pattern
         realized by the model testing machine

This is a very complex problem and we believe that the combination of
model test stand and simulator constitutes the best way to compare
different designs of existing prostheses and also to develop the criteria necessary to optimize the tribological behaviour of knee-joint
prostheses.

REFERENCES

Morrison, J.B. (1970) The mechanics of the knee joint in relation to
normal walking. J. Biomechanics, 3, 51-61.
Nietert, M. (1977) Das Kniegelenk des Menschen als biomechanisches Problem. Biomedizinische Technik, 22, 13-21.
Seireg, A. & Arvikar R.J. (1975) The prediction of muscular load sharing
and joint forces in the lower extremities during walking. J. Biomechanics,8
89-102.
Stallforth, H. & Ungethüm M. (1977) Systematisierung künstlicher Kniege-
lenke unter Berücksichtigung von am natürlichen Kniegelenk abgeleiteten
konstruktiven Merkmalen. Arch. orthop. Unfall-Chir. 89, 227-237.
Ungethüm, M. (1978) Technologische und biomechanische Aspekte der Hüft-
und Kniealloarthroplastik, Aktuelle Probleme in Chirurgie und Orthopädie,
Band 9, Verlag Hans Huber, Bern.

Biomaterials 1980
Edited by G. D. Winter, D. F. Gibbons, and H. Plenk, Jr.
© 1982 John Wiley and Sons Ltd.

TRIBOLOGICAL PROPERTIES OF CARBON MATERIALS IN ARTIFICIAL JOINTS

K. J. Hüttinger*, H.-J. Mäurer

* Institut für Chemische Technik der Universität Karlsruhe,
7500 Karlsruhe, FRG
Schunk & Ebe GmbH, 6300 Gießen, FRG

SUMMARY

Two very hard, strong carbon materials were developed for the use as sliding components in artificial joints. The tribological properties of both materials, an isotropic carbon and a SiC/C-composite material, were examined using ring-on-disk- and ball-in-socket-arrangements. The all-carbon sliding combinations show lower wear rate and friction compared with clinically applied prostheses.

INTRODUCTION

Carbon shows excellent performance as a biomaterial (Weber, 1980). Pyrolytic carbons are clinically accepted in the USA and are used extensively in construction of cardiovascular prosthetic devices. Over 35000 artificial heart valves have been implanted since the introduction in 1969 (Bokros et al, 1977). It is also well known, that carbon is an excellent bearing material, especially under conditions of dry friction or in chemically aggressive media (Savage and Schäfer, 1956, Midgley and Teer, 1963, Bowden and Tabor, 1964). These properties suggest that carbon materials should perform well as the sliding components in artificial joints. None of the commercially available grades of carbon is acceptable for joint replacements, either because of insufficiency in strength or size.

The demands for the components of joint prostheses are quite severe (table 1). The hip joint experiences a maximum load of about four times of the body weight (Pauwels, 1973). The relative sliding speed of the surfaces is about 0,05 m/sec and is characterized by instantaneous changes in direction of motion. Under these conditions, the lubricating film may break down and direct contact between the two sliding surfaces may occur. To achieve a life time of 30 to 40 years, the wear rate must be less than 50 μm/year. Nevertheless, the coefficient of friction of the sliding surfaces should be below 0,1, because the friction of the head in the cup will lead to a torque, which is transmitted to the bone/implant interface.

177

TABLE 1. Requirements for the sliding components

load an the hip joint	~ 4-times body weight
low sliding speed	~ 0,05 m/sec
low wear rate	< 50 μm/year
low coefficient of friction	< 0,1

MATERIALS AND METHODS

Two very hard, strong carbon materials were developed (Brückmann, 1980). Fig. 1 shows an optical micrograph taken with reflected polarized light of one of these materials, a high strength isotropic carbon. It shows a finegrain polycrystalline material of high optical isotropy. This material is porous and available in dimensions required for joint replacements.

Fig. 2 shows an optical micrograph of an other carbon material, a SiC/C-composite. This material is manufactured by impregnating a graphite with liquid silicon at temperatures of about 2,000 $^{\circ}$C. Silicon was chosen due to its ability to form a chemically resistant, biocompatible and wear resistant carbide. The resulting composite material consists of two phases, 60 vol.-% SiC and 40 vol.-% graphite.

The wear behaviour of the materials was examined with a ring-on-disk-test (Fig. 3). The ring oscillates ± 30 degree around its axis on a stationary flat plate. The wear is measured by the depth of penetration of the ring into the disk. Fig. 3 shows the results for a SiC/C-ring on isotropic carbon. After a short running-in period, where the microroughness of the sliding surfaces is worn down, a low constant wear rate is found.

The wear rate of isotropic carbons shown in Fig. 3, strongly depends on the heat treatment temperature of the carbon. Fig. 4 shows, that the constant wear rate exhibits a minimum after a heat treatment at 1,100 $^{\circ}$C which coincides with a maximum hardness. As the treatment temperature is increased to 3,000 $^{\circ}$C, the wear rate increases by approximately 20 times. This correlates with the reduction of the hardness due to the graphitization of the carbon. On the other hand the coefficient of friction shows only a small decrease with increasing heat treatment temperature. At the minimum wear rate the coefficient of friction is approximately 0,05.

Fig. 5 shows the wear rate and coefficient of friction as a function of load for SiC/C - carbon and SiC/C - SiC/C pairs. The two upper curves show, that in the range 10 - 30 MN/m^2 the wear rates increase linearly, which indicates that there is no change in the mechanism of wear. The coefficient of friction exhibits the same behaviour as a function of load.

Both of these sliding combinations exhibit very low wear rates. Table 2 compares these results with wear rates obtained with Al_2O_3 on Al_2O_3. The data for alumina (Hinterberger and Ungethüm, 1978) were obtained using slightly different test conditions, therefore the data requires that the depth of penetration be first compared in terms of number of cycles and second the sliding distance. The carbon combination shows a lower wear rate when compared by either criteria.

TABLE 2. Comparison of wear rates in ring-on-disk-test of
isotropic C - SiC/C and Al_2O_3 - Al_2O_3
(Hinterberger and Ungethüm, 1978)

	Al_2O_3 - Al_2O_3	isotropic C - SiC/C
__test conditions__		
specific load	20 MN/m^2	20 MN/m^2
frequency/rotation	1 Hz/$\pm$ 25 ^{0}	2 Hz/$\pm$ 30 ^{0}
ring ϕ inner	14 mm	13 mm
ring ϕ outer	20 mm	19 mm
lubricant	Ringer's solution	Ringer's solution
distance/cycle	14,8 mm	16,7 mm
distance/test	6,4 x 10^3 m	12 x 10^3 m
test duration	120 h	87 h
__test results__		
depth of penetration per 10^7 cycles	6,2 /um	4,3 /um
depth of penetration per 100 km	4,2 /um	2,6 /um
coefficient of friction	0,3 - 0,2	0,06 - 0,05

In order to test the carbon materials under more practical conditions, experiments were carried out using the ball-in-socket-method. Fig. 6 shows the experimental arrangement used in these studies. The ball oscillates ± 30 degree round the vertical axis and the socket oscillates by the same angle round the horizontal axis.

Fig. 7 shows experimental results with a SiC/C-ball and an isotropic C-socket. After a short running-in-period a very low, constant wear rate is obtained. The wear of the socket and ball were nearly equivalent inspire of the difference in hardness. Almost identical results were obtained using a socket of SiC/C instead of isotropic carbon.

The wear of the carbon joints were compared analytically with those used clinically by using the relationship developed by HERTZ (Timoshenko, 1934) under an applied stress of 6,6 MN/m^2 or a load of 2,500 N. The Figures 8 and 9 show these comparisons as penetration depth of the ball into the socket as a function of the number of cycles. Both of these conditions show the carbon combinations to be superior. On the basis of this analytical comparison with clinically used prostheses one can predict that the wear rates in vivo for the carbon joints should by approximately 1 μm/year. The all-carbon-joint-prostheses therefore should markedly increase prosthesis life time controlled by wear.

ACKNOWLEDGEMENTS

Research work has been sponsored by Grant of the German Minister of Research and Technology (M T 207).

REFERENCES

Bokros, J. C., Akins, R. J., Shim, H. S., Haubold, A. O. Agerwal, N. K., (1977) Chemtech. 1, 40

Bowden, F. P. & Tabor, D. (1964) The friction and lubrication of Solids II, Oxford University Press

Brückmann, H. & Hüttinger, K. J. (1980) Biomaterials, Vol 1, 73 - 81

Hinterberger, N. & Ungethüm, N. (1978) Z. Orthopädie, 116, 249

Midgley, J. W. & Teer, D. G. (1963) Transact. of ASME, 12, 488

Pauwels, F. (1973) Atlas zur Biomechanik der gesunden und kranken Hüfte, Springer-Verlag, Berlin

Savage, R. H. & Schäfer, D. L. (1956) Journal of Appl. Phys. 27, 136

Timoshenko, S. (1934) Theory of Elasticity, Mc.-Graw-Hill, New York

Weber, U. (1980) Thesis submitted for the certificate of habilitation, University Gießen

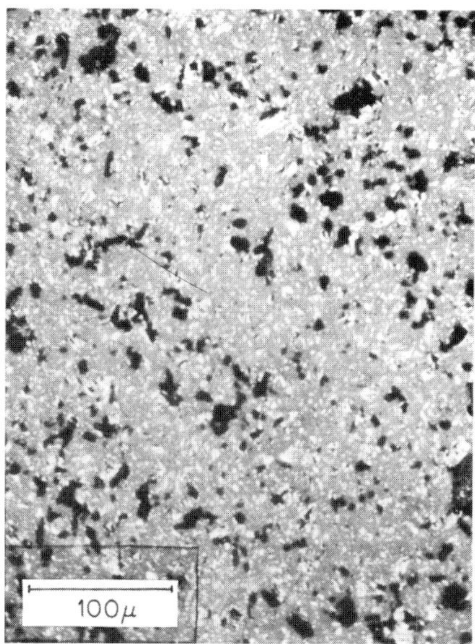

Fig. 1. High strength isotropic carbon, polarized light

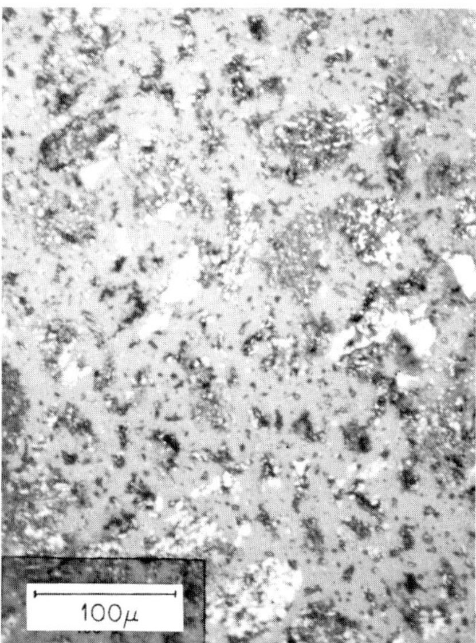

Fig. 2. Siliconcarbide/carbon-composite, (SiC/C), polarized light

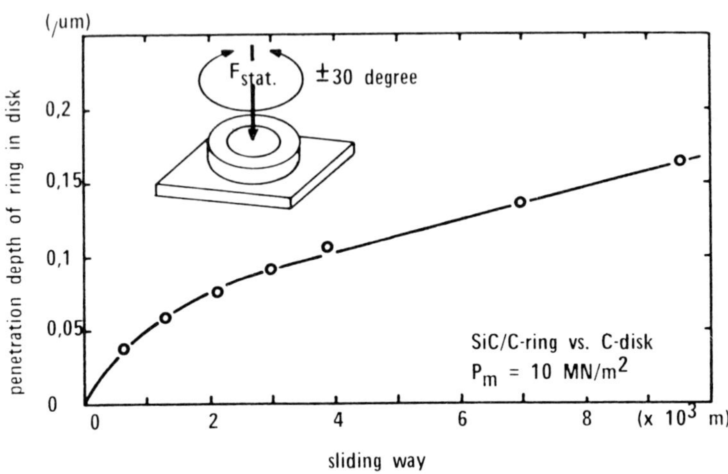

Fig. 3. Depth of penetration of a SiC/C-ring into a disk of isotropic carbon (HTT = 1,200 °C), ring-on-disk-arrangement

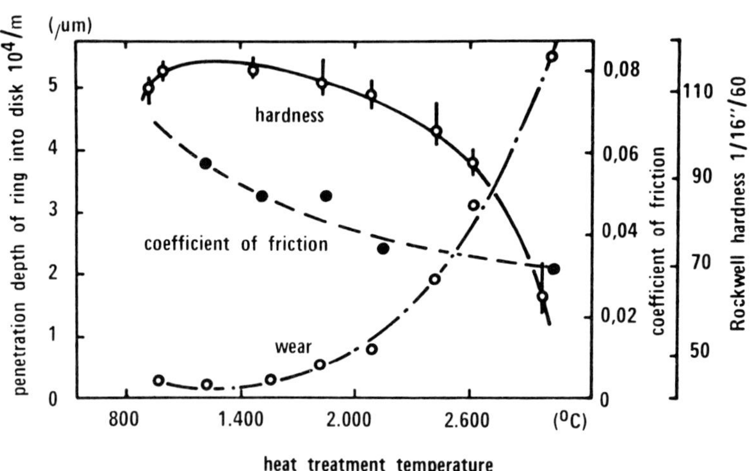

Fig. 4. Penetration depth of SiC/C-ring into isotropic carbon, coefficient of friction and hardness of isotropic carbon versus HTT of the isotropic carbon

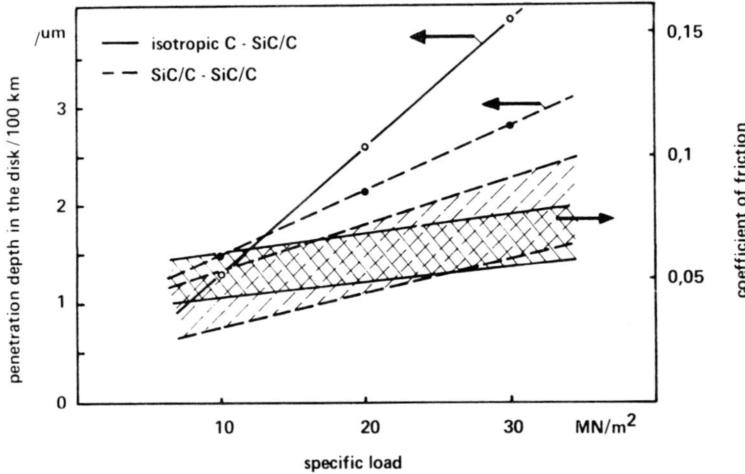

Fig. 5. Wear of the disk (isotropic carbon resp. SiC/C) and coefficient of friction versus specific load, SiC/C-ring

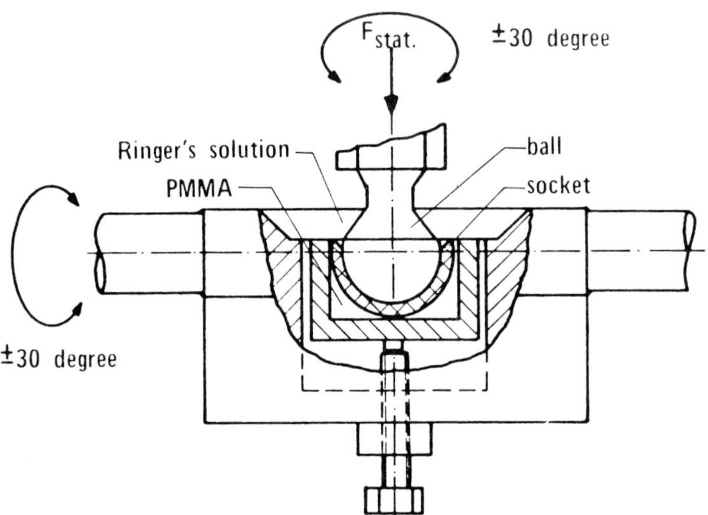

Fig. 6. Ball-in-socket-arrangement

                     K. J. Hüttinger and H.-J. Mäurer

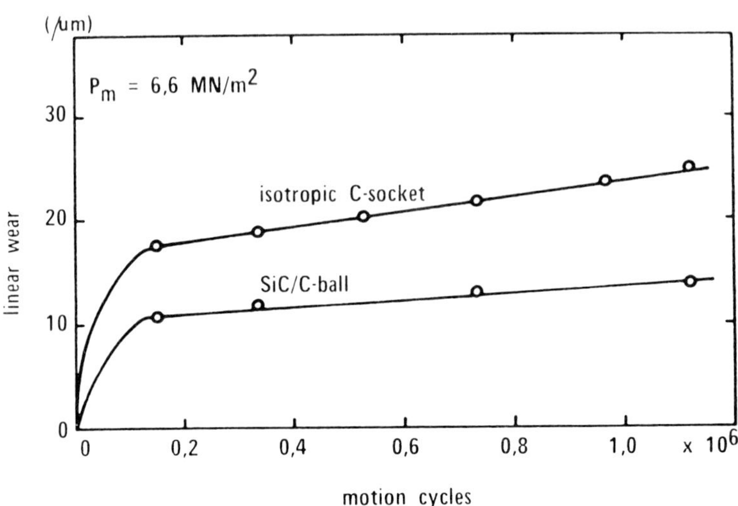

Fig. 7. Increase in depth of the isotropic C-socket and decrease in height of the SiC/C-ball versus motion cycles

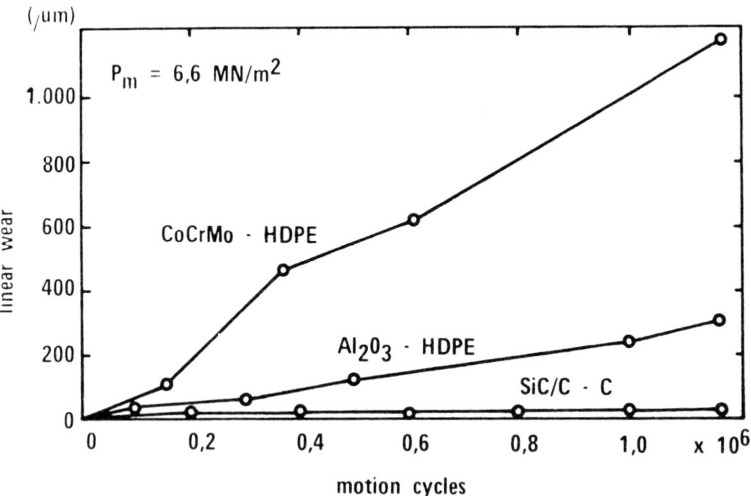

Fig. 8. Wear of different artificial cups versus motion cycles, maximal pressure of all prostheses 6,6 MN/m^2

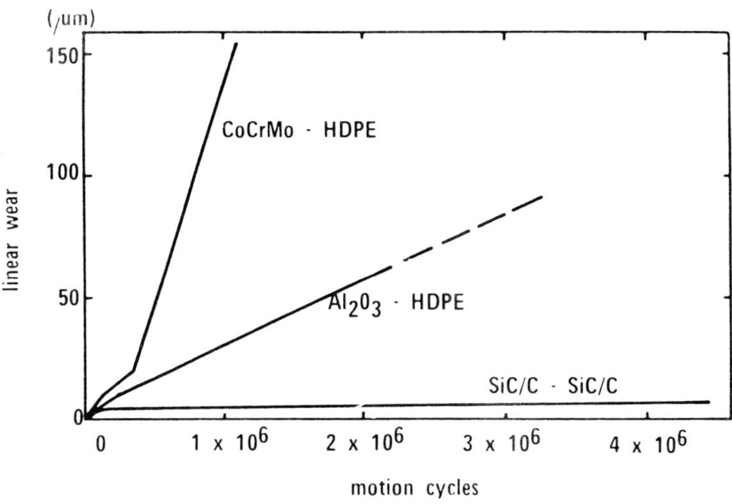

Fig. 9. Wear of different artificial WAGNER-cups versus motion cycles, applied load 2,500 N

Biomaterials 1980
Edited by G. D. Winter, D. F. Gibbons, and H. Plenk, Jr.
© 1982 John Wiley and Sons Ltd.

WEAR OF ALUMINA-CERAMIC HIP JOINTS: SOME
CLINICAL AND TRIBOLOGICAL ASPECTS

W. Plitz and H.U. Hoss

Orthopadische Klinik und Poliklinik der Universitat
München (Direktor: Prof. Dr. A.N. Witt)
Labor fur Biomechanik, Harlachingerstr. 51,
D 8000 München 90, West Germany.

SUMMARY

We analysed 17 endoprostheses having Al_2O_3 ceramic bearing surfaces
which had to be removed from patients for various reasons including
loosening of one or more components. Despite claims to the contrary
we find that considerable wear of the Al_2O_3 ceramic bearing surfaces
of hip joint prostheses can occur in patients as well as in hip
joint simulators.
The results of scanning electron microscope studies lead us to conclude
that the starting point for surface destruction is always a grain
excavation. The loose fragment, caught between the moving surfaces,
causes further grain excavations and an avalanche-like acceleration
of wear.

INTRODUCTION

In the past 10 years arthroplasty of the hip joint has made progress
and has taken new directions. One of these directions concerned the
search for highly wear-resistant materials which would satisfactorily
perform their function for decades despite the extremely severe
conditions encountered in the artificial joint. The ideal bearing
material appeared to have been found with the introduction of the
high purity alumina ceramic.
This paper concerns a critical examination of 17 cases of endoprosthesis with articulating bearing surfaces of Al_2O_3 ceramic which were
removed for various reasons after different implantation periods.

METHODS

The position of the prostheses and any loosening of the stem or cup was
evaluated from post-operation and pre-retrieval radiographs. The
following methods were used to investigate the prostheses that had been
removed from patients. After identifying zones of wear by macroscopic
and steremicroscopic examination they were studied in the scanning
electron microscope (SEM). Some specimens were subjected to thermal
etching ($1500°C$, 5h., normal atmosphere) and then examined in the SEM
to determine the grain size distribution and the structure of the

alumina ceramic. The sphericity of the bearing surfaces was
measured and the depth of any worn zones calculated.

RESULTS

Extensive wear of the Al_2O_3 head of a femoral prosthesis which had
to be removed 3 years after implantation because the stem became
loose is illustrated in Figure 1. The maximum material loss in the
center of the load transmission zone amounts to about 0.9 mm. The
destroyed area comprises approximately 650 square mm, almost two-
thirds of the available bearing surface. The scanning electron microscope (SEM) surface analysis (Figure 2) indicates massive surface
area destruction. Figure 2 (E) shows the frequently observed
phenomenon of a grain excavation which is probably the initial phase
of the total destruction process. The arrow (E) points to a crack
which can be recognised as the originating point of another grain
excavation which is just beginning. Regarding the clinical aspect of
this case, no signs of an intra-operative fault can be found to
explain this excessive amount of wear. The post-operative radiographs show perfect fit and the patient's post-operative progress was
absolutely normal.

Figure 3 illustrates another instance of wear on a prosthesis from
another manufacturer, showing that manufacturer-specific variations
in material are not the cause of these types of wear. Essentially
the same manifestations of destruction occur in the sockets as in the
heads, but the destroyed surface area is always less on the sockets.
This is illustrated by two examples of damage to the surfaces of the
head and socket of removed prostheses (Figures 4 & 5).

Parallel to this self-destruction of the surface area seen macroscopically as filed-down areas, thin and extremely thin wearing away
occurs. The surface structure in these areas is largely preserved.
However, material denudation of 5 microns and more has been proved.
These zones appear optically dark compared with the otherwise light
intact surface area. It is not clear to what extent this mild wear
either initiates or is a prerequisite for more extensive destruction.

DISCUSSION

As has been substantiated by numerous authors (Hinterberger & Ungethum,
1978; Willert & Semlitsch, 1976; Willert et al., 1978) basically
every wear particle produced in the artificial joint has a detrimental
effect on the long-term function. The amount of wear per unit of
time and the form and size of the wear particles are considered to be
the decisive factors in the functional deterioration of the artificial
joint system. Because of their chemical structure the wear particles
were thought to be bio-inert, but this has proved to be untrue. One
of the causes of failure is now recognised to be an extensive flooding
of the joint's interior by the wear particles. This results in an
overburdening of the body's own ability to deal with this debris, that
is to store and to eliminate it. The presence of these particles in

the joint results in a renewed tissue loss and consequent loosening
of the prosthesis components. A direct functional deterioration of
the prosthesis components themselves, perceived first of all by an
increase in friction, is not attributed to the use of hard against
soft materials because the softer wear particles generally left the
hard bearing partner intact. The use of two identical materials as
bearing couplings always presents a risk when viewed from a tribological standpoint. This is especially so when, because of an
adverse stress/movement relationship, as in artificial hip joints,
the hydrodynamic lubricating conditions are unreliable. If bearing
surface geometry is precise, as is usually the case, the pressure at
the surface is so low that the material is unlikely to be damaged,
but there are already minute trouble spots in the surface because of
the required high sphericity of the head and socket. These trouble
spots constitute the starting point for a progressively developing
surface destruction of the brittle Al_2O_3 material.

CONCLUSIONS

Our hypothesis concerning this wear phenomenon is that the starting
point for surface destruction is always a grain excavation. Figure
6 (B) shows such a grain excavation. 6 (A) shows the undamaged
surface; 6 (C) and 6 (D) show damaged surface and grain excavation.
The generally sharp-cornered fragment is released into the space
between the surfaces which are moving under a load. This causes the
fragment to move and consequently causes further damage to the
regions which have considerably increased the maximum load on this
fragment (Figure 7). The result is an avalanche-like acceleration
of further grain excavations and finally the destruction of whole
surface areas. A damaged area is compared with the original surface
in Figure 8.

There can be various reasons why the initial grain excavation occurs
at all (Figures 9 & 10). In general, grain excavation from an
intact surface is always possible when a mechanical overload exceeds
either the trans-crystalline or the inter-crystalline strength of the
material. This strength may already be reduced because of a course-
grained structure or by contamination of the materials. Figure 11
shows clearly visable grain boundaries on an air-corroded surface of
a removed socket. The large grain in (B) measures approximately
45 microns across. Excessive local surface pressure can arise from
too large a deviation in sphericity and/or inferior surface finish.
An additional cause of excessive surface pressure can be increased
stress which occurs perhaps at a sublaxation or when the head and
socket are adversely positioned. Each of these possible causes do
not generally occur in isolation but may exist simultaneously,
whereby their adverse effects are additive. Because of this we have
consciously refrained from a statistical enumeration and classification of individual cases because the total picture is still not clear.
Considering the large number of hip endoprostheses with the ceramic-
ceramic bearing surfaces that have been implanted, the number of
failures we have experienced appears to be minimal. It is premature
to state a percentage failure rate at this time because reliable
figures are not available for either the implanted or the removed

cases. The observations reported in this paper prove that the alumina ceramic coupling, contrary to constantly asserted claims by manufacturers, is not absolutely free of wear. Further critical studies are required.

ACKNOWLEDGEMENT

These investigations were supported by a grant from the Bundesministerium fur Forschung und Technologie (MT 267).

REFERENCES

Hinterberger, J. & Ungethum, M. (1978) Untersuchungen zur Tribologie und Festigkeit vin Aluminiumoxidkeramik-Huftendoprothesen. Z. Orthop. 116, 294-303.
Willert, H.G., Semlitsch, M., Buchhorn, G. & Kriete, U. (1978) Materialverschleiss und Gewebereaktion bei kunstlichen Gelenken. (Histopathologie, Biokompatibilitat, biologische und klinische probleme). Orthopade, 7, 62-83.
Willert, H.G. & Semlitsch, M. (1976). Tissue reactions to plastic and metallic wear products of joint endoprostheses. In: Total hip prosthesis. (Eds. Gschwend & Debrunner). Hans Huber Publishers, Bern, Stuttgart, Vienna.

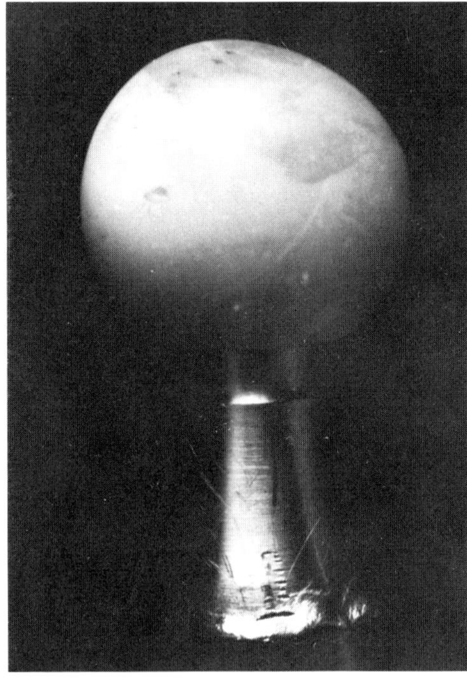

Figure 1. Worn head of an Al_2O_3 ceramic hip joint prosthesis removed after 3 years

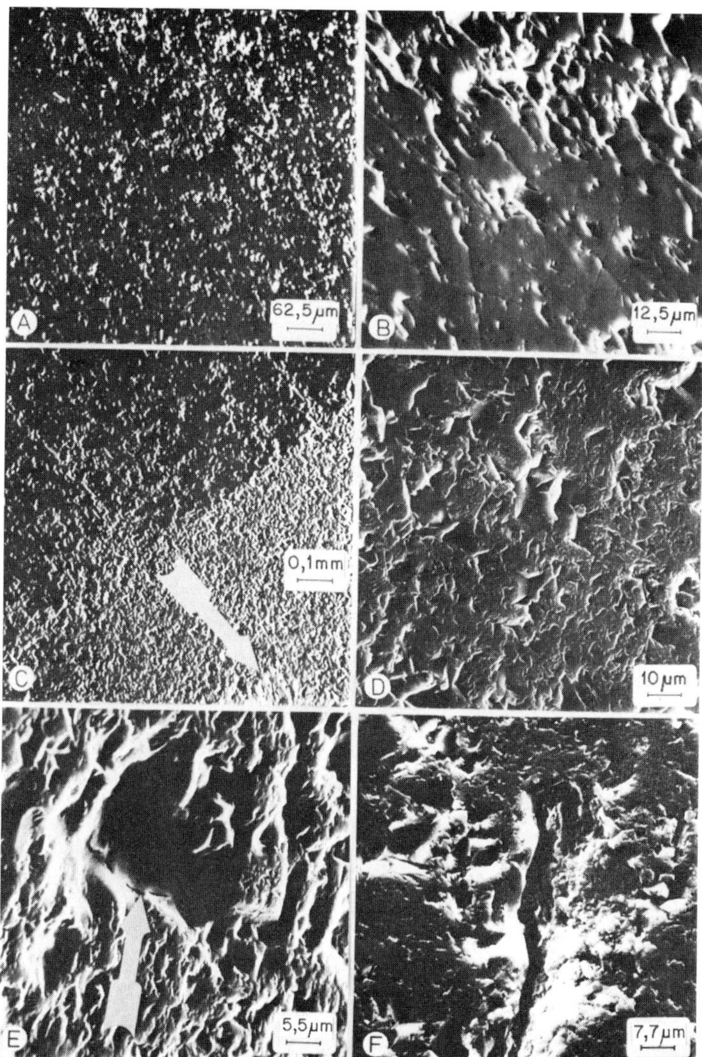

Figure 2. SEM analysis of the head of the prosthesis illustrated in Figure 1. (A) and (B): undamaged surface area; (C) damaged/undamaged area. Arrow indicates zone of very high roughness; (D) section of damaged area; (E) and (F) grain excavation hole and cracked surface.

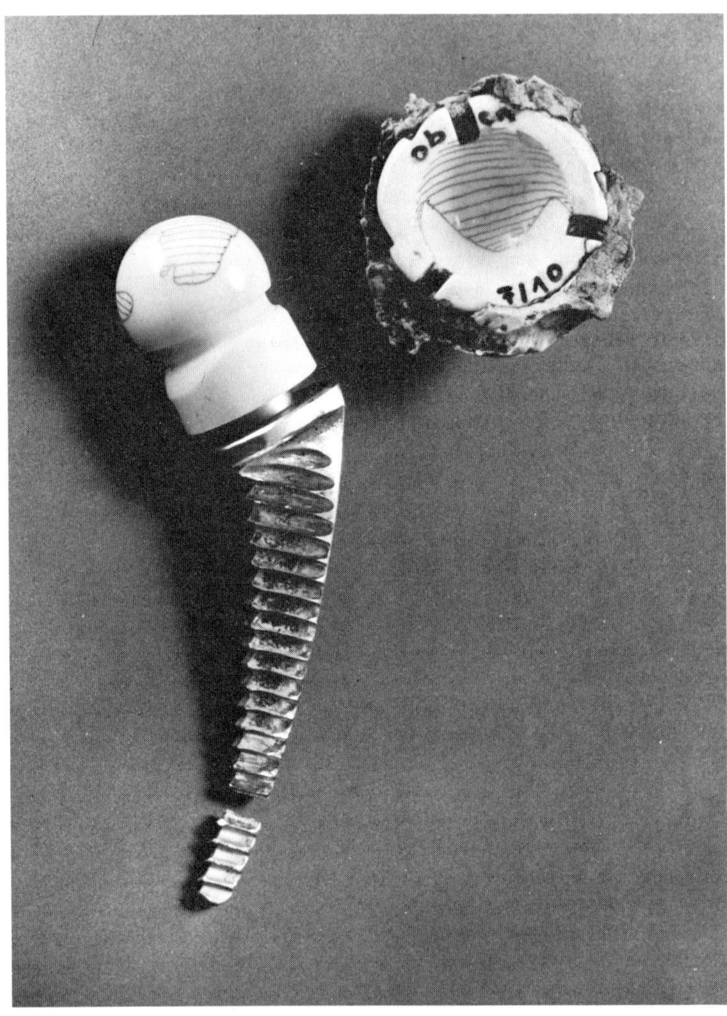

Figure 3. Removed prosthesis (period of implantation –
2½ years). Worn area has been marked.

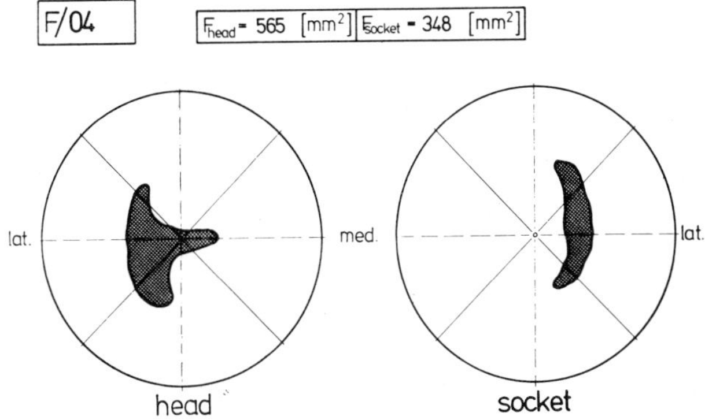

Figure 4. Destroyed surface area on the alumina-ceramic prosthesis removed after 3 months

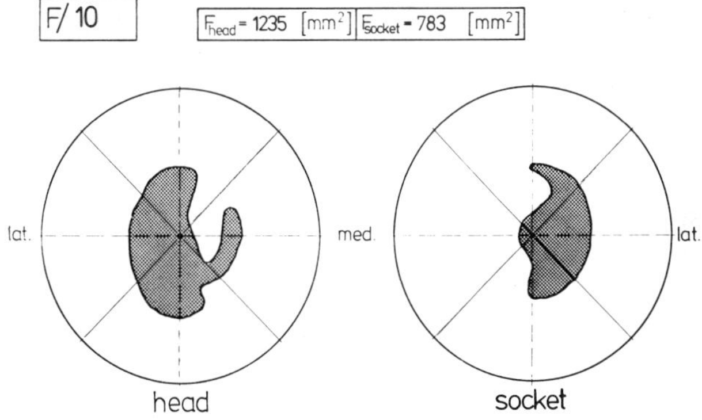

Figure 5. Destroyed surface area on the alumina-ceramic prosthesis illustrated in Figure 3, removed after 2½ years

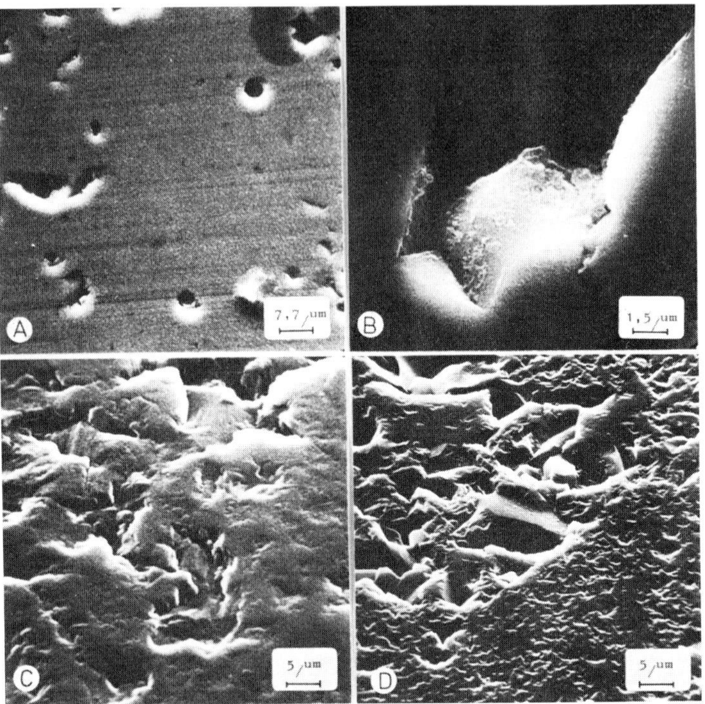

Figure 6. Surface with grain excavation from the head of
the prosthesis shown in Figure 3

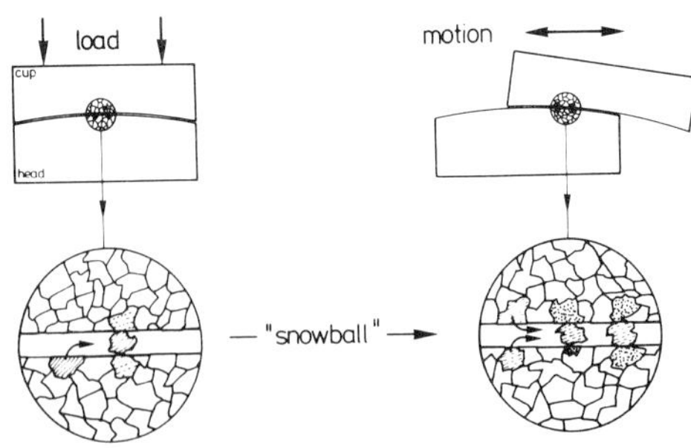

Figure 7. Suggested mechanisms of destruction of Al_2O_3
bearing surfaces

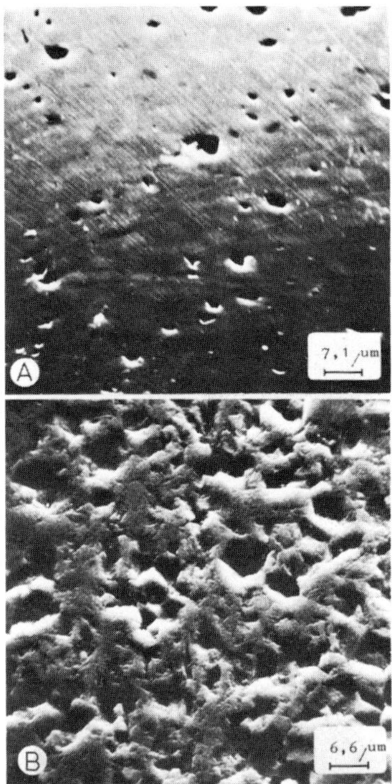

Figure 8. Comparison at similar magnification of the worn surface with an area of normal surface on the head of the alumina-ceramic prosthesis shown in Figure 3.

Schematic draft of Al_2O_3-bearing-surface destruction

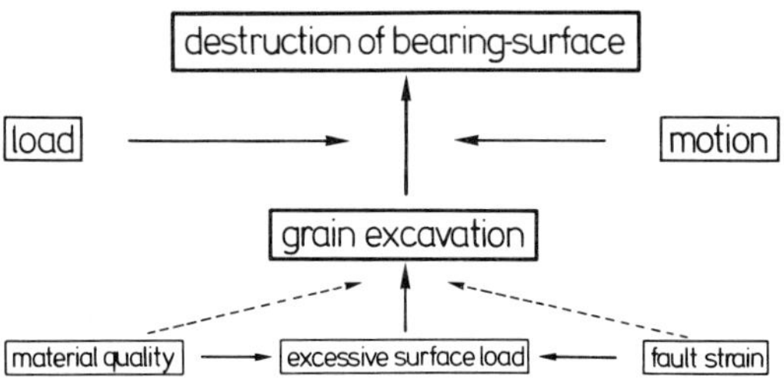

Figure 9. Mechanism of destruction of Al_2O_3 bearing surfaces in hip joints

                    W. Plitz and H.U. Hoss

<u>Al₂O₃ bearing-surface destruction factors</u>

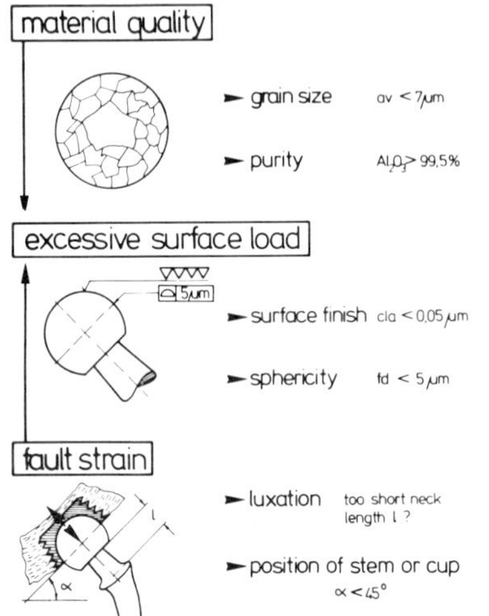

Figure 10. Possible causes of wear of the surfaces of Al_2O_3 prostheses

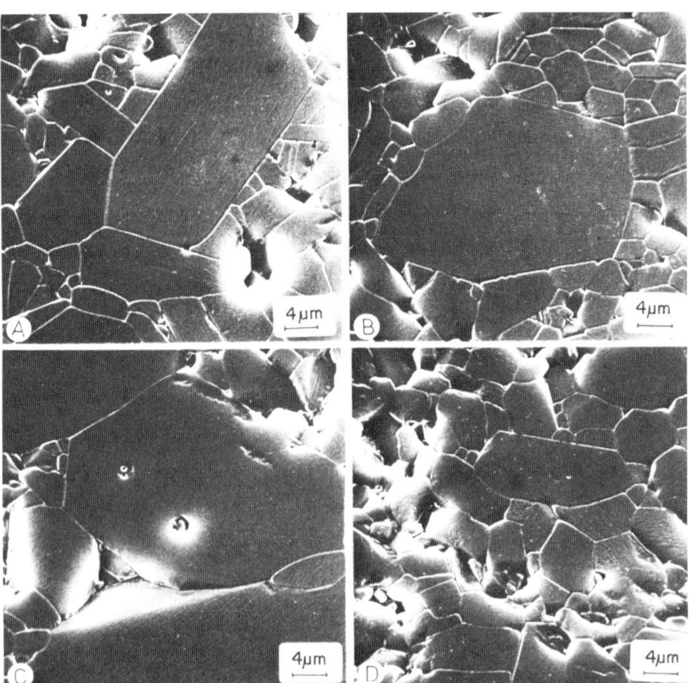

Figure 11. Air-corroded specimen from a socket

Biomaterials 1980
Edited by G. D. Winter, D. F. Gibbons, and H. Plenk, Jr.
© 1982 John Wiley and Sons Ltd.

TISSUE TOLERANCE OF WEAR DEBRIS FROM ARTHROPLASTIES

J.L. Leray and P. Christel

I.N.S.E.R.M. - U. 18, Pavillon Ollier, Hôpital Cochin
27, rue du Fg. St-Jacques - 75674 Paris Cédex 14, France.

SUMMARY

Human tissues explanted at revision of arthroplasties with metal-
metal, metal-polyethylene and alumina-alumina pairs of sliding
materials are examined with conventional histology and ion microprobe
elementary analysis.
Comparison of tissue reactions to particulate materials shows that
abundant release of any foreign material leads repeatedly to excessive
foreign body reaction and necrosis. At moderate concentrations
of wear material, the alumina crystallites are not so susceptible to
fragmentation and further degradation as particulate metallic alloys
and do not alter the general appearance of the host tissues. Since
the wear rate of alumina surfaces is lower than for other material
combinations investigated, this ceramic combination should exhibit
a superior long term tissue tolerance if catastrophic failures can be
avoided by careful manufacture of the sliding parts.

INTRODUCTION

It has been recognized from early experience in total hip replacement
(Charnley 1970) that the release of wear debris from sliding
surfaces was a critical factor for the long-term behavior of such
arthroplasties. High concentration of small polytetrafluorethylene
(PTFE) particles or metallic grains released from plastic-metal and
metal-metal sliding pairs triggered early loosening of implants through
inflammation, fibrosis and necrosis of periprosthetic tissues. Because
of this, high density polyethylene (HDPE) replaced PTFE for the
acetabular cup material (Charnley 1970). More recently, to further
reduce the wear of sliding parts, sintered alumina has been introduced
for the femoral head and acetabular cup in combination with titanium
alloy for the femoral stem (Boutin 1972), while a Al_2O_3 - HDPE
combination has been incorporated in a modified version of the Charnley-
Müller design.
We have had the opportunity to examine the periprosthetic tissues
retrieved during revision of five patients with Boutin prostheses. In
this report, we compare these cases to similar ones with metal-metal
and metal-HDPE sliding pairs.

HISTOLOGICAL TECHNIQUES

Soft tissues from the regenerated capsule were fixed in Bouin fixative and hard bony explants in buffered formalin. The samples were then dehydrated in alcohols, embedded in polymethyl-methacrylate and sectioned to 5-8 micron slices. The plastic embedding medium was removed by soaking in 2-methoxyethylacetate and the sections stained with hematoxylin-eosin (H.E.) and by the Goldner trichrome and Giemsa methods. Microscopic examination was carried out under natural and polarized illumination with the light microscope. Some typical sections have been analysed with an ion microprobe to verify the chemical nature of foreign particles within the tissues but the rapid etching of the sections under ion bombardment did not permit quantitative analysis of the inclusions.

PATIENT HISTORY

Three of the five ceramic prostheses were removed because of loosening of the stem-head assembly and subsequent breakage of the head and two because of loosening of the acetabular cups which had been inserted without cement. The time of implantation ranged from 5 months to 7 years (average 3.5 years) and the patients' ages were between 45 and 76 years.

The HDPE-metal prosthesis was removed because of abnormal wear of the polyethylene cup, implanted for 4 years in a young patient suffering from osteoarthritis.

The metal-metal prostheses were cobalt-chrome alloy sliding pairs in one elbow prosthesis, one McKee-Farrar hip prosthesis and one Postel hip model (grooved metallic cup). The age of the patients ranged from 70 to 76 years and the implantation time from 5 to 8 years.

RESULTS

The tissue response is reported in three steps according to the scale of observation for the three combinations alumina-alumina (Ceramic), HDPE - metal (Plastic) and metal-metal (Metal).

Macroscopic scale (x 1, x 2.5) - Fig. 1.

Ceramic (Fig. 1a) : Sclerotic and dark tissues are densely infiltrated with black debris from the metallic stem (Ti 90%, Al 6%, V 4%). Some necrotic zones; mostly located close to the implant, are densely invaded with black metal while the tissues within the areas with lower contamination maintain a normal appearance with a population of viable cells (observed at x10 magnification). Several empty spaces lined with giant cells correspond to lumps of bone cement which have been removed during the histological preparation.

They are often surrounded with sclerotic and scar tissues. In one case significantly discolored zones are absent but dense non metallic granules are clustered close to well cellularized areas within connective and scar tissues.

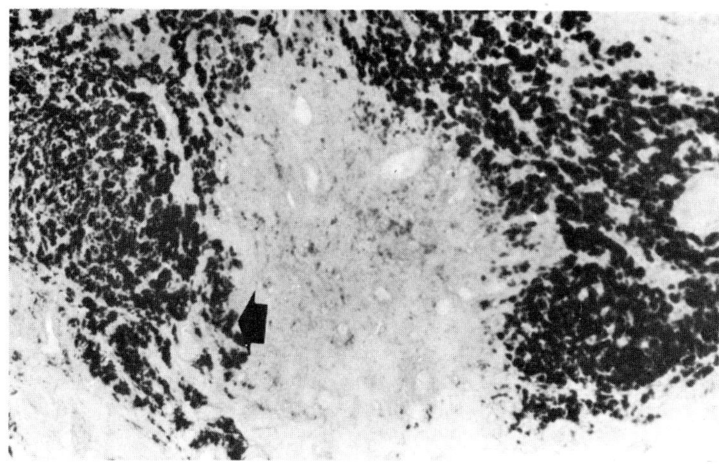

Fig. 1a. Sclerotic darkly stained tissue from the vicinity
of a ceramic-titanium alloy hip joint implanted for 5 years
and revised for loosened stem-head assembly. Note presence
of opaque particles ($\uparrow$) identified as Ti and Al by electron
probe analysis in macrophages. x 2.5 - H.E. stain.

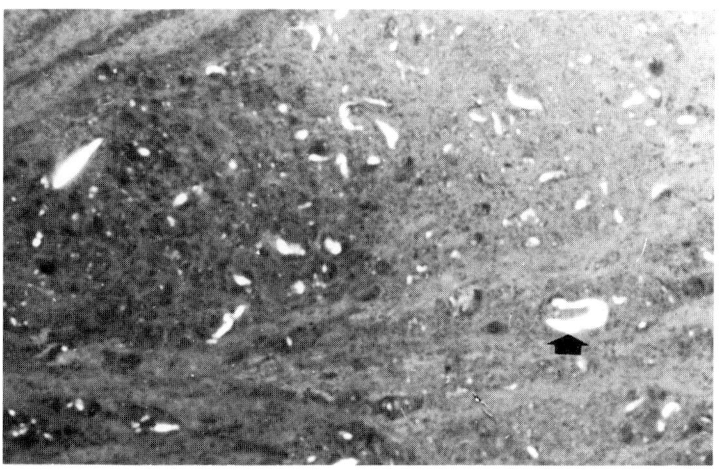

Fig. 1b. Connective tissue from newly formed capsule around
a HDPE-metal hip prosthesis implanted for 4 years. Nodules
of giant cells around PE flakes ($\uparrow$). x 2.5 polarized light -
Trichrome.

Plastic (Fig. 1b) : No appreciable metal infiltration is noted, however lumps of both polyethylene and bone cement are found at a distance from the implant. Plastic chips are also present around the femoral component, surrounded by nodules of giant cells. Around the newly formed capsule, sclerotic and even necrotic areas alternate with hemorrhagic ones. A restricted area is infiltrated with eroded metallic grains.

Metal (Fig. 1c) : In the specimens from 2 patients, most tissues are necrotic with a few enucleated cells displaying a granulated cytoplasm. Some zones are well cellularized and vascularized with a prominent lympho-plasmocytic reaction and granulations (Fig.1d).

Intermediate scale (x 25, x 40 objectives) - Fig. 2.

Ceramic (Fig. 2a, 2b) : The tissues infiltrated exclusively with transparent, strongly birefringent particles of sintered alumina do not show fibrosis or necrosis. The reaction is predominantly histiocytic with no apparent morphological damage (Fig. 2a). Some histiocytes migrate far away along connective or muscular fibers. The larger crystallites, 3 to 6 micron wide, are released presumably from fractured and crushed fragments and found both intra- and extra-cellular. The smaller ones less than 1 micron diameter, originating from the sliding surfaces and resulting from wear proper are mostly phagocyted by histiocytes. These loaded macrophages are clustered around capillaries which most probably they cannot enter because of their size. No giant or polymorphonuclear cells are found.
When metallic wear is predominant, the reaction specific to the titanium alloy is elicited, leading to granuloma and necrosis. Giant cells are present as well as thickening of capillary walls (Fig. 2b).

Plastic (Fig. 2c) : The giant cells are remarkably wide to engulf the plastic flakes and contain several vacuoles and pale nuclei. They are often found in clusters which tend toward necrosis. Some mononucleated macrophages located in the marrow of cancellous bone are filled with birefringent granules which absorb the various stains. These granules might very well be identified with particular polyethylene.

Cell morphology (x 100 objective) - Fig. 3.

Ceramic (Fig. 3a, 3b) : The ceramic loaded macrophages (Fig. 3a) found in the alumina invaded areas between acetabular cup and bone contrast with the metal and ceramic loaded multinucleated cells (Fig. 3b) found in areas contaminated with metal as well. However both cell types are normal in appearance and do not show any damage at this magnification. Only slight inflammation was seen. Vascular lesions and necrosis were observed only in areas of excessive accumulation of metal.

Plastic : The macrophages containing berefringent polyethylene are found close to the wear surfaces and far away from it as well, trapped within the bone-prosthesis interface as has been frequently observed (Willert and Schreiber 1969).

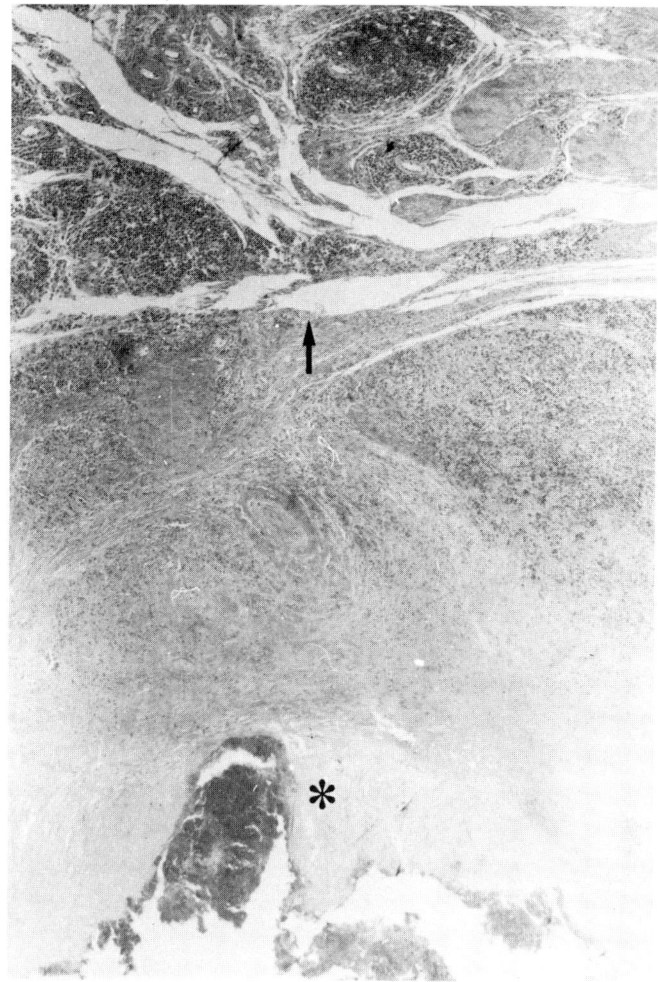

Fig. 1c. Sclerotic (↑) and necrotic (✳) zones in tissue
located around a metal-metal (CoCr alloy) elbow prosthesis
implanted for 4 years. In the upper zone, dense infiltration
of plasmocytes (visible with x 25 objective).

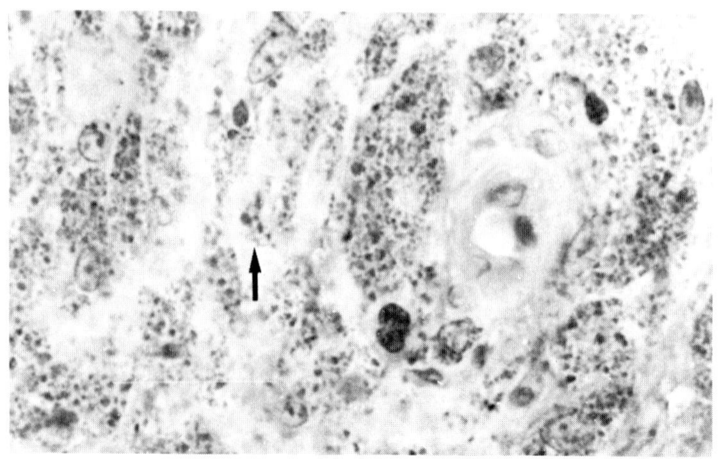

Fig. 1d. Connective tissue from newly formed capsule around
a metal-metal hip prosthesis (Postel) implanted for 7 years:
metal loaded, lysed histiocytes (↑) around a vessel with
thickened walls. x 40,Giemsa stain.

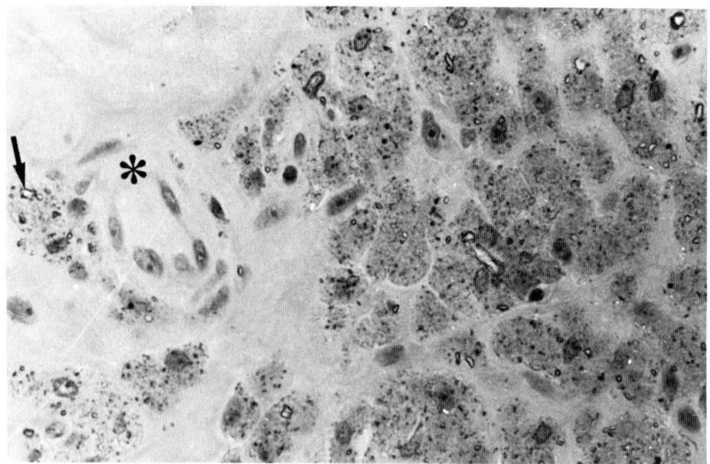

Fig. 2a. Connective tissue around ceramic-titanium prosthesis
implanted for five years and revised for protruding cemented
cup : macrophages containing alumina particles (↑) in the
vicinity of a capillary vessel (✻). x 25, trichrome stain.

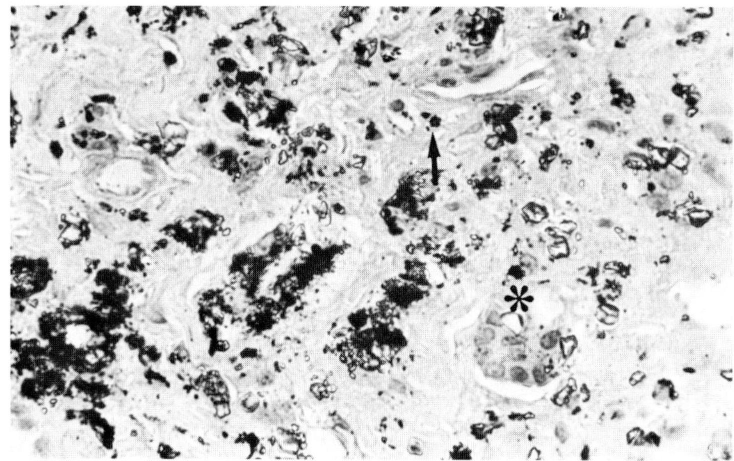

Fig. 2b. Connective tissue from same patient as Fig. 1a.
Note infiltration with dark particles of titanium alloy (↑)
and transparent alumina crystallites (✷). x 25, Trichrome
stain.

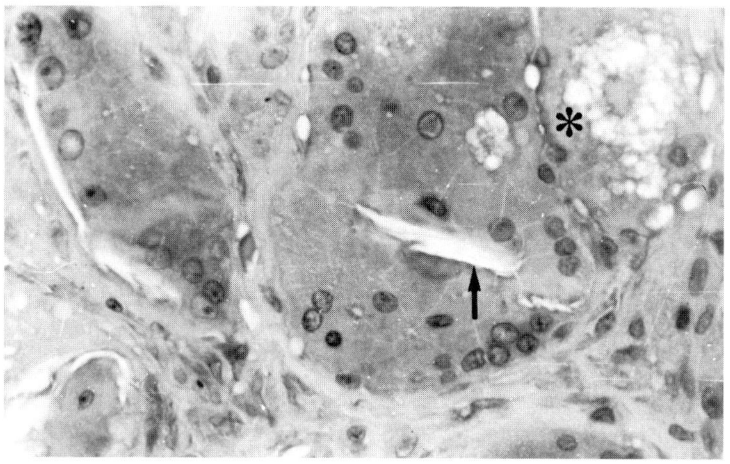

Fig. 2c. Same patient as Fig. 1b : giant cells loaded with
PE flakes (↑) and vacuoles (✷). x 25, Giemsa stain.

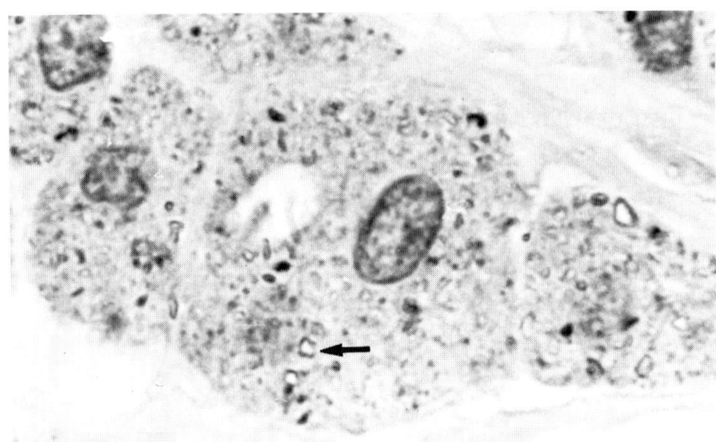

Fig. 3a. Same patient as Fig. 2a : histiocyte with alumina granules (↑). x 100, H.E. stain.

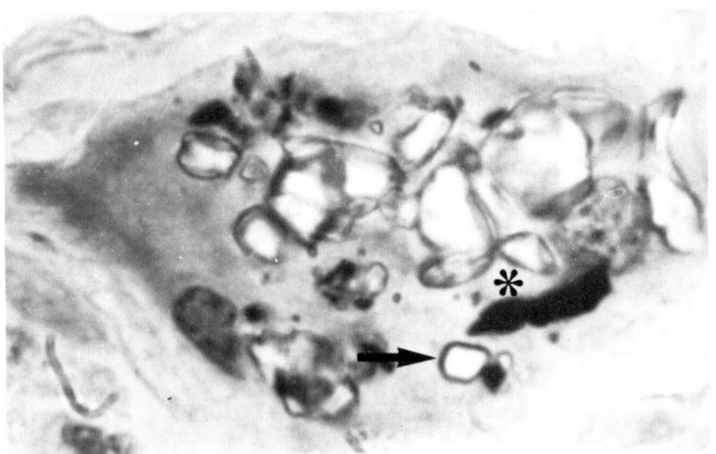

Fig. 3b. Giant cell containing both alumina crystals (↑) and titanium alloy chips (✻) in tissue close to broken ceramic head of hip prostheiss implanted for 6 months. x 100, Trichrome stain.

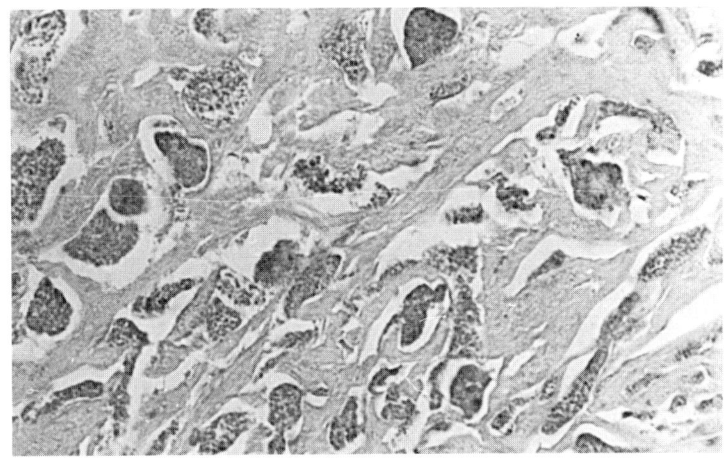

Fig. 3c. Same patient as Fig. 1c : necrotic tissue filled
with densely granulated cells. x 40, Giemsa stain.

Metal (Fig. 3c) : Varying with the patient various types of
cells predominate, either plasmocytes with a few macrophages or polymorphonuclear leucocytes or densely granulated cells (Winter 1974).

Ion and electron microprobes : The images with SEM and ion
microprobes confirm the presence of titanium and aluminium in the
blackened areas of the tissue specimen (ceramic case) and enhanced
concentration of calcium in the same areas.

DISCUSSION

Study of catastrophic failures, which might be regarded as accelerated
wear testing of sliding material combinations may give some clues on
the long term behavior of periprosthetic tissues under normal clinical
conditions. In the earlier versions of ceramic prosthesis investigated here, the stem-head assembly involved a female threaded metallic
part brazed inside the ceramic head which unscrewed in vivo from the
metal stem. After breakage of the ceramic parts, the massive amounts
of alumina and titanium alloy powder which were produced subsequently
might be considered as human implantation of divided materials, providing information complementary to the animal experimentation (Griss
et al 1974, Harms and Maüsle 1979).

Broadly speaking, significant accumulation of debris within connective
tissue leads to thickening of capillaries and necrosis, regardless of
chemical composition of the foreign bodies.

When the release rate of toxic products is not significant, the tissue
reaction depends largely on the size and concentration of infiltrated
debris. Smaller particles are phagocyted by histiocytes, larger lumps

are excluded functionally by a fibrous capsule.

While the eluted material from titanium alloy does darken the tissues without eliciting any inflammation at moderate concentrations of debris, abrasion of Co-base alloys at similar concentration levels produces sometimes granuloma with accumulation of plasmocytes and other immuno competent cells which are indicative of sensitization and allergy-like systemic processes.

The mild reaction observed with relatively high concentration of alumina crystallites might be traced back to their slow rate of dissolution, since the alumina crystallites found in the tissues retain a shape and size similar to the grains of the original sintered alumina. Even when the crystallites are crushed by the wear processes, the resulting high specific area (area per unit weight) exposed to body fluids does not lead to an overall chemical activity which might elicit adverse reactions, as observed with metallic particles. It has been suggested the absorbed substances - water essentially - at the crystal surface screen the material from further interaction with body fluids (Dawihl and Dorre 1980).

In conclusion, if catastrophic failures of the composite alumina-titanium alloy prostheses are avoided by care in the manufacture and surgical techniques, the wear of sintered alumina should be well tolerated. In this respect, the alumina-alumina combination is superior to the other sliding material pairs examined.

ACKNOWLEDGEMENTS

We thank very kindly Mrs. M. Hott who carried the histological work and prepared the microphotographs and Mrs. M. Henry-Amar for typing the manuscript.

REFERENCES

Boutin, P. (1972) Arthroplastie totale de la hanche par prothèse en alumine frittée. Revue de chirurgie Orthopédique, 58, 229-246.
Charnley, J. (1970) Total hip replacement for low friction arthroplasty. Clinical Orthopaedics and Related Research, 72, 7-21.
Dawihl, W. & Dörre, E. (1980) Absorption behaviour of high density alumina ceramics exposed to fluids. in Evaluation of Biomaterials (Eds., Winter, Leray & de Groote), 239-245. Wiley, London.
Griss, P., Krempien , B., Andrian-Werburg, H., Heimke, G., Fleiner, R. & Diehm, T. (1974) experimental analysis of ceramic-tissue interactions. A morphologic, fluorescenceoptic and radiographic study of dense alumina oxide in various animals. Journal of Biomedical Materials Research Symposium, 5, 39-48
Harms, J. & Mäusle, E. (1979) Tissue reaction to ceramic implant material. Journal of Biomedical Materials Research, 13, 67-87.
Willert, H.G. & Schreiber, A. (1969) Unterschiedliche Reaktionen von Knochen und Weichteillager auf autopolymerisierende Kunststoffimplanate. Zeitschrift f. orthopedie, 106, 231-252.
Winter, G.D. (1974) Tissue reactions to metallic wear and corrosion products in human patients. Journal of Biomedical Materials Research Symposium, 5, 11-26.

Biomaterials 1980
Edited by G. D. Winter, D. F. Gibbons, and H. Plenk, Jr.
© 1982 John Wiley and Sons Ltd.

EVALUATION OF CRITICAL AND SUBCRITICAL CRACK
EXTENSION PARAMETERS WITH BIOCERAMICS

A. Bornhauser, K. Kromp and R.F. Pabst

Max-Planck-Institut fuer Metallforschung, Institut
fuer Werkstoffwissenschaften, Stuttgart, F.R.G.

<u>SUMMARY</u>

Subcritical (n,A) and critical (K_{IC}) crack extension parameters were
measured with an Al_2O_3 bioceramic to determine the life time t_f under
an applied load σ_a. The subcritical parameters were evaluated from
double torsion experiments (macrocrack extension) and, for comparison,
by dynamic fatique in a compact bending test (microcrack extension).
K_{IC} were measured in vacuum in a four-point-bending-test. The high
standard deviation of the results is due to the inhomogeneous microstructure of the ceramic used. Life time predictions must therefore
be cautiously handled.

<u>INTRODUCTION</u>

The use of bioceramic joint substitutes requires a material specific
strength characterisation which is independent of specimen size and
test procedure. This is best effected by using fracture mechanics,
where the strength behaviour is described by stress intensity factors
(Pabst 1972).
Although ceramic materials are very brittle, subcritical crack
extension in moist environments is of great importance. In order to
obtain life time predictions of ceramic joint substitutes under load
in a physiological environment, the subcritical crack extension
parameters n and A and the critical stress intensity K_{IC} are needed.
This paper deals with the determination of n, A and K_{IC} and the life
time t_f for an applied stress σ_a.

MATERIAL

The material properties are given in table 1.

TABLE 1: Material Properties

Quality	Density	$\overline{d}$	Youngs Modulus E
% Al_2O_3	g/cm^3	μm	GN/m^2
99.7	3.95	3	391

$\overline{d}$ = average grain size

A pure, dense commercial material was used. This material contains holes of average diameter 30 μm which influenced the homogenity of the microstructure (Fig. 1).

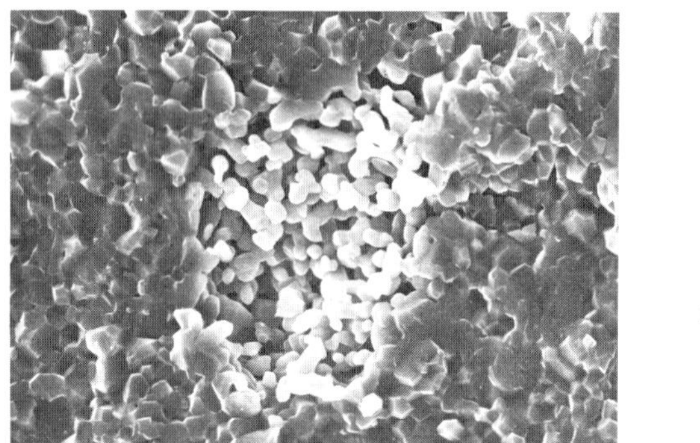

Fig. 1. Material with hole.

FORMALISM

The following relations were used to characterize strength behaviour and life time (Bornhauser, 1980).

1. For subcritical crack extension

$$v = AK_I^n \tag{1}$$

v = crack velocity, K_I = stress intensity factor

A, n = subcritical crack extension parameters

2. For critical crack extension

$$K_{IC} = \sigma_{IC} \sqrt{a_c} \cdot Y \qquad (2)$$

K_{IC} = critical stress intensity factor,

σ_{IC} = inert strength (vacuum strength),

a_c = critical crack length, Y = geom. correction function.

3. For life time

$$t_f = \frac{2 \cdot \sigma_a^{-n}}{(n-2) \cdot A \cdot Y^2} \cdot \left(\frac{\sigma_{IC}}{K_{IC}}\right)^{n-2} \qquad (3)$$

σ_a = applied stress

EXPERIMENTAL

The crack extension parameters were obtained in two different ways (Bornhauser, 1980).

1. Directly, by observing a single, well defined macroscopic crack in a double torsion specimen.(DT specimen) (Evans, 1972; Outwater, 1974). Fig. 2 shows a DT specimen.
9 DT specimens were used and tested in distilled water.

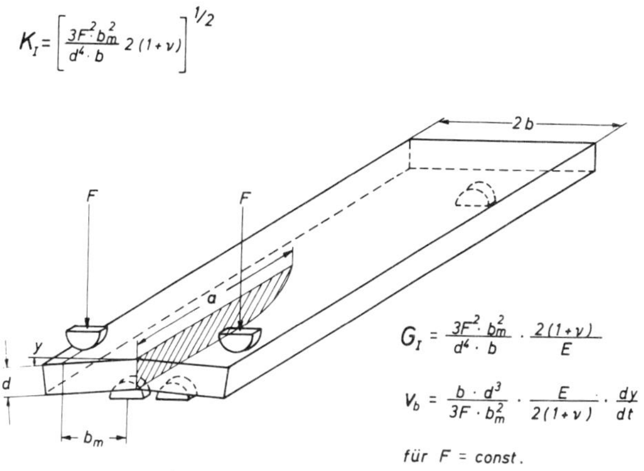

$$K_I = \left[\frac{3F^2 b_m^2}{d^4 \cdot b} 2(1+v)\right]^{1/2}$$

Fig. 2.   Double torsion specimen.

     A. Bornhauser, K. Kromp and R. F. Pabst

2. Indirctly, by measuring the extension of undefined microcracks
   in compact bending specimens by dynamic fatique.

   34 specimens were used and tested in distilled water at five

   different loading rates $\dot{y}$ (Jakus, 1978).

The inert strength σ_{IC}, needed for evaluating t_f, was obtained by
measuring the bend strength in vacuum (2×10^{-5} Torr).

14 four-point-bend-specimens were used in this experiment.

The K_{IC} values were measured in a four-point-bend-test where a well-
defined slit of length a_c = 0.5 - 1.0 mm and width of 80 µm was

introduced with a diamond saw.

9 specimens were used and tested in vacuum.

The dimensions of the specimens were: a) DT specimens: L = 80 mm,

2b = 25 mm, d = 2 mm. b) Four-point-bend-specimens: L = 40 mm,

b = 7 mm, d = 2 mm.

RESULTS AND DISCUSSION

1. Results of n, A, K_{IC} and σ_{IC} measurements.

The results of n and A, evaluated from a DT-test are given in Fig. 3.

A and n may be determined from a v-K_I diagram in a logarithmic plot:

$\log v = n \cdot \log K_I + \log A$.

The values n = 50 ± 17 and log A = -29 ± 14 show a high standard

deviation, revealing an inhomogeneous microstructure. For comparison

the parameters n and A were also determined by a "mean-value-plot",

measured with four-point-bending-specimens. The results are: n = 56

and A = 3×10^{-26} (Fig. 4).

The value of n is higher than with DT specimens, indicating a

difference in the extension behaviour between microcracks and

macrocracks, but nevertheless within the errors of the DT test.

The four-point-bend-test in vacuum gives K_{IC} values of 5.8 ± 0.6
$MN/m^{3/2}$.

2. Life time prediction.

The results of life time t_f as a function of the applied stress

σ_a are given in Fig. 5.

The following data were used to evaluate t_f:

$K_{IC} = 5.8 \pm 0.6$ MN/m$^{3/2}$, $\sigma_{IC} = 497,5 \pm 35$ MN/m^{2}, $n = 50 \pm 17$, log A = -29 ± 14. For Y the correction factor of a four-point-bending-specimen was inserted.

The deviation of life time t_f corresponds to the standard deviation of n and K_{IC}. It indicates the difficulties in life time prediction if an inhomogeneous ceramic material is used.

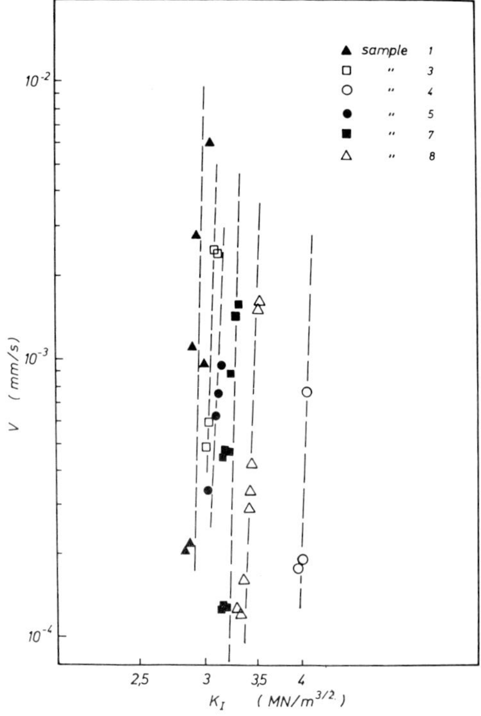

Fig. 3. v-K_I diagram

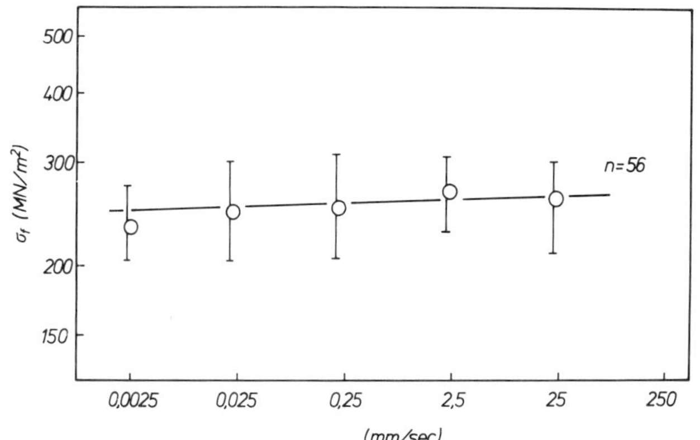

Fig. 4.

Mean-value-plot

     A. Bornhauser, K. Kromp, R.F. Pabst

CONCLUSION

The strength characterisation of an alumina bioceramic material
reveals critical and subcritical strength parameters with high
standard deviations. This is due to an inhomogeneous microstructure
of the material used, which leads to irrational predictions of the
life time t_f.

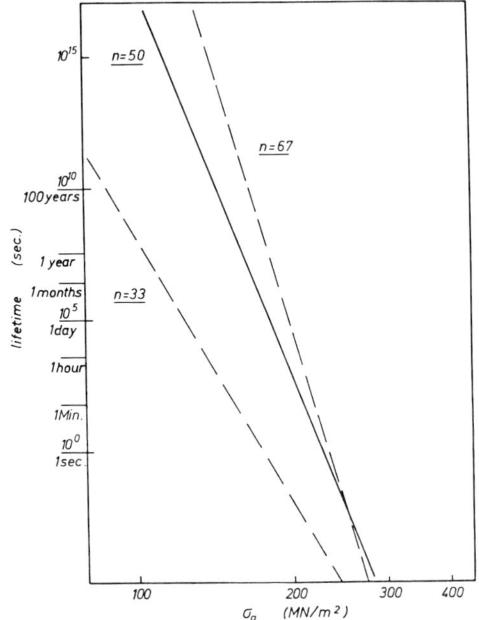

Fig. 5.

Life time diagram

REFERENCES

Bornhauser, A. (1980) Master Thesis, Univ. Stuttgart

Evans, A.G. (1972) A method for evaluating the time dependent
failure characteristics of brittle materials... J.Mat.Sc. 7 1137-46

Jakus, K. (1978) Analysis of fatique data for life time
predictions for ceramic materials. J.Mat.Sc. 13

Outwater, J.O. (1974) Double torsion technique as a universal
fracture toughness test method. ASTM,STP, 2071-2080.

Pabst, R.F. (1972) Dissertation, Univ. Stuttgart.

Biomaterials 1980
Edited by G. D. Winter, D. F. Gibbons, and H. Plenk, Jr.
© 1982 John Wiley and Sons Ltd.

ON THE STRUCTURAL SAFETY OF CERAMIC HIP-JOINT HEADS

U. Seidelmann, H. Richter, U. Soltész

Fraunhofer-Institut für Werkstoffmechanik, Freiburg, GFR

SUMMARY

For safety and life-time predictions of ceramic hip-joint heads the
stress distributions are calculated by the method of finite elements.
Permanent "frozen" stresses caused by a relative sliding motion on
the conical interface between head and stem are considered as well
as the stresses due to alternating external loads distributed over
different areas on the sphere. Based on fracture mechanics maximum
allowable flaw depths for given life times are evaluated using these
stress distributions and the known slow crack growth behaviour of
different bioceramics. Under normal loading conditions a flaw depth
up to 500 μm can be accepted for an appropriate life time, whereas
assumming an accumulation of disadvantageous conditions the flaws
should not exceed 100 μm. For detecting such flaws a proof-testing
configuration is discussed.

INTRODUCTION

Due to their outstanding biocompatibility and wear resistance, ceramic heads are increasingly used in total hip-joint replacement. For
this application maximum possible safety against mechanical failure
must be ensured. Since the structural reliability for long times cannot be estimated with sufficient accuracy by statistically determined
strength values, more refined methods have to be employed which ex-
plicitly take into account the fact that the failure behaviour depends not only upon the applied stresses, but also on the size and
location of defects and the materials resistance to crack propagation.

STRESS DISTRIBUTIONS IN THE HEAD

The most common design for ceramic heads is a sphere which is attached to a metal stem via a conical interface. When this structure is
loaded in clinical applications two effects arise. First the sphere
will slide down on the cone and the enlargement of its diameter will
cause hoop stresses. Second, the shell at the end of the conical hole
will be subjected to bending deformation. In order to estimate the
influence of these effects finite-element (FE) calculations have been
performed with different models in which the different boundary conditions have been simulated. In all the cases investigated the tensile stresses – which are the most dangerous for ceramics – are grea-

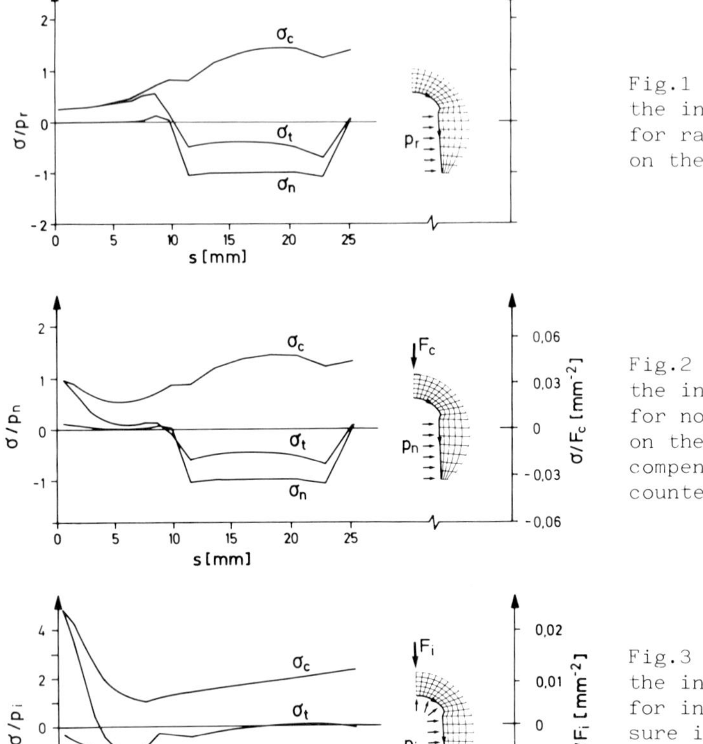

Fig.1 Stresses on the inner surface for radial pressure on the cone

Fig.2 Stresses on the inner surface for normal pressure on the cone and a compensating axial counterforce

Fig.3 Stresses on the inner surface for internal pressure in the hole and a concentrated axial counterforce

test at the surface of the conical hole. Therefore, only these surface stresses are considered in this paper. The part of the surface in question for each case is marked by a thick line on the FE-meshes shown in figures 1-7 along with the stress distributions. For every distribution the path s starts at the axis of symmetry.

Axial symmetric loading cases. The most important axial loading effect is produced by the relative sliding motion between sphere and stem. It can be assumed that the maximum relative motion will occur on overloading and that the sphere will remain in this position due to adhesive friction, thus producing a permanent "frozen" stress field. This case can be simulated by a constant radial pressure (p_r) on the inner cone surface (Fig.1). The circumferential stress (σ_c) which is generated reaches a maximum in the lower part of the cone and then decreases to about one fifth of this value towards the center of the upper shell. The tangential stresses (σ_t) are tensile and approximately equal to σ_c on the shell but change to compression on the cone. The normal stresses (σ_n) are determined by the boundary conditions.

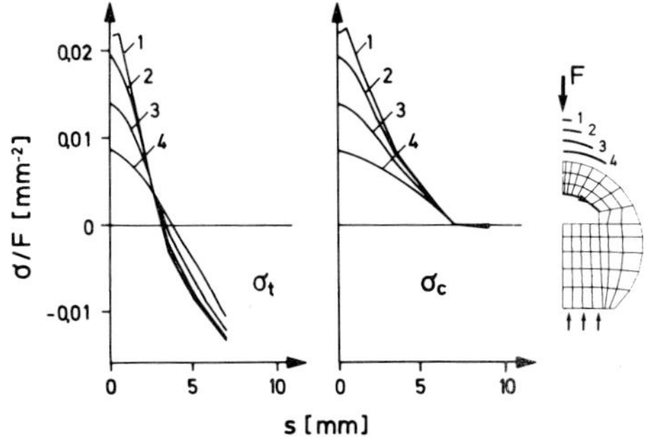

Fig.4 Tangential and circumferential stresses on the shell for
axial loading of different areas
– axial symmetric model

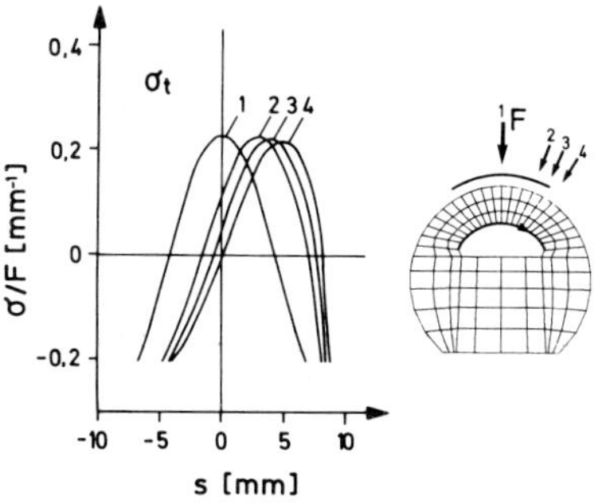

Fig.6 Tangential stresses on
the shell for different loading
directions

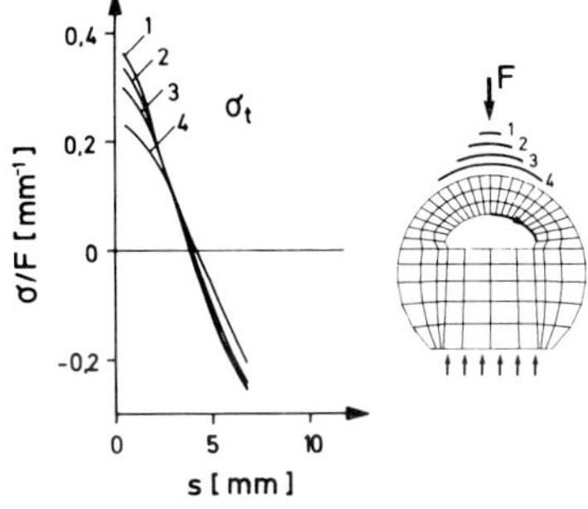

Fig.5 Tangential stresses on the
shell for symmetric loading of
different areas – plane model

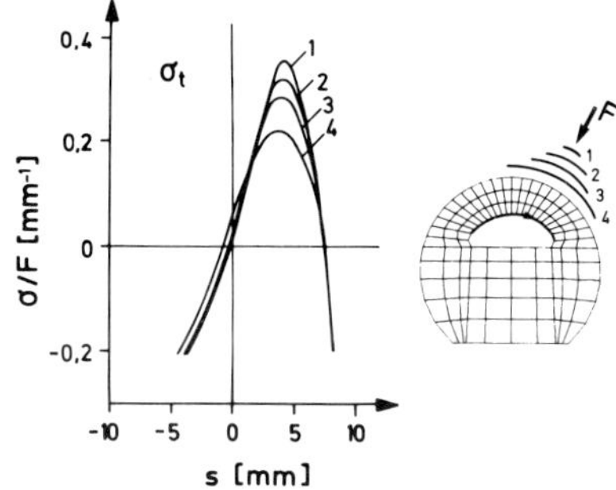

Fig.7 Tangential stresses on
the shell for oblique loading
of different areas

If we assume an average set of clinical parameters (a body weight
of 750 N and normal walking with an intensification factor of 4.5
due to inertial effects (Paul, 1976)) and a realistic friction coefficient of .65, a maximum σ_c of about 12 N/mm^2 will arise. Under extreme conditions (body weight 1000 N, intensification of 12 by a
jump) σ_c can increase to about 42 N/mm^2 and if in addition we assume
a very low friction coefficient of .2, a maximum σ_c of 135 N/mm^2 may
be achieved. In this case the tensile stresses on the shell surface
would be between 24 and 34 N/mm^2.
To check the influence of an additional bending of the shell the same
model has been examined with constant normal pressure (p_n) on the
cone and an axial counterforce F_c outside on the sphere (Fig.2)
which compensates the axial components of p_n. The resulting stress
profiles are similar to those in Fig.1 except for the region just
below the external force F_c. Here the stresses σ_c and σ_t are different, especially in the center where the stresses are higher by
about a factor of 4. This means that an external load has a considerable influence only on the stresses on the inside of the shell and
not an the cone. These results are in good agreement with those of
Maier et al. (1978) computed under similar assumptions.

A third case has been calculated with this model with the aim of obtaining an appropriate testing configuration in which the realistic conditions could be simulated. A constant hydrostatic pressure (p_i) is applied in the hole and the resulting component of force in the axial direction is compensated by a concentrated axial counterforce F_i (Fig.3). This leads to similar tensile stresses on the cone (compared with Fig.2) but to distinctly higher stresses on the inside of the shell.

In order to study the influence of pure bending for different load distributions, other structures have been generated in which the counterpart of the metal stem is also represented. In the FE-mesh stem and sphere are connected so that sliding cannot occur. But to allow all other real displacements, except sliding, the connection is made only at the nodes which transfer compression normal to the interface. Fig.4 shows the resulting circumferential and tangential stresses for different loaded areas on which the total force F is parabolically distributed. With decreasing area the stresses increase strongly; they are more than doubled going from the largest to the smallest area. These extreme areas roughly approximate the contact zones for combinations of the ceramic head with a polyethylene and a ceramic cup respectively.

Oblique loading. In the realistic application the head is loaded obliquely. To study the change of the stress distributions under these conditions plane strain models have been considered which represent sections of the sphere. Fig.5 shows once more the symmetric loading case now applied to this model. The plotted stresses are calculated for a variation of loaded areas comparable to those shown in Fig.4. Because of the two-dimensional idealization and the linear variation of the areas in Fig.5 as opposed to the real three-dimensional case with quadratic area variation in Fig.4, the stress levels cannot be compared. Furthermore, a circumferential stress does not exist in the plane model. It is obvious, however, that the shapes of the curves are very similar so that the ratios of the stresses in both models can be used as factors to transfer the results of one model to the other. By means of these factors the stresses in the real three-dimensional case can at least be estimated from results for oblique loading in the plane model.

Fig.6 shows the tangential stresses for different loading angles but with equal areas. The curves for σ_t are very similar in height and shape and are only shifted following the center of the applied load. In Fig.7 the stresses are plotted for different loading areas with an angle of 27° between the normal and the applied force, which is approximately the normal physiological position. The maximum values change in practically the same manner as for symmetric loading (Fig.5). From these results it can be concluded that the maximum tensile stresses in the real three-dimensional structure under oblique loading are essentially the same as for axial loading, but that the position of the highly stressed region changes corresponding to the loading angle.

LIFE TIME CALCULATIONS

These computed stress distributions are used to calculate maximum

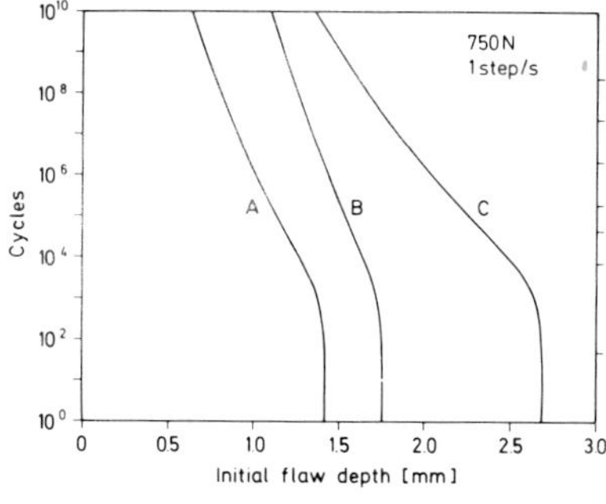

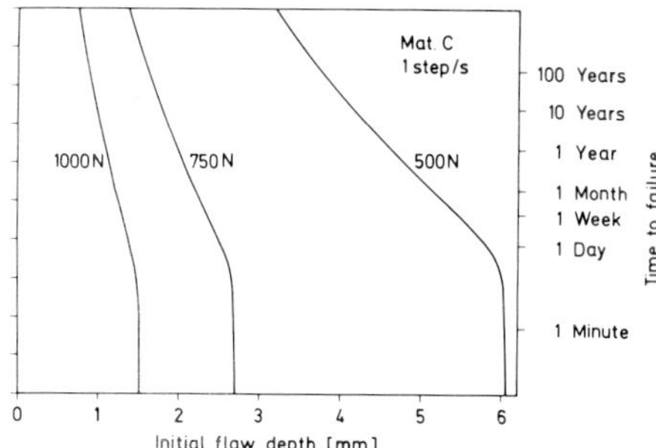

a. Influence of material   b. Influence of body weight

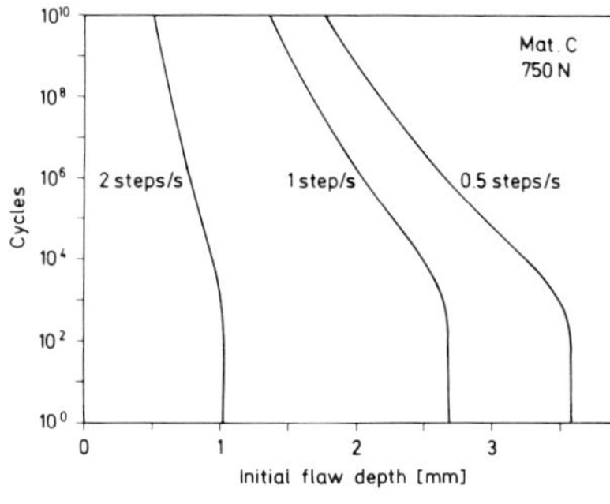

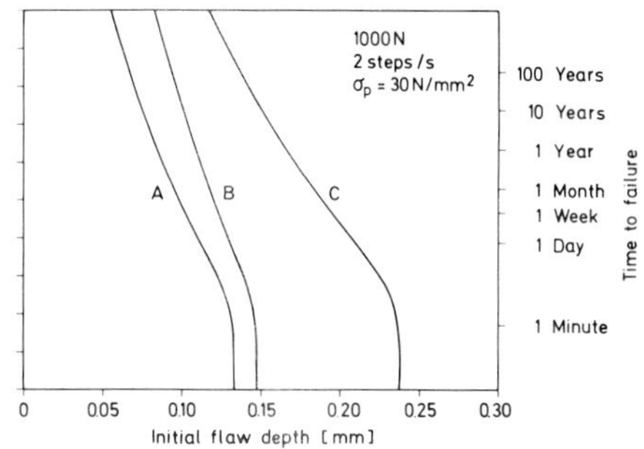

c. Influence of walking speed   d. Extreme conditions

Fig.8 Calculated life times for different bioceramics and different
      loading conditions

allowable flaw depths to achieve given life times, using a fracture
mechanics model and the experimentally measured dependence of slow
crack propagation rate on the loading conditions (Richter et al.,
1977). Details of the procedure have been described earlier (Seidelmann et al., 1978). For the "frozen" stresses caused by the relative
sliding motion, i.e. for constant load conditions, the allowed flaw
depths for a life time of 100 years are in the range of 1 mm or more
for the different bioceramics; this is even true in the extreme case
of 135 N/mm^2. Such flaws could be detected by normal inspection.

For external loading a time dependence must be considered. For these
calculations a load function was assumed which idealizes the physical
conditions during walking as described by Paul (1976). Fig.8 shows
several results for varying loading conditions. In each diagram the
life time in walking cycles (and in years assuming 2 hours walking
per day) is plotted against the maximum allowable initial flaw depth.
All curves are calculated for a semielliptical flaw, which describes
the most probable shape, and for the highest stresses according to
Fig.4, i.e. for a very small contact zone of head and cup. In Fig.8a
the influence of material is demonstrated under normal conditions
which are defined by a body weight of 750 N and a normal walking
speed of 1 step per second. Three different high density alumina are
considered which are produced as bioceramics by three German manu-
factureres. Fig.8b gives an example of the influence of body weight

and Fig.8c of the walking speed in comparison with the normal case. Under all these conditions the allowable flaw depth for long times to failure is greater than 500 um which should not appear in a standard quality product so that there should be no risk of failure. In Fig.8d an accumulation of disadvantageous conditions is assumed: high body weight, fast walking, and an additional frozen stress of $30N/mm^2$ in the shell region which was estimated as the mean value under the extreme assumptions of symmetrical axial loading. Under these conditions the flaw depths to achieve long life times become smaller than 100 um at least for two materials which is a range where flaws cannot be found by normal inspection; i.e. although such faults are not very probable there remains a risk.

PROOF TESTING

In order to avoid any remaining risk of failure proof tests can be performed (Evans & Wiederhorn, 1974). This means that the heads should be loaded statically in such a way that all regions in which tensile stresses are caused in the real application, are stressed with a similar distribution. The load level must be chosen so that all heads with flaws deeper than a maximum value obtained from the life time calculations for a desired life time, will be destroyed. For all heads surviving this test a minimum life time will be guaranteed. An appropriate proof configuration would be a test with internal pressure in the conical hole as shown in Fig.3. This configuration is similar to that proposed by Maier et al. (1978) which is, however, restricted to proof against failure resulting from the "frozen" stresses. With an arrangement such as that shown in Fig.3, it is possible to test also against failure by the external loads,which is more dangerous. Furthermore, in this arrangement the proof stress level in the shell can easily be adapted to the corresponding level in practice by choosing the right loading area for the counterforce F.

REFERENCES

Evans, A.G.; Wiederhorn, S.M. (1974): Proof Testing of Ceramic Materials - An Analytical Basis of Failure Prediction, Int.J.Fracture 10, 379-392
Maier, H.R.; Stärk, N.; Krauth, A. (1978): Reliability of Ceramic-Metallic Hip Joints Based on Strength Analysis, Proof- and Structural Testing, 3rd Conf. on Mat. for Use in Medicine and Biology, Mechanical Properties of Biomaterials, Keele, UK
Paul, J.P. (1976): Loading on Normal Hip and Knee Joints and on Joint Replacements, in Advances in Artificial Hip and Knee Joint Technology (Eds. M. Schaldach, D. Hohmann) Springer, Berlin/Heidelberg/New York
Richter, H.; Seidelmann, U.; Soltész, U. (1977): Slow crack growth and failure for alumina in simulated physiological media, 1st Europ. Conf.on Evaluation of Biomaterials, Strasbourg
Seidelmann, U.; Richter, H.; Soltész, U. (1978): Failure of ceramic hip endoprostheses by slow crack growth - predictions of life-time, Congr.on Biomaterials and Biomechanics, Brussels

This work has been sponsored by the German Ministry for Research and Technology (BMFT).

Biomaterials 1980
Edited by G. D. Winter, D. F. Gibbons, and H. Plenk, Jr.
© 1982 John Wiley and Sons Ltd.

LONG LIFE CERAMIC-METAL HIP JOINTS

H.R. Maier, A.Krauth, N.Stärk, A. Zeibig

Rosenthal AG, Institut für Werkstofftechnik
Rosenthal Technik AG, Werksgruppe III
Wittelsbacher Str. 49, D 8672 Selb

SUMMARY

The objective is to prolong the life time of endoprostheses to much greater than ten years by application of ceramic materials. The long life mechanical reliability of ceramic components can be secured by proof testing. A method which achieves this goal is described for a cone fitted cast CoCrMo stem-alumina sphere-polyethylene cup prosthesis (fig.1), however it may be applied in a similar manner to more sophisticated alternatives.

INTRODUCTION

The weak links in the reliability chain concerning lifetime of conventional systems are stem loosening and subsequently stem failure, which are accompanied by bio-responses to the wear and corrosion products (Ungetühm 1980), (Semlitsch, 1978), (Friedebold, 1978), (Vernon-Roberts, 1978). A prerequisite for taking full advantages of the excellent friction, wear, corrosion and biocompatibility properties of alumina is however the longterm reliability of the ceramic sphere and its fixation to the metallic stem. The topics addressed in this paper are pointed out in fig. 1.

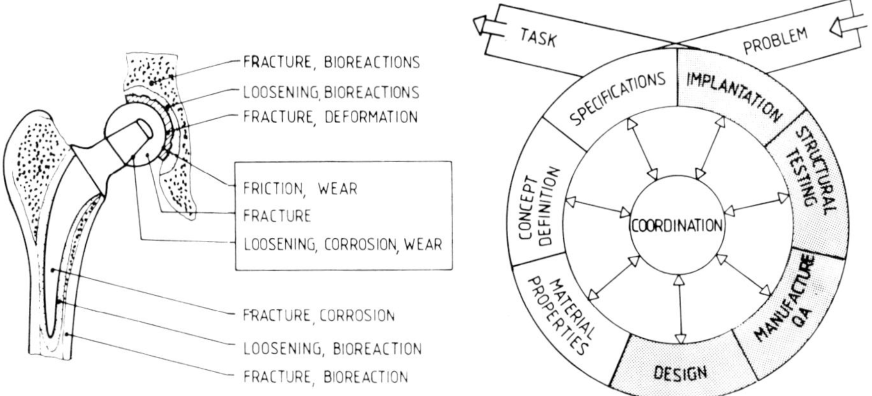

Fig. 1: CoCrMo stem-alumina sphere-polyethylen cup
Failure modes and quality assurance cycle

SPECIFICATIONS

The following requirements refer to the metal stem-ceramic sphere-polyethylene cup prosthesis:
life time much greater than 10 years
maximum load 9000 N (5000 N for metal stem)(Semlitsch, 1978)
variable load between 1000 and 9000 N
reliable fixation of sphere to stem
minimum friction and wear between sphere and cup

CONCEPT DEFINITION

The ceramic sphere-polyethylene cup concept is not only applicable to a
stem prosthesis but also to ceramic femoral head resurfacing prostheses
(Wagner, 1978). An alternative approach to improvement of wear and
friction is the ceramic sphere-ceramic cup concept.
The solide cone fixation methode produces very unfavourable tensile
stresspattern within the ceramic sphere, requires high precision for cone
dimensions and makes a hot sterilization difficult. However it has the
advantage of restricted micromovement, which could causes wear and
corrosion problems.

MATERIAL PROPERTIES

Alumina: Most alumina materials employed nowadays exceed the German
Standard DIN 58835 Teil 1 and the corresponding ISO-draft. For the calculation of dimensions and lifetime of alumina spheres however we need
additional characteristics (Maier, 1978).
- statistical values in Ringer's solution (σ_{ov} = 560 N/mm^{-2}, m = 12.5)
- fracture thoughness in air as proof test (K_{IC} = 4.1 MNm$^{-3/2}$)
- subcritical crack growth in Ringer's solution
   (n = 63, -log a = 418 for crack velocity in m/s)

Interface alumina sphere-polyethylene cup: The wear rate of the polyethy-
lene/alumina interface is about 1/10 th if compared with the polyethyle-
ne/metal concept. Even better results are obtained however with the combination alumina/alumina (Dörre, 1978). Results of (Ungethüm, 1978),
(Wright, 1978), (Blanquaert, 1978), differ from each other, but when
applied properly, alumina can improve lifetime and clinical success.

Interface alumina sphere-metal stem: Permanent "frozen" stress incor-
peration after removing external load has been measured by strain gauges
(fig. 2 left). Micromovement and corrosion effects are very small for
the solid cone fixation (fig. 2, right), (Thull, 1980).

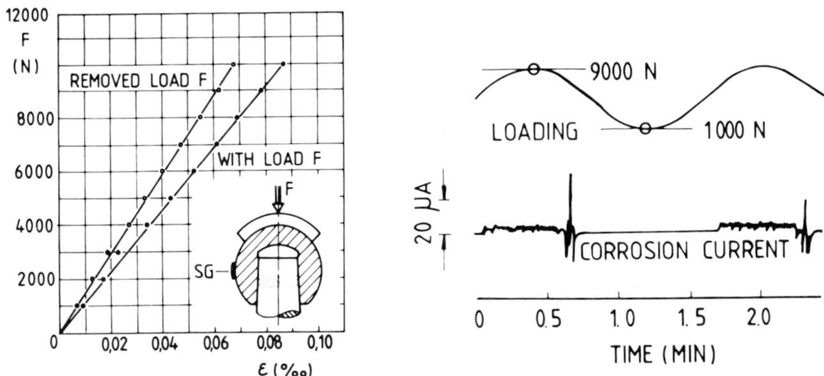

Fig. 2: Permanent strain and corrosion measurement

DESIGN

The design criteria, including size effect (statistics), fracture mechanics, subcritical crack growth and combinations of those points are discussed in (Maier, 1978). The principle loading conditions for a sphere with an outer diameter of 32 mm and their resultant surface hoop stresses σ_u are shown in fig. 3. The finite element calculations were confirmed by strain gauge measurements at the outer meridian surface. The additional risk caused by inclined loading may be compensated by a suitably higher proof testing level. Based on the data at page 2 a life time of much more than 10 years has been predicted (Maier, 1978). The assumption of the applied hypotheses are summerized in (Johnson, 1979), (Evans, 1974).

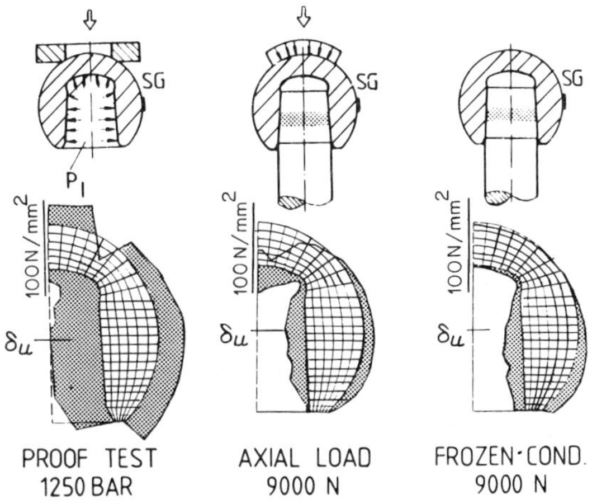

Fig. 3: Distribution of surface hoop stresses

MANUFACTURING AND QUALITY ASSURANCE

<u>Mechanical reliability of spheres.</u> In order to assure mechanical reliabili-
ty of alumina spheres it is necessary to take into account e.g. residual
stresses, anisotropic structures and mechanical respectivly thermal overloading during fabrication and handling. Therefor careful proof testing procedures have been developed.
1. The dome base region unter axial cycling load, fig. 3 middle.
2. The cone region after removed axial load, fig. 3 right.
The objective is to eliminate all outliers (anomalies) with undetectable
flaws above a certain size by internal pressure overloading, fig. 4. The
following points are of prime importance:
- the maximum applied stress profile σ_a s known
- the proof stress profile σ_p is similar to σ_a (fig. 3)
- the minimum quality is given by the proof testing level
- the risk of predamaging during proof testing is controlled by a tandem
  procedure with a second level reduced by 20 %
- the ratio of σ_p / σ_a depends on subcritical crack growth and also on the
  considerable number of unknown effects.
Proof testing is most suitable for keeping down the manufacturing costs
(process control) to guarantee a certain quality level (final and acceptance control) and to calculate the distribution of the occupied spheres to the
failed ones.

<u>Friction and wear properties.</u> The friction and wear properties are ensured
by control of the microstructure (DIN 58835, Teil 1), surface raughness
(CLA < 0.025 /um) and deviation from sphericity (< 3 /um).

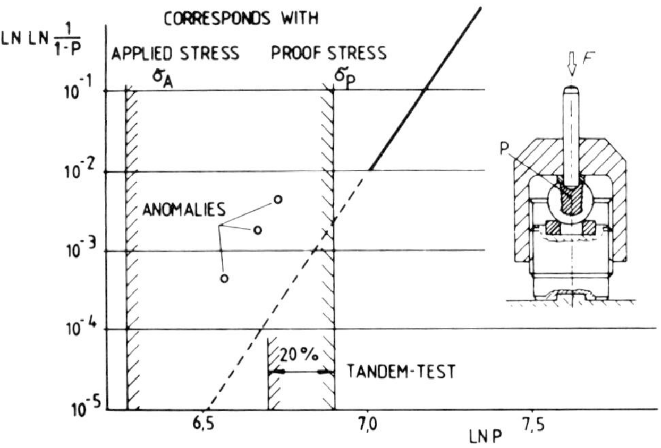

Fig. 4: Principle of tandem proof testing

MECHANICAL TESTING

It has been shown that it is relativly simple to calculate reliability and
lifetime of ceramic components according to certain assumptions
(Maier, 1978). However there are also a large number of interacting
factors, e.g. statistics (Johnson, 1979), fracture mechanics and proof
testing (Evens, 1974). The obvious solution is: simulation testing before "in vivo" application.

Static and impact axial cone loading. The loading capacity of cone fitted
spheres has been demonstrated by static cone loading with mean fractur-
re loads up to 52000 N. Peak loads of the same region (48000 N) have
been measured in an impact test be releasing a mass of 3 kg from a
heigth of 1m. In comparsion to the maximum loading capacity of metal
stems (about 5000 N) the mean quality of alumina spheres is outstanding. The only problem is the "outlier", e.g. 1 out of 1000.

Quick motion mechanical cycling of prostheses. The influence of inclined loading (23 degrees between load
and cone axis) has been tested by a
specially developed double unit device
fig. 5. More than 20 original prostheses were tested under the following
conditions:
- proof testing at 1250 bar after firing
- sinoidal cycling between 1000 and
  9000 N
- 10^6 up to 10^7 cycles with 37 Hz
- in Ringer's solution at 25-37 $^\circ$C
All prostheses survived the cycling
test without any damage. After
cycling the prostheses were stressed
with increasing load up to fracture
which was greater than 35 KN. There
is therefor no major effect caused by
inclined loading.

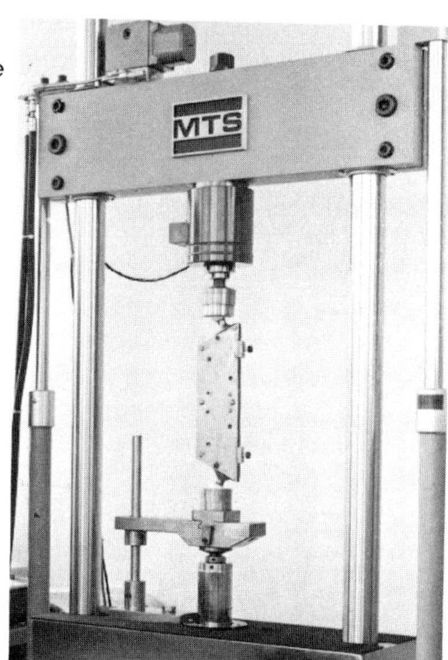

Fig. 5: Double unit cycling of
original prostheses

COMBINED STATIC-CYCLING TEST OF PROSTHESES.

The time load sequence starts with the implantation technique and subsequently on the activity of the patient. This implies a combination of "frozen" stresses in the cone region (relaxed human body, fig. 2 left and fig. 3 right), and random cycling stresses in the base of the dome region of the sphere (fig. 3 middle). With these concepts in mind the following tests have been initiated for a period of five years.

Preliminary tests. Three lots of spheres with 100 % final proof testing of the cone region at levels of 900, 1000 and 1250 bars have been wetted with Ringer's solution before fitting to original stems and axial loading up to 9000 N.

Static-cycling test no. 1. Proof test level 900 bar, 8 prostheses. Alternation of quick motion cycling (37 Hz, 10^4 cycles) between 1000 and 9000 N and storage in Ringer's solution at 37 $^{\circ}$C for about two weeks ("frozen"condition without external load).
Result: 2.2×10^5 cycles during 45 weeks without any fracture.

Static-cycling test no. 2. Proof test level 1250 bar, 3 prostheses. Identical with test no. 1. Result: 2.2×10^6 cycles during 45 weeks without any fracture.

Static-cycling test no. 3. Proof test level 1250 bar, 7 prostheses. Similar to test no. 1 Result: 10^5 cycles (during 22 weeks) between 1000 and 20000 N after 1.2×10^5 cycles (during 23 weeks) between 1000 and 9000 N.

Static-cycling test no. 4. Proof test level 1000 bar, 8 prostheses. Alternation of quick motion cycling (37 Hz, 10^4 cycles) between 1000 N and stepwise increased upper load (fig. 5) and storage in Ringer's solution for one or two weeks Result: First fracture after 13 weeks (1.1×10^5 cycles) during cycling at 22000 N. Subsequent alternation at a cyling level of 23000 N, 1.5×10^4 cycles, during 32 weeks without additional fracture.

Static-cycling test no. 5. Proof test level 1250 bar, 4 prostheses. Similar to test no. 3. Result: First fracture after 38 weeks (2.9×10^5 cycles) during cycling at 40000 N. Second fracture after 41 weeks (3.1×10^5 cycles) during storage after cycling at 39000 N. Subsequent alternation at a cycling level of 39000 N, 2×10^4 cycles during 7 weeks without additional fracture.

The test arrangement for storage in Ringer's solution ("frozen" condition without external load) and the sequence of test no. 4 is given in fig. 6. Result: Although strain gauges measurements have indicated a decrease of "frozen" condition with time fracture may be caused without external load if no or not sufficient proof testing is applied.

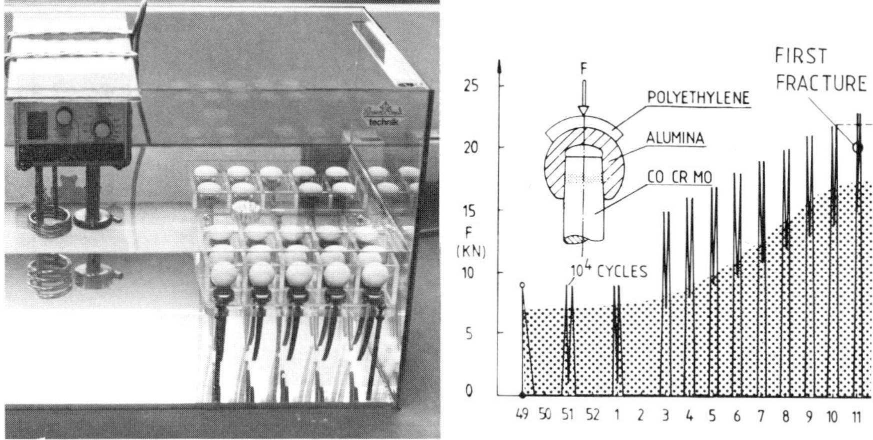

Fig. 6: Combined static-cycling test no. 4

IMPLANTATION

There is a need for a defined implantation procedure in order to secure a reliable cone fixation of sphere to stem and to avoid a one-peak-over-loading, for instance by hammering in of the prostheses. A compound hot-sterilisation is impossible because of the different thermal expansion coefficients.

CONCLUSIONS

Structural reliability of alumina spheres depends primarily on the absolute elimination of outliers and not on the mean quality of alumina. It is easier to define a certain quality of the ceramic component by proof testing than to define an absolute upper limit of the applied stress. Compared to these facts, subcritical crack growth of alumina which occurs considerably below a ratio of σ_p / σ_a 1.3 - 1.5 (fig. 4) is of less importance: A proof test level of 1000 bar at a maximum load of 9000 N corresponds to a "safty ratio" σ_p / σ_a > 2.3 and in comparsion with the maximum load of 5000 N for a metallic stem (Semlitsch, 1978), there is no risk of rupture for proof tested ceramic spheres. If, at the beginning of human implantations in 1976, a quality assurance procedure as described, would have been available in combination with certain implantation instructions, we would be in the position to present a much more successful balance than 6 known catastrophic failures out of about 2000 delivered alumina spheres.

ACKNOWLEDGEMENT

This study is supported by the German Federal Ministry of Research and Technology under Grant No. 01 VG 119 - ZK/NT/MT 290

REFERENCES

Blanquaert, D. (1978) Evaluation of wear and frictional torque on hip prosthesis with different simulators. Comparsion of various materials combinations, including alumina-alumina combination, in Advances in Biomaterials, Mechanical Properties of Biomaterials (Eds., Hastings & Williams). Wiley, London. In press.

Dörre, E. & Dawihl, W. (1978) Mechanische und tribologische Eigenschaften keramischer Endoprothesen. Biomed. Techn. 23, 305-310.

Evans. A.G. & Wiederhorn, S.M. (1974) Proof testing of ceramic materials - an analytical basis for failure prediction. International Journal of Fracture, 10, 379-392.

Friedebold, G. & Kölbel, R. (1976) State of the art of hip and knee joint replacement, in Artifical Hip and Knee Joint Technology (Eds., Schaldach & Hohmann), 3-24. Springer, Berlin.

Johnson, C.A. (1979) Fracture statistics in design and applications. Reprint. Agard-Structure and Panel, Specialists Meeting on Ceramics for Turbine Engine Applications. DFVLR, Cologne.

Maier, H.R., Stärk, N. & Krauth, A. (1978) Reliability of ceramic-metallic hip joints, based on strength analysis, proof and structural testing, in Advances in Biomaterials, Mechanical Properties of Biomaterials (Eds. Hastings & Williams). Wiley, London. In press.

Semlitsch, M. & Panic, B. (1978) Corrosion fatique testing of femoral head prostheses made of implant alloys of different fatique resistance, in Advances in Biomaterials, Mechanical Properties of Biomaterials (Eds., Hastings & Williams). Wiley, London. In press.

Thull, R. & Schaldach, M. (1980) Mechanische und elektrochemische Ausfallmechanismen orthopädischer Gelenkimplantate, in Implantatbrüche, 1. Vortragsreihe des Arbeitskreises Implantate, DVM, Berlin.

Ungethüm, M. Hinterberger, J. & Plitz, W. (1978) Tribological Properties of Al_2O_3-ceramics, in Advances in Biomaterials, Mechanical Properties of Biomaterials (Eds., Hastings & Williams). Wiley, London. In press.

Ungethüm M. (1980) Ursachen von Prothesenschaftbrüchen und Möglichkeiten zu deren Vermeidung, in Biomed. Techn., to be published.

Vernon-Roberts, B. & Freeman, M.A.R. (1976) Morphological and analytical studies of the tissues adjacent to joint prosthesis: investigations into the causes of loosening of prostheses, in Artifical Hip and Knee Joint Technology (Eds. Schaldach & Hohmann). 148-186. Springer Berlin.

Wagner, H. (1978) Surface replacement orthroplasty of the hip. Clinical Arthopedics and Related Research, Vol. 134, 102 - 1380.

Wright, K.W. J. & Scales, H.J. (1978) Wear and friction studies on materials and total hip prostheses, in Advances in Biomaterials, Mechanical Properties of Biomaterials (Eds. Hastings & Williams). Wiley, London. In press.

Corrosion of metallic implants

Biomaterials 1980
Edited by G. D. Winter, D. F. Gibbons, and H. Plenk, Jr.
© 1982 John Wiley and Sons Ltd.

FACTORS AFFECTING THE CORROSION OF SURGICAL IMPLANTS

M. T. Shepherd* and R. Wilkinson

Bioengineering Unit, University of Strathclyde,
Wolfson Centre, 106 Rottenrow, Glasgow G4 ONW, U.K.

SUMMARY

Results from an examination of retrieved surgical implants are presented.
A method for assessing contact corrosion on steel implants is described and used
to assess the influence of various factors on the observed corrosion.   Chemical
compositions outside BS 3531 have been found in 8/43 components, inclusions
containing calcium and aluminium have been shown to reduce corrosion resistance
as has increased (although within specification) silicon.   Different patterns of
corrosion incidence have been observed in different classes of implant.

INTRODUCTION

Ever since man first attempted to use implanted artificial materials to repair the
human body, interactions between implant and body have been a problem.
Stainless steel is a commonly used metal in orthopaedic surgery since it is
relatively cheap and easy to work but suffers the disadvantage of liability to
contact corrosion (Cohen and Hammond, 1959, Scales, 1959, Scales, 1961,
Weinstein et al, 1973).   Crevice, galvanic, pitting and fretting mechanisms
have all been suggested (How and Mears, 1966, Williams and Roaf, 1973,
Jordan, 1976).

Poor heat treatment, allowing the steel to remain in the 'sensitisation' range of
$500^{\circ}C$ to $950^{\circ}C$, may cause precipitation of chromium carbide in the grain
boundaries and consequent loss of protective chromium oxide in the adjacent
grain unless the carbon content is lowered below 0.03% (Cahoon and Paxton,
1968, Hughes and Jordan, 1972).   Other inclusions and their effects on
corrosion have not been extensively studied in type 316 stainless steel, although
some data does exist for other steels (Jordan, 1976, Galante and Rostoker, 1972,
Baltitude and Morris, 1972, Smialowska, 1972).

This paper seeks to assess the effects of different inclusions on the corrosion
resistance of stainless steel and to identify other factors such as chemical
composition or implant design which may be manipulated to reduce observed
corrosion.

* Present address – Deloro Surgical
Swindon, England

227

METHOD

Multi-component implants removed at surgery were collected, assayed for bacterial contamination, autoclaved, washed and dried.   Details of age and sex of patient, duration and site of implantation, reason for removal and antibiotics administered within 72 hours of surgery were supplied by the hospital. Devices had been used for fracture fixation or sometimes osteotomy of the long bones.   Each component was examined visually and corrosion on any surface noted.   The Vickers hardness number was determined.   One hundred and seventy-one screw heads were mounted for examination in a Philips SEM 500 fitted with peak energy dispersive X-ray analysis facilities.   Polished sections were prepared from 44 randomly selected screws and samples for microprobe analysis from a random selection of 37 screws and 6 plates used in a different study.

A number of corroded areas were photographed in the SEM and 20 areas ranging from barely detectable to the maximum observed corrosion arranged in rank order and assigned a grade number from 1 to 20.   Each corroded surface was examined and the area corresponding to a particular grade estimated, the corrosion rating (Corr) was then calculated as:-

$$\text{Corr} = 0.1 \sum_1^{20} A_1 G_1 + \ldots A_n G_n \ldots + A_{20} G_{20}$$

where A = area in μm^2,   and G = grade.

Inclusions visible in a randomly selected area of 2,500 sq. μm on the polished sections were identified and measured using the PSEM 500.   Wavelength dispersive analysis was used to determine chemical composition of the matrix to avoid problems with the simultaneous presence of molybdenum and sulphur. Carbon analysis could not be carried out on the small amount of available material using University equipment.   The results were statistically analysed using the SPSS package on an IBM 370 computer.

RESULTS

Typical examples of mild (grade 2) and severe (grade 16) corrosion are shown in Figs. 1 and 2 respectively.

Incidence of corrosion was tabulated for each countersink of 4 classes of device, rigid hip nails, sliding hip nails, variable angle hip nails and straight fracture plates; in each case hole 1 was proximal.   From Table 1 it can be seen that the pattern of corrosion varies between the four groups.   The relatively high incidence of corrosion on variable angle hip nails and the fact that the proximal hole is most likely to be corroded in sliding hip nails but least likely in variable angle hip nails are worthy of note.

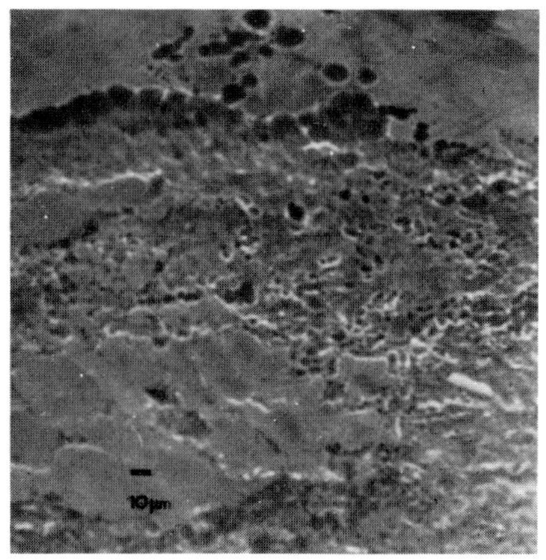

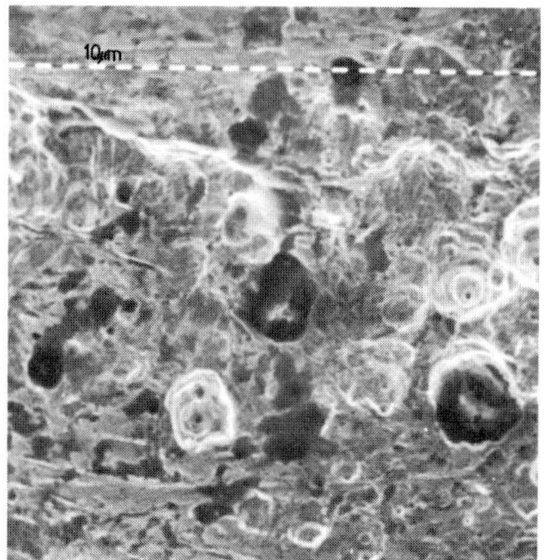

Fig. 1 A typical example
of mild (grade 2) corrosion

Fig. 2 A typical example
of severe (grade 16) corrosion

TABLE 1. Incidence of corrosion on four classes of implant

Hole number	1	2	3	4	5	6	7	8	Last
Sliding hipnail	100%	50%	40%						50%
Rigid hipnail	66%	75%	50%	66%					50%
Variable angle hipnails	71%	100%	100%	100%	100%	100%	100%		100%
Tibial plates	82%	68%	55%	69%	61%	39%	75%	57%	41%

Examination of mean values of different variables (Table 2) shows that on
average plates were softer than screws by 50–60 VPN although in individual
cases plates may be harder than screws, explaining the large standard deviation
in VHDiff.   None of the values measured on the SEM has a normal distribution
but aluminium-containing inclusions represent the largest volume fraction.

After microprobe analysis, six components were found to have nickel contents
less than British Standard and 2 components had manganese contents higher than
British Standard allowing for a 10% error in the values obtained.

Regression analysis showed that only three results significantly affected the
corrosion rating, calcium and aluminium inclusions and silicon content.

The equation produced was:-

$$\text{Corr} = 1.47 \text{ Ca Inc} + 802\% \text{ Si} + \text{Al Inc}$$

where Ca Inc = calcium inclusion, Al Inc = aluminium inclusion

The equation is probably of more value in indicating significant variables rather than any interpretation of the coefficients.

TABLE 2. Means of variables

Variable	No. of Cases	Mean	Std. Dev.
Time	147	32.5	37.1
Age	148	43.6	24.1
VHScrew	171	316.2	34.8
VHPlate	138	248.8	60.1
VHDiff	136	55.6	58.9
Corr	163	76.4	170.0
Inc Rat	44	186.2	169.6
% Cr	37	18.0	0.42
% Ni	37	12.0	1.51
% Mo	37	2.73	9.23
% Mn	37	1.71	0.21
% Si	37	0.42	0.12

DISCUSSION

The first problem when discussing factors affecting the corrosion of retrieved implants is to define and measure 'corrosion'.   Incidence of corrosion is relatively easy to assess reproducibly but severity is more difficult. Weight loss and volume loss are not applicable to retrieved implants from a clinical situation and some form of grading system is often used.   Such systems are essentially subjective although often reproducible for a single observer.   The system used in this study attempted to reduce the element of subjectivity by adapting standard photographs which could be employed by different observers.   However the method of converting grade to rating presupposes a linear scale which cannot be checked, departures are more likely at the higher end.

Explanations for the changes in patterns of corrosion are not easy to find but may be in the realm of interfacial stress between screw and plate. Hardness and hardness difference did not significantly affect corrosion. It is suggested that the effects of small changes in electrode potential caused by work hardening are masked by other uncontrolled variables in a clinical situation.

Small changes in chemical composition may affect corrosion resistance. The increased corrosion found in implants with more aluminium and calcium inclusions (probably from deoxidation procedures) suggests that better quality control is needed. This is borne out by the 8/43 components outside British Standard specification, 6 of which were low nickel concentrations. Low nickel predisposes to δ-ferrite formation and further investigations are planned. The effect of silicon needs further investigation since it may be possible to further reduce silicon concentration in stainless steel by changing steel-making practice.

Thus improvements in corrosion resistance may be possible by better specification and quality control.

ACKNOWLEDGMENTS

This work was supported by the Science and Medical Research Councils. The assistance of Glasgow Royal Infirmary and Gartnavel General Hospital in supplying the implants and the University of Edinburgh in providing X-ray facilities is greatly appreciated.

REFERENCES

Bultitude, F.W. & Morris, J.R. (1972) The corrosion of surgical implants. Laboratory study of the corrosion of implants. DHSS project A101, A.W.R.E. GR0/44/83/29.
Cahoon, J.R. & Paxton, H.W. (1968) Metallurgical analysis of failed orthopaedic implants. J. Biomed. Mater. Res. 2, 1-22.
Cohen, J. & Hammond, G. (1959) Corrosion in a device for fracture fixation. J. Bone Jt. Surg. 41A, 524-34.
Galante, J. & Rostoker, W. (1972) Corrosion related failures in metallic implants: an experimental study. Clin. Orthop. Rel. Res. 86, 237.
Hoar, T.P. & Mears, D.C. (1966) Corrosion resistant alloys in chloride solutions: materials for surgical implants. Proc. Roy. Soc. A294, 486-510.
Hughes, A.N. & Jordan, B.A. (1972) Metallurgical observations on some surgical implants which failed in vivo. J. Biomed. Mater. Res. 6, 33-48.
Jordan, B.A. (1976) The characteristics of fretting and fretting corrosion damage in surgical implant materials. DHSS project A129, A.W.R.E. 44/83/18.
Kinoshita, N., Ohashi, N. & Takeda, M. (1976) Effect of the composition of

non-metallic inclusions on the rusting of ferritic stainless steels. Trans Iron Steel Inst. Japan 16, 251-7.

Scales, J.T., Winter, G.D. & Shirley, H.T. (1959) Corrosion of orthopaedic implants - screws, plates and femoral nails. J. Bone Jt. Surg. 41B, 810-20.

Scales, J.T., Winter, G.D. & Shirley, H.T. (1961) Corrosion of orthopaedic implants - Smith-Peterson type hip nails. Brit. Med. J. 2, 478-82.

Smialowska, Z.S. (1972) Influence of sulphide inclusions on the pitting corrosion of steels. Corr. 28, 388-96.

Weinstein, A., Amstutz, H., Pavan, G. & Franceschini, V. (1973) Orthopaedic implants: a clinical and metallurgical analysis. J. Biomed. Mater. Res. Symp. 4, 297-325.

Williams, D.F. & Roaf, R. (1973) Implants in Surgery, W.B. Saunders & Co.

Biomaterials 1980
Edited by G. D. Winter, D. F. Gibbons, and H. Plenk, Jr.
© 1982 John Wiley and Sons Ltd.

INFLUENCE OF FORGING AND HEAT TREATMENT ON FATIGUE-
CORROSION BEHAVIOUR OF TI 6-4 TITANIUM ALLOY
Application for total hip prostheses

SUTTER, E.M.M., CORNET, A.

Ecole Nationale Supérieure des Arts et Industries
24 Bld de la Victoire F 67000 STRASBOURG

JAEGER, J.H., Centre de Traumatologie and MUSTER, D.,
Lab. Chir. Maxillofaciale

Groupe d'Etudes de Biomécanique Ostéo-Articulaire de
Strasbourg.

SUMMARY

With the Ti 6-4 titanium alloy, we have investigated the effect of
forging conditions ($\alpha + \beta$ or β) and thermal treatments on the fatigue
limit under rotating bend stresses, in air and in simulated
biological solution. The fatigue behaviour depends more on the metallurgical structure of the alloy than on its environment.

INTRODUCTION

In the recent years, Ti 6-4 titanium alloy (which contains 6 %
aluminium and 4 % vanadium) was demonstrated as an especially
attractive material for total hip prostheses, with regard to its
mechanical properties and to its corrosion behaviour (Steinemann,
1980, Cornet et al, 1978, Cornet et al, 1979, Muster et al, 1979).

When submitted to electrochemical corrosion in a simulated biological environment, this material shows a remarkable corrosion resistance which is reflected in the current-potential curves (Fig. 1).

Knowledge of the fatigue limit is needed because of the different
forging conditions and the various heat treatments that this alloy
may undergo. Table I indicates the structures and the usual industrial treatments for Ti 6-4. Our fatigue tests were performed on
these different structures and treatments. All the samples used in
our experiments were obtained from the same initial ingot. These
fatigue tests have been performed under rotating bend stresses in
air or in the Ringer's solution. (Table II).

MATERIAL AND METHODS

Auvinet et al (1973), Stubbington and Bowen (1974), Hempel and
Hillnhagen (1966) have reported the Wöhler S-N curves of the TI 6-4
alloy in $\alpha + \beta$ or β forging conditions.
These curves show the variation of the stresses as a function of
the number of cycles which are applied in rotating bend tests.
Because of the relatively low number of samples (we had four samples
for each type of heat treatment in each type of environment) we used
the Locati method to determine the fatigue limit. This method
consists in an application of loading steps during a given number of

cycles (10^5) and in calculation of the cumulated damages using the most likely Wöhler's curves. Whe have also submitted some samples to constant loads, either under the presumed fatigue limit, or in the range of high stresses, in order to readjust if necessary the Wöhler curves found in the literature.

Fatigue tests :

The samples were tested according to the diagram given in Fig. 2 and the central region was polished with 6/0 abrasive paper strips in order to avoid the working scratches which may result in an incipient crack.

The test machine used is a Schenck rotating bend machine at 3,000 rpm (Fig. 2.) A pledget of cotton impregnated with Ringer's solution comes into contact with the central region of the sample where the solution drips on to the specimen.

RESULTS

The corrected Wöhler's curves which were used for the calculation of the cumulated damages are given on Fig. 3 and 4 for all the $\alpha + \beta$ forged samples and for all the β forged samples.
Table III indicates the mean values of the fatigue limits calculated for each type of heat treatment and for each environment.
It appears that :

A) all the $\alpha + \beta$ forged samples show a better fatigue limit than the β forged samples

B) for each type of forging, the quenched and tempered state allows one to obtain a fatigue strength slightly higher than in the annealed state

C) there is no significative difference for the same type of heat treatment between the tests performed in the open air or in the simulated biological environment.
It must be underlined that during the tests under corrosion, 50 % of the samples broke out of the zone in contact with the Ringer's solution. This fact seems to confirm that the Ti 6-4 alloy is poorly sensitive to corrosion in biological environment.

DISCUSSION

We have compared our results with other data found in the literature and obtained in similar test conditions.

Laziou (1976) evaluates the mechanical tensile characteristics of the Ti 6-4 alloy, with regard to the heat treatment and finds the best tensile strength characteristics for the quenched state, whether followed by annealing or not. However, the ductility characteristics appear rather weak for this type of treatment.

In general the fatigue limit varies in a similar way to that of the tensile strength and this fact seems well confirmed by our measurements.

Stubbington and Bowen (1974) observe a better fatigue behaviour of the $\alpha + \beta$ forged alloys in comparison with β forged alloys. The initiation of the cracks in the later case, which is corresponds to an acicular structure, would seem to be faster than in a equiaxial structure (Laziou, 1976, Bevalot, 1975, Hadj Sassi and Lehr, 1977) but their propagation seems slower.

Smith and Hughes (1978) have perfomed comparative fatigue tests in open air and in 3,5 % NaCl solutions and they do not observe any significative difference for the fatigue strength between the two environments.

It must be emphasised out that in performing our tests we always used samples obtained from the same ingot, consequently with the same degree of working. This factor seems to influence considerably the value of the fatigue limit and we have observed during our experiments that for the same heat treatment there could be significantly different fatigue limits for samples machined from two different ingots. A more accurate study of the influence of the amount of working for the Ti 6-4 alloy has been perfomed by Stubbington and Bowen (1974) who demonstrated that the fatigue limit is increased when the amount of working increases.

CONCLUSION

Titanium alloy Ti 6-4 is a very suitable material for the design of endoprosthesis because it has good mechanical properties, a good corrosion behaviour and a good interfacial stability with the bone (Muster et al, 1980).
However it is important to note that these optimal properties can only be obtained by use of careful industrial techniques similar to those used in the aerospace industry.

TABLE I. Types of heat treatment

1)	forged and annealed	forging at 930° - 950° C	- annealing 1 hr at 730°C - air cooling
2)	forged, quenched and tempered	forging at 930° - 950° C	
3)	forged and annealed	forging at 1110° - 1130° C	
4)	forged, quenched an tempered	forging at 1110° - 1130° C	

TABLE 2. Composition of the Ringer's solution

NaCl : 8 $CaCl_2$: 0,2   KCl : 0,2 $NaHCO_3$: 0,2   Glucose : 1

TABLE 3. Mean values of the fatigue limits calculated for
each sample types in open air and in biological
environment

Type of treatment	Fatigue limits in open air M Pa	Fatigue limits in biological environment MPa	Tensile Strenghs M Pa
annealed	510 ± 20	540 ± 20	1000
quenched and tempered	560 ± 20	570 ± 20	1150
annealed	355 ± 20	345 ± 20	925
quenched and tempered	450 ± 20	440 ± 20	975

REFERENCES

Auvinet, J., Leleu, G., Notton, G., Marquier, G. (1973),
Mem. Sc. Rev. Metall., 11, 809-821.

Bevalot, J (1975), Mat. et Techn., 5, 203-212.

Cornet, A., Orlhac, A., Jaeger, J.H., Muster, D., Kempf, I. (1978)
'Meeting of the European Society of Biomaterials', Brussels May
22-27.

Cornet, A., Muster, D., Jaeger, J.H. (1979); Biomat. Med. Dev. and
Artif. Organs, 7, 155-167.

Daubertès, C., Renout, M., Cazaud, R. (1958), Rev. Metall. , 11,
1048-1056.

Hadj Sassi, B., Lehr, P. (1977), J.Less-Common Met., 56, 157-165.

Hempel, M., Hillnhagen, E. (1966), Arch. Eisenhüttenwesen, 3,263-274.

Laziou, J.C. (1976), J.Less-Common Met., 46, 229-249.

Muster, D., Bouzouita, M., Burggraf, C., Cornet, A., Jaeger, J.H.
(1979) 'Gordon Res. Conf. Biomaterials, Tilton July 16-20.

Muster, D., Jaeger, J.H., Bouzouita, M., Burggraf, C. (1980), to be
pres. at Biomaterials in Stomatology and Implantology, Kyot. June
9-11.

Smith, C.J.E., Hughes, A.N. (1978), Engin. in Medic., 3, 158-171.

Steinemann, S.G. (1980), Chapter 1, in : 'Evaluation of Biomaterials',
(Eds, Winter, Leray, De Groot) J. Wiley & Sons, Chichester, U.K.

Stubbington, C.A., Bowen, A.W. (1974), J. Mater. Sci., 9, 941-947.

8
6
4
2
0
-2
-4
-6
CURRENT DENSITY x 10⁻⁶ A.cm⁻²
$1,7 \times 10^{-7}$ A.cm⁻²
TITANIUM ALLOY TA6V
-400
0
400
800
1200
POTENTIAL mV_H

Fig.1.

65
96
65
12 n6
Ø 7.52
25
Test-piece
A
P₁
P₂
B
Electric motor
G₁
G₂
G₃
A
P₁
P₂
B
Moment
diagram
G₁ balancing weight
G₂ adjustable   "
G₃ additional   "

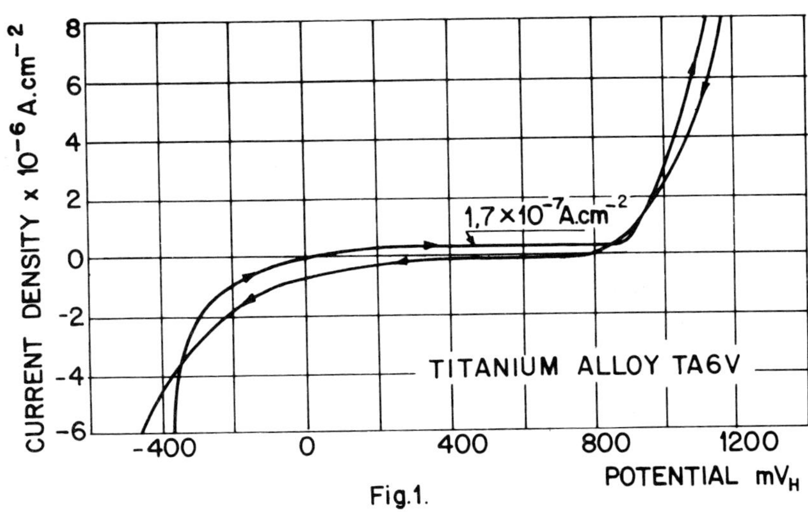

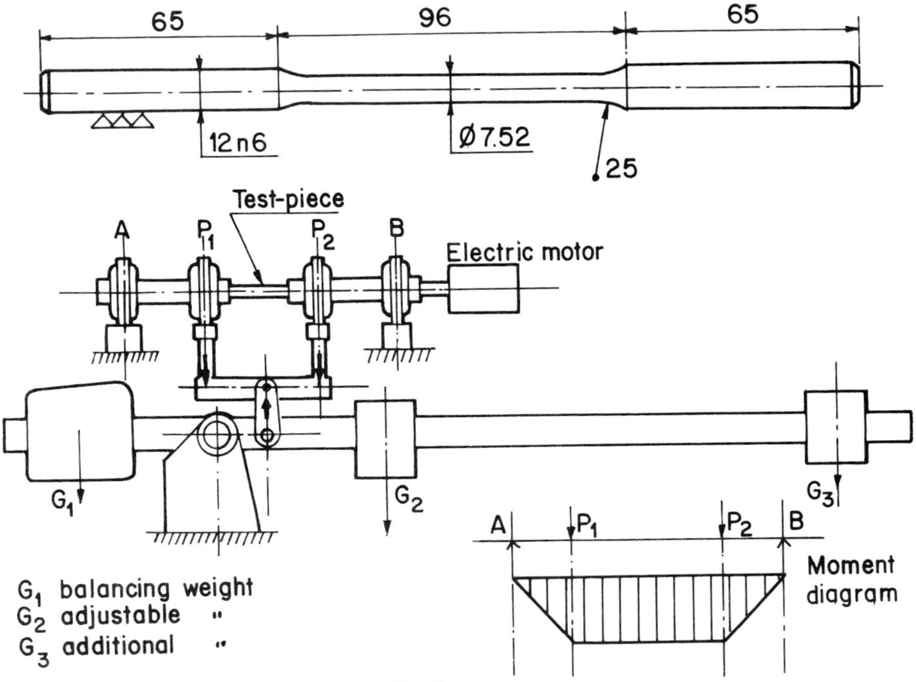

Fig.2.

TA6V-α+β
Our results
Stubbington 90:1
8:1
Auvinet
Hempel et al.
σ MPa
800
700
600
500
10^4
10^5
10^6
10^7   N.CYCLES

Fig. 3.

TA6V-β
Our results
Stubbington
σ MPa
600
500
400
300
10^4
10^5
10^6
10^7   N.CYCLES

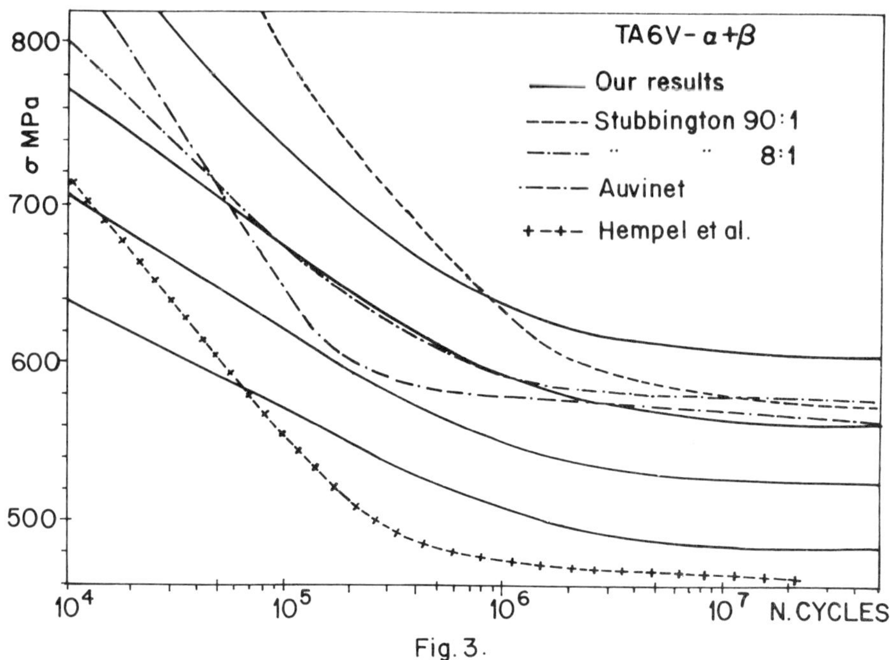

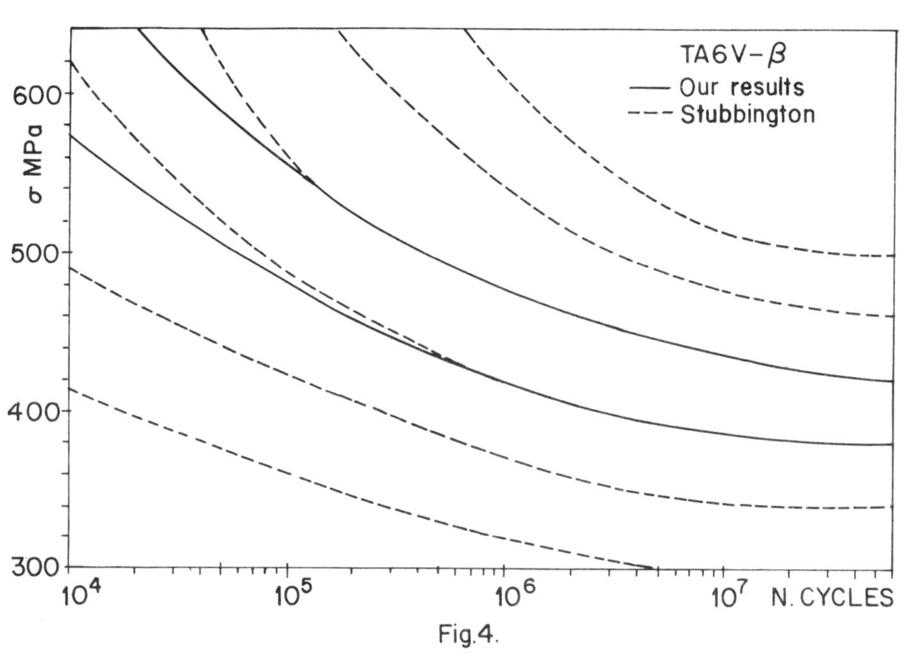

Fig.4.

Biomaterials 1980
Edited by G. D. Winter, D. F. Gibbons, and H. Plenk, Jr.
© 1982 John Wiley and Sons Ltd.

FAILURE ANALYSIS OF METALLIC SURGICAL IMPLANTS

H. Zitter and D. Schaschl - Outschar

Institut fuer Allgemeine und Analytische Chemie
Montanuniversitaet Leoben
Leoben, Austria

SUMMARY

Failure of surgical implants made from austenitic stainless steels
due to corrosion fatigue, pitting, fretting and crevice corrosion
depends on the chemical analysis of the steels, in particular on the
contents of chromium and molybdenum. Failure reduction could be
achieved by increasing the contents of these elements and, to
approach fully austenitic structure, of nickel.

INTRODUCTION

The purpose of this paper is to present a statistical evaluation of
failures based on the examination of more than 100 implants which had
been judged in the past ten years by various surgeons to be unsatisfactory. These failed implants represent, as Cohen (1966) stated in a
similar evaluation, an unknown percentage of an unknown total. Thus
the percentage of a particular failure can be related only to the sum
of all failures. The following implants fabricated primarily from
austenitic stainless steels have been studied:
     80 screws
     23 plates
      8 tri-fin nails
     18 intramedullary nails type Kuentscher
     33 elastic nails type Ender-Simon-Waidner
      4 different prostheses
     11 other implants.
Implant failures are classified according to the following most frequently observed types of corrosion:
     1) fretting and crevice corrosion
     2) pitting corrosion   and
     3) corrosion fatigue.
Alloys which are standardized for implants today owe their corrosion
resistance exclusively to passivity which is determined primarily by
the chromium and molybdenum content. Since iron alloys are most sensitive to passivation by alloying elements, the following statements
will be restricted to their properties.

<u>FAILURE ANALYSIS</u>

Pitting has occured in several chromium-nickel-molybdenum-steel implants and is characterized by small, deep pits (figure 1).

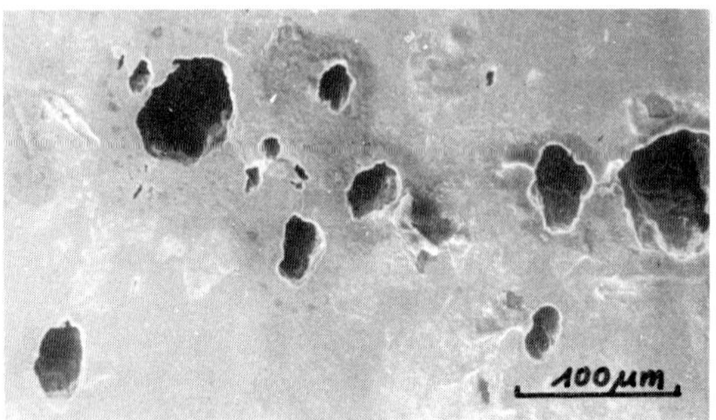

Fig. 1. Pitting of a CrNiMo type Kuentscher intramedullary nail

Pitting occurs only within the passive range above a certain potential, the so called pitting potential (determination see e. g. Kuron, Graefen, 1977), which is directly influenced by the contents of the passivating elements chromium and molybdenum. The "effective sum" of these elements is generally defined as the percentage of chromium + 3 times the percentage of molybdenum (Lorenz, Medawar, 1969;Horn, Kuron, Graefen, 1979) and calculated from chemical analysis. We adopted this "effective sum" in order to recognize the influence of the composition of the steels on the occurence of pitting and crevice corrosion. Our analysis (figure 2) shows a marked reduction of failure by pitting

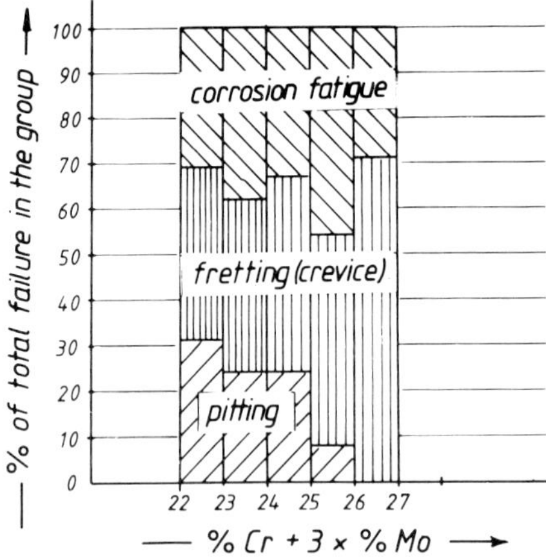

Fig. 2. Mode of failure of stainless steel implants

from approximately 30 % in the group with an effective sum of 22 to 0 % in that with an effective sum greater than 26. That limit of 26

signifies a molybdenum content of 2.7 % for steels containing 18 %
of chromium.
Because stress corrosion cracking in surgical implants can be completely excluded on the basis of many experiments and careful investigations of fractured surfaces (Zitter, Oberndorfer, Schaschl-Outschar,
1978) all brittle fractures of implants have to be classified as
corrosion fatigue. In our example (figure 3), a tri-fin nail, corro-

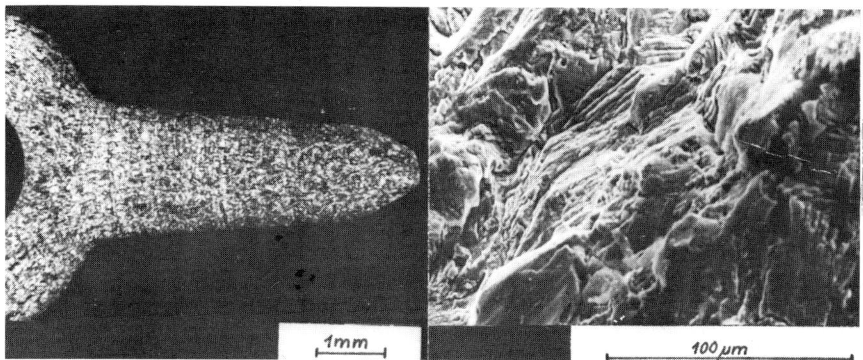

Fig. 3. Corrosion fatigue of a tri-fin nail

sion fatigue had its origin at the tip of one lamella and led to the
fracture of the nail. The broken surface showed typical fatigue stri-
ations and only a few square millimeters of fracture by violence.

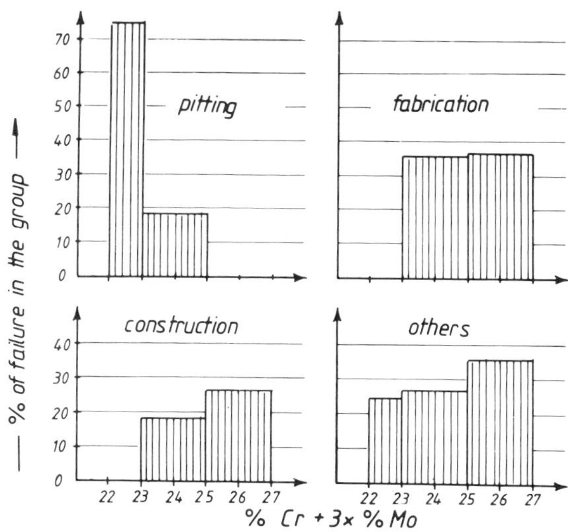

Fig. 4. Causes of corrosion fatigue on stainless
steel implants

We therefore investigated the causes of corrosion fatigue (figure 4)
of more than 30 implants. In the group with the poorest passivability

three quarters of all fractures were initiated by pitting. This is
simply and very easily explained by the fact that faults in construction and fabrication do not originate as critical notches as does
pitting.

DISCUSSION OF RESULTS

Since corrosion fatigue has the most dangerous consequences,measures
taken to reduce failure should begin here. Reduction of corrosion
fatigue failure can be achieved in two ways:

1) Improvement of shape and surface conditions which may be
   achieved by changes in construction and fabrication
2) Elimination of local corrosion, especially pitting, by
   enhancement of the passivation characteristics by
   alloying with chromium and molybdenum.

The second, generally efficient measure should be employed in all
circumstances because the best construction can be destroyed by the
action of local corrosion.

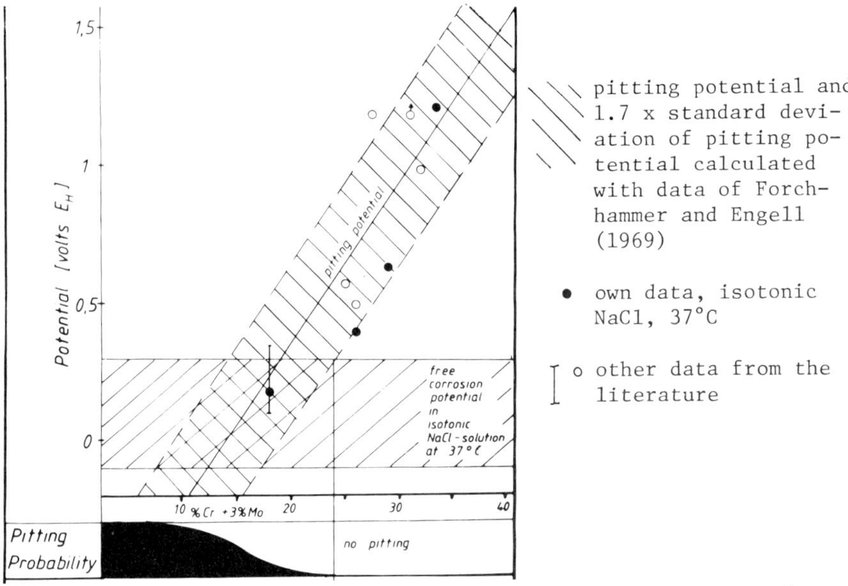

pitting potential and
1.7 x standard devi-
ation of pitting po-
tential calculated
with data of Forch-
hammer and Engell
(1969)

• own data, isotonic
  NaCl, 37°C

o other data from the
  literature

Fig. 5.   Pitting potential and free corrosion potential vs.
effective sums of chromium and molybdenum (% Cr + 3 x % Mo)

It has been shown as summarized by Horn, Kuron and Graefen (1977)
that there is an upper limiting potential to the region of passivity
in the presence of chloride ions. Thus the pitting potential increases with the effective sum of chromium and molybdenum (% Cr + 3 x
% Mo). This dependence is plotted in figure 5 for literature data in
sea water at room temperature (e. g. Forchhammer, Engell, 1969; Lorenz, Medawar, 1969) and our own data in isotonic salt solution at

37°C. These media have corresponding corrosivity because the higher
chloride content of sea water is compensated by the higher temperature of the isotonic salt solution. In these media the free corrosion
potential of stainless steels is not influenced by their composition.
Security against pitting exists, when the pitting potential is more
positive than the free corrosion potential of the passive alloy.
Where these two potentials which are additionally influenced by texture, segregation, sulfur content and surface, overlap, pitting will
occur with variable probability.
For crevice corrosion, local activation is less pronounced but is in
principle equally dependent on the alloying elements which promote
passivity (Baeumel, 1980).
According to laboratory pitting experiments (see figure 5) no pitting
occurs above 25 (% Cr + 3 x % Mo) and corrosion fatigue failure due
to pitting (see figure 4) ceases at about the same value.

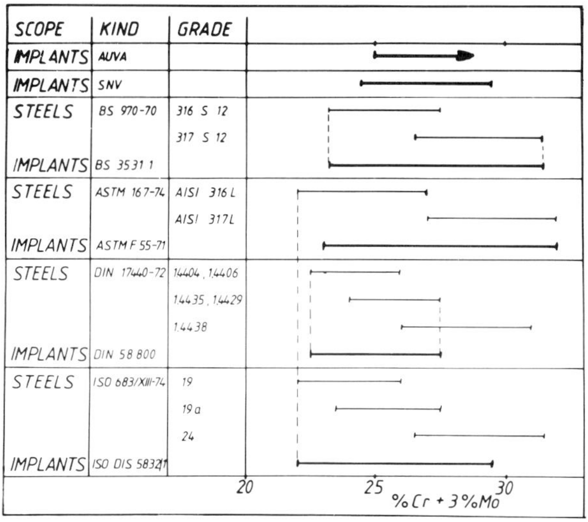

SCOPE	KIND	GRADE
IMPLANTS	AUVA	
IMPLANTS	SNV	
STEELS	BS 970-70	316 S 12
		317 S 12
IMPLANTS	BS 3531 1	
STEELS	ASTM 167-74	AISI 316 L
		AISI 317L
IMPLANTS	ASTM F 55-71	
STEELS	DIN 17440-72	1.4404 , 1.4406
		1.4435 , 1.4429
		1.4438
IMPLANTS	DIN 58 800	
STEELS	ISO 683/XIII-74	19
		19 a
		24
IMPLANTS	ISO DIS 5832 1	

Scale axis: 20 · · · 25 · · · 30 %Cr + 3%Mo

AUVA: Allgemeine Un-
fallversicherungsan-
stalt (Austrian stan-
dard for implants)

SNV: Schweizer Nor-
menvereinigung

BS: British Standard

ASTM: American Socie-
ty for Testing and
Materials

ISO: International
Organisation of
Standardisation

DIN: Deutsches Insti-
tut fuer Normung

Fig. 6.   Comparison of standards for steels and implants

A comparison with the composition of present day standard steels used
for implants shows that the failures observed are to be expected. On
the other hand the comparison of figure 6 demonstrates that there are
steels available, even within the limits of several standards for implants, which would prevent pitting corrosion.

CONCLUSION
<u></u>

The relation of the composition of present day surgical implants to
the occurrence of pitting reveals that this type of corrosion and
corrosion fatigue due to pitting could be minimized by the use of
steels with higher chromium and molybdenum contents. We therefore
suggest an increase of the lower limits of these elements to an
"effective sum" of at least 25 (% Cr + 3 x % Mo). As a consequence

of this modification one needs to stabilize the austenitic structure
by increasing the contents of nickel or nitrogen.

ACKNOWLEDGEMENTS

This research has been partially supported by the "Fonds zur Foerde-
rung der wissenschaftlichen Forschung, Wien" and the "Allgemeine Un-
fallversicherungsanstalt, (AUVA), Wien".

REFERENCES

Baeumel, A. (1980). "Spaltkorrosion an temporaeren Implantaten."
Vortraege der 1. Sitzung des Arbeitskreises Implantate, medizinisch
technische Zusammenarbeit, des Deutschen Verbandes fuer Materialprue-
fung e. V., 28./29. Februar 1980, Berlin, DVM 1980 / 300.
Cohen, J. (1966). "Performance and Failure in Performance of Surgical
Implants in Orthopedic Surgery." Journal of Materials 1, 354-365
Forchhammer, P. & Engell, H.-J. (1969). "Untersuchungen ueber den
Lochfrass an passiven austenitischen CrNi-Staehlen in neutralen
Chloridloesungen." Werkst. u. Korrosion 20, 1-12.
Frank, E. & Zitter, H. (1971). Metallische Implantate in der Knochen-
chirurgie. Springer, Wien - New York, ISBN 3-211-81002-1 and
ISBN 0-387-81002-1.
Horn, E.-M.; Kuron, D. & Graefen, H. (1977). "Lochkorrosion an passi-
ven Legierungssystemen der Elemente Eisen, Chrom und Nickel."
Z. Werkstofftech. 8, 37-55.
Horn, E.-M.; Kuron, D. & Graefen, H. (1979). "Korrosion von nicht-
rostenden austenitischen Staehlen in halogenidhaltigen waessrigen
Loesungen." Werkst. u. Korrosion 30, 723-724
Kuron, D. & Graefen, H. (1977). "Lochkorrosion an passiven Legierungssystemen der Elemente Eisen, Chrom und Nickel. Teil 2: Pruef-
verfahren zur Ermittlung der Lochkorrosionsbestaendigkeit-Chemi-
sche Pruefungen- elektrochemische Untersuchungen."
Z. Werkstofftech. 8, 182-191
Lorenz, K. & Medawar, G. (1969). "Ueber das Korrosionsverhalten
austenitischer Chrom Nickel (Molybdaen) Staehle mit und ohne Stick-
stoffzusatz unter besonderer Beruecksichtigung ihrer Beanspruchbar-
keit in chloridhaltigen Loesungen." Thyssenforschung 1, 3, 97-108.
Zitter, H.; Oberndorfer, M. & Schaschl - Outschar, D. (1978).
"Stress Corrosion Cracking (SCC) - A Cause of Failure of Surgical
Implants ?" Lecture held at the Meeting of the Working Party "Stress
Corrosion Test Methods" of the European Federation Corrosion, 1978.
Sept. 19 - 22, Firminy, France.

Biomaterials 1980
Edited by G. D. Winter, D. F. Gibbons, and H. Plenk, Jr.
© 1982 John Wiley and Sons Ltd.

ORGANOMETALLIC CORROSION PRODUCTS OF 316L SS AND HS-21 IN SERUM: IN VITRO AND IN VIVO COMPARISON IN AN ACUTE RAT MODEL

J.L. Woodman, J. Black and S. Jimenez

Department of Orthopaedic Surgery, Department of
Bioengineering, University of Pennsylvania
Philadelphia, Pennsylvania

SUMMARY

The purpose of this research was to detect blood borne organometallic compounds that may arise from the corrosion of metals used in orthopaedic prosthetic devices. Two models were chosen for this procedure. The in vivo model consisted of a rat which was implanted with spherical powders of 316L and HS-21 alloys with the size of -270 to +375 mesh. In the in vitro model the same alloys were incubated with fresh human serum. The results of this study indicate significant elevations in chromium, nickel and cobalt due to corrosion of the two alloys.

INTRODUCTION

The history of the application of metals in the repair of the human body spans the last 400 years during which time virtually every known engineering and precious metal has been tried. Most metals have proven inadequate for implantation purposes owing to their inability to satisfy necessary requirements in the biological environment particularly the strength of corrosion resistance. That corrosion is a phenomenon common to all currently used implant metals exposed to the hostile biological environment has been well substantiated in the literature. Equally as popular in terms of biomaterials research is the local tissue reaction elicited by the implant and its secondary corrosion complexes. In contrast there exists little information even remotely directed to the question of possible long term systemic consequences of metallic implantation.

Historical Review. "There probably does not exist a single enzyme-catalyzed reaction in which either substrate, product, enzyme or some combination within this triad is not influenced in a very direct and highly specific manner by the precise nature of inorganic ions which surround or modify it" (Plaut, 1969). Numerous metal ions at physiological levels (10^{-6} to 10^{-12} gm/gm wet wt tissue) play a significant role in normal metabolic processes. Increases in these levels beyond physiological limits often upset the precise biochemical balance with consequent toxicity. Whether or not toxic levels of metal ions are obtained is a function of inherent toxicity of the metal involved, the amount absorbed and the rate at which the body detoxifies or excretes

                    J.L. Woodman, et. al.

it. The systemic effects of implant corrosion can be grouped into
four main categories: metabolic, immunological, bacteriologic and
carcinogenic.

Since cobalt, chromium, iron, molybdenum and nickel have all been shown
to participate in metabolism (Rheinhold, 1975), intakes exceeding the
amount required for metabolic activity, either by ingestion, inhalation,
or corrosion may produce pharmacological actions and these are followed
by toxic effects if still larger amounts are taken (Underwood, 1971).

Foussereau and Laugier (1966) have found allergic eczemas from implanted foreign bodies. Jones et. al., (1975) has described seven
cases of metal sensitivity. Once the implants are removed the allergic reactions resolve. Merritt, et. al. (1979) reported an in vitro
leukocyte migration inhibition in agarose (MIF test) for metal sensitivity. Of 61 patients whose orthopaedic prosthesis were removed, 60
percent of 20 patients with metallic screws were reacting and 35 percent were sensitive.

For several years it has been recognized that a host's response to
bacterial invasion is a reduction in the serum iron content of the
blood (Weinberg, 1974). Recently, the mechanism of this reduction has
been identified as a suppression of intestinal assimilation of iron
concurrent with an increased storage of iron in the liver, the net effect being to make growth essential non-heme iron less available to
microbial invaders and thus manifest a so-called "nutritional immunity"
for the host. (Kochan, 1973).

Cobalt, chromium and nickel are all on the list of materials which have
proven to be carcinogenic. Hueper (1958) and Heath (1957) found sarcomas associated with the implantation of these metals in powder form.
Oppenheimer et. al., (1956) induced sarcomas with Vitallium and stainless steel foils implanted subcutaneously. The positive results for
both powders and foils indicates in addition to possessing the ability
to promote foreign body carcinogenesis, the alloy has the intrinsic
property of chemical carcinogenesis.

Objectives. The objectives of this study are four-fold. First, it is
necessary to prove the existence of blood borne corrosion products.
Secondly, once their existence has been proven, the form of these corrosion products must be elucidated. That is, in what form (free ion,
hydroxide or complexed with serum proteins) are these corrosion products transported in the blood. Third, can any correlation be made
from a comparison of the in vivo or in vitro results. Lastly, can
these corrosion products be produced in sufficient quantity to allow
further characterization.

MATERIALS AND METHODS

The first model examined is a short term rat model. Spheres of 316L
SS and Haynes Stellite 21 were implanted in the surpaspinatus muscle
of 150 gram Sprague-Dawley rats. The size of these spheres is -270 to
+325 mesh. A calculation was performed to determine the surface area

to body weight ratio of total hip prosthesis in a human. That figure
of 2.9 cm^2/kgm body weight was then increased by factors of 10, 100
and 1000 times to increase the amount released. After ten days the
serum was harvested.

The in vitro model consisted of incubating the same powders with the
same acceleration factors for a period of five days, at a standard (1x)
surface area to body fluid volume ratio equalling 1.74 cm^2/liter.
Penicillin, streptomycin and an antifungal agent were added to inhibit
microbial growth. The experiment was performed in a 5 percent CO_2 incubator at 37°C with constant but gentle agitation, and pH determinations
were made daily. The pH remained at 7.4 for the duration of the experiment.

The sample analysis consisted of three parts. First, a wet digestion
matrix modification with perchloric acid - H_2O_2 was done. Secondly,
atomic absorption spectroscopy was performed for Cr and Ni in 316L SS
and Co and Ni in HS-21 using a Perkin Elmer Model 360 with burner assembly replaced by a HGA-2100 Graphite Furnace. Additionally aliquots of
serum were analyzed for protein content using the Lowry procedure. As
all of the metal was found associated with serum proteins this standardization was necessary to remove any inconsistencies in protein
concentration. This conclusion was based on an ultrifiltration technique which excluded all molecular species above 1000 in molecular
weight. No metal was found in this small molecular weight fraction.

DISCUSSION

The results shown on Table 1 indicate that only chromium and nickel concentrations were raised significantly in the rat model. A 1.13 x indicates an increased concentration over normal by a factor of 1.13.

The in vitro date is represented on Table 2. It can be clearly seen
that cobalt as well as chromium and nickel concentrations are increased
significantly. It is important to note a disparity in the serum nickel
concentrations between the two alloys. Nickel concentration in the serum
derived from the 316L SS alloy is much greater than the nickel concentration in the serum from the HS-21 alloy. This was not seen in the in
vivo model.

As the metal concentration was determined from daily samples in the in
vitro experiment, it is possible to graph concentration as a function of
time. The results of this analysis for chromium indicate the steady
state concentration attained in serum is a function not only of time
but also of the surface area to unit fluid volume ratio present. The
same behavior is not seen in saline. (Figure 1).

Cobalt concentration is shown on these graphs to be independent of the
surface area ratio for both serum and saline. (Figure 2).

Nickel concentration in serum from the 316L SS alloy again show a strong
dependence on the surface area ratio of the powder. (Figure 3).

the graph obtained for nickel in serum from HS-21 alloy shows a similar
dependence on the surface area ratio although these concentrations do
not attain the same equilibrium levels as from the 316L SS alloy. This
may be indicative of the lower activity of nickel in the parent alloy,
being only 2-5 weight percent in HS-21 compared to 10-14 weight percent in the 316L SS alloy. (Figure 4).

Conclusions. The difference in dependence on the surface area to unit
fluid volume ratio indicates that complexing of the metal ions released
through corrosion occurs at two different locations. Chromium and
nickel complex with serum proteins at the metal sphere-serum protein
interface, thus giving rise to dependence on the surface area of powder
present. Cobalt, however, apparently complexes in solution and therefore is independent of the surface area present.

These graphical representations also allow for the establishment of a
functional relationship between concentration and time. From these
relationships corrosion rates may be determined. When applied to the
in vivo model, these rates predict concentrations very similar to those
actually measured.

The corrosion rates are derived from the slope of the logic curve selected from the family of sigmoid curves which was determined by the
least squares method. This curve is a four parameter equation in the
general form of:

$$y(t) = y\ min + \frac{(y\ max - y\ min)}{1 + e^{k[t_{1/2} - t]}}$$

Where: y min = minimum value approached asymptotically by y(t)
         y max = maximum value approached asymptotically by y(t)
         $t_{1/2}$ = value of t at which y(t) is halfway between y max and y min
         k = $\frac{4y(t_{1/2})}{[y\ max - y\ min]}$ where $y(t_{1/2})$ is the slope of the curve at $t_{1/2}$

In conclusion, the two models in this study proved that blood borne
corrosion products can be determined, and that metal ions are indeed
complexing with serum proteins. It is possible to correlate the results of the models. Also the in vitro model provides the vehicle for
production of sufficient quantities or organometallic complexes for
further consideration.

The results of this study indicate significant elevations in chromium,
nickel and cobalt due to the corrosion of 316L SS and HS-21. These
corrosion products could in turn significantly alter many trace-element
catalyzed reactions as their concentrations rise in the serum.

ACKNOWLEDGEMENTS

This study was in part supported by NIAMDD Training Grant AM-17132-04
and NIH Research Grant AM25752.

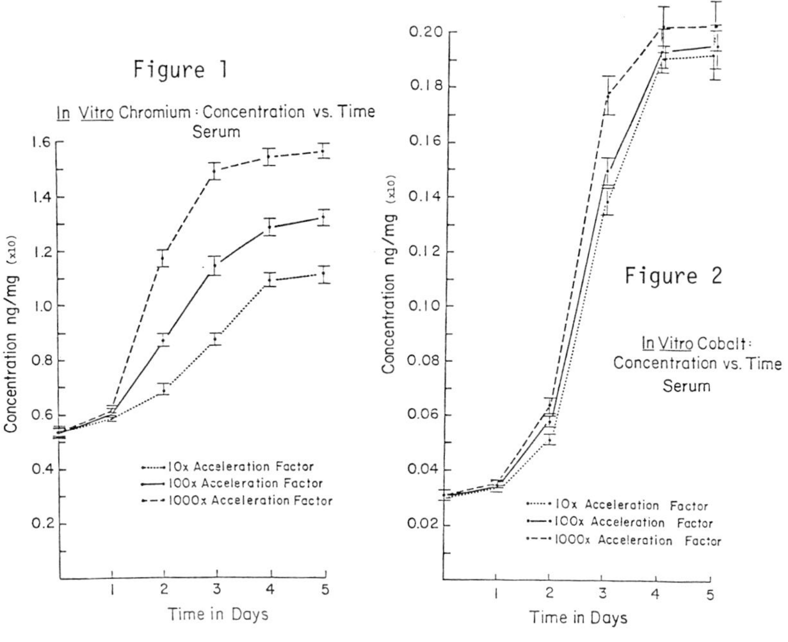
Figure 1
In Vitro Chromium: Concentration vs. Time
Serum
Concentration ng/mg (x10)
1.6
1.4
1.2
1.0
0.8
0.6
0.4
0.2
10x Acceleration Factor
100x Acceleration Factor
1000x Acceleration Factor
1
2
3
4
5
Time in Days

Figure 2
In Vitro Cobalt:
Concentration vs. Time
Serum
Concentration ng/mg (x10)
0.20
0.18
0.16
0.14
0.12
0.10
0.08
0.06
0.04
0.02
10x Acceleration Factor
100x Acceleration Factor
1000x Acceleration Factor
1
2
3
4
5
Time in Days

Figure 3
In Vitro Nickel: Concentration vs. Time
Serum 316LSS Spheres
Concentration ng/mg (x10)
10.0
9.0
8.0
7.0
6.0
5.0
4.0
3.0
2.0
1.0
0.5
10x Acceleration Factor
100x Acceleration Factor
1000x Acceleration Factor
1
2
3
4
5
Time in Days

Figure 4
In Vitro Nickel: Concentration vs. Time
Serum HS-21 Spheres
10x Acceleration Factor
100x Acceleration Factor
1000x Acceleration Factor
Concentration ng/mg (x10)
7.0
6.0
5.0
4.0
3.0
2.0
1.0
0.5
1
2
3
4
5
Time in Days

250   J.L. Woodman, et. al.

TABLE I

RAT

METALS		ACCELERATION FACTORS		
Normal Serum (ng/mg protein)		10X	100X	1000X
Cr:	0.408 (316L SS)	1.13X	1.16X	1.19X
Co:	0.054 (HS-21)	1.04X	1.07X	1.05X
Ni:	0.715 (316L SS)	1.31X	1.32X	1.05X
Ni:	0.715 (HS-21)	1.25X	1.31X	1.53X

TABLE II

IN VITRO

METALS		ACCELERATION FACTORS		
Normal Serum (ng/mg protein)		10X	100X	1000X
Cr:	0.539 (316L SS)	1.84X	2.45S	3.24X
Co:	0.0306 (HS-21)	6.31X	6.47X	6.67X
Ni:	0.741 (316L SS)	6.79X	9.38X	12.27X
Ni:	0.741 (HS-21)	5.24X	6.71X	8.22X

REFERENCES

Foussereau, J. & Laugier, P. (1966) Allergic Eczemas from Metallic Foreign Bodies. Transactions of the St. John's Hospital Dermatology Society, 52, 220.

Heath, J.C. (1957) The Production of Malignant Tumors by Cobalt in the Rat. British Journal of Cancer, 18, 261.

Hueper, W.C. (1958) Experimental Studies in Metal Cancerigenesis: IX. Pulmonary Lesions in Guinea Pigs and Rats Exposed to Prolonged Inhalation of Powdered Metallic Nickel. Archives of Pathology, 65, 600.

Jones, D.A., Lucas, H.K., O'Driscoll, M., Price, C.H.G. & Wibberley, B. (1975) Cobalt Toxicity after McKee Hip Arthroplasty. The Journal of Bone and Joint Surgery, 57B, 289.

Kochan, I. (1973) The Role of Iron in Bacterial Infections with Special Consideration of Host-Tubercle Bacillus Interaction. Current Topics in Microbiology and Immunology, 60, 1.

Merrit, K., Mayor, M.B. & Brown, S.A. (1979) Evaluation of Sensitivity to Metallic Implants. Advances in Biomaterials, John Wiley and Sons, London.

Oppenheimer, B.S., Oppenheimer, E.T., Danishefsky, I., & Stout, A.P. (1956) Carcinogenic Effects of Metals in Rodents. Cancer Research, 16, 43

Plaut, D. (1969) Timely Topics in Clinical Chemistry: Toxicology of Trace Metals II. American Journal of Medical Technology, 35, 652.

Rheinold, J.B. (1975) Trace Elements - A Selective Survey. Clinical Chemistry, 21, 476.

Underwood, E.M. (1971) Trace Elements in Human and Animal Nutrition, Academic Press, New York.

Weinberg, E.D. (1974) Iron Susceptibility to Infectious Disease. Science, 184, 952.

Biomaterials 1980
Edited by G. D. Winter, D. F. Gibbons, and H. Plenk, Jr.
© 1982 John Wiley and Sons Ltd.

AN ION RELEASE STUDY
OF COMMONLY USED IMPLANT ALLOYS

R. W. Treharne[+] and M. Marek[++]

[+]Richards Manufacturing Company, Inc.
Memphis, Tennessee, USA

[++]Georgia Institute of Technology
Atlanta, Georgia, USA

SUMMARY

The chromium and nickel ion release rates from 316L Stainless Steel*
and MP35N®** shavings immersed in 37°C Ringer's solution has been
studied. The release rates of chromium from the two alloys were
found to be within experimental error of being identical. The release rates of nickel from the two alloys were also found to be nearly identical. The main difference for these two ions was that the
chromium release rates were approximately two orders of magnitude
lower than the nickel. These results could not have been predicted
based solely upon the chemical composition of the two alloys.

INTRODUCTION

The reactions taking place on the surfaces of man-made materials implanted in the human body are the subject of great interest. In
metals these reactions are generally electrochemical or corrosive in
nature. This corrosion release rate must be sufficiently low to
avoid any harmful physiological reactions. Therefore, the release
of metal ions to the body fluids and tissues is of importance.

Two commonly used elements in metallic implants are chromium and
nickel. If present in sufficient quantity, some released metallic
elements may cause physiological effects. Hence, the rate of release
of chromium and nickel ions from alloys implanted in the human body
may be important parameters in the evaluation of alloys for medical
applications.

MATERIALS AND METHODS

In this study, the chromium and nickel ion release rates of 316L
Stainless Steel and an alloy designated MP35N was studied. The

*This material is described by ASTM Standard F138, Grade 2.

**MP35N, a trademark of SPS Technologies, Inc., is described
by ASTM Standard F562.

percent chromium and nickel in these two commonly used implant alloys
is shown in Table 1.

TABLE 1. Alloy Composition

Alloy	% Chromium	% Nickel
316L	17 – 20	12 – 14
MP35N	19 – 21	33 – 37

EXPERIMENTAL PROCEDURE

The experiments were performed in the following manner: first, each
metal sample was cut to make shavings. The reason for this process
was to make the surface area-to-volume of liquid ratio as high as
possible. These samples were then passivated per ASTM Standard F86.
The surface area was determined by a low temperature physical adsorption technique using krypton gas.

Greatly simplified, this procedure involves degassing of the metal
surface in a high vacuum and introducing inert krypton gas in a
series of controlled steps at a low temperature. The amount of the
gas required to form a monolayer is then determined from the pressure
readings, and the surface area is calculated using the cross-sectional
area of the krypton gas molecules.

The metal shavings were then immersed in 37°C Ringer's solution.
Periodically, some of the solutions were analyzed for Cr and Ni ions
by flameless atomic absorption spectrophotometry. The advantages of
the flameless atomic absorption technique are that a very small
amount of solution is needed, the systems are not disturbed very
much, and the sensitivities are usually higher than those obtained
by other methods of analysis.

RESULTS

The result for nickel is shown in Figure 1.

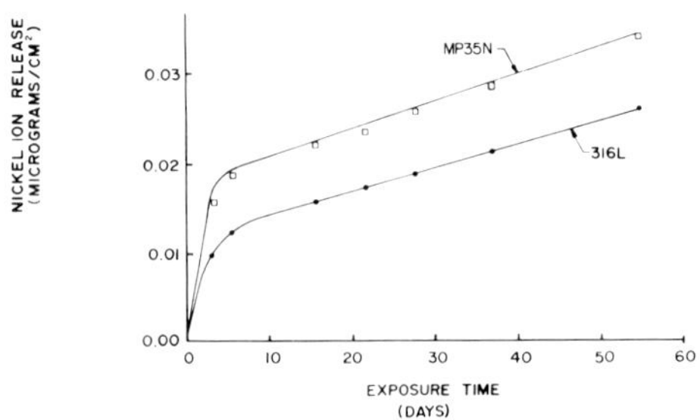

Figure 1. Rate of dissolution of nickel from MP35N alloy
and 316L Stainless Steel. Reproduced with permission from the Orthopaedic Research Society.

In both cases, the dissolution rate rose rapidly for about five days. The dissolution rate then slowed to a constant rate for the next 50 days. A similar curve was found for the chromium release for these two alloys, except that the chromium release rate was about two orders of magnitude lower than nickel. Within experimental error the chromium release rates were identical for both implant alloys.

DISCUSSION

The results show that the rate of release of a specific element is not simply a function of the composition of the alloy. (See Table 1) This finding is the same as that reported previously by Ferguson et al. (1960). Two factors apparently play major roles. The first is the corrosion resistance of the alloy. The second is the selectivity of the corrosion process with respect to the ions.

Some caution must be exercised in predicting the behavior of the materials in the human body on the basis of this in vitro test. For instance, the much more complicated environment of the body and events caused by the surgery could cause a more substantial change in the reported dissolution rates. Further, formation of localized corrosion cells or destruction by any means of the protective film which is responsible for the good corrosion resistance of these alloys could dramatically alter both the dissolution rates and the number of ions being released. It must be emphasized that these experiments only measured the amount of "free" chromium and nickel ions released into the fluid by the metallic shavings. Ions that formed compounds that precipitated from the solution were not measured in this analysis.

CONCLUSIONS

For these experiments 316L Stainless Steel and MP35N alloy were found to have approximately the same release rates for chromium and nickel ions. These results were not proportional to their chemical composition indicating that metallic ion release rate cannot be predicted based solely upon chemical composition.

REFERENCE

Ferguson, A. B., Laing, P. G., & Hodge, E. S. (1960) The Ionization of Metal Implants in Living Tissues. J. Bone Joint Surg., 42-A, 77-90.

Biomaterials 1980
Edited by G. D. Winter, D. F. Gibbons, and H. Plenk, Jr.
© 1982 John Wiley and Sons Ltd.

METAL ION RELEASE AFTER TOTAL HIP REPLACEMENT

H.S. Dobbs[1] and M.J. Minski[2]

[1]The Institute of Orthopaedics
Royal National Orthopaedic Hospital
Brockley Hill, Stanmore, Middlesex.

[2]University of London Reactor Centre
Silwood Park, Ascot, Berks.

SUMMARY

The concentration of cobalt (Co), chromium (Cr), molybdenum (Mo),
nickel (Ni), iron (Fe), and zinc (Zn) in tissue taken from an 81 year
old female at necropsy, was measured using neutron activation
analysis. The patient had bilateral cobalt-chromium-molybdenum
(Co-Cr-Mo) total hip replacements : one, a metal-on-metal had been in
place for 14 years, the other a metal-on-plastic for 5.5 years.
Although the metal-on-metal side had become painful, the patient
remained active until she died. The measurements indicated that the
concentrations of Co and Cr in the lung, kidney, liver and spleen
were up to fifty times "Standard Man" values. High values occurred
also in the urine and in the hair. The tissue adjacent to the
metal-on-metal joint was heavily laden with metal wear debris,
whereas that adjacent to the metal-on-plastic joint was relatively
free of debris. Cobalt predominated in the urine, whereas chromium
predominated near the implants. The existence of such high levels,
especially in the organs, is a possible cause for concern.

CLINICAL DETAILS

In February 1965, the patient had a total hip replacement in her
right side. She was 67 years old and had bilateral osteo-arthritis.
The component was a Co-Cr-Mo Stanmore metal-on-metal total hip
replacement of very early design (Mk 1). It consisted of a femoral
component with Eicher type head of 41.5mm diameter, and an acetabular component with cup and separate liner. The stem was
attached with acrylic bone cement, and the cup was pinned into the
ilium, ischium and pubis. At operation both components were firmly
attached. Post-operatively the patient made a normal recovery. She
had good range of movement and walked with crutches. After a few

255

years there was a suggestion of looseness, accompanied by noise
and pain. At this time she was still satisfied with the result,
but later (in 1977) she was not.

In August 1973, when she was 75 years old, she had a total hip
replacement on her left side. This was a Stanmore metal-on-plastic
total hip replacement of recent design (Mk7) and consisted of a
Co-Cr-Mo stem, a 25mm head, and a polyethylene (RCH 1000) cup. Both
components were attached with acrylic bone cement. A year later she
was satisfied with both her hips and walked over a mile a day using
elbow crutches. She did her own gardening and housework. In
January 1979, she died of a heart attack at which time the former
joint had been in place for 14 years and the latter for five and a
half years.

At necropsy both femora and acetabula were excised. On opening the
metal-on-metal joint it could be seen that the head and cup were
highly polished where the surface was worn, and the surrounding
joint capsule and tissue were a shade of pale green. There was an
extensive granuloma, also discoloured, extending along the psoas
tendon. The cup was loose and one of the pins had pierced the
acetabulum, and had protruded into the abdominal cavity. Some dark
fluid was aspirated from the joint. On opening the metal-on-plastic
joint there was nothing abnormal to be seen. Both components were
firmly fixed and there was no evidence of metallic wear debris or of
discolouration, although the rim of the cup had worn slightly where
it had impinged on the neck of the femoral component. There was no
thickening of the fibrous capsule and no free fluid within the joint.
Next the abdomen and thorax were opened and the spleen, the right
kidney, a lobe of lung and a piece of liver were removed. All the
removed material was stored in separate containers in formal saline
(10% formaldehyde in normal saline). A urine sample was taken from
the bladder and a hair sample from the head.

METHOD

Four days after necropsy the material was removed from the formal
saline. Samples of tissue were prepared using a titanium knife.
Samples of bone and acrylic bone cement were prepared using a hand
saw and were then trimmed with the knife to remove possible contamination from the saw. All the samples were weighed before and
after drying - the wet weight was approximately one gramme in each
case. They were dried either by air drying in an incubator at 37°C
or by freeze drying. Samples were also prepared from 1ml of the
joint fluid, from 10ml of the urine and from 10ml of the formal
saline. A sample of hair, approximately half a gramme in weight,

and untreated after removal from the scalp was prepared. Metal
samples were also taken from each of the prostheses.

All the samples were stored in small plastic containers and were
irradiated in the University of London Consort Reactor for 100 hours
at a neutron flux of ~ 1 x 10^{12} n $cm^{-2}s^{-1}$ together with standards.
After a decay period of five days the samples were transferred to
clean containers and analysed by gamma spectrometry using a Ge (Li)
semi-conductor detector, resolution 2.2 keV at 1322 keV, connected
to a 4000 channel analyser. Counting times were between 2-3 hours
per sample. Peak analysis was by the Covell method (Covell 1959).

The detection limit in ppm for irradiation of a sample weighing one
gramme was as follows : 0.003 Co, 0.03 Cr, 0.04 Mo, 0.4 Ni, 5 Fe
and 0.1 Zn.

RESULTS

The chemical composition of the Co-Cr-Mo prostheses (two stems and
one cup) was found to be similar and complied with the relevant
British Standard (BS 3531, 1962 and 1968). The following composition was the average of the three components ; Co 59%, Cr 30%,
Mo 9%, Ni 1.5%. The ratio of Co to Cr was approximately 2:1. Fe
and Zn were not detectable.

The following analysis was obtained for the formal saline sample
before storage (ppm) : 0.001 Co, 0.006 Cr,<0.03 Mo, 0.003 Ni, 0.09
Fe and 0.07 Zn from which it was concluded that the tissue samples
could be stored in formal saline, without significant contamination.

In the following tables the concentrations are given in ppm or more
precisely in µg/g for the tissue or in µg/ml for the fluids. For
the tissues the concentrations are as a function of the wet weight,
but the factor needed to convert from ppm wet weight to ppm dry
weight is also given, this factor being the ratio of the wet weight
to the dry weight.

Tables 1 and 2 give the values of Co, Cr, Mo, Ni, Fe and Zn (also
the Co:Cr ratio) in the immediate vicinity of the metal-on-metal
and metal-on-plastic joints respectively. Values are given for the
following : joint fluid, joint capsule and granuloma (both adjacent
to the joint), tissue from the neck of femur (5cm from joint), from
the mid-femur (15cm away), bone (5cm away) and bone cement (adjacent
to the rim of the plastic cup). The following results can be
noted:-

TABLE 1. Metal concentration on the metal-on-metal side (ppm wet weight)

Sample	Joint Fluid	Joint Capsule	Granuloma	Tissue (mid femur)
Co	12.9	62.6	193.1	6.9
Cr	63.3	327.2	322.8	5.5
Mo	3.97	6.6	<0.03	0.74
Ni	1.29	2.78	3.18	0.40
Fe	11.6	158.3	320.9	32.5
Zn	4.1	16.8	91.8	8.7
Factor	–	3.1	5.0	2.3
Co:Cr	0.2:1	0.2:1	0.6:1	1.3:1

TABLE 2. Metal concentration on the metal-on-plastic side (ppm wet weight)

Sample	Joint Capsule	Tissue (neck)	Tissue (mid femur)	Bone	Bone Cement
Co	0.61	1.34	0.21	0.56	0.12
Cr	0.90	1.04	0.34	8.32	<0.01
Mo	0.44	0.59	0.14	<0.03	<0.03
Ni	1.83	0.42	0.27	<0.4	<0.4
Fe	222.9	115.0	23.2	159.2	6.7
Zn	7.4	5.5	7.9	61.6	3.9
Factor	3.2	3.6	2.7	1.4	1.1
Co:Cr	0.7:1	0.6:1	1.3:1	0.1:1	>12:1

Note: Tables 1-4 reproduced from Dobbs,H.S. & Minski,M.J., Biomaterials 1980,1,pp 193-198. by premission of the publishers, IPC Business Press Ltd. C.

1. For the metal-on-metal side, very high levels occurred for Co
    and Cr, and to a lesser extent for Mo and Ni, suggesting that
    the tissue and joint fluid were heavily laden with wear debris.

2. For the metal-on-plastic side, relatively low levels occurred
    suggesting that the metal may have been released by corrosion
    rather than wear.

3. For both sides the levels of Co, Cr, Mo and Ni in the immediate
    vicinity of the joint were higher than those at the mid-femur
    position, suggesting that the levels decreased with distance
    from the joint.

4. For both sides Cr was more plentiful than Co in the immediate
    vicinity of the joint.

Fig. 1 is a photomicrograph of a stained histological section of the
granuloma on the metal-on-metal side at a magnification of 800 X.
The tissue consists largely of macrophages inundated with wear debris,
each particle being one micron or less in size. These observations
are in agreement with previous work on the tissue response to Co-Cr-
Mo implants by Winter (1974) who observed both the fine size of the
wear debris and the incidence of granuloma.

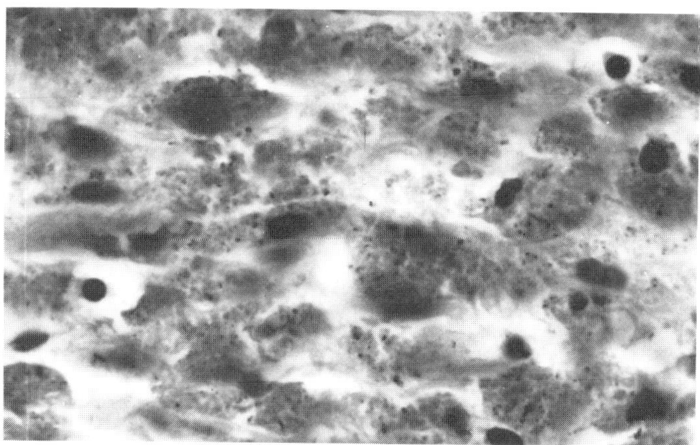

Fig. 1. Section of the granuloma showing particulate
wear debris; haematoxylin and eosin (x 800).

Table 3 gives the concentration of Co, Cr, Mo, Ni, Fe and Zn (also
the Co:Cr ratio) in the samples of the organs, hair and urine. For
comparison the table includes the mean value of the concentration of
the metals in normal tissue, the values given being the "Standard Man"
values (ICRP 23, 1975) obtained from various sources (Tipton and Cook,
1963; Parr and Taylor, 1964; Sunderman et al, 1972; Mitman, et al,
1975). The following results can be noted:

                    H.S. Dobbs and M.J. Minski

TABLE 3. Metal concentration in the organs, hair and urine
          (ppm wet weight).

Sample	Lung	Kidney	Liver	Spleen	Hair	Urine
Co	0.24 (0.02)*	0.31 (0.013)	0.47 (0.06)	0.23 (0.035)	0.68 (1.0)	0.07 (0.02)
Cr	0.18 (0.09)	0.39 (0.01)	0.61 (0.009)	0.56 (0.007)	1.39 (0.25)	0.04 (0.006)
Mo	0.12 (0.03)	0.16 (0.35)	0.68 (1.0)	0.23 (0.06)	$<$0.03 (−)	$<$0.03 (0.01)
Ni	0.39 (0.05)	0.15 (0.05)	0.64 ($<$0.06)	$<$0.4 (0.06)	1.46 (0.5)	0.01 (0.01)
Fe	181.5 (360.0)	77.3 (74.2)	488.4 (177.8)	321.7 (272.2)	34.9 (2.0)	1.08 (0.07)
Zn	6.3 (11.0)	15.4 (48.4)	35.9 (47.2)	12.8 (17.8)	193.5 (17.0)	0.39 (0.13)
Factor	6.3	3.8	4.0	4.3	−	−
Co:Cr	1.3:1	0.8:1	0.8:1	0.4:1	0.5:1	1.75:1

* Figures in parenthesis are metal concentrations in normal
  human tissue and urine, ppm wet weight, from ICRP publication
  23, "Standard Man".

TABLE 4. Metal concentration in normal human organs, "Standard
          Man" 80% range values from ICRP Publication 23, (ppm
          wet weight).

Sample	Lung	Kidney	Liver	Spleen
Co	−	−	−	−
Cr	−	0.001 − 0.048	0.001 − 0.044	0.001 − 0.045
Mo	−	0.21 − 0.58	0.4 − 1.8	0.04 − 0.07
Ni	0.04 − 0.23	0.05 − 0.14	0.05 − 0.17	0.05 − 0.08
Fe	−	38.7 − 119	72.2 − 322	122 − 667
Zn	−	35.5 − 80.6	27.2 − 77.8	13.9 − 27.2

1. For the organs the levels were considerably raised for Co and
    Cr (up to fifty times normal values), slightly raised for Ni
    and Mo, unchanged for Fe and decreased for Zn.

2. For the hair the level of Cr was considerably raised; the level
    of Co, namely 0.69 ppm, was a factor of ten greater than the
    value for this patient obtained ten years earlier by Coleman,
    Herrington and Scales (1973), namely 0.06 ppm.

3. For the urine the values of Co and Cr were raised as compared
    with normal values.

4. Cr was more plentiful in the organs and in the hair, but Co was
    more plentiful in the urine and lungs.

COMPARISON WITH PREVIOUSLY PUBLISHED RESULTS

Our study of metal sequestration in the organs following total hip
replacement is, we believe, the first of its kind with the exception
of the study of cobalt by Jones et al (1975). Our values for this
element are comparable with theirs and our values for Co, Mo and to
a lesser extent Ni are of particular interest because of the high
levels obtained.

Our results for Co, Cr and Mo in the tissue adjacent to the metal-
on-metal joint are comparable in magnitude to previously obtained
values (Evans et al, 1974; Jones et al, 1975; Smethurst and Waterhouse, 1977; Postel and Langlais, 1977).

Our values for Co and Cr in the hair and urine are greater than
those obtained by Coleman, Herrington and Scales (1973). Our value
for Cr in the hair is similar to the value reported by Owen, Meachim
and Williams (1976), but is greater than the value of 0.96 ppm obtained for females by Schroeder and Nason (1969).

Our results for the dependence of the Co:Cr ratio on location suggests
that Co is more mobile than Cr, which is consistent with previous
findings (Ungethüm and Zenker, 1973; Coleman, Herrington and Scales,
1973; Taylor, 1973). Our results, however, demonstrate for the first
time that Co and Cr are both absorbed by the tissue at a considerable
distance from the implant. Such mobility had previously been
ascribed to Co, but not to Cr. Thus it was thought that Co exhibited
high mobility but was readily excreted rather than absorbed, whereas
Cr exhibited low mobility and, although it was excreted, it remained
essentially local to the implant. No longer can these views be
considered correct.

Our results for the biological trace element Zn are in keeping with
those of Lux and Zeisler (1974) who noted a marked decrease of this
element in "metallosis" tissue, i.e. tissue affected by metal released from an implant, in their case stainless steel. They
suggested that this decrease may result from a displacement of the

enzyme bonded Zn by the components of the implant, causing changes in
the enzymatic processes governing the development of metallosis. This
decrease they associated with an increase in iron, but our results
imply that it may be associated with other elements as well.

DISCUSSION

The values reported for the organs are of particular interest as
stated above because of the high levels obtained. But were these
levels the normal levels for this person? It must be recognised
that for any normally occurring metal in any tissue the values observed in a population of normal people will vary over a considerable range and it has been suggested as a working rule that the
upper limit of the range will be three times the mean (Perry et al,
1962). This being so the values for Co and Cr obtained in this study
are typically one order of magnitude greater than the upper limit of
the range, and would not normally occur by chance. This conclusion
is supported by "Standard Man" data given in Table 4, showing the
range of values occurring in normal people.

What then is the significance of such high levels? There is relatively little information on the pathological effects in man of
increases in the systemic load of metals, whether physiologically
important or not. Certain well known cases are often cited in the
literature, namely the Co-related myocardiopathy in beer drinkers
(Sullivan et al, 1969) and the high concentrations of Fe in Bantu
tribesmen (Wintrobe, 1967). Also certain diseases are thought to be
associated with high concentrations of metal, namely for Co : thy-
roid hypofunction, polycythaemia and myocardiopathy, for Cr : liver
and kidney disease and carcinoma, and for Fe : haemochromatosis,
refractory anaemia and siderosis. Low concentrations of Zn have
been associated with growth retardation. Ni and Mo are thought to be
relatively non-toxic, though a high incidence of respiratory tract
neoplasia has been observed among workers in nickel refineries and
Ni has been implicated as a pulmonary carcinogen in tobacco smoke
(Taylor 1973; Underwood, 1977).

In view of the general lack of information, the amount of Co and Cr
which can be taken with impunity by normal individuals cannot yet be
specified, nor can the risk associated with the levels existing
after long term implantation. In view of this state of uncertainty
and until further research has been carried out, a cautious approach
can be recommended.

ACKNOWLEDGEMENTS

We are grateful to the following at the Institute of Orthopaedics and
the Royal National Orthopaedic Hospital: Professor J.T. Scales, Dr.
K.W.J. Wright, Miss Mary Wait, Mrs Sheila Barnett, Dr. G.D. Winter,
Mr. J. Fincham, Dr. J. Cook, Mrs Lesley Davis, Mr. E. Andrews, Miss
Beverley Coates, Miss Linda Adams, the Department of Medical Photo-
graphy, the Institute Librarian and the Department of Medical Records.

We are also grateful to Mr. M. Kerridge, Director of the University of London reactor centre. Finally, we are grateful to Mr. J.N. Wilson for allowing us to review this case and to the patient's relatives whose interest and generosity made this research possible.

REFERENCES

Coleman, R.F., Herrington, J. and Scales, J.T. (1973) Concentration of wear products in hair, blood and urine after total hip replacement. British Medical Journal, 1, 527-9.

Covell, D.F., (1959) Determination of gamma ray abundances directly from the total absorbtion peak. Analytical Chemistry, 31, 1785-1790.

Evans, E.M. et al. (1974) Metal sensitivity as a cause of bone necrosis and loosening of the prosthesis in total joint replacement. Journal of Bone and Joint Surgery, 56-B, 4, 626-642.

ICRP 23 (1975) International Commission on Radiological Protection, publication 23, Report of the task group on reference man, Pergamon Press, Oxford.

Jones, D.A., et al. (1975) Cobalt toxicity after McKee hip arthoplasty. Journal of Bone and Joint Surgery, 57-B, 289-296.

Lux, F. & Zeisler, R. (1974) Investigation of the Corrosive deposition of components of metal implants. Journal of Radio-analytical Chemistry, 19, 289-297.

Mitman, F.W., et al. (1975) Urinary chromium levels of nine young women eating freely chosen diets. Journal of Nutrition, 105, 64-8.

Owen, R., Meachim, G. & Williams, D.F. (1976) Hair sampling for chromium content following Charnley hip arthroplasty. Journal of Biomedical Materials Research, 10, 91-9.

Parr, R.M. & Taylor, D.M. (1964) Concentrations of Co, Cr, Fe and Zn in some normal human tissues. Biochemical Journal, 91, 424-431.

Perry, H.M., et al. (1962) Variability in metal content of human organs. Journal of Laboratory and Clinical Medicine, 60, 245-253.

Postel, M. & Langlais, F. (1977) L'usure des prostheses totales de hance enstellite. Rev. Chir. Orthop. (Suppl. II), 63, 84-94.

Schroeder, H.A. & Nason, A.P. (1969) Trace metals in human hair. Journal of Investigative Dermatology, 53, 71-78.

Smethurst, E. & Waterhouse, R.B. (1977) Causes of failure in total hip prostheses. Journal of Materials Science, 12, 1781-1792.

Sullivan, J.F., et al. (1969) Myocardiopathy in beer drinkers. Annals of Internal Medicine, 70, 277-282.

Sunderman, F.W., et al. (1972) Nickel metabolism in health and disease. Annals of the New York Academy of Sciences, 199, 300-312.

Taylor, D.M. (1973) Trace metal patterns and disease. Journal of Bone and Joint Surgery, 55-B, 422.

Tipton, I.H. & Cook, M.J. (1963) Trace elements in human tissue. Health Physics, 9, 103-145.

Underwood, E.J. (1977) Trace elements in human and animal nutrition. 4th Edition, Academic Press, New York.

Ungethüm, M. & Zenker, H. (1973) Abrieb-und Oberflachenumtersuchung bei einer Total endoprothese nach McKee-Farrar. Arch. Orthop. Unfall-Chir., 76, 212-219.

Winter, G.D. (1974) Tissue reactions to metallic wear and corrosion products. Journal of Biomedical Materials Research, 8, 11-26

Wintrobe,M.M. (1967) Clinical Haematology, Kimpton, London.

Fracture fixation and ligament reconstruction

Biomaterials 1980
Edited by G. D. Winter, D. F. Gibbons, and H. Plenk, Jr.

THE MECHANICS OF INTRAMEDULLARY NAILING

David Seligson, T. Scott Stanwyck and Malcolm H. Pope

University of Vermont College of Medicine
Department of Orthopaedic Surgery
Burlington, Vermont 05404

SUMMARY

An investigation was made of the biomechanical principles of
intramedullary nailing by bench testing intramedullary nails in tibiae
obtained from amputations. Three-and four-point bending tests of the
bone-nail composite showed a stiffness the same as the bone alone.
Only when the stiffness of the bone was decreased by making a sawcut
did the nail have an effect. Strain gauges were placed on the surface
of the bone and the effect of driving Küntscher nails and Schneider
nails was observed. The maximum elastic hoop strain was greater for
the reamed K-nail ($200\mu\epsilon$) than for the Schneider nail ($50\mu\epsilon$). These
experiments show that sufficient gliding takes place in the bone-nail
system to prevent compound beam behavior; however, the nail does expand
the cortex elastically as described by Küntscher. The complex bone-nail
interaction is the subject of continuing study.

INTRODUCTION

Gerhard Küntscher (1940) developed the method of stable osteosynthesis
for diaphyseal fractures by the use of a thick intramedullary nail
placed in an enlarged medullary cavity. He emphasized three principles: use of a nail of adequate size and strength, elastic adherence
of the nail within marrow space and case selection by fracture type
and location.

It is clear that Küntscher (1967) understood the relationship of nail
size to bending strength for bone and also the possibility that an
open section nail could be jammed into the fractured bone. The
mechanical characteristics and the optimum configurations for insertion of nails have been studied (Soto Hall & McCloy 1953, Lawrence
et al. 1967, Allen et al. 1968). As expected, larger diameter nails
are more rigid and bending configurations which maximize area moment
of inertia maximize stiffness. However, the studies were done in
bone and intramedullary nails separately, although Lindahl (1962)
and Lawrence et al. (1967) did test the composite in torsion comparing
the behavior of the bone-nail system to other forms of osteosynthesis.
Bourgois and Burny (1972) considered the relationship of strain in
an intramedullay nail to fracture healing. Obara (1979) implanted
strain gauge instrumented medullary nails in goats and reported not

only the load characteristics of the nail in gait, but also the reduction in nail strain with fracture healing. Cordey (1980) is
conducting studies of nail and bone deformation at the Laboratorium
Für experimentelle Chirurgie.

This paper concerns the mechanical principles of intramedullary
nailing by measuring the bending rigidity of various bone-nail
composites and making strain gauge measurements of the effect of
nailing on bone. In particular, the importance of 'fit' on rigidity
is considered.

METHODS

Four test situations were employed to investigate the biomechanical
principles of intramedullary nailing of human tibiae; these are:

1. Control: bending stiffness of nails and bone separately (three-
and four-point).

2. Bending stiffness of bone (unbroken) with nails in place (three-
and four-point).

3. Bending stiffness of bone with transverse sawcut, on tension side,
through half-diameter. This was done to simulate a pathological
fracture (four-point).

4. Strain measurement during nailing and extraction by means of
strain gauges attached to the anterior and posterior surfaces of the
tibia segment.

Diaphyseal tibial segments were obtained from surgical amputation
specimens and stored at $-20^{\circ}C$ in Ringer's lactate, a procedure known
not to affect the mechanical properties of bone (Sedlin and Hirsch
1966). The surrounding tissue was removed and the bone tested with an
Instron machine, care being taken to keep the tissue moist at all times.
The crosshead applied a load via an indenter of generous radius in
either three- or four-point bending at a crosshead speed of 1/2 mm per
second. All nails were placed using normal clinical technique, and
standard reaming procedures were followed where appropriate.

Nail insertion experiments were carried out in a jig with a pendulum
hammer so that each impact would be the same. Removal was done at a
constant rate of 5 mm/sec while extraction force was measured with a
load cell. Strain gauges were bonded to the surface using a
modification of the technique of Lanyon (1973).

RESULTS

1. The results of the four test configurations are as follows:

1. Three- and four-point bending of Schneider, Hansen-Street and Küntscher nails (K-nails) with our equipment agreed with previous workers (Allen, Heiple and Burstein, 1978). The stiffness of the 11 mm Küntscher nail was the same as the 11 mm Schneider nail at 3×10^3 Nm/m. Bending of cloverleaf nails showed the expected increase in stiffness with increasing nail size; a 13 mm K-nail approximately the stiffness of the tibia at 10^4 Nm/m.

2. Insertion of Küntscher nails in the two clinical configurations (hand-fitted or reamed and jammed), or of Hansen-Street or Schneider nails into intact tibial segments did not significantly change the bone's stiffness except for the occasional observation of an increase in rigidity with the tightly jammed K-nails. For example, the stiffness of an intact tibia was increased from 12×10^3 Nm/m to 17×10^3 Nm/m when a tightly jammed 11 mm K-nail was inserted. When this same specimen was reamed to 12 mm, a 12 mm K-nail did not change the composite stiffness above that of the control (un-nailed) stiffness.

3. In tibia specimens whose stiffness was reduced by making a sawcut, an increase in bending stiffness with nailing was observed. Each of the four samples studied displayed a behavior of its own. In general, a tight K-nail increased the stiffness of the reamed and weakened bone more frequently than did the Schneider or Hansen-Street (Fig. 1).

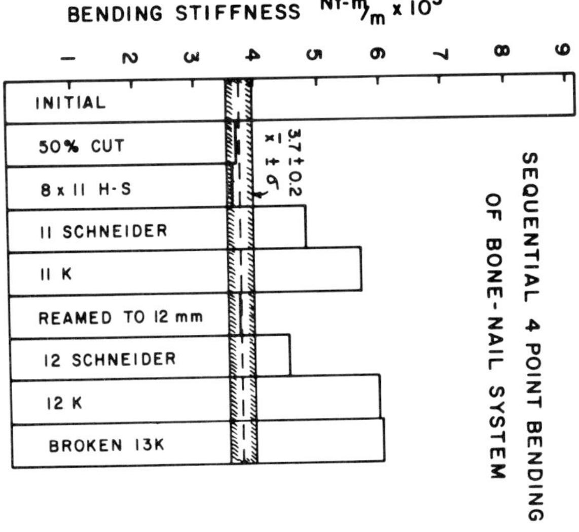

Fig. 1. Sequential 4 point bending of bone-nail system.

4. During controlled nail insertion, peak strains were observed at
the moment of impulse. These exceed the maximum elastic hoop strain
in the range of 200$\mu\epsilon$ for reamed, fitted K-nails and 50$\mu\epsilon$ for
Schneider nails (Fig. 2). Upon removal of the nail five minutes after
insertion, no permanent strain relief was observed. During removal
the pattern of strain relief varied as the nail renegotiated the
medullary canal.

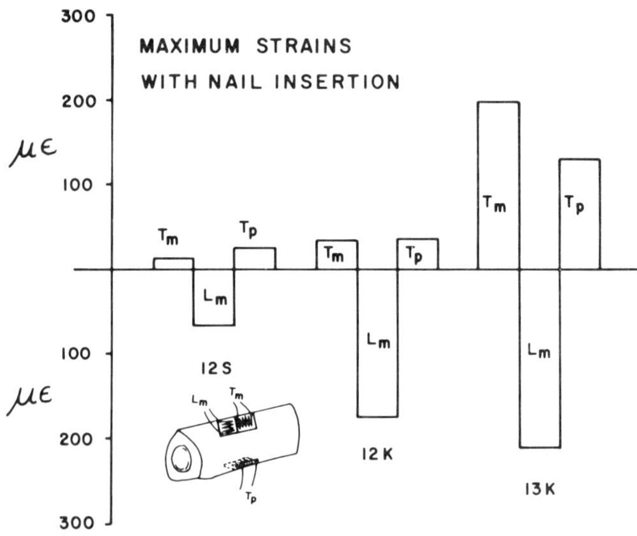

Fig. 2.   Maximum strains with nail insertion.

<u>DISCUSSION</u>

The tests of nailed intact bone demonstrate sufficient gliding of the
bone-nail system to prevent compound beam behavior. This effect is
also seen in a weakened bone simulating an impending pathological
fracture. Therefore, situations must be introduced to increase the
surface interaction between bone and nail if stable osteosynthesis
is to be achieved. This can be accomplished by either increasing
the normal force between the bone and nail, by increasing bone-nail
interface, or by increasing the amount of friction at the interface.
Thus the factors promoting rigidity are at least those identified
by Küntscher.

Our strain gauge experiments demonstrate that elastic adherence does

take place, although this can vary relative to the position of the
intramedullary canal as demonstrated by the removal experiment.
Closed configurations which reduce nail elasticity may trade bending
stiffness of the composite for torsional rigidity by the introduction
of cutting flutes. In addition, a nail may also act elastically between distant contact points in the canal as emphasized by Rush (1955).
These experiments do not exclude the possibility that bending of the
nail as it glances against the cortex plays an important role in its
clinical effect.

The precise relationship between optimum insertion pressure as
measured by surface strain, rigidity in bending and torque, and the
fracture properties of bone needs to be further studied. Clearly
peak insertional strains are capable of initiating cracks in the
critical longitudinal axis of long bones as discussed by Pope &
Outwater (1972).

We are currently examining changes in ambulatory strain with _in vivo_
nailing of sheep tibiae, looking at surface effects in relation to
driving and extraction forces.

<u>REFERENCES</u>

Allen, W. C., Piotrowski, G., Burstein, A. H., & Frankel, V. H.
(1968) Biomechanical principles of intramedullary fixation. <u>Clin.
Orthop</u>. 60, 13-20.
Allen, W. C., Heiple, K. G., & Burstein, A. H. (1978) A fluted fem-
oral intramedullary rod. <u>J. Bone Joint Surg</u>. 60-A, 506-515.
Bourgois, R., & Burny, F. (1972) Measurement of the stiffness of
fracture callus <u>in vivo</u>. A theoretical study, <u>J. Biomech</u>. 5, 85-91,
Cordey, J. (1980) Personal communication.
Küntscher, G. (1940) Die marknagelung von knochenbruchen, <u>Arch. f.
klin. chir</u>., 200-443.
Küntscher, G. (1967) Practice of Intramedullary Nailing, Charles
Thomas, Springfield, Illinois.
Lanyon, L. E. (1973) Analysis of surface bone strain in the calcaneus
of sheep during normal locomotion, <u>J. Biomech</u>. 6, 41-49.
Lawrence, M., Freeman, M. A. R., & Swanson, S. A. V. (1967)
Engineering considerations of internal fixation, <u>J. Bone Joint Surg</u>.
51-B, 754-768.
Lindahl, O. (1962) Rigidity of immobilization of transverse fractures,
<u>Acta Orthopaedica Scand</u>. 32, 237-246.
Obara, T. (1979) A biomechanical study on the fracture treatment,
<u>J. Jap. Orthop. Assoc</u>. 53, 199-212.
Pope, M. H. & Outwater, J. O. (1972) The fracture characteristics
of bone substance, <u>J. Biomech</u>. 5, 457-465.
Rush, I. V. (1955) <u>Atlas of Rush Pin Techniques</u>, Berivon, Meridian,
Mississippi.

Sedlin, E. & Hirsch, C. (1966) Factors affecting the determination of the physical properties of femoral cortical bone, _Acta Orthop. Scand._ 37, 29-48.
Santo-Hall, R. & McCloy, N. P. (1953) Cause and treatment of angulation of femoral intramedullary nails, _Clin. Orthop. 2_, 66.

Biomaterials 1980
Edited by G. D. Winter, D. F. Gibbons, and H. Plenk, Jr.
© 1982 John Wiley and Sons Ltd.

BIODEGRADABLE COMPOSITES FOR INTERNAL FIXATION

P. Christel[*+], F. Chabot[++], J.L. Leray[+], C. Morin[+], M. Vert[++]

* Laboratoire de Recherches Orthopédiques (Pr. J. Witvoët)
  Faculté de Médecine Lariboisière-Saint-Louis,
  10, avenue de Verdun - 75010 Paris.

+ I.N.S.E.R.M. U. 18 - Hôpital Cochin - Paris.

++ E.R.A. 471 - C.N.R.S., Université de Haute Normandie,
   76130 Mont-Saint-Aignan.

SUMMARY

The potential applications of biodegradable implants for osteosynthesis present many advantages over conventional metallic devices.
After biological, chemical and mechanical testing, poly-L-lactic acid
was selected as a candidate. In vivo implantations showed the necessity to reinforce this polymer with fibers. Biodegradable fibers made
of polyglycolic acid were embedded within massive poly-L-lactic acid
to construct composite internal fixation plates which gave promising
results when implanted on sheep tibias.

INTRODUCTION

Metal implants are usually used for internal fixation of fractures.
However, metals are very stiff compared to cortical bone and thus
strongly disturb bone remodeling. Furthermore, another surgical
procedure is very often required to remove the appliance after bone
healing. For several years, many attempts have been made to avoid such
phenomena by developing metallic plates with variable stiffness
(Meyrueis et al 1978) or such composite materials as methacrylate-
carbon (Woo et al 1974), polycarbonate-glass fibers (Tonino 1974),
carbon fiber reinforced carbon (Fitzer et al 1978) and poly-L-lactic
acid-carbon (Alexander et al 1978). The use of bioresorbable materials
for osteosynthesis should lead to several improvements. The implant
might provide the fixation required at the early stage of fracture
healing. Later it should progressively degrade and, therefore,
gradually restore stresses to the bone. The osteosynthesis device,
once degraded, need not be removed, thus avoiding the risks and the
cost of a secondary surgical procedure.

In order to produce biodegradable materials, adequate for human long
bone osteosynthesis, we selected poly-α-hydroxy acids, a class of
polyesters, the main polymers of which are polyglycolic acid (PGA)
and polylactic acid (PLA). These polymers have been known for sometimes (Higgins 1954, Lowe 1954, Fouty 1969) but their biological
applications are relatively recent (Kulkarni et al 1966, Schmitt and
Polistina 1967).

These polymers have demonstrated a very good biocompatibility and are
biodegradable in vivo (Kulkarni et al 1971, Cutright et al 1974)
essentially through a hydrolitic process (Brady et al 1973, Salthouse
and Matlaga 1976), although enzymatic degradation has also been
proposed (Williams and Mort 1977). They are routinely used as surgical
sutures (Dexon[R], Vicryl[R]) and are progressively replacing catgut.
Orbital floor reconstruction (Cutright and Hunsuck 1972) and osteosynthesis of mandible fracture (Getter et al 1972) in monkeys have
been reported with total resorption of the implants. Despite these
promising results no further developments in the field of orthopaedic
surgery have been published.

In the past years, we have undertaken a systematic study of biodegradable rates and mechanical properties of poly-α-hydroxy-acids especially prepared for orthopaedic applications. The compatibility of massive
implants with bone and marrow was first investigated (Leray et al
1977, Sedel et al 1978) and our results have confirmed the outstanding
tolerance of these compounds (Kulkarni et al 1966, Brady et al 1973).
We have also shown that biological and mechanical properties of poly-
α-hydroxy-acids depend on several parameters (molecular weight, molecular weight distribution, presence of low molecular weight compounds
including water, processing conditions) (Chabot et al 1978, Vert et
al 1980).

In this paper, we wish to report the results of our recent attempts
to fabricate internal fixation parts which may fulfill the requirements for safe osteosynthesis of long bone.

MATERIALS AND METHODS

The study was carried out with poly-L-lactic acid (PLA 100), stereocopolymers of D and L-lactic acid (PLA X) where X is the percentage
of L-lactic units and copolymers of lactic acid (D and L) with
glycolic acid (PLA X - PGA Y) where Y is the percentage of glycolic
units in the polymer, which were especially prepared according to
already reported processes (Leray et al 1976, Chabot et al 1978).
The implants were formed using compression moulding technique with
careful control of moulding temperature. Molecular weights of processed polymer materials were assayed by gel permeation chromatography
and viscosimetry.
Sterilization either with dry heat or autoclave caused thermal
degradation and have been precluded (Chabot et al 1978). The effects
of β or γ radiations and ethylene oxide sterilization on the viscosity
of poly-L-lactic acid are exemplified in Table 1. Only ethylene oxide
did not alter the polymers and no ethylene oxide gas was detectable
from carefully vacuum degassed implants.

TABLE 1. Effects of the sterilization mode on viscosity of poly-L-lactic acid.

Sterilizing agent	(η) viscosity ($100\ cm^3\ G^{-1}$)		
	Initial	After sterilization	
		β radiation	γ radiation
Irradiation	0.97	0.8	0.56
(4 Mrad)	1.1	0.7	0.7
Ethylene oxide	1.58	1.59	
	1.56	1.60	

Table 2 exhibits some thermal characteristics as obtained by differential thermo-analysis for our samples of PLA 100 , PGA and several copolymers and stereocopolymers. These results well agree with those recently reported in the open literature (Gilding and Reed 1979).

TABLE 2. Differential thermo-analysis of polymers PLA, PGA, copolymers and stereocopolymers.

% L-lactic	% DL-lactic	% Glycolic	TDA° C
100	0	0	Tf^1 = 174°
75	25	0	Tg^2 = 60°
50	50	0	Tg = 60°
25	75	0	Tg = 59°
0	100	0	Tg = 59,5°
0	0	100	Tf = 218°
25	0	75	Tg = 44°
50	0	50	Tg = 44°
75	0	25	Tg = 52°
0	25	75	Tg = 43°
0	75	25	Tg = 54°

[1]Tf = Melting point

[2]Tg = Glassy transition point

Three series of in vivo implantations were performed to evaluate both material resorption and mechanical degradation.

1. <u>Cylinders and dice</u> (Fig. 1.)

The resorption rate was first studied with 80 cylinders (5 x 5 mm) inserted within the lateral cortex of sheep femora and with 15 x 10 x 2 mm dice drilled with one hole and screwed on the femoral diaphysis of sheep. Both types of implants were made from different polymers : PLA 100 , PGA, PLA X - PGA Y . Implant resorption and tissue response were appraised with microradiographs of thick sections (200 microns) and conventional histology on 5-6 microns sections of explants embedded in methylmethacrylate.

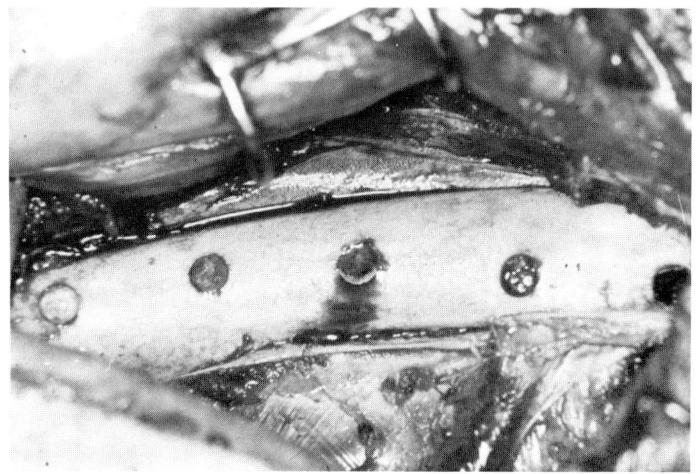

Fig.1. Cylindrical implants (5 x 5 mm) inserted within the lateral cortex of a sheep femur.

2. <u>PLA 100 plates</u> (Fig. 2.)

Twelve 6-hole osteosynthesis plates (90 x 15 x 4 mm) were compression moulded from PLA 100 and screwed with stainless steel screws without osteotomies on sheep tibias. Molecular weights were evaluated for various implantation times on the whole sample, on the outer part underneath the surface and on inner core material.

2. <u>Composite plates</u> (Fig. 3.)

The melting point of highly crystalline PGA (228° C) lies about 50° C above that of PLA 100 . That difference allows to construct a composite material with a PGA renforcing fabric embedded in a PLA 100 matrix by compression moulding (Vert et al 1978). Composite plates were prepared by combining a PLA 100 matrix with plies of two dimensionally woven fabrics of PGA threads (0.1 mm in diameter). By passing the fibers around plate holes and excellent adhesion between fibers and matrix insured high strength to the end product. A typical

improvement of the mechanical behavior of the composite material is
shown in Table 3. Seven composite six-hole plates, the same size as
pla 100 plates, were implanted in sheep tibias.

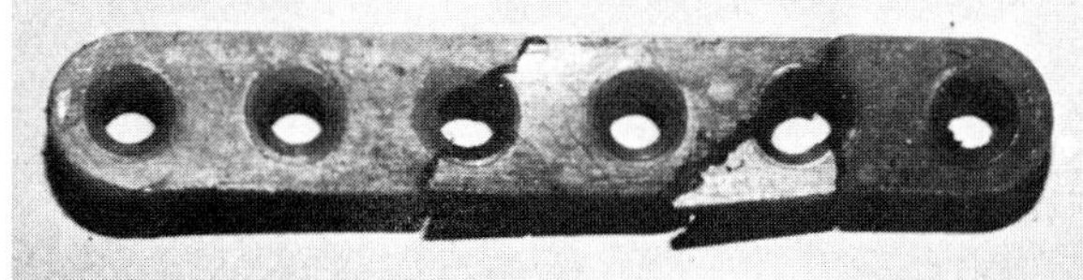

Fig. 2. Broken PLA 100 plate after 4 month implantation
on a sheep tibia without osteotomy.

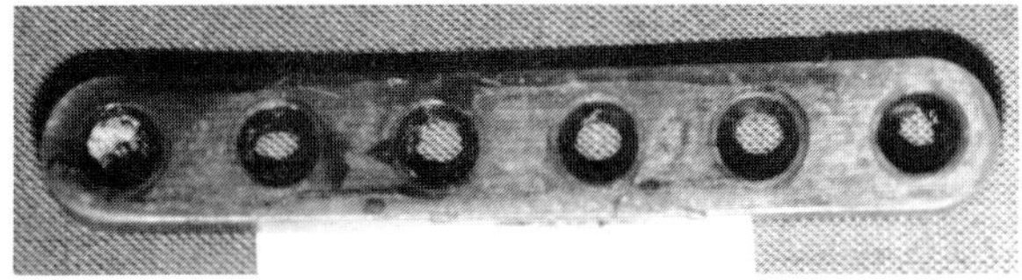

Fig. 3. Composite osteosynthesis plate made of PLA matrix
reinforced with PGA fibers implanted for 7 months on a sheep
tibia without osteotomy : unlike the non reinforced plate
shown in Fig. 2. this suffered only limited damage.

TABLE 3. Comparison between mechanical properties of PLA 100
and PLA 100 reinforced with PGA fibers.

Material	Young modulus bending (GPa)	Elongation %	Resilience	
			Tensile impact test (kj/m^2)	Per notch length (j/m)
PLA 100	4	2	5.2	Raw 30-35 Heat treated 79
PLA 100 + PGA fibers (12 layers of fabric)	6	—	10 to 35	229

                                    Christel et al

RESULTS

1. Implanted cylinders

No appreciable resorption occurred for PLA 100 at 12 months (Fig.4a),
whilst the PGA implant was completely resorbed and the material was
replaced by bone at 4-5 months.

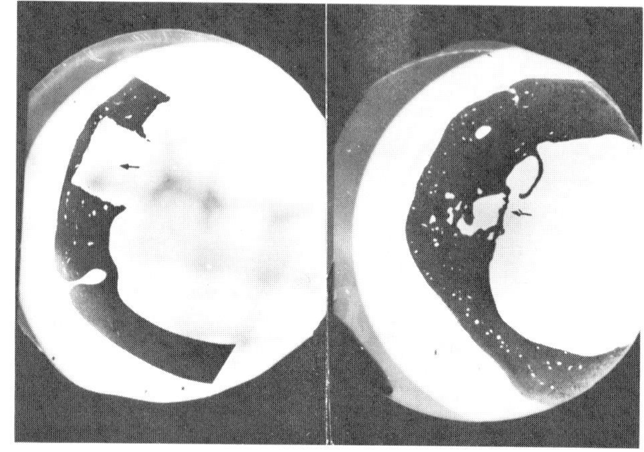

Fig. 4a   Fig. 4b

Fig. 4. Resorption of cylindrical implants.

a : PLA 100 homopolymers after one year. Arrow indicates the
    implant which has maintained its initial shape.
    Radiomicrograph 200 μm section.

b : PLA 25 - PGA 75 copolymers after 6 months. Arrow indicates
    site of implant which is resorbed and replaced by bone.
    Radiomicrograph 200 μm section.

As the rate of degradation of PLA X - PGA Y copolymers increases rapidly
with amount of PGA in the copolymer (Fig. 4b), it should be possible
to adjust approximately rate of degradation to potential use. However,
amorphous copolymers PLA X - PGA Y degrade too fast and have glass
transition too close to 37° C (Table 2), to provide safe fixation for
the healing period. Consequently only highly crystallinic PLA 100 and
PGA where Tg is in the 60° C range were considered for further
investigations. PGA displayed good initial properties : ultimate
tensile strength (UTS) = 57 MPa, Young's modulus E = 6.5 GPa and
elongation ΔL/L = 0.7 % but it was brittle, degraded quickly and was
found inadequate for osteosynthesis. PLA 100 displayed about the same
initial properties : UTS = 59 MPa, E = 4 GPa, ΔL/L = 2.1 % and its
degradation, judging from histology, was slow enough to consider this
polymer as a potential candidate for osteosynthesis material.

2. PLA 100 plates

The initial molecular weight (Table 4) lay around 21×10^4 as referred by GPC to polystyrene standards and circa 12×10^4 as referred to viscosity (Vert et al 1978).

TABLE 4. Degradation of PLA 100 osteosynthesis plates implanted on sheep tibia, with time, as measured by fall in molecular weight.

Duration of implantation	Molecular weight of the whole plate	Molecular weight of the core	Molecular weight of the periphery
0	21×10^4	21×10^4 19×10^4	21×10^4 22×10^4
5 weeks	19×10^4 18×10^4	–	–
6 weeks	21×10^4 21×10^4	–	–
2 Mo 2 w	21×10^4 21×10^4	–	–
3 Mo	–	22×10^4	22×10^4 22×10^4
4 Mo	–	19×10^4	19×10^4 18×10^4
5 Mo	–	22×10^4	18×10^4 18×10^4
13 Mo	–	16×10^4	16×10^4 16×10^4

While no significant change in GPC molecular weight was detected at
the plate surface after 4-5 month implantation (18×10^4), the
molecular weight began to drop in the whole plate after one year
implantation (16×10^4). Initial resilience was 5.2 kj/m^2 and
decreased to 3.2 kj/m^2 after two months in vivo. Animals are still
running with PLA 100 plates, and molecular weight distribution will
be studied up to 3 years. Thus the chemical stability appears to be
adequate compared to fracture healing rate. Although we achieved a
poly-L-lactic acid having lower degradation rates than reported by
others for similar products, the mechanical properties of PLA 100
still appeared as too low. All the explanted plates were broken
(Fig. 2) even after one month implantation probably because of
stresses brought by metal screws. This led us to reinforce PLA 100
with fibers to form a composite material.

3. <u>Composite plates</u>

The five plates without osteotomies, implanted for 1 to 7 months did
not break but exhibited cracks initiated at some screw holes, where
stress concentrations occur (Fig. 3). These cracks allow quick
hydrolysis of the PGA fabric, which was no longer isolated from body
fluids. Two plates were implanted on osteotomized tibias : one broke
one month later, the other one is still under test.

DISCUSSION

Biodegradability alone does not insure the successful use of resorbable materials, which should exhibit characteristics required
specifically by the end use. Earlier attempts to use biodegradable
materials in reconstructive surgery (Cutright and Hunsuck 1972, Getter
et al 1972) were unsuccessful because of the inadequate mechanical
behavior of the materials. The increase in molecular weight of PLA 100
achieved by us, improves significantly the mechanical properties
however this homopolymer alone is not strong enough for internal
fixation of long bones.

When this material is reinforced, composite biodegradable bone plates
show promising mechanical characteristics and a rate of degradation
compatible with the pace of fracture healing. The use of high modulus
carbon fibers embedded within a PLA matrix (Alexander et al 1978) did
not provide a fully resorbable device but underlined the necessity
to reinforce the PLA matrix. With completely resorbable materials the
forming processes are very critical and are certainly not yet
optimized. Fibers size, orientation and distribution should be further
adapted to the end use of the material. Additional investigations will
be carried out using both biodegradable matrix and fibers for plates,
intramedullary nails and screws.

ACKNOWLEDGEMENTS

The authors thank MM. de Charentenay and Dewas (University of
Technology of Compiègne) for mechanical and physical testings,
Mrs Hott for histology, MM. Masingue and Rouse (IFT-Nord) for weaving
PGA and Mrs Henry-Amar for typing the manuscript.
Grants D.G.R.S.T. n° 75 7 1183, 75 7 1184, 75 7 1185, 75 7 1186,
78 7 1021 and 79 7 0311.

REFERENCES

Alexander, H., Strauchler, I., Weiss, A.B., Mayatt, C. & Parsons, J.
(1978) Carbon polymer composites for tendon and ligament replacement.
Proceedings of the 4th Annual Meeting Society for Biomaterials, 123.
Brady, J.M., Cutright, D.E., Miller, R.A. & Battistone, G.C. (1973)
Resorption rate, route of elimination and ultrastructure of the
implant site of polylactic acid in the abdominal wall of the rat.
Journal of Biomedical Materials Research, 7, 155-166.
Chabot, F., Vert, M. & Selegny, E. (1978) Final report DGRST : Polymè-
res nouveaux et améliorés. Grant n° 75 7 1185, avail. CDST-CNRS.
Chabot, F., Vert, M. & Selegny, E. (1980) Action concertée DGRST :
Matériaux et pièces pour ancrage de prothèses osseuses et ostéo-
synthèses. Grant n° 78 7 1021, avail. CDST-CNRS.
Cutright, D.E. & Hunsuck, E.E. (1972) The repair of fractures of the
orbital floor using biodegradable polylactic acid. Oral Surgery, 33,
28-34.
Cutright, D.E., Perez, B., Beasley, J.D., Larson, W.J. & Posey, W.R.
(1974) Degradation rates of polymers and copolymers of polylactic and
polyglycolic acids. Oral Surgery, 37, 142-152.
Fitzer, E., Hutlner, W., Manocha, L.M., Wolter, D., Claes, L.E. &
Kunzl, L. (1978) Carbon fiber reinforced composites as material for
internal bone plates. Proceedings of the 5th London Carbon and
Graphite Conference, 1, 454.
Fouty, D.J. (1969) Preparation of high molecular weight poly-lactide.
Canadian Patent, March 18, 808 731.
Getter, L., Cutright, D.E., Bhaskar, S.N. & Ausburg, J.K. (1972)
Fracture fixation using biodegradable material. Oral Surgery, 30,
344-348.
Gilding, D.K. & Redd, A.M. (1979) Biodegradable polymers for use in
surgery - polyglycolic - polylactic acid homo- and copolymers : 1.
Polymer, 20, 1459.
Higgins, N.A. (1954) Condensation polymers of hydroxyacetic acid.
U.S. Patent, 2 676 945.
Kulkarni, R.K., Pani, K.C., Neuman, D. & Leonard, F. (1966) Polylactic
acid for surgical implants. Archives of Surgery, 93, 839.
Kulkarni, R.K., Moore, E.G., Hegyeli, A.F. & Leonard, F. (1971)
Biodegradable poly (lactic acid) polymers. Journal of Biomedical
Materials Research, 5, 181-191.
Leray, J., Vert, M. & Blanquaert, D. (1976) Nouveau matériau de
prothèse osseuse et son application. French Patent appl., n° 76 28163.
Leray, J.L. (1977) Final report DGRST : Matériaux et pièces pour
ancrage de prothèse osseuse et ostéosynthèse. Grant n° 75 7 1183,
avail. CDST-CNRS.

Lowe, C.E. (1954) Preparation of high molecular weight polyhydroxy-acitic ester. <u>U.S. Patent</u>, 2 668 162.

Meyrueis, J.P., Bonnet, G., de Bazelaire, E. & Zimmerman, R. (1978) Ostéosynthèses par plaques à flexibilité variable. Etude théorique et expérimentation physique. <u>Revue de Chirurgie Orthopédique</u>, 64, 108-112.

Salthouse, T.N. & Matlaga, B.F. (1976) Polyglactin 910 suture absorption and the role of cellular enzymes. <u>Surgery , Gynecology</u> & <u>Obstetrics</u>, 142, 544-550.

Schmitt, E.E. & Polistina, R.A. (1967) Surgical sutures. <u>U.S. Patent</u>, 3 297 033.

Sedel, L., Chabot, F., Christel, P. de Charentenay, X., Leray, J. & Vert, M. (1978) Les implants biodégradables en chirurgie orthopédique. <u>Revue de Chirurgie Orthopédique</u>, 64, Suppl. II, 92-96.

Tonino, A.J. (1974) Operatieve fractuur fixatie met plastic. <u>Thesis</u>, Amsterdam.

Vert, M., Chabot, F., Leray, J. & Christel, P. (1978) Nouvelles pièces d'ostéosynthèse ; leur préparation et leur application. <u>French Patent appl.</u>, n° 78 29878.

Vert, M., Chabot, F., Leray, J. & Christel, P. (in press) Stereo-regular bioresorbable polyesters for orthopaedic surgery. <u>Macromole-cular Chemie</u>.

Williams, D.F. & Mort, E. (1977) The effects of some enzymes on synthetic polymers. <u>Journal of Bioengineering</u>, 1, 231.

Woo, S. L-Y., Akeson, B., Levenetz, B., Coutts, R.D., Matthews, J.V. & Amiel, D. (1974) Potential application of graphite fiber and methyl methacrylate resin composite as internal fixation plates. <u>Journal of Biomedical Materials Research</u>, 8, 321-328.

Biomaterials 1980
Edited by G. D. Winter, D. F. Gibbons, and H. Plenk, Jr.
© 1982 John Wiley and Sons Ltd.

MECHANICAL BEHAVIOR OF BICOMPONENT BRAIDS AS POTENTIAL SURGICAL IMPLANTS

Elizabeth E. Fitzgerald, C.C. Chu*, and David Buchanan

Department of Design and Environmental Analysis
Martha Van Rensselaer Hall, Cornell University
Ithaca, New York 14853, USA

SUMMARY

The concept of bicomponent braids was introduced for the design of more durable surgical implants particularly anterior cruciate ligament. Two sets of tubular bicomponent braid samples from Dacron, Kevlar, and Lycra, differing in construction and composition were made and their mechanical properties were evaluated. Kevlar/Dacron braids exhibited higher tensile strength than the Dacron control braid. They possess sufficient strength to withstand functional forces on the ACL at various activities. However, only the L2 braid withstood most of these loads. A variety of material-structural combinations still remain to be investigated as potential surgical implant; and additional tests are needed for justifying the feasibility of applying this new concept of design of prosthetic devices to surgical implantation.

INTRODUCTION

Injury to the ligaments of the knee joint results in knee laxity and leads to the degenerative joint diseases of articular cartilage, meniscial damage and synovial change. The synthetic prosthetic materials that are currently used for anterior cruciate ligaments replacement are knitted, woven, meshed or in other configurations (Meyers 1979; Grood 1976; James 1977; Rubin 1975). Success in reconstruction has been limited by inherent differences between the mechanical and structural properties of the ACL and the replacement material and the difficulty of permanent implantation (Kennedy 1974).

The purpose of this report is to introduce a new design concept--bicomponent braids--into the search for more durable synthetic materials for better prosthetic construction. In the bicomponent braid as shown in Figure 1, two different synthetic materials are braided tubularly together; the tube may or may not contain a core of a third, filamentary material.

MATERIALS AND METHODS

Three types of fibrous polymers of different denier (d) were used. Kevlar 29 is a high-strength, high-modulus fiber. It has excellent stress relaxation behavior and dynamic and static fatigue resistance. Dacron 52 is a high tenacity industrial yarn. Reconstruction of a canine anterior cruciate ligament using a Dacron velour showed minimal

* To whom all correspondence should be addressed.

tissue reaction and deterioration in strength when implanted in soft tissues (Bruck 1973). Lycra, a polyester-based urethane fiber, is notable for its high elongation and rate of recovery after loading.

Two sets of tubular bicomponent braids, differing in construction and composition, were manufactured. One set of Kevlar (1000 d)/Dacron (1000 d) braids differed in braid construction and contained a 220 denier Dacron core. The other set of Lycra (420 d)/Dacron (440 d) braids differed in the proportions of the component yarns and contained no core. Table 1 summarizes structural characteristics of each braid set.

The test specimens were autoclaved for 30 minutes and then immersed in 0.9% (w/w) saline solution at 37.5°C for periods of 1, 2, 10, 30, 60, and 120 days. Mechanical testing was performed at 21°C $\pm$ 1°C and 65% $\pm$ 2% RH. The gauge length was 3 inches for all tests, and strain rates were 33.3%/minute for Kevlar/Dacron and 333%/minute for Lycra/Dacron samples. For tensile recovery tests, samples were loaded to 40 pounds, maintained at this load for 30 seconds, and then unloaded at the same rates. Each test was repeated five times.

RESULTS

Stress-stain parameters of all test specimens are shown in Table 2. The sterilization process significantly decreased all mechanical properties associated with tensile strength including initial modulus, yield stress, and tenacity. This may be attributed to the shrinkage of braids and hence the denier of the braid increases correspondingly. It is expected that the components of braid don't shrink to the same extent. To minimize shrinkage, other sterilization techniques should be explored.

The weave or construction of the Kevlar/Dacron appears not to effect the mechanical properties greatly. Braids K1, K3, and K4 exhibit similar initial moduli, yield stresses, tenacities, and breaking elongations in ambient and sterilized conditions, as shown in Figure 2. However, the bicomponent braids K1, K3, K4, all possessed higher tensile strength than the Dacron control braid. Braid K4 exhibited a higher tenacity than the rest. On the other hand, the percentage of elongation of the bicomponent braids was smaller than that of the Dacron control braid. It is believed that the breaking strain of a bicomponent braid is mainly controlled by the least ductile component. In the Lycra/Dacron bicomponent braid systems, initial modulus, yield stress, and tenacity increased proportionately with the percentage of Dacron in the Lycra/Dacron braids, as shown in Figure 3.

Mechanical properties of the bicomponent braids were not adversely affected by long-term immersion in normal saline. Tenacity of the Kevlar/ Dacron braids (K1, K3, K4) increased slightly and leveled off after 30 days' exposure in a saline environment. There was no apparent effect on the tenacity of the Lycra/Dacron braids after 60 days' immersion.

Table 3 lists parameters of recovery for tested braids loaded to 40
pounds and then unloaded. Tensile recovery, defined as the percent
of the original elongation recovered after the removal of tensile
stress, was approximately 33% in the K braids and varied in the other
set of braids with the proportion of Lycra to Dacron. The K braids
exhibited 88% hysteresis; the L braids varied. K braids exhibited
slightly greater energy losses with time over periods up to 10 days
in normal saline. This was also true of the L braids, with the exception of the L4 braid which could not support a 40 pound load.

DISCUSSION

The most important characteristic of our design that is different from
current prosthetic devices is the use of bicomponent braids with or
without a core. Different mechanical behaviors of braids were observed due to different components, compositions of the components, and
constructions of braids. Stress-strain curves of the 100% Dacron
braids illustrate the contribution of that component yarn to each of
the bicomponent braids. Even though Dacron 52 is a high-tenacity yarn,
it serves to diminsh the rigidity of K braids. In combination with
Lycra, Dacron is the more rigid component, and increases the tensile
strength of the braid proportionately with the percentage of Dacron
in the braid.

What interests us most is how the mechanical properties of these braids
are different from other prosthetic devices, and how closely they can
reproduce the stress-strain behavior of the human ACL. Noyes reported
failure of the ACL at 1730 N (392 lbs) for young adult specimens, and
at 734 N (166 lbs) for older specimens (Noyes 1976). Other breaking
tensile strengths of ACL specimens such as 625 N (141 lbs) and 285 (56
lbs) to 1,718 N (389 lbs) have also been reported (Kennedy 1976; Trent
1976). Breaking tensile strength of the K braids in this study was approximately 880 N (199 lbs) in the ambient condition and 600 N (136 lbs)
after sterilization. Failure of all L braids occurred below 300 N (68
lbs) in both ambient and sterilized conditions.

The question remains whether a prosthesis should closely duplicate
functional and/or ultimate mechanical properties of the ACL. Morrison
calculated the functional forces on the ACL at various activities and
they ranged from 27 N (6 lbs) while ascending a 9.45° ramp to 445 N
(101 lbs) while descending stairs (Morrison 1969). All of the K braids
tested possess sufficient strength to withstand these loads. Of the
other braids, only the L2 braid will withstand most of these loads, but
will fail under the stresses applied while descending stairs. Since
the yield points of both of the above sets of braids are low compared
with that of the ACL, permanent deformations would occur in the K
braids at stresses exceeding 74 N (17 lbs) and in the strongest of the
L braids at 48 N (11 lbs). The stresses exceeding this yield point in
the K braids occur during level walking and descension of stairs. The
only stress which does not exceed the yield point of the L braids occurs during ascension of a 9.45° ramp. The 100% Dacron control braids
(K2 and L1) exhibit yield stresses of 117 and 56 N (27 & 13 lbs), respectively.

Controversial data about biocompatibility of Kevlar have been reported. In two studies, Kevlar exhibited similar tissue reactivity to
Dacron (King 1977; Huxster 1977). The biocompatibility of Kevlar
should not discourage any further development of bicomponent braids
made of other biocompatible materials for designing more satisfactory
surgical implants. Further research seeking even better structural
combinations and using implant grade materials should be conducted to
assess the feasibility of this new design concept.

ACKNOWLEDGMENTS

We wish to thank the College of Human Ecology, the Department of Design and Environmental Analysis of Cornell University, the Cortland
Cable and Line Company and F.R.L. for their support.

REFERENCES

Bruck, S.D., (1973). "Polymeric Materials: Current Status of Biocom-
patibility", Biomat. Med. Devices, and Artificial Organs, 1:79-89.
Grood, E.S., Noyes, F.R., (1976). Cruciate Ligament Prosthesis:
Strength,Creep,& Fatigue Properties, J. Bone & Joint Surg., 58A:1083.
Huxster, R.H., Jaeger, S.H., and Hunter, J.M., (1977). New Core for
Active Tendon Prosthesis, 23rd Annual Meeting Orthopaedic Research
Society, Las Vegas, Nevada, Feb. 1-3, p. 108.
James, S.L., Woods, G.W., Homsy, C.H., Prewitt, J.M., and Slocum,
D.B., (1979). Cruciate Ligament Stents in Reconstruction of the Un-
stable Knee, Clin. Orthop. and Related Res., 143:90.
Jenkins, D.H.R., Forster, I.W., McKibbin, B., and Ralis, Z.A., (1977).
Induction of Tendon and Ligament Formation by Carbon Implants,
J. Bone and Joint Surg., 59A:53.
Kennedy, J.C., Weinburg, M.C., and Wilson, A.S., (1974). The Anatomy
and Function of the Anterior Cruciate Ligament, J. Bone and Joint
Surg. 56A:233.
Kennedy, J.C., Hawkins, R.J., Willis, R.W., and Danylchuk, K.D.,
(1976) Tension Studies of Human Knee Ligaments - Yield Point, Ultimate
Failure and Disruption of the Cruciate and Tibial Collateral Liga-
ments, J. Bone and Joint Surg. 58A(3):350.
King, R.N., McKenna, G.B., and Statton, W.O., (1977). Novel Uses of
Fibers as Tendons and Bones. J. Appl. Polym. Sci.: Appl. Polym. Symp.
#31, p. 335.
Meyers, J.F., Grana, W.A., & Lesker, P.A., (1979). Reconstruction of
the Anterior Cruciate Ligaments in the Dog, Am. J. Sports Med.,7(2):85.
Morrison, J.B., (1968). Bioengineering Analysis of Force Actions
Transmitted By the Knee Joint, J. Biomech., 3:167
Noyes, F.R., and Grood, E.S., (1976). The Strength of the Anterior
Cruciate Ligament in Humans and Rhesus Monkeys, J. Bone and Joint
Surg., 58A:1074.
Rubin, R.M., Marshall, J.J., and Wang, J., (1975). Prevention of Knee
Instability Experimental Model for Prosthetic Anterior Cruciate Liga-
ment, Clin. Orthop., 113:212.
Trent, P.A., Walker, P.S., & Wolf. B., (1976). Ligament Length Pat-
terns, Strength and Rotational Axes to the Knee Joint, Clin. Orthop.
117:263.

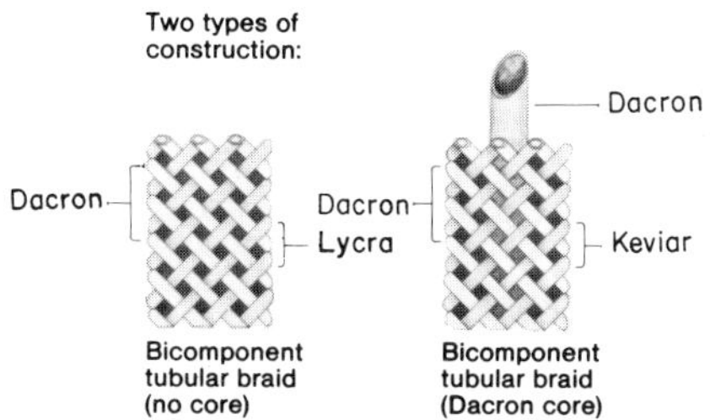

Fig. 1. Schematic drawing of two types of braid construction

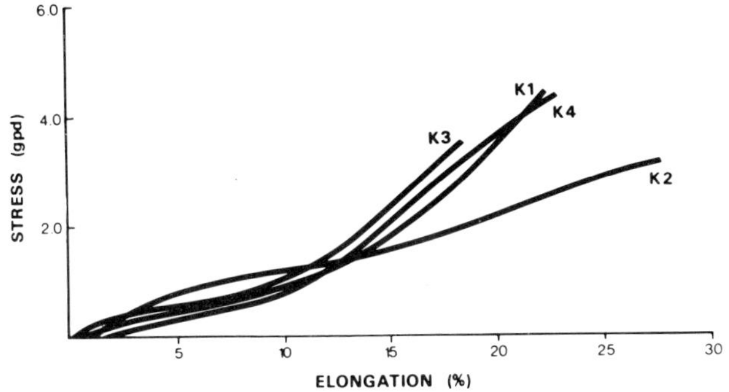

Fig. 2. Stress-strain curves of Kevlar/Dacron braids

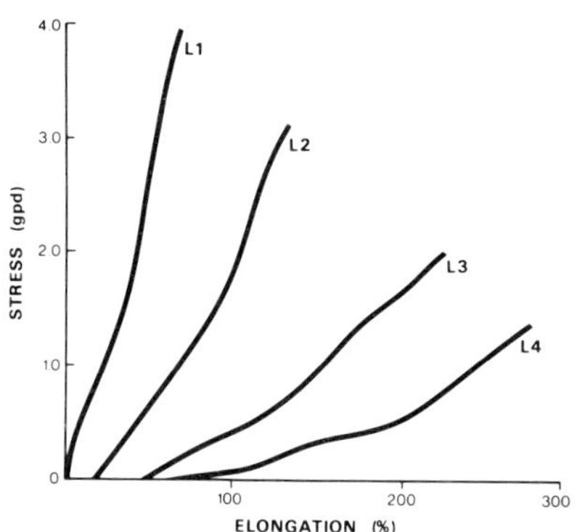

Fig. 3. Stress-strain curves of Lycra/Dacron braids

E. E. Fitzergald, C. C. Chu, and D. Buchanan

TABLE 1. Structural Characteristics of Braids

Braid	Carrier*	Weave[+]	Yarn Composition	Core	Braid Denier
K1	12	$\frac{1}{1}$	50% Dacron 52 50% Kevlar 29	Dacron 52	1.37×10^4
K2	12	$\frac{1}{1}$	100% Dacron 52	Dacron 52	1.45×10^4
K3	12	$\frac{2}{2}$	50% Dacron 52 50% Kevlar 29	Dacron 52	1.36×10^4
K4	12	$\frac{2}{1}$	50% Dacron 52 50% Kevlar 29	Dacron 52	1.33×10^4
L1	16	$\frac{2}{2}$	100% Dacron 52	none	$.868 \times 10^4$
L2	16	$\frac{2}{2}$	75% Dacron 52 25% Lycra 126	none	$.876 \times 10^4$
L3	16	$\frac{2}{2}$	50% Dacron 52 50% Lycra 126	none	$.896 \times 10^4$
L4	16	$\frac{2}{2}$	25% Dacron 52 75% Lycra 126	none	$.777 \times 10^4$
L5	16	$\frac{2}{2}$	100% Lycra 126	none	$.543 \times 10^4$

* The # of bobbins in the braiding machine that carry & feed yarns for making braids.
[+] (x/y) An identification system indicates that the x # of strands passes over & then under y # of another strand of the opposing group.

TABLE 2. Stress-Strain Parameters for Kevlar/Dacron & Lycra Braids

Braid	Initial Modulus (gpd)	Yield Stress (gpd)	Breaking Strain (%)	Tenacity (gpd)
K1	1.00 (0.16)	- (0.48)	9.39 (23.98)	6.35 (4.32)
K2	0.57 (0.32)	0.75 (0.76)	12.75 (27.31)	4.07 (3.21)
K3	0.98 (0.17)	- (0.45)	8.86 (18.0)	6.25 (4.03)
K4	1.00 (0.20)	- (0.55)	9.39 (23.01)	6.99 (4.46)
L1	4.77 (4.87)	- (0.58)	48.6 (86.0)	5.07 (3.5)
L2	1.67 (1.85)	- (0.47)	111.3 (145.6)	3.54 (2.48)
L3	0.72 (0.78)	- (0.42)	197.2 (229.8)	2.46 (1.90)
L4	0.32 (0.33)	- (0.30)	272.8 (326.8)	1.67 (1.31)
L5	0.14 (-)	- -	645.7 (-)	0.55 (-)

Data inside the parentheses are from sterilized specimens while others are from unsterilized specimens.

TABLE 3. Recovery Parameters for Kevlar/Dacron and Lycra/Dacron Braids

Braid	Tensile Recovery (%)	Work Recovery[+] (%)	Hysteresis[§] (%)
K1	35.4 (2.7)	12.0 (1.22)	88.0 (1.22)
K2	33.8 (5.02)	12.6 (1.34)	87.4 (1.34)
K3	33.4 (1.82)	10.6 (.55)	89.4 (.55)
K4	32.4 (1.14)	14.2 (1.64)	85.8 (1.64)
L1	85.0 (2.60)	14.8 (4.2)	85.2 (4.2)
L2	45.5 (3.7)	5.5 (2.2)	92.7 (2.2)
L3	52.0 (1.4)	5.5 (0.71)	94.0 (0.71)
L4*	-	-	-

* Maximum load of 40 pounds exceeds capacity of this braid.
[+] Defined as the fraction of total work done in extension that has been recovered & is measured by $\frac{\text{area under recovery curve}}{\text{area under elongation curve}} \times 100$.
[§] Defined as the proportion of total work dissipated as energy & is equal to (1 - work recovery) x 100.

Biomaterials 1980
Edited by G. D. Winter, D. F. Gibbons, and H. Plenk, Jr.
© 1982 John Wiley and Sons Ltd.

TRAP-DOOR FIXATION OF BRAIDED CARBON FIBRE KNEE JOINT LIGAMENT PROSTHESES

R. Neugebauer, C. Burri, L. Claes
and G. Helbing

Department of Traumatology
University of Ulm, W-Germany

SUMMARY

To obtain a ligament prosthesis with some elastic
properties a carbon fibre strand with a braid angle
of 43 degrees and 32 tows was developed. Two different anchorage systems were tested on cadaveric human
knees. A trap-door anchorage was studied in vivo on
sheep knees. In the in vitro studies on the trap-
door- and the bone channel-anchorage almost the same
resistance to tensile forces was found as on the normal human medial collateral ligament. The in vivo
studies on sheep knees showed a good biocompatibility with ingrowth of connective tissues around the
single carbon fibres. Carbon fibres were also found
embedded in newly formed bone. The trap-door anchorage attained 60 % of the strength of the normal medial ligament after 3 months.

INTRODUCTION

Late reconstruction of knee ligaments is still a
problem and the search for a suitable alloplastic
replacement continues. Recently carbon fibres were
introduced as a new biomaterial (Jenkins and
De Carvalko, 1977; Wolter et al. 1978). They are
suitable because of their good biocompatibility
and their high resistance to tensile forces

(Helbing et al., 1977). To function satisfactorily
the material should have properties similar to the
natural ligament. To increase the elasticity of a
carbon fibre strand a ligament was developed consisting of 32 tows with a braid angle of 43 degrees
(Claes et al., 1979). To prevent immobilization-
damage to the joint early motion is necessary and
so primary stability of the reconstruction of the
knee ligaments is desirable. To achieve this two
different anchorage systems were investigated in
a tensile force test on human cadaveric knees. We
also studied the biological and biomechanical behavior of the carbon fibre strand implanted into
sheep knees.

MATERIAL AND METHODS

For the in vitro test 16 fresh-frozen human cadaveric knees were used. In 8 knees the carbon fibre
strand was inserted under a shelf of bone, simulating a "trap-door". In the second group the carbon ligament was pulled through a V-shaped bone-
channel in the area of the ligament insertion and
then fixed to cortical bone by screw and washer.
Then a tensile force test was performed with the
Instron material testing machine. The force used
to break the normal human collateral ligaments was
also measured.

The in vivo studies were done on eleven 2 year old
sheep weighing 50-55 kg. The medial collateral ligament was resected and replaced by a carbon fibre
strand. The ends were put under a trap-door in the
area of the ligament insertion. The bone shelf then
was refixed by screw and washer. Postoperatively
the knee-joint was not immobilized. After 3 months

the animals were examined clinically and then
killed. Both joints were excised. On 8 specimen
a biomechanical strength test was performed. The
ligament prostheses of 3 knees were fixed in
formalin and embedded in paraffin, for histological examination.

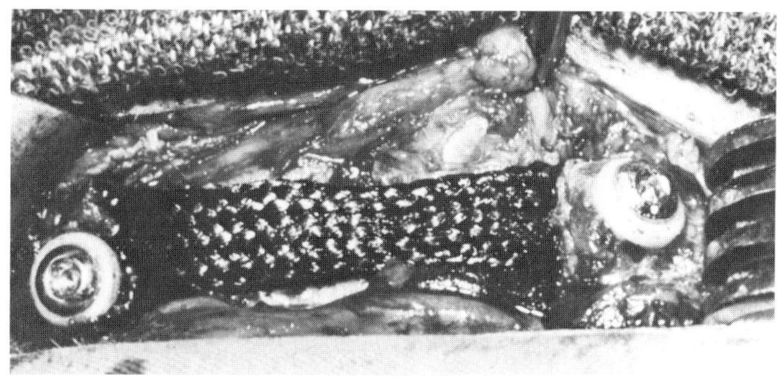

Fig. 1.   Carbon fibre strand as medial
collateral ligament replacement in the
sheep knee. Trap-door anchorage on the
right.

CLINICAL AND MACROSCOPIC FINDINGS

After a few days non-weight bearing all the animals
walked normally. At all times the knee-joints were
stable and there were no signs of inflammation. In
dissecting the specimen it was observed that connective tissue surrounded the carbon fibre strand and
the anchorage to bone was firm. Signs of tissue overgrowth or inflammation were absent. The joint was intact and no cartilage damage or excessive amount of
synovial fluid was observed. The synovia were not
irritated.

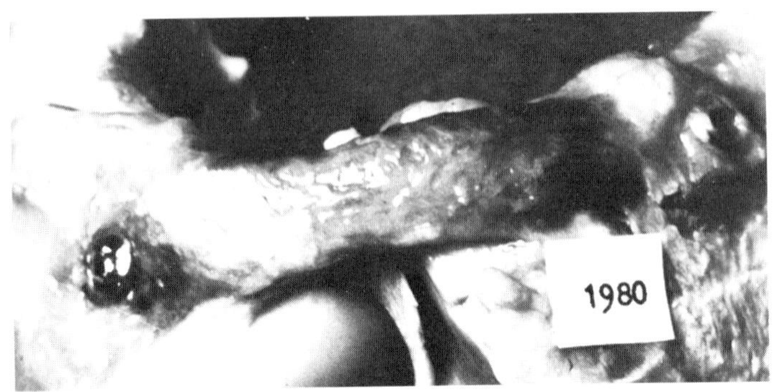

Fig. 2.   Carbon fibre - connective tissue composite ligament 3 months after operation.

BIOMECHANICAL RESULTS

TABLE 1.   Breaking strength of knee ligaments and anchorage systems.

	No. of Specimen	rupture force	
human med. coll. lig.	8	650.8 ± 154	Newton
human lat. coll. lig.	8	354 ± 139.2	Newton
trap-door anchorage	8	434 ± 122	Newton
channel anchorage	8	583 ± 125	Newton
med. coll. lig. sheep	8	590 ± 204	Newton
trap-door anchorage sheep	8	294 ± 60	Newton

The human medial collateral ligament broke at a tensile force of 650.8 ± 154 Newton, the lateral at 354 ± 139.2 Newton. To tear the carbon strand out of

the trap-door anchorage a force of 434 $\pm$ 122 Newton
was necessary. The carbon ligament was pulled out of
the channel at 583 $\pm$ 125 Newton.

The natural medial collateral ligament of the sheep
knee burst at a force of 590 $\pm$ 204 Newton. The ligament prosthesis slipped out of the trap-door at a
force of 294 $\pm$ 60 Newton.

HISTOLOGICAL RESULTS

Around the carbon ligament prosthesis there was a
fibroblast rich granulation tissue at days. Single
carbon fibres were broken. Multinucleated giant cells
were seen in close present contact with the carbon
fibre particles. Collagen fibres developed in and
around the ligament prosthesis. There were many collagen fibres in areas with numerous carbon fibres.
The collagen fibres were orientated in the longitudinal axis of the implant. A new tendon-like tissue
was formed.

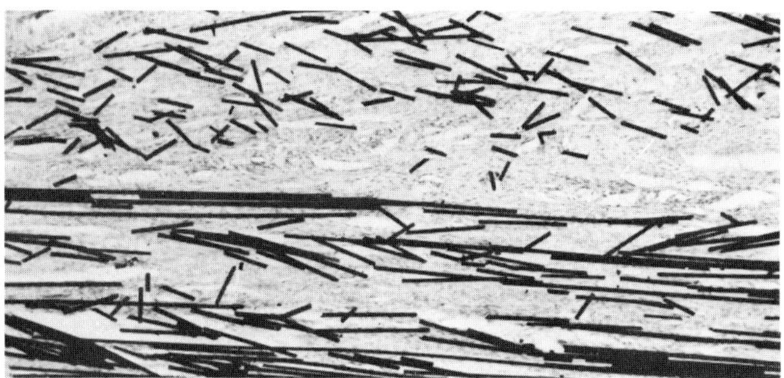

Fig. 3.   Cross section of the carbon prosthesis three months after implantation
showing cell rich connective tissue and
collagen fibres, many of which are broken.
HE; 60 x

                R. Neugebauer et al

Under the bone shelf most of the carbon fibres were
embedded in fibrous connective tissue. At the periphery of the implant, single carbon fibres were found
closely embedded in newly formed bone.

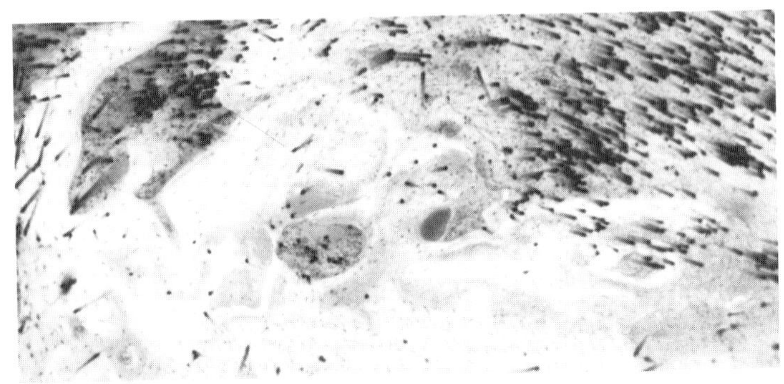

Fig. 4.   Carbon fibres in cancellous bone
and single fibres embedded in newly formed
bone. Undecalcified, cut 60 μ m, 60 x

DISCUSSION

Braided carbon fibre strands can be anchored firmly
to bone to allow early joint motion. This avoids im-
mobilization-damage to the cartilage, ligaments and
muscles. The ingrowth to connective tissue and development of orientated collagen fibres within the implant provides a ligament-like composite of carbon
and collagen fibres which can take up all stresses to
the joint. The observation, in the study, of newly
formed bone around single carbon fibres indicates a
good anchorage, as required for a long lasting ligament replacement. After three months the braided carbon fibre ligament anchored by the trap-door technique
attained 60 per cent strength of the natural ligament
in the sheep knee. If fragmentation of carbon fibres

occurs, the new formed collagen fibres take over
function. Small carbon fibre fragments migrate the
parenchymal organs, but there was no toxic or
granulous reaction to the particles. No damage
to the joint-cartilage or other tissues was seen.

REFERENCES

Claes, L., Burri, C., Neugebauer, R., Wolter, D. &
Rose, P. (1979). The elasticity of various carbon
fibre ligament prostheses, in Conference digest,
2nd Meeting of the European Society of Biomechanics,
Strasbourg.
Helbing, G., Burri, C., Mohr, W., Neugebauer, R. &
Wolter, D. (1980). The reaction of tissue to carbon
particles, in:Evaluation of Biomaterials, (Eds.
Winter, Leray, de Groot) Wiley, U.K., pp 313-380.
Jenkins, G.M.& De Carvalko, F. (1977) Biomedical
applications of carbon fibres reinforced carbon in
implanted prostheses. Carbon 15, pp. 33-37.
Wolter, D., Burri, C., Fitzer, E., Helbing, G. &
Müller, A. (1978). Der alloplastische Ersatz des
medialen Knieseitenbandes durch beschichtete Kohlen-
stoffasern. Unfallheilkunde 81, 390-397.

Biomaterials 1980
Edited by G. D. Winter, D. F. Gibbons, and H. Plenk, Jr.
© 1982 John Wiley and Sons Ltd.

REPLACEMENT OF THE ANTERIOR CRUCIATE LIGAMENT IN THE DOG KNEE WITH A CARBON FIBER IMPLANT

J. Béjui, J. Tabutin and F. Pérot

Service Professeur H. Dejour
Hôpital Edouard Herriot, 69374 Lyon Cédex 2,
France

SUMMARY

A carbon fiber implant was used to replace the anterior cruciate ligament in seven knees of beagle dogs. Clinical results were good seven months after implantation but at necropsy it was discovered that a majority of the implants had broken. The expected fibrous tissue substitution was poor in quantity and quality and cartilage damage and synovial reaction was common. The biological bonding of the implant to bone was efficient although some resorption was apparent and carbon deposits were found histologically in the synovium and regional lymph nodes. The implant did not appear to be suitable for this application.

INTRODUCTION

Ligamentous damage in the knee joint is very frequent and difficult to repair especially when the central pivot (cruciate ligament) essential for the stability of the knee is damaged. A large number of surgical techniques in use today try to repair or replace a torn or absent cruciate ligament. Many surgeons have attempted to use prosthetic material, i.e., Dacron (Renaud, 1978) or polyethylene (Blazina, 1975) but breakage and reactive synovitis are common sequelae. Recently, carbon fiber implants have been reported to be biocompatible and of sufficient strength to warrant a study of the possibilities of using this material for replacement of the anterior cruciate ligament.

METHODS

The implant consists of a plaited bundle of seven micrometer, high strength carbon fibers, the mechanical charac-

          J. Béjui, J. Tabutin and F. Pérot

teristics of which are detailed in Table 1. Additionally,
it has been coated with vapour phase deposited pyrocarbon
to prevent fragmentation without fusing the fibers together.

TABLE 1. Mechanical characteristics carbon fiber
implant

Cylindrical plait   48,000 filaments
Filaments diameter   7 μm
Composition   more than 99.5 % carbon
Total diameter   2.8 mm
Total length   200 to 250 mm
Usable length   150 mm
Ultimate tensile stress   1000 N
Ability to lengthess   10 %

Seven adult two years old range male beagle dogs weighing
15-18 kg were used as the test system. The surgical technique involved an anterolateral approach to the knee with
medial dislocation of the patella. The anterior cruciate
ligament was resected as completely as possible and replaced with the carbon fiber implant following MacIntosh's
"over the top" procedure (MacIntosh, 1974) with the addition of femoral and tibial bone tunnels. Fixation of the
device to bone was accomplished by knotting the proximal
end of the device above a specially designed ring, also
made of carbon composites. A conical bearing device secured
the distal end. The stability of the joint was tested immediately. The knee was immobilized with a splint for three
weeks post-operatively. After seven months the animals were
sacrificed and the knee examined clinically and radiologically. At necropsy special note was made of the cartilage
and synovium. These structures were also studied microscopically. Any regional migration of carbon was noted. Any
changes seen in the normal structures were compared to that
which occurs when the anterior cruciate ligament is
resected and not replaced as determined in another study.

RESULTS

Full weight bearing and range of motion with no noticeable
limp on the operated leg occurred within five to six weeks
after surgery. Radiologically the amount of anterior drawer
present at seven months was 7.1 mm on the operated knee

compared to a normal of 6.6 mm. No radiological sign of
arthrosis was seen.

At necropsy three joints had significant hydroarthrosis.
The synovium was colored black in all cases. In two, a
"bucket handle" tear of the medial meniscus was present
(Fig. 1).

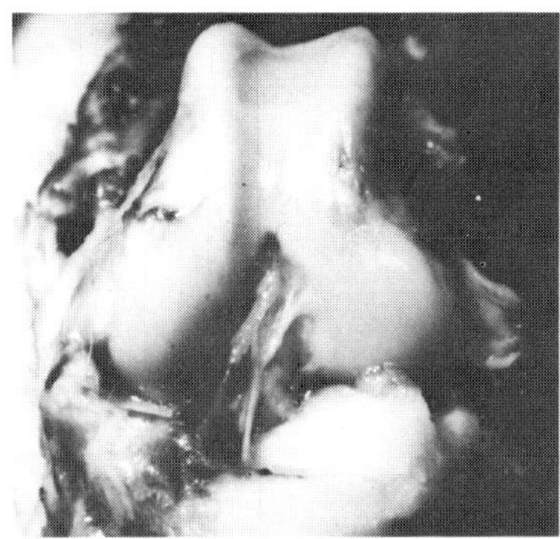

Fig. 1. Right knee : rupture of the implant
"bucket handle" tear of the medial meniscus.

The implant was broken in every case usually in its middle
intra-articular portion. A whitish fibrous tissue surrounded the broken ends, uniting them in all but two cases.
This tissue, however, was very fragile with an ultimate
tensile strength under 100 newtons. The parts of the
implant within bone were well incorporated with no motion
apparent between the implant and bone. Black colored
fibrous tissue was commonly found around the proximal end.
Significant synovial congestion (hyperplasia) with minimal
to no osteophytosis and a diffuse chondromalacia and fissuration were present in all operated knees (Table 2).

J. Béjui, J. Tabutin and F. Pérot

TABLE 2. Fissure formation, osteophytes and synovitis after anterior cruciate ligament replacement

	DOG	1	2	3	4	5	6	7	UNOPERATED
FISSURATION %	Patella	5	5	0	0	5			0
	Trochlea	5	10	5	20	20	20	20	0
	Med. Cond.	30	40	30	5	40	20	20	5
	Lat. Cond.			20	5	10	5	10	0
	Med. Plat.	60	60	30	30	65	60	60	20
	Lat. Plat.	70	50	20	20	50	40	40	5
Osteophytosis		±	0	0	±	0	0	0	0
Synovitis		+	±	+	+	±	±	0	0

Conditions of knees of 7 beagle dogs after implantation of carbon fiber ligament prosthesis for seven months (Technique after Meachim, 1972)

There appeared to be a good correlation between fissuration and the anterior drawer sign. These changes were similar to those observed in a knee in which the anterior cruciate had been cut three to four months previously with regard to the amount of chondromalacia and fissuration (Fig. 2), but osteophytosis and synovitis were less after prosthetic replacement of the anterior cruciate ligament.

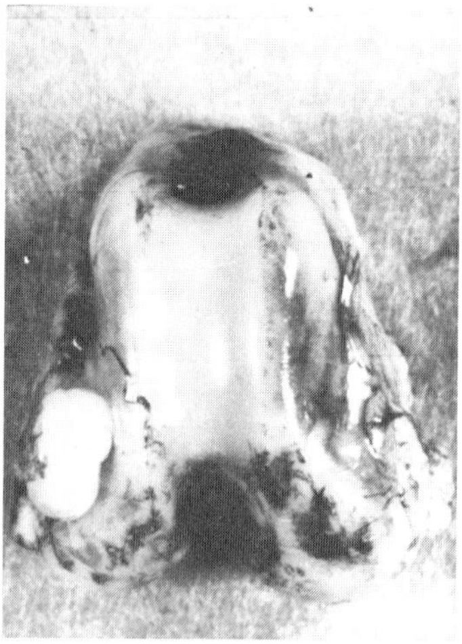

Fig. 2. Significant fissuration mainly at the condylo-trochlea ridge.

Histologically, the synovium was hyperplastic and containing many multinucleated giant cells (Fig. 3).

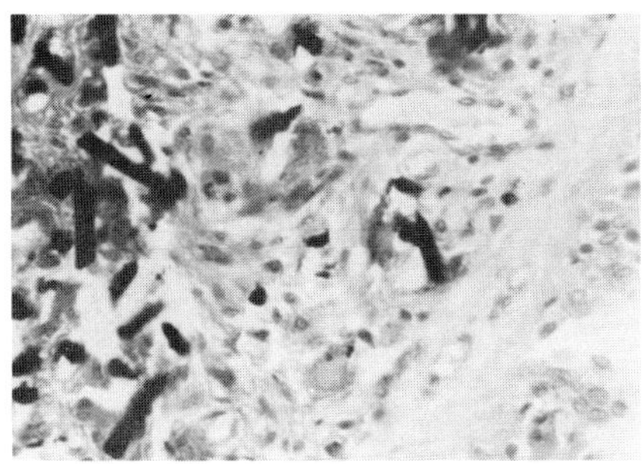

Fig. 3. Synovial hyperplasia. Carbon fragments
totally and partially included in giant cells.

Resorption granulomas were frequently observed around
three types of carbon elements : large long fragments
which were partly included in giant cells; small fragments
totally located inside giant cells; very small fragments
within histiocytes. These patterns were found in the synovium, bone and covering tissue. In the intercondylar notch,
the implant and surrounding tissue demonstrated some con-
tinuity : orientated collagen fibers were present between
the broken ends of the implant. In this area remaining
carbon fibers were separated by collagen bundles and were
covered by a synovial membrane. Numerous giant cells were
again present. The medullary cavity near the tibial and
femoral bone tunnels was no longer present. Carbon fibers,
collagen and giant cells were plentiful between the bone
trabeculae. Resorption of bone and replacement with collagen fibers was the main phenomenon observed. The muscle
adjacent to the implant distally was undergoing fibrosis
and contained numerous histiocytes but no giant cells were
present. The muscle proximally was surrounded by a hyperplastic synovial membrane containing oriented collagen fibers. The inguinal lymph nodes contained carbon in three
cases usually within histiocytes. Lung biopsies were all
normal.

DISCUSSION

Since all implants disrupted and the operative technique was presumed to be adequate, the most likely cause for disruption, in the opinion of the authors, is that the mechanical properties of the implant were not suitable for this application. The ultimate strength of the repair should come from tissue ingrowth and substitution of the carbon fibers. Although some fibrous tissue was seen in place of the implant that did contain oriented collagen fibers in a synovial coating, this tissue did not have the required mechanical properties to function as an anterior cruciate ligament. However, the lesions were much less serious than after simple section of the ligament. This means that either the implant was efficient during a certain amount of time or that the tissue which formed between its broken ends had some mechanical value. Bonding of the implants to bone seemed to be reliable as the trans-osseous tunnels provided secure fixation. Fixation devices were unnecessary once bonding to bone was achieved. The implants did undergo marked fragmentation with resultant migration of carbon to regional lymph nodes and caused a severe synovial reaction. Although no real sign of toxicity was demonstrated, it appears that carbon fiber ligaments may not be applicable to the intra-articular environment.

Ruptures of this and other inert anterior cruciate ligament prostheses may be due either to a lack of elasticity of the material (Beaucham et al, 1979) or to the fact that the normal ligament has several parts, functional at different times, depending on the type of movement; behaviour which cannot be realized by an implant.

ACKNOWLEDGEMENTS

We thank M. Arlot, L.N. Patricot and E. Vignon for their outstanding assistance.

REFERENCES AND BIBLIOGRAPHY

Beaucham, P., Laurin, C.A. & Baillon, J.P. (1979) Etude des propriétés mécaniques des ligaments croisés en vue de leur remplacement prothétique. Revue de Chirurgie Orthopédique, 65, 197-207.

Blazina, M.E.S. & Kennedy, J.C. (1975) Surgical technique for prosthetic cruciate ligament replacement (Eds., Richards Manufactoring Co Inc.) Memphis, USA.

Jenkins, D.H.R., Forster, I.W., McKibbin, B. & Raliz, Z.A. (1977) Induction of tendon and ligament formation by carbon implantation. The Journal of Bone and Joint Surgery, 59B, 53-57.

Jenkins, D.H.R. (1978) The repair of cruciate ligament with flexible carbon fiber. The Journal of Bone and Joint Surgery, 60B, 520-522.

Lawrin, C.A. (1973) Prosthetic replacement of the cruciate ligaments. The Journal of Bone and Joint Surgery, 55A, 1771.

Lawrin, C.A. & Saidi, K. (1973) Prosthetic replacement of the anterior cruciate ligament. The Journal of Bone and Joint Surgery, 55A, 652.

MacIntosh, D.L. (1974) The anterior cruciate ligament "over the top repair". The Journal of Bone and Joint Surgery, 56B, 591.

Meachim, G. (1972) Light microscopy of Indian ink preparation of fibrillated cartilage. Annals of the Rheumatic Diseases, 31, 457-464.

Neugebauer, R., Burri, C. & Wolter, D. (1979) The replacement of ligaments with carbon fibers in the knee joint. Paper read at the First Congress of the International Society of the Knee, Lyon, France.

O'Donoghue, D., Frank, G.R., Jeter, G.L., Johnson, W., Zeiders, J.W. & Kenyon, R. (1971) Repair and reconstitution of the anterior cruciate ligament in dogs. The Journal of Bone and Joint Surgery, 53A, 710-718.

Renaud, F. (1978) Etat actuel de nos tentatives d'implantation de ligaments croisés prothétiques. Chirurgie du Genou (Eds., Simep), pp 99. Lyon.

Woods, G.W. (1979) Cruciate ligament prosthesis : five years of development. Paper read at the First Congress of the International Society of the Knee, Lyon, France.

Bone cement

Biomaterials 1980
Edited by G. D. Winter, D. F. Gibbons, and H. Plenk, Jr.
© 1982 John Wiley and Sons Ltd.

EPR STUDIES OF PMMA BONE CEMENT

J.B. Park,* M.A. Ackley,* and R.C. Turner**

*Department of Interdisciplinary Studies
**Department of Physics and Astronomy
Clemson University, Clemson, SC 29631, USA

SUMMARY

Radiolucent and radiopaque surgical bone cements were used to monitor
the number of free radicals during polymerization and curing by using
EPR spectroscopy in vitro conditions. It was found that the general
shape of the free radical concentration curves are similar for both
types of cements. The number of free radicals does not increase until
after the first 6 minutes and reaches maximum at about 15 minutes.
The free radicals then decay very slowly over a period of many days.

INTRODUCTION

Polymethylmethacrylate (PMMA) bone cement is being used widely for
fixation of orthopedic implants (Charnley, 1972; Eftekar, 1978; Park,
1979; Schaldach and Hohmann, 1976). Although this material has been a
subject of many studies (Hass, et al., 1975; Lautenschlager, et al.,
1974; Lee, et al., 1975) the polymerization process at the molecular
level is not well understood (Meyer, et al., 1973).

Electron paramagnetic resonance (EPR) spectroscopy is a tool which can
be used to detect unpaired electrons or free radicals in materials.
EPR has been utilized extensively in determining chemical structure
(Campbell, 1976) and the structure-property relationship of both biological (Feher, 1970; Swartz, et al., 1972) and non-biological materials such as synthetic polymers (Kausch and DeVries, 1975; Keller and
Turner, 1972, Park, et al., 1978a, 1978b; Turner and Keller, 1972).

Recently we have utilized the EPR technique to study polymerization
behavior of PMMA bone cement and found that an observable number of
free radicals are generated during polymerization after mixing the
polymer powder and monomer liquid (Park, et al., 1980). The present
preliminary study is concerned with the aging of bone cement in vitro
at room temperature in air and at 37°C in saline solution.

MATERIALS AND METHODS

Radiolucent and radiopaque Surgical Simplex® P bone cements (Howmed-
dica, Inc., Rutherford, NJ) were used for this study.

303

The cement was mixed according to the instructions of the manufacturer and the starting time was noted. After throroghly mixing the powder and monomer for two minutes, the dough was inserted into a 0.28 cm diameter 7.5 cm long quartz tube which in turn was inserted into the microwave cavity of an EPR spectrometer. The spectrum was measured at room temperature using a Varian E3 spectrometer. The concentration of polymerization radicals was measured continuously for 30 minutes and intermittently after that.

The samples were removed from their quartz tubes 45 minutes after mixing and were then stored either in a dessicator at 22°C or in a 37°C 0.9% NaCl solution bath in between measurements in order to see the effect of temperature and saline solution on the decay of the free radicals.

RESULTS AND DISCUSSION

Figure 1 shows a typical EPR absorption spectrum of radiolucent bone cement. The main difference between radiolucent and radiopaque cement is the presence of sterilization radicals superimposed onto the PMMA polymerization spectrum for the radiopaque bone cement (Park, et al., 1980). The sterilization radicals are apparently present in the $BaSO_4$ in the polymer powder and do not decay away after polymerization with

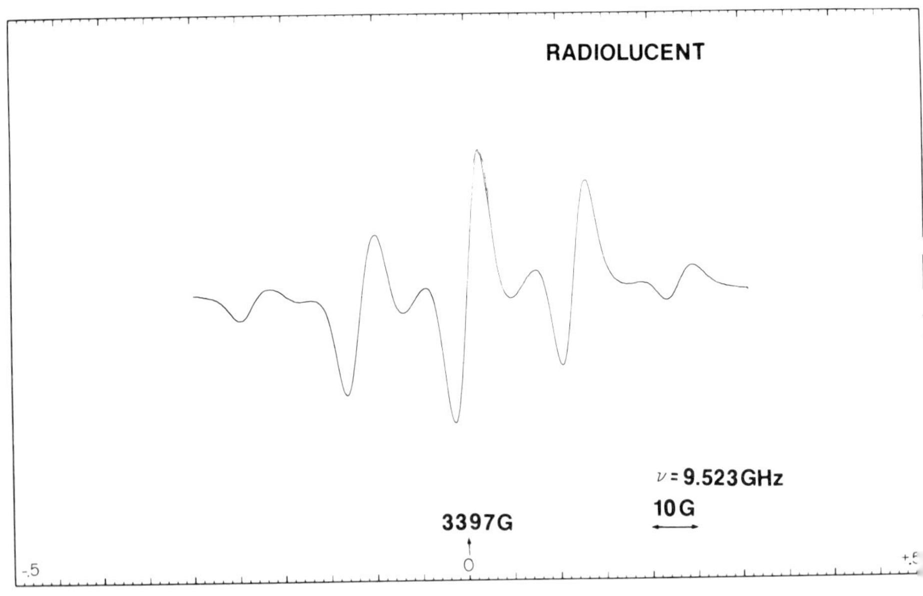

Figure 1. Typical EPR spectrum of the polymerization radical in radiolucent bone cement after mixing polymer powder and monomer liquid.

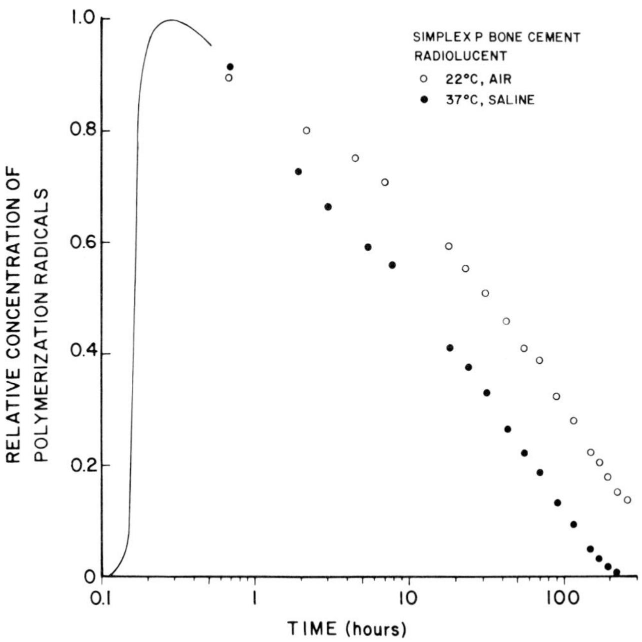

Figure 2. Relative free radical concentrations vs time after mixing polymer powder and monomer liquid of radiolucent cement.

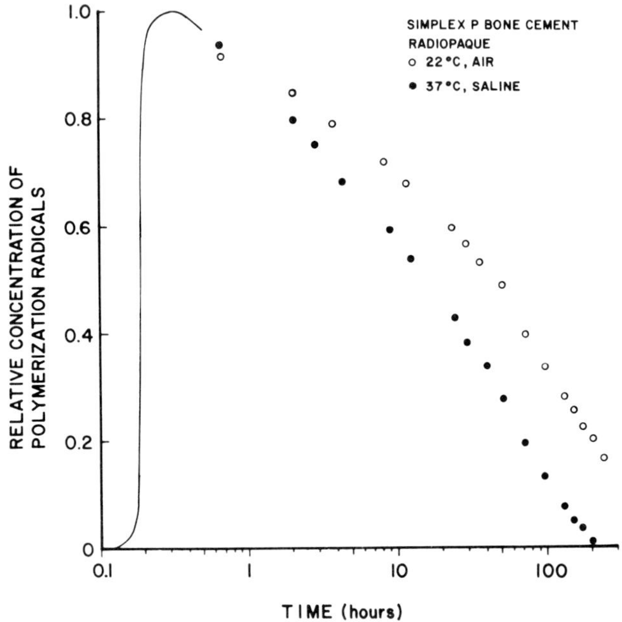

Figure 3. Relative free radical concentrations vs time after mixing polymer powder and monomer liquid of radiopaque cement.

liquid monomer. They are found to be quite stable up to 100°C, however, and do not seem to interfere with the polymerization process
(Park, et al., 1980).

Figures 2 and 3 show the results of the growth and decay of the polymerization radicals of radiolucent and radiopaque bone cement. Some
observations can be made:

(1) The general shape of the concentration curves are the same for
both radiolucent and radiopaque bone cement whether aged in air or
saline solution. Both the growth and decay occur slightly more rapidly in the radiolucent cement. Apparently the $BaSO_4$ present in the
radiopaque cement delays the reaction, probably by diluting the concentration of reactants.

(2) The number of free radicals does not increase with time for about
the first 6 minutes. The rapid rise in the number of free radicals
after about 10 minutes coincides with the rise in temperature after
mixing (Turner, et al., 1980). It is likely that the increasing temperature may be "auto-accelerating" the polymerization process
(Turner, 1977).

(3) The number of free radicals does not decay rapidly after reaching
the peak concentration but decays quite slowly. Although the decay
rate is faster when stored in the saline solution (see Figures 3 and
3), the complete disappearance of the free radicals still takes a very
long time (hundreds of hours). If the implication of this result can
be extrapolated to the in vivo circumstance, then the free radicals
may have time to diffuse out of the bone cement as do the monomers
(Homsy, 1971). However, it is not yet understood whether this process
is clinically significant or not.

ACKNOWLEDGEMENT

The project was supported in part by the FRC grant of Clemson University and by the Departments of Interdisciplinary Studies and Physics
and Astronomy. The help of Mr. F.B. White is gratefully acknowledged.
This manuscript was typed by Mrs. Nancy Looney.

REFERENCES

Campbell, D. (1976) Electron spin resonance of polymers. J. Poly.
Sci. - D, 4, 91-181.
Charnley, J. (1972) Acrylic cement in orthopedic surgery. Williams
and Wilkins Col, Baltimore.
Eftekar, N.S. (1978) Principles of total hip arthroplasty. C.V. Mosby,
St. Louis.
Feher, G. (1970) Electron paramagnetic resonance with application to
selected problems in biology. Gordon and Breach, New York.
Hass, S.S., Braner, G.M. & Dickson, G. (1975) A characterization of
polymethylmethacrylate bone cement. J. Bone Joint Surg., 57A, 380-
391.

Homsy, C.A. (1971) Current research on the in vitro stabilization of skeletal prosthetic elements. Biomaterials, (ed. Bement, A. L.), pp 135-155, U. of Washington Press, Seattle.

Kausch, H.H. & DeVries, K.L. (1975) Molecular aspects of high polymer fracture as investigated by ESR techniques. Intern. J. Fract., 11, 727-759.

Keller, F.J. & Turner, R.C. (1972) An ESR study of thermal degradation of polyethylene terephthalate. Bull. Am. Phys. Soc., 17, 341.

Lautenschlager, E.P., Moore, B.K., & Schoenfeld, C.M. (1974) Physical characteristics of setting of acrylic bone cements. J. Biomed. Mat. Res. Symp. No. 5 (Part 1), 185-196.

Lee, A.J.C., Ling, R.S.M. & Wrighton, J.D. (1973) Some properties of PMMA with reference to its use in orthopedic surgery. Clin. Orth. Rel. Res., 95, 281-287.

Myer, P.R., Lautenschlager, E.P. & Moore, B.K. (1973) On the setting properties of acrylic bone cement. J. Bone Joint Surg., 55A, 149-156.

Park, J.B. (1979) Biomaterials, an introduction, Plenum Publishing Co., New York.

Park, J.B., DeVries, K.L. & Statton, W.O. (1978a) Chain rupture during tensile deformation of nylon 6 fibers. J. Macromol. Sci., B15, 205-227.

Park, J.B., DeVries, K.L. & Statton, W.O. (1978b) Structure changes caused by strain annealing of nylon 6 fibers. J. Macromol. Sci., B15, 409-420.

Park, J.B., Turner, R.C. & Atkins, P.E. (1980) EPR study of free radicals in PMMA bone cement: a feasibility study. Biomat. Med. Dev. Art. Org., 8, 23-33.

Schaldach, M. & Hohmann, D. (1976) Advances in artificial hip and knee joint technology, Springer-Verlag, Berlin.

Swartz, H.M., Bolton, J.R. & Borg, D.C. (1972) Biological application of electron spin resonance. J. Wiley, New York.

Turner, D.T. (1977) Autoacceleration of free radical polymerization 1. the critical concentration. J. Macromol., 10, 221-226.

Turner, R.C., Atkins, P.E., Ackley, M.A. & Park, J.B. (1980) Molecular and macroscopic properties of PMMA bone cement: free radical generation and temperature change versus mixing ratio. submitted to the J. Biomed. Mater. Res.

Turner, R.C. & Keller, F.J. (1972) An ESR study of thermal and radio-active decomposition of polyethylene terephthalate. Bull. Am. Phys. Soc., 17, 201.

Biomaterials 1980
Edited by G. D. Winter, D. F. Gibbons, and H. Plenk, Jr.
© 1982 John Wiley and Sons Ltd.

A METHOD FOR IN VIVO OBSERVATION OF THE
CEMENT-BONE INTERFACE

T. Albrektsson and L. Linder

The Laboratory of Experimental Biology, Dept of
Anatomy, University of Gothenburg and the
Institute for Applied Biotechnology, Mölndal,
Sweden

SUMMARY

A method for long-term *in vivo* observation of rabbit bone is presented.
A modification of the technique allows direct observation of the bone
reaction following application of bone cement. Grave acute local
tissue injury was obvious but no long-term adverse reactions were
detected by this method.

INTRODUCTION

The events taking place in bone after insertion of an implant have so
far been described only in histological sections taken at serial intervals. Continuous observation of the tissue reaction round the same implant has not been possible.

This paper will describe a new method of continuous observation of the
same bone compartment over long periods of time, before and after application of an implant material in contact with the tissue. The
method is not limited to any specific type of implant material. The
recordings are made by vital microscopy of bone tissue, a method which
is sensitive in the detection of tissue injury and which, in bone,
allows study of repair and remodelling phenomena (Albrektsson 1980).

METHODS

The experiments are carried out in rabbits. Each animal receives in
one tibial metaphysis a titanium chamber as described by Albrektsson
and Albrektsson (1978). In principle the chamber consists of a screw-
shaped titanium frame containing two quartz glass rods. Between the
rods there is a space of 100 microns. As the chamber heals into the
tibia, bone grows into this space. By transilluminating the chamber
this "living histological specimen" can be studied in the vital microscope. After installation of the chamber the skin is closed, but by
making small skin incisions at the chamber ends, the tissue in the
chamber can be studied at repeated intervals over periods of months -
years.

The chamber described in this paper contains a canal along the top
glass rod, reaching the edge of the test tissue. At the time of
chamber installation this canal is occupied by a titanium pin, which
later is removed and substituted for by the test substance. This
substance then reaches the test tissue and remains in contact with
the tissue until the experiment is terminated. Fig. 1 represents a
schematic drawing of the titanium chamber.

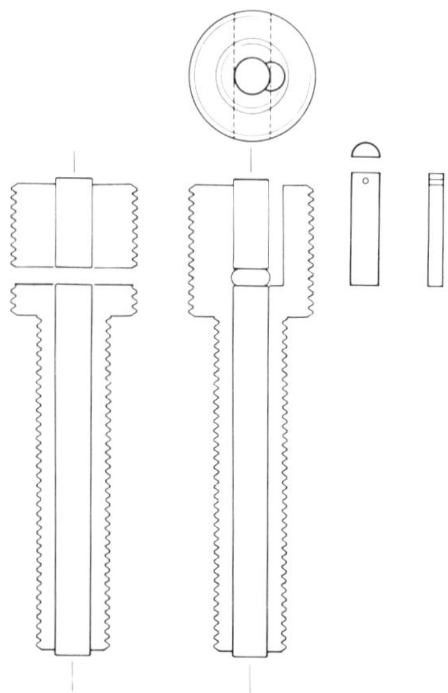

Fig. 1. Total length of the titanium frame is 27 mm,
outer diameter 7 mm and 4,5 mm, respectively, and
glass rod diameter 2 mm. After chamber installation
bone grows into the space between the glass rods and
can be observed in the microscope through transillumi-
nation of the chamber.

The installation of the chamber and the subsequent recordings are
made under general anaesthesia and aseptic conditions. After installation the chamber is allowed to heal into the bone for about 6 weeks.
At this interval the chamber tissue is examined in the microscope. Two
weeks later the test substance is applied following another examination. These observations are made to ensure that a steady state has
been reached in the chamber tissue. Immediately following the application of the test substance, its acute effects on the tissue are recorded. Further recordings are made weekly until a new steady state has
developed.

In fig. 2 the principles of the present experiment are exposed.

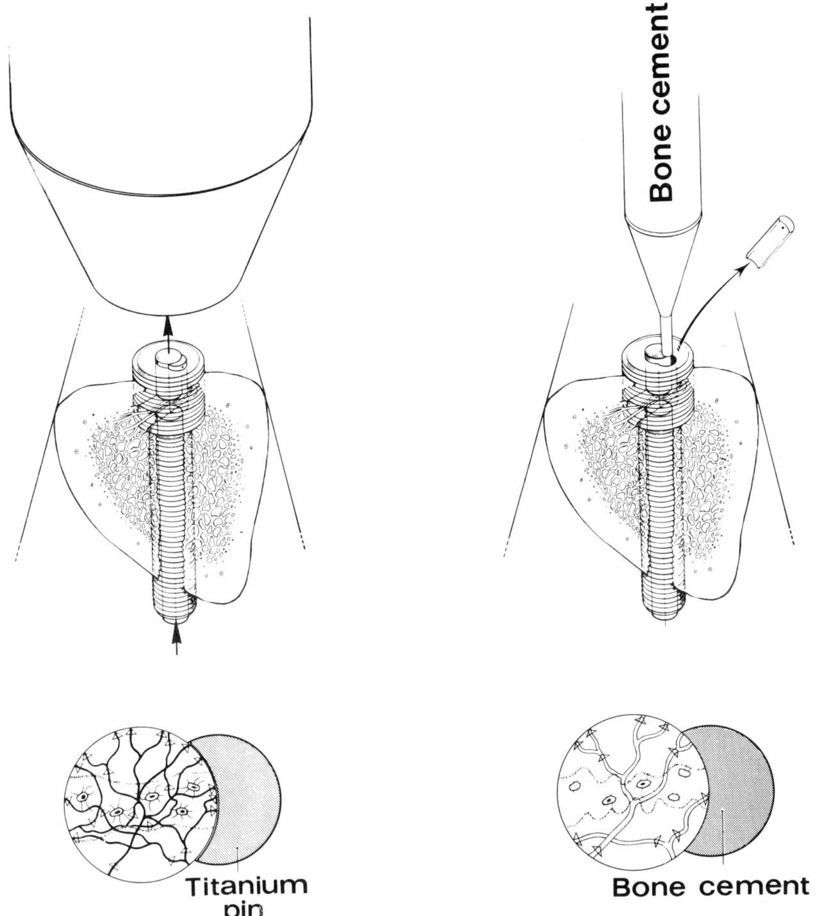

Fig. 2. The chamber is filled with living bone. The titanium plug is removed, giving access to the chamber tissue with minimal trauma. Bone cement or monomer is applied to the edge of the living tissue and the subsequent reactions at the interface are studied intravitally.

Methods of recording are colour slides, cine film and video tape.
After animal sacrifice the test tissue is removed, decalcified in
formic acid and sectioned for histology and stained as appropriate.

To test the applicability of the method, pilot experiments have been
done with bone cement. Palacos-R dough has been implanted 3 minutes
post-mixing. Palacos-R monomer has been applied in the form of a
monomer-soaked piece of paper. Also, to study the mechanical effect
of pressing a doughy material down the canal of the chamber, a third
experiment with silicone rubber as test material has been performed.

RESULTS AND DISCUSSION

Bone cement (Palacos-R) and its monomer were tested in pilot experiments with the purpose of exploring the potential of the vital microscopic method. The aim of these experiments was to define qualitatively the tissue injury caused by the methyl methacrylate, while the
purpose of future experiments will be to quantatively determine the
degree of tissue damage. The parameters tested are defined in earlier
vital microscopic experiments (Linder and Romanus, 1976, and Albrektsson, 1979), and include possible acute vascular influences such as
heamolysis, cessation of blood flow and corpuscular extravasation or
long-term reactions such as vessel reorientation, caliber or flow
changes. Fat cells have been shown to be resorbed following tissue
injury caused by ischaemia (Albrektsson, 1979) or irradiation
(Albrektsson, Jacobsson and Turesson,1980). Bone resorption may
also occur for the same reasons, although bone remodelling is a slow
process and does not occur at all in cases of poor and disturbed
vascularization.

Our experiments with Palacos-R cement gave rise to all the reactions
listed above. Both acute and long-term injuries were registered. By
6 weeks the peak of observeable changes had been reached, and vascular,
fat cell and bone regeneration processes were evident.

Experiments with the monomer-soaked piece of paper pressed into the
test canal showed severe tissue damage with haemolysis as well as
rapid bone and fat cell resorption. In a specimen processed for
histology, an acute inflammatory reaction was present, dominated by an
abundance of polymorphonuclear granulocytes.

The pilot experiments demonstrate that the titanium chamber provides
new possibilities to study the tissue repair dynamics after a defined
bone injury, as well as the phenomena taking place at the interface
after implant insertion. No other method allows repeated in situ observations of bone cement and its adverse effects at the tissue level,
but the method is not limited to bone cement and in principal any
topically used substance can be studied.

REFERENCES

Albrektsson, T. & Albrektsson, B. (1978) Microcirculation in
grafted bone. A chamber technique for vital microscopy of rabbit
bone transplants. Acta Orthop Scand, 49, 1-7.
Albrektsson, T. (1980) Repair of bone grafts. A vital microscopic
and histological investigation in the rabbit. Scand J Plast Reconstruct Surg, 14, 1-12.
Albrektsson, T., Jacobsson, M. & Turesson, I. (1980) Irradiation
injury of bone tissue. A vital microscopic method. Acta Radiologica,
in press.
Linder, L. & Romanus, M. (1976) Acute local tissue effects of poly-
merizing acrylic bone cement. Clin Orthop, 115, 303-311.

Biomaterials 1980
Edited by G. D. Winter, D. F. Gibbons, and H. Plenk, Jr.
© 1982 John Wiley and Sons Ltd.

PHARMACOKINETICS AND TOLERANCE OF GENTAMICIN-POLYMETHYLMETHACRYLATE-BEADS IN BEAGLE DOGS

E. Dingeldein[1], R. Bergmann[1], H. Wahlig[1],
A. Metallinos[2], Z. Simane[3] and P. Hermanek[4]

Department of Medical Microbiology[1], Institute
for Toxikology[2], Department of Medical Biochemistry[3], E. Merck, Darmstadt
Department of Clinical Pathology[4], University
Erlangen, Fed. Rep. of Germany

SUMMARY

11-17 Gentamicin-PMMA-Beads (GB) were implanted into
the femoral cavity of beagle dogs for a time period
of 6 months. During that time 70 % of the primarily
incorporated gentamicin amount, but only 0,4 % of
Methylmethacrylate content were released from the beads.
While gentamicin concentrations in serum and urine were
extremely low, which excludes side-effects, in bone
tissues even after 6 months antibiotic concentrations
were measured still sufficiently high to control
pathogens. These findings correspond very well with
results from pharmacokinetic studies in patients.
Excellent tolerance has been shown, both in a test for
tissue tolerance in cell cultures and in dogs after
implantation of the GB. Histologically no foreign body
reactions were observed. Studies in hematology, urinalysis and radiology revealed results within the
normal range.

INTRODUCTION

Gentamicin-PMMA-beads* (GB) are a further development of
gentamicin loaded bone cement. The clinical indications
are posttraumatic osteomyelitis, hematogenic osteomyelitis, infected osteosynthesis, infected pseudarthro-
sis, infected total hip arthroplasty and soft tissue
infections. This novel therapeutic concept for the local
treatment of infections, which was first applied by
Klemm (1977) is considered to be an alternative to both
irrigation suction drainage and systemic antibiotic
treatment. After thorough debridement of the infected
area, the resulting bone cavity is completely filled

* Septopal[R], E. Merck, Darmstadt, in collaboration with Kulzer,
+ Co.GmbH, Bad Homburg v.d.H.,F.R.Germany.

with GB. After insertion of an overflow drainage, the
wound should be completely closed. The beads are usually
removed 10-14 days after implantation.

The purpose of this paper is to report upon pharmacokinetic studies concerning gentamicin concentrations in
body fluids and bone tissues after implantation of GB,
as well as upon the local and general tolerance of the
implanted GB.

METHODS

GB have a diameter of 7 mm and a weight of 0.2 g. They
are fixed on a multistranded stainless steel wire in the
form of chains. Each bead contains 4.5 mg gentamicin
base and 20 mg zirconium dioxide as radiopaque material.
GB of the batch No. E 66/48 were used.

The gentamicin concentrations in phosphate buffer,
serum, urine and tissue homogenates were measured by
the agar diffusion test, using B. subtilis ATCC 6633 as
the test bacterium (Wahlig et al, 1972).

All dogs used were beagle dogs about one year old. For
implantation of the GB the medullary cavity was opened
from the trochanteric fossa. The marrow was removed,
the cavity reamed, and 11-17 GB were implanted. After
the operation samples of serum were obtained at various
times and all the urine was collected. From day 11 to
day 173 after the operation, samples of urine were
taken without measurement of the volume (see Table 1).
6 months after implantation samples of fibrous tissue
and cancellous bone from the vicinity of the GB and
of renal tissues were taken, both for the evaluation
of the gentamicin concentration and the histological
examination. In order to obtain an indication of the
local and general tolerance of the beads, studies in
hematology, urinalysis and radiology were done at
various times over a period of 6 months.

RESULTS

Gentamicin is released from the beads by diffusion.
Initially the amount of gentamicin base released per
bead is 400-600 µg per day. Around the 10th day 120 µg
are detectable and even on day 80 10 µg of gentamicin
base are still released.

The diffusion of gentamicin out of the beads leads in
vivo to high antibiotic concentrations in the infected
area. In serum and urine, however, only low concentrations were observed. Peak serum concentrations of up
to 0.3 µg/ml were measured 2 to 4 h after operation.

Peak urine concentrations ranged between 1.5 and
20 µg/ml immediately after the operation (Table 1).
Since gentamicin is eliminated via the kidneys it
was possible to detect gentamicin in the urine
throughout the whole observation time.

TABLE 1. Gentamicin concentrations in canine
serum and urine and renal excretion
after implantation of gentamicin-
PMMA-beads

Serum	hours				days		
µg/ml	1	2	6	24	2	6	20
Mean	0.10	0.16	0.11	0.05	<0.05	<0.05	0
SD	0.05	0.07	0.04	0.02			

Urine	days						
µg/ml	1	5	10	20	61	104	173
Mean	8.9	1.9	1.9	1.9	1.2	0.8	0.4
SD	5.4	0.6	0.5	0.9	0.3	0.3	0.3

Accumulative renal excretion mg	days						
	1	2	3	4	6	8	10
Mean	1.8	3.6	5.3	6.7	9.1	12.1	14.3

Renal excretion during 10 days was 10 to 18 mg. Also in
renal tissues gentamicin was observed at the end of the
implantation period (Table 2). The tissue concentrations,
however, were only 1/3 of those achieved after one
single i. m. injection of 2 mg/kg (Wahlig et al, 1974).

TABLE 2. Gentamicin in canine renal tissue
and bone tissue

	Renal tissue (mg/g)		Bone tissue (mg/g)	
	medulla	cortex	fibrous tissue	cancellous bone
Range	5.5 - 11.0	7.0 - 15.0	1.5 - 35.0	0.4 - 16.3
Mean	8.04	10.3	9.26	4.45
SD	1.7	2.4	9.6	4.8

Even 6 month after the implantation of GB gentamicin
concentrations in bone tissues were high, exceeding
the minimal inhibitory concentrations of pathogens
(Table 2).

Studies in hematology, urinalysis and radiology
during a follow up period of 6 months revealed results
within the normal range. Urinalysis considering renal
tolerance gave no indication for nephrotoxic reactions.
No protein or blood cells and tubular cells were
detectable in spite of long lasting gentamicin
concentrations in the renal tissue.

In the bone cavities the beads were surrounded by
fibrous tissue and the spaces between the beads were
filled with newly formed cancellous bone within six
months. Histologically no foreign body reactions
were observed.

Assaying the gentamicin concentrations of the explanted
beads after 6 months it was observed that 70 % of the
primarily incorporated gentamicin amount was released
from the beads during that time (Table 3).

TABLE 3.   Content (%) of gentamicin, methyl-
             acrylate (MA), and methylmethacry-
             late (MMA) in gentamicin-PMMA-beads

	Gentamicin	MA	MMA
before implantation (mean)	100	<0.1	3.4
after 6 months implantation (mean)	30.3	<0.1	3.0

The amount of methylmethacrylate of the beads, origi-
nally as low as 3.4 %, was further deminished only by
0.4 % during the implantation period of 6 months
(Table 3).

DISCUSSION

Although the gentamicin concentrations in serum and
urine were extremely low, in bone tissues even 6 months
after implantation of GB gentamicin concentrations were
sufficiently high to control pathogens.

These findings correspond to results from pharmacokinetic studies in patients. After implantation periods
of 30, 40 and 70 days in tissue samples derived from
patients again high gentamicin concentrations were

observed. The amounts range from 9.1 to 33.5 µg/g in
connective tissue and thus were distinctly higher than
the corresponding values in dogs. In specimens of
cancellous bone, taken in a distance of 5 to 10 mm
from the beads concentrations between 1.6 and 4.3 µg/g
were measured. Even in the cortical bone gentamicin
was detectable in concentrations ranging from 0.6 to
3.0 µg/g (Wahlig, 1979).

Due to high and prolonged gentamicin concentrations
favourable clinical results were obtained in more
than 1500 patients with chronic bone and soft tissue
infections (Grieben, 1980).

Due to low gentamicin levels in serum and urine the
risk of side effects after implantation of GB is extremely small.

The excellent tolerance of GB in bone tissues in dogs
correspond to results obtained in a test for tissue
tolerance in cell cultures: the fibroblasts from
rabbit kidneys grew just as well on gentamicin-PMMA
as on the bottom of conventional culture dishes
(Wahlig et al, 1978).
In Patients, histologically, only slight foreign body
reactions were described. In general a rapid and
undisturbed wound healing was observed (Böhm and
Hörster, 1979).

<u>REFERENCES</u>

Böhm, E. u. Hörster, H.-G. (1979) Histologische
Verlaufsuntersuchungen bei der lokal mit Gentamycin
behandelten chronischen Osteomyelitis, in <u>Aktuelle
Probleme in Chirurgie und Orthopädie, Bd. 12</u> (Eds.,
Burri, Herfarth u. Jäger), pp 182-186. Huber, Bern,
Stuttgart, Wien.
Grieben, A. (1980) Results of Septopal in more than
1500 cases of bone and soft tissue infections. A
review of clinical trials. <u>Journal of Bone and Joint
Surgery, 62-B,</u> 275.
Klemm, K. (1977) Die Behandlung chronischer Knochen-
infektionen mit Gentamycin-PMMA-Ketten und -Kugeln.
<u>Unfallchirurgie, Sonderheft,</u> 20-25.

Wahlig, H., Hameister, W. u. Grieben, A. (1972)
über die Freisetzung von Gentamycin aus Poly-
methylmethacrylat I. Experimentelle Untersuchungen
in vitro. Langenbecks Archiv für Chirurgie, 331,
169-192.
Wahlig, H., Metallinos, A., Hameister, W.u. Bergmann, R. (1974) Gentamycin-Konzentrationen in
Geweben und Körperflüssigkeiten von Versuchstieren.
International Journal for Clinical Pharmacology, 10,
212-229.
Wahlig, H., Dingeldein, E., Bergmann, R. a. Reuss, K.
(1978) The release of gentamicin from polymethylmethacrylate beads. -An experimental and pharmacokinetic study. Journal of Bone and Joint Surgery,
60-B, 270-275.
Wahlig, H. (1979) Experimentelle Grundlagen für
die Anwendung von antibiotikahaltigem Polymethyl-
methacrylat, in Aktuelle Probleme in Chirurgie und
Orthopädie, Bd. 12 (Eds., Burri, Herfarth u. Jäger),
pp 102-112. Huber, Bern, Stuttgart, Wien.

Dental materials

Biomaterials 1980
Edited by G. D. Winter, D. F. Gibbons, and H. Plenk, Jr.
© 1982 John Wiley and Sons Ltd.

A CELL CULTURE METHOD FOR SCREENING THE BIOCOMPATIBILITY
OF DENTAL MATERIALS

G. Schmalz

Dental School of Medicine, University of Tubingen
D-7400 Tubingen, West-Germany

SUMMARY

A cell culture technique for use as a standard procedure for biocompatibility testing of dental materials was evaluated, eluates of different materials were tested on L-929 cells. Toxicity was evaluated
by the slope of the dose response curves. The technique was easy to
perform, was not expensive and yielded measurable, reproducible and
statistically treatable results. This test method should be considered as part of a standardized programme for biocompatibility testing
of dental materials.

INTRODUCTION

Many different cell culture techniques for testing the biocompatibility of dental materials have been published but only a few have been
adopted into national or international standardized testing protocols
(American Dental Association, 1979; Fédération Dentaire Internationale, 1980). The reason is that a standard cell culture method has to
fullfill special requirements (Autian and Dillingham, 1978):
- it should be reasonable in cost,
- all components should be easily available through commercial sources,
- the procedure has to be so clear and easy, that it can be performed
  by average laboratory personnel,
- the recording should be done systematically, either by grading or
  measuring,
- the results must be reproducible, statistically significant, and
  quickly available,
- the results should have a definite relationship to animal and human tissue compatibility.
The purpose of this investigation was to further develop and evaluate
a cell culture technique for biocompatibility testing of dental materials which meets these specifications.

MATERIALS AND METHODS

Thirty eight test materials (Table 1) were investigated. These were
mixed according to the manufacturer's instructions and separate specimen were aged for 1 hour and 24 hours at 37°C and 100% relative humidity. Samples of the aged materials, each weighing 4.0 g, were in-

cubated in BME cell culture Medium (GIBCO, Nr. A988450/D132) at 37°C.
After 24 hours the medium was decanted, filtered under sterile conditions and diluted with conc. BME medium according to the following
scheme: 1:0, 1:1, 1:7, 1:31.

TABLE 1:   Test materials

A: Summary of the 38 test materials

impression materials	filling materials
silicones	amalgams
polysulphides	composites
ZnO/E pastes	phosphate cem.
tooth pastes	silicophosphate cem.
endodontic materials	copper cement

B: Specifications of materials specially mentioned

Code-Nr.	Name	Manufacturer	batch-Nr.
G-66	Guttapercha	DeTrey/W.Ger.	RA 4
G-80	Chloropercha	OY Dental/Finnl.	10,6
G-91	Jodoform	A.Haupt/W.Ger.	n.i.[+]
G-92	N 2	Dr.Sargenti	n.i.[+]
G-100	Diaket	ESPE/W.Ger.	75324
G-162A	Ledermix	Cyanamid/W.Ger.	557/9771

[+]No information (n.i.) was available about batch-Nrs for
G-91 and G-92. Both materials were purchased Feb. 1977

Cultures of L-929 mouse fibroblasts were grown in BME medium, supplemented with foetal calf serum (GIBCO, No. HL590101S) to 5%. One ml of
a cell suspension containing 2×10^5 cells/ml together with one ml of
the diluted test solution was put into a sterile test tube. These
cell suspensions were incubated at 37°C, in an atmosphere of 5% CO_2
and 100% relative humidity for 72 hours. For the control cultures the
cell suspension was mixed with regular medium instead of the test solution. One set of the controls was kept at 4°C (0 hour control), the
other set was incubated like the test cultures (72 hours control).
The test cultures were performed with 10 replicates, the control cultures with 20.

The growth of the cultures was evaluated by the LOWRY protein determination (Oyama and Eagle, 1956). The relative growth of the test
cultures was calculated as the percentage of the maximum growth, represented by the 72 hours controls (Dillingham et al., 1973). The
95% confidence interval for the average relative growth was calculated by a computer programme (Schmalz, 1981). For each material and
each aging period dose response curves were derived with the different concentrations of the extracts as doses. From the regression of
each curve according to the equation $y = e^{-ax}$, the slope ($-a$) was used
as an indicator for the biocompatibility of the respective material.
The slopes were compared for significant differences by the Fischer-test (Miller, 1966).

<u>RESULTS</u>

The linear calibration curve of the LOWRY protein determination
against cell count (Fig. 1) indicates good agreement between both
methods which corresponds to results in other laboratories (Dillingham et al., 1973). The growth curve of the 72 hours control cultures
(Fig. 2) shows that in our system the test is performed during the
logarithmic growth phase, therefore monitoring the influence of toxi-
cants upon growth kinetics. This is a better test than one in which
only cell lysis is measured (Autian, 1970). Typical dose response
curves are demonstrated in Figures 3 and 4. The endodontic filling
material N2 (G-92) proved to be one of the most toxic substances in
the test series showing very steep dose response curves (Fig. 3). A
chloropercha sealer (G-80) was only slightly toxic and decreases in
toxicity after 24 hours aging (Fig. 4).

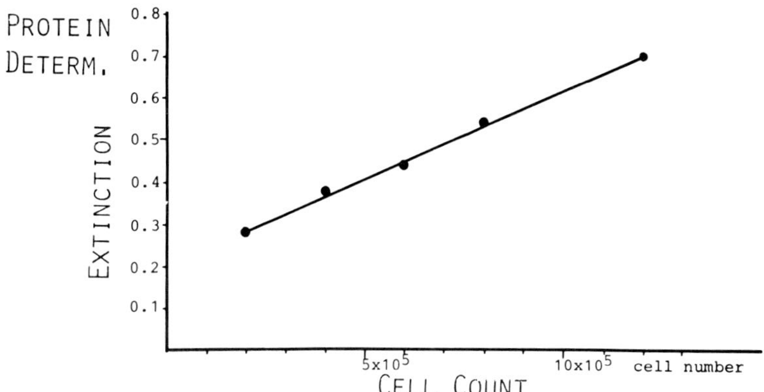

Fig. 1. Calibration curve of LOWRY protein determination
against cell count

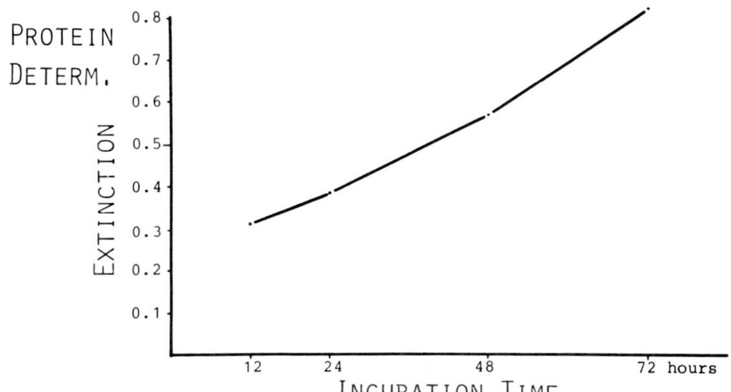

Fig. 2. Growth curve of the 72 hours control cultures

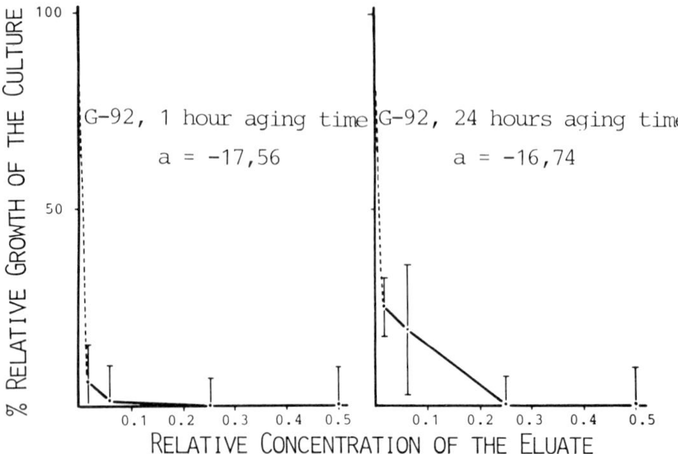

Fig. 3. Influence of material G-92, defined in table 1, upon the growth of L-929 cells. a=slope; regression model: $y=e^{-ax}$

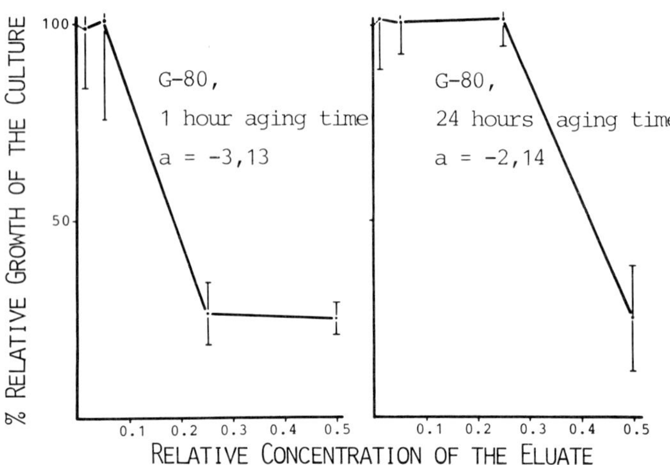

Fig. 4. Influence of material G-80, defined in table 1, upon the growth of L-929 cells. a=slope; regression model: $y=e^{-ax}$

The reliability of our results was evaluated by comparing them with corresponding reports in the literature about in vitro and in vivo findings. I am well aware that because of the lack of standardization, different results were reported for the same materials (Langeland and Klötzer, 1971; Schmalz, 1981). However a critical review of the literature (Schmalz, 1981) shows with two exceptions (silicophosphate- and copper cement), that there is good agreement between these results and those of other investigators and fewer discrepancies than with the diffusion test (Autian, 1970) using the same materials.

The reproducibility of the results obtained by our test method was
evaluated by repeating the same experiment with 5 materials in the
same laboratory, but with different personnel, different commercial
sources for the cells and with a time lapse of 12 months between the
respective experiments. The results (Tab. 2) show that $\beta=1.00$ and
$\alpha=0.3$ almost optimal reproducibility, optimum being characterized by
$\beta=1$ and $\alpha=0$ (Moran, 1971). The 95% confidence intervals are high because only a small number of experiments were done.

TABLE 2. Test of reproducibility

test materials	slope of the dose response curves	
	1	2
G-92	-17.56	-16.40
G-91	-14.25	-15.10
G-162A	- 7.23	- 8.41
G-100	- 7.04	- 6.81
G-66	- 2.96	- 2.10

statistical analysis (Moran, 1971)

general equation	calculated equation
$y = \beta x + \alpha$	$y = 1.00\ x + 0.03$

95% confidence limits: 0.2 - 5.3 (for β)

Materials, defined in Table 1, were aged one hour,
1 = result of initial test; 2 = result of similar test
12 months later

According to the Fischer-test the least significant difference between two slopes was 3.5 (95% confidence), where the original data
for the slopes ranged from 0 to -18.

DISCUSSION

Examining this method in the light of the criteria for standardized
cell culture testing published by Autian and Dillingham (1978), the
test under discussion is lower in cost than the Cr^{51} release test
(Spangberg, 1973) which was proposed for the same purpose (Fédération
Dentaire Internationale, 1980), because the latter needs scintillation equipment and radiochemicals.

All components of our test are easily available. Problems of safety
when handling radiochemicals needed with the Cr^{51}-test are avoided.
The test was performed by average laboratory personnel. Working with
gamma-emitters like Cr^{51} is more complicated and requires specially
trained personnel.

The recording of the experimental data by photometric readings is
more objective than the diffusion method described by Autian (1970),
in which the cell response is graded by the investigator. The method
generates dose response curves which are more reliable than the single data points obtained by the diffusion method and the Cr^{51}-release
test. In our hands there were larger variations in the results when
cells were counted, probably because of problems in taking aliquots.

                                    G. Schmalz

The data are available within 4 days, which is longer than with the
Cr^{51}-test (1 day) and the diffusion test (1 day), but this length of
time still seems reasonable.

It may be argued that a disadvantage of this method is, that there is
no direct cell/material contact (Spangberg, 1973). However, based on
earlier investigations (Schmalz, 1978) in which the results of in vitro tests on the materials themselves and different eluates were compared, it is thought that acute toxicity testing of dental material
eluates is justified if the eluation is performed in the nutritient
medium for the cell culture. Using eluates instead of the material
itself, antibiotics in the nutritient cell medium are avoided and
dose response curves are easily established.

The results of this investigation suggest that the test method described might be a useful addition to established standard testing
procedures.

REFERENCES

American Dental Association (1979). American National Standards In-
stitute/American Dental Association Document No. 41 for Recommended
Standard Practices for Biological Evaluation of Dental Materials.
J. Amer. Dent. Ass. 99, 697-698
Autian, J. (1970). The use of rabbit implants and tissue culture tests
for the evaluation of dental materials. Int. dent. J. 20, 481-490
Autian, J. & Dillingham, E.O. (1978). Overview of general toxicity
testing with emphasis on special tissue culture tests, in In vitro
toxicity testing (Eds. Berky, J. & Sherrod, C.), p 24-49
Dillingham, E.O., Mast, R.W., Bass, G.E. & Autian, J. (1973). Toxi-
city of methyl- and halogen-substituted alcohols in tissue culture
relative to structure activity models and acute toxicity in mice.
J. Pharm. Sci. 62, 22-30
Fédération Dentaire Internationale (1980). Recommended standard prac-
tices for biological evaluation of dental materials. Int. dent. J.
30, 140-188
Langeland, K. & Klötzer, W.T. (1971). Verfahren zur Prüfung der bio-
logischen Eigenschaften zahnärztlicher Werkstoffe. Dtsch. zahnärztl.
Z. 26, 298-315
Miller, R.G. (1966). Simultanous statistical interference. p 90,
McGrawhill, New York
Moran, P.A.P. (1971). Estimating structural and functional relation-
ships. J. multivariate analysis 1, 232-248
Oyama, V.I. & Eagle, H. (1956). Measurement of cell growth in tissue
culture with a phenol reagent (Folin-Ciocalteu). Proc. Soc. Exper.
Biol. Med. 91, 305-311
Schmalz, G. (1978). Ein Vergleich zweier Eluationsverfahren zur bio-
logischen Materialprüfung. Dtsch. zahnärztl. Z. 33, 850-855
Schmalz, G. (1981). Zellkulturen als Standardverfahren zur Prüfung
der Gewebeverträglichkeit zahnärztlicher Materialien. Georg Thieme
Verlag, Stuttgart, in press
Spangberg, L. (1973). Kinetic and quantitative evaluation of material
cytotoxicity in vitro. Oral Surg. 35, 389-401

Biomaterials 1980
Edited by G. D. Winter, D. F. Gibbons, and H. Plenk, Jr.
© 1982 John Wiley and Sons Ltd.

NEW COPPER-RICH DENTAL AMALGAMS

W. Kraft and G. Petzow

Max-Planck-Institut für Metallforschung,
Institut für Werkstoffwissenschaften,
Stuttgart-80, Federal Republic of Germany

SUMMARY

The phase-boundaries of copper-rich dental amalgames to phase-equilibria, which contain neither the corrodible $Sn_{7-8}Hg$-phase (γ_2) nor liquid mercury, were estimated by studying the isothermal section Ag_3Sn (γ_o)-Cu_3Sn (ε)-Hg at 37°C in the system silver-copper-tin-mercury. It is shown that amalgams with 43 to 45 wt % Hg are γ_2-free and contain no liquid mercury, if the composition of the pre-alloyed powder is within the two-phase equilibrium γ_o and ε with 8 to 38 wt % Cu in the system silver-copper-tin. Because of these investigations also the phase relations in two commercially sold copper-rich amalgams can be explained, which were developed only empirically.

Hardening of silver-copper-tin-amalgams involves negative and/or positive volume changes depending on the chemical composition of the pre-alloyed powders. By mixing and varying the ratios of the pre-alloys a superposition of their properties is obtained and it is possible to control the volume changes and the phase equilibrium. A powder mixture with the composition Ag 33.3 Cu 33 Sn 33.7 and amalgamated with 50 wt % Hg shows almost no final volume change and has no free mercury at the end of hardening.

INTRODUCTION

Amalgams are mercury based alloys used in dentistry. They are produced by mixing mercury with pre-alloyed powders, mainly Ag-Cu-Sn-powders. During the hardening complicated reactions take place which involve both positive and negative volume changes.

In conventional amalgams with silver and tin the intermetallic phase $Sn_{7-8}Hg$ (γ_2) is formed after mixing with mercury. This γ_2-phase corrodes very easily (Jørgensen and Saito, 1970; Otani et al., 1973; Wagner, 1962) and causes a contraction in the final stage of hardening (Aldinger et al., 1976). For the clinical practice this is a disadvantage, as gaps are formed between the amalgam and the dental enamel increasing the susceptibility to corrosion. Alloying of copper to the silver-tin-powders prevents the formation of the γ_2-phase (Asgar, 1974).

                    W. Kraft and G. Petzow

The main purpose of this study was to determine which compositions of
Ag-Cu-Sn-alloys prevent the formation of the γ_2-phase after mixing
with mercury. Therefore the phase equilibria of the quaternary system
have to be determined. Another reason for this study is to establish
the compositional regions which do not contain any free mercury.

CONSTITUTION

An isothermal section of a quaternary system is a three-dimensional
space. The most common representation is the equilateral tetrahedron
(Fig. 1) in which the apexes represent the pure components - in this
case silver, tin, copper and mercury - the edges represent the six
binary systems, the triangular faces represent the four ternary systems, an the interior of the tetrahedron represents the quaternary
system. It is useful to investigate an isothermal tetrahedron by any
kind of plane sections through the tetrahedron. In this study a plane
has been investigated which con-
tains the three points Hg,
Ag₃Sn (γ_0), and Cu₃Sn (ε) (Fig. 1).
Pre-alloys containing γ_0 and ε in
the two-phase field of the ternary
system Ag-Cu-Sn (Fig. 2) avoid the
appearance of (ß)-Ag-Sn-phase
which is unfavorable to the volume
changes (Aldinger et al., 1976).
Furthermore there are hints from
previous studies, that the formation of the γ_2-phase does not
take place in the composition
plane chosen (Aldinger et al.,
1977). This section was selected
because it includes all alloys
which can be prepared simply by
mixing different amounts of mercury with ternary silver-tin-
copper pre-alloys with variable
copper content. In order to investigate this plane three pre-
alloyed powders (Table 1, Fig.1,2)

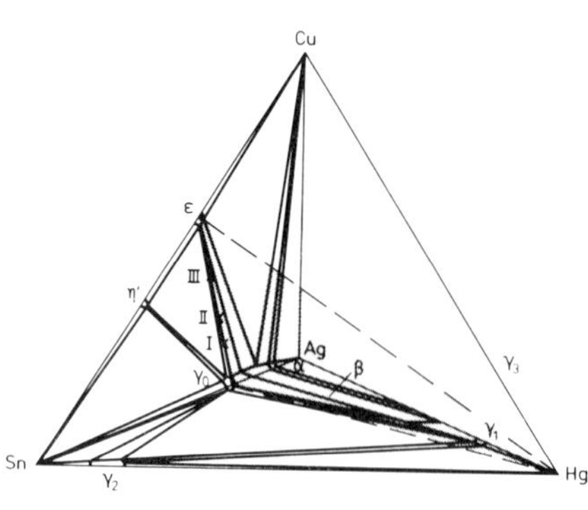

Fig. 1. The tetrahedron of the
system silver-copper-mercury-
tin (37°C) and the plane
Ag₃Sn (γ_0)-Cu₃Sn (ε)-Hg (by wt%)

were prepared and mixed with different amounts (10-70 wt%) of mercury (Table 1). The mixtures were compacted by isostatic pressing
and were equilibriated for at least six weeks at 37°C and were subsequently investigated by means of optical microscopy, X-ray studies
and electron microprobe as well as chemical analysis.

From the results (Table 1) the phase diagram in Fig. 3 was constructed.
It can be seen, that at 37°C the range of composition used technically
(43-45 wt% Hg) (shadowed region in Fig. 3) consists mainly of the uni-
variant equilibrium Ag₃Sn (γ_0) + Ag₃Hg₄ (γ_1) + Cu₃Sn (ε) + Cu₆Sn₅ (η')
and the neighbouring three-phase equilibria and the phase equilibria
contain neither γ_2 nor liquid mercury.

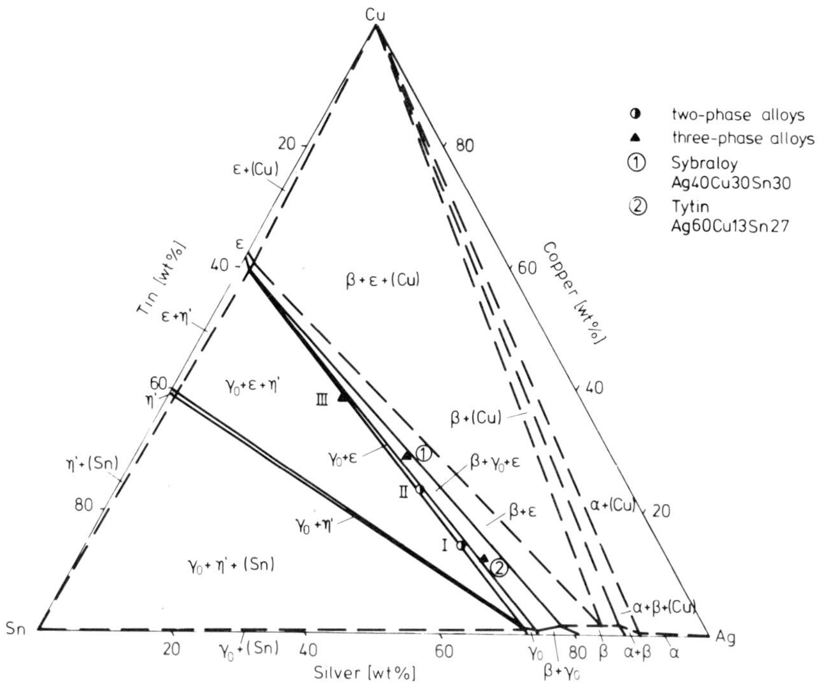

Fig. 2. Isothermal phase diagram Ag-Cu-Sn at 37°C (by wt%)

TABLE 1. Results of the phase studies

Mercury content (wt%)	PRE-ALLOY (wt%)		
	Ag55Cu15Sn30 I	Ag45Cu24Sn31 II	Ag26Cu39Sn35 III
0	$\gamma_0+\varepsilon$	$\gamma_0+\varepsilon$	$\gamma_0+\varepsilon+\eta'$
10	$\gamma_0+\gamma_1+\varepsilon$	$\gamma_0+\gamma_1+\varepsilon+\eta'$	$\gamma_0+\gamma_1+\varepsilon+\eta'$
20	$\gamma_0+\gamma_1+\varepsilon+\eta'$	$\gamma_0+\gamma_1+\varepsilon+\eta'$	$\gamma_0+\gamma_1+\varepsilon+\eta'$
30	$\gamma_0+\gamma_1+\varepsilon+\eta'$	$\gamma_0+\gamma_1+\varepsilon+\eta'$	$\gamma_0+\gamma_1+\varepsilon+\eta'$
35	–	–	$\gamma_1+\varepsilon+\eta'$
40	$\gamma_0+\gamma_1+\varepsilon+\eta'$	$\gamma_0+\gamma_1+\varepsilon+\eta'$	$\gamma_1+\varepsilon+\eta'$
45	–	$\gamma_0+\gamma_1+\varepsilon+\eta'$	$\gamma_1+\varepsilon+\eta'+Hg$
50	$\gamma_0+\gamma_1+\varepsilon+\eta'$	$\gamma_1+\varepsilon+\eta'$	$\gamma_1+\varepsilon+\eta'+Hg$
55	$\gamma_1+\eta'$	$\gamma_1+\varepsilon+\eta'+Hg$	–
60	$\gamma_1+\gamma_2+\eta'+Hg$	$\gamma_1+\varepsilon+\eta'+Hg$	$\gamma_1+\varepsilon+\eta'+Hg$
70	$\gamma_1+\gamma_2+\eta'+Hg$	$\gamma_1+\varepsilon+\eta'+Hg$	–

330   W. Kraft and G. Petzow

Within this shadowed region quaternary amalgams are formed from ternary pre-alloys and mercury, if the pre-alloyed powders consist of γ_o- and ε-phase and the copper-content is between 8 and 38 wt%.

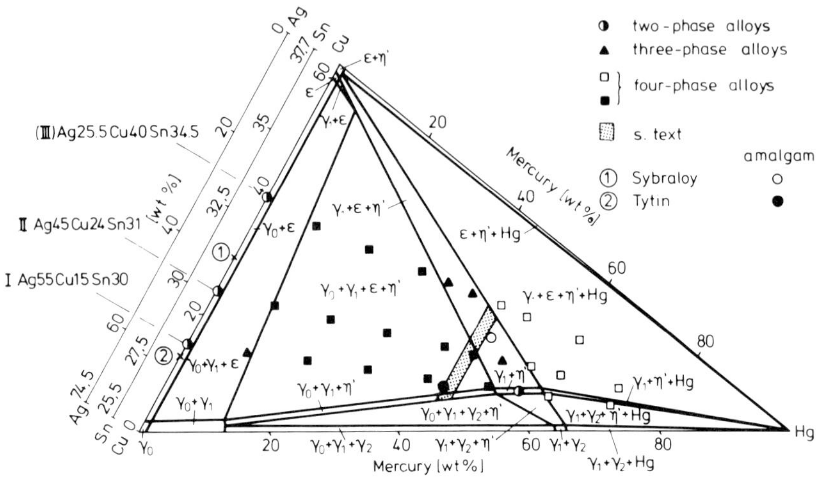

Fig. 3. Isothermal section (37°C) Ag₃Sn (γ_o)-Cu₃Sn (ε)-Hg of the quaternary system Ag-Cu-Hg-Sn

This new phase diagram explains also the phase relations in the commercially sold amalgams, which were developed only empirically. Tytin (S.S. White Dental Products International, Philadelphia) a ternary pre-alloy, is nearby the two-phase equilibrium $\gamma_o + \varepsilon$ at the ß-side (Fig. 2, point 2). The addition of prescribed 43 wt% Hg forms a quaternary amalgam located in the four-phase equilibrium $\gamma_o + \gamma_1 + \varepsilon + \eta'$ nearby the three-phase equilibrium $\gamma_o + \gamma_1 + \eta'$ and within the shadowed region (Fig. 3). Investigations of Tytin-amalgams with 49.5 and 51.6 wt% Hg have shown the formation of the γ_2-phase including γ_1, η', and γ_o (Malhotra and Asgar, 1978). The reason for formation of the γ_2-phase is to be seen in the investigated section (Fig. 3): Amalgams with this composition form the four-phase equilibrium $\gamma_o + \gamma_1 + \gamma_2 + \eta'$.

As with Tytin, Sybraloy (Kerr Manufacturing Co., Romulus, Michigan) with a higher copper content of 30 wt% in the pre-alloyed powder (Fig. 2, point 1), no γ_2-phase forms after mercury addition. As the phase diagram in Fig. 3 shows, the amalgam with a content of 46 wt% Hg (added by the producer) is in the three-phase equilibrium $\gamma_1 + \varepsilon + \eta'$ nearby the shadowed region.

DIMENSIONAL CHANGE DURING HARDENING

Hardening of Ag-Cu-Sn-amalgams usually involves volume changes. The knowledge of these changes is important because a too large expansion will cause the tooth to fracture while on the other hand a contraction over the whole hardening time involves a loosening of the amalgam in the cavity.

Fig. 4 shows the volume changes of the amalgams mixed from the pre-alloyed powder I and II (Table 1 and Fig. 1, 2) with 50 wt% Hg. The dilatometer curves are divided in three principle branches: 1. shrinkage, 2. swelling and 3. the final reaction. The final result is different for amalgams of the pre-alloyed powder I, where a shrinkage appears (curve a in Fig. 4) and amalgams of the powder III, where a swelling is observed (curve b in Fig. 4).

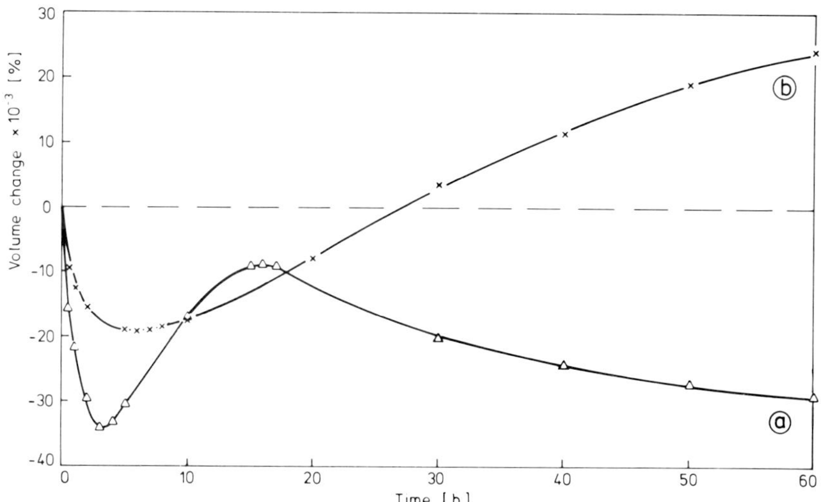

Fig. 4. Volume changes of amalgams with 50 wt% Hg
a) Ag55Cu15Sn30 (I);   b) Ag26Cu39Sn35 (III)

The mechanisms have been investigated which involve these volume changes during hardening (Kraft, 1979). The results yield a clear association with mechanisms which may occur, namely liquid phase sintering (shrinkage), formation of the intermetallic phases γ_1 and η' (swelling) and solid phase sintering (shrinkage at the end of hardening).

The amalgams made from alloy III with 50 wt% Hg have no shrinkage at the end of hardening. This is explained by the fact that liquid mercury is present in the equilibrium state (Table 1) and therefore no solid phase sintering occurs. The alloy cannot be used in dentistry.

On the other hand amalgams made from alloy I and 50 wt% Hg contain
no liquid mercury (Table 1), but shrink during the whole hardening
time, and the amalgam is not anchored in the cavity.

By mixing the pre-alloyed powders I and III a superposition of their
properties is obtained. In Fig. 5 it can be seen that with increasing
amount of alloy III in the mixture the shrinkage at the beginning of
hardening decreases and the subsequent swelling is prolonged at the
expense of the final shrinkage phase (curve c and d).

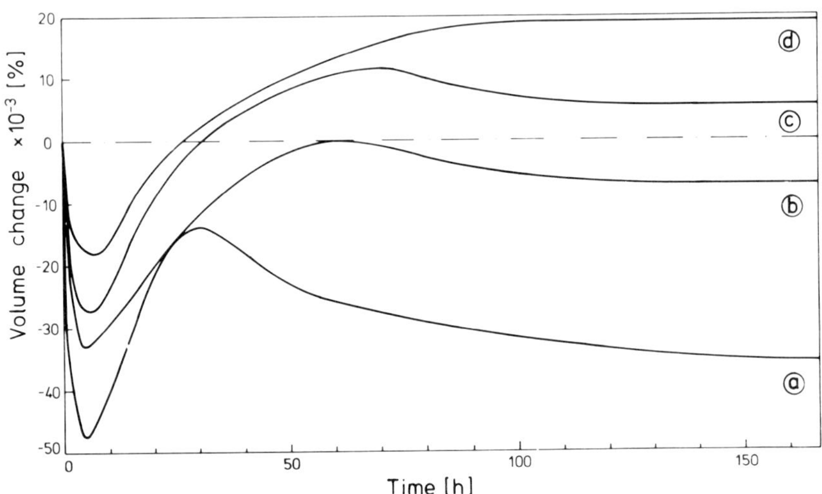

Fig. 5. Volume changes of amalgams with various mixture of pre-
alloyed powders I and III with 50 wt% Hg. Ratio of mixture I:III
a) 1:1; b) 1:2.3; c) 1:3; d) 1:4.

The contraction at the end of hardening cannot be avoided because only
the amalgam mixture I:III = 1:4 mercury exists. In contrast the
mixture I:III = 1:3 with the gross compound of Ag33.3Cu33Sn33.7 and
50 wt% Hg (curve c in Fig. 5) consists only of solid phases and the
shrinkage is a minimum.

ACKNOWLEDGEMENT

The authors thank the DEGUSSA Pforzheim for providing the silver-
copper-tin powders.

REFERENCES

Aldinger, F., Schuler, P. & Petzow, G. (1976). Reaktionsmechanismen beim Erhaerten von Silber-Zinn-Amalgamen. Z. Metallkde., 67, 625.
Aldinger, F., Kraft, W. & Petzow, G. (1977). Constitution of Quaternary Silver-Tin-Copper-Amalgams. J. Dent. Res., 56, IADR Abstracts 1977, 145.
Asgar, K. (1974). Amalgam Alloy with a Single Composition Behavior Similar to Dispersalloy. J. Dent. Res., 53, IADR Abstracts 1974, 60.
Jørgensen, K.D. & Saito, T. (1970). Structure and Corrosion of Dental Amalgam. Acta Odont. Scand., 28, 129.
Kraft, W. (1979). Reaktionskinetik in quaternaeren Dentalamalgamen. Thesis, Universitaet Stuttgart.
Malhotra, M. & Asgar, K. (1978). Investigation of Metallurgical Phases in High Copper Amalgams Containing Varying Mercury. J.Dent. Res., 57, IADR Abstracts 1978, 194.
Otani, H., Jesser, W. & Wilsdorf, H. (1973). The in vivo and in vitro Corrosion Products of Dental Amalgams. J. Biomed. Mat. Res., 7, 523.
Wagner, E. (1962). Beitrag zur Klaerung des Korrosionsverhaltens der Silber-Zinn-Amalgame. Dtsch. Zahnaerztl. Z., 17, 99.

Biomaterials 1980
Edited by G. D. Winter, D. F. Gibbons, and H. Plenk, Jr.
© 1982 John Wiley and Sons Ltd.

CHARACTERISTICS OF THE REACTION ZONES OF SOME Cu-RICH AMALGAMS

Grayson W. Marshall, Jr. and Sally J. Marshall

Department of Biological Materials,
Northwestern University, Chicago, Illinois, USA

SUMMARY

Many clinically successful Cu-rich amalgams contain reaction zones around the Cu-rich particles which vary considerably in microstructure. However, many of these systems have received little attention. This investigation sought to analyze the nature of the reaction zones in five blended and one single particle Cu-rich amalgam systems. SEM and x-ray microanalysis were combined with x-ray diffraction studies to determine the nature and quantities of phases present for each system. The compositions of the zones varied widely from system to system. Based on this information and the diffraction results, estimates of the volume fraction of each phase in each zone were made. In all cases at least three phases were found with the γ_1 and Cu_6Sn_5 phases common to all systems. In three systems Cu_3Sn was also present. The quantities of these phases varied widely and it is suggested that such variations are significant in efforts to understand the correlation of properties with clinical performance.

INTRODUCTION

It is well established that a number of Cu-rich amalgams offer superior marginal integrity as compared with conventional Ag-Sn amalgams. (Mahler, et al, 1973; Osbourne and Gale, 1979). The reaction zone surrounding the Ag-Cu eutectic particles in a blended Cu-rich amalgam, Dispersalloy, is predominantly Cu_6Sn_5 with some γ_1-Ag-Hg (Mahler, et al, 1975; Marshall, et al, 1977; Okabe, et al, 1977). In a large number of other blended and single particle Cu-rich systems, Cu_6Sn_5 has been shown (Marshall and Marshall, 1979) to result from amalgamation, but the microstructures of the reaction zones vary considerably (Marshall, et al, 1977). Many of the systems have received little attention, even though considerable variations in composition, mechanical properties (Eames and MacNamara, 1976) and clinical performance exist (Osbourne and Gale, 1979). This investigation sought to analyze the nature of the reaction zones in a number of these systems in order to: 1) establish if there are differences in the nature of phases present and 2) determine the quantities of the phases in the reaction zones of these amalgams.

MATERIALS AND METHODS

Six amalgam systems were chosen for study based on the nature of the
reaction zone surrounding the copper rich particles. All the reaction
zones contained phases which could not be analyzed separately with
electron induced x-ray spectra. The amalgams were assigned code letters as shown in Table 1. Standard test cylinders were prepared following manufacturer's directions for alloy to mercury ratio and trituration time and were condensed according to ADA Specification No. 1.
All samples were stored for a minimum of one month prior to metallographic polishing and SEM/EDS analysis. Additional amalgam samples
for x-ray diffraction were triturated in the same way and hand condensed into dies to form disk shaped samples 1.3 cm in diameter and 1
mm thick. Metallographically polished amalgam alloy pellets were also
studied.

TABLE 1. Amalgam systems

Code	Brand name	Manufacturer
C	Cupralloy	Weber
D	Dispersalloy	Johnson & Johnson
E	Ease	L. D. Caulk Co.
M	Micro II non-Zn	L. D. Caulk Co.
P	Phasealloy	Phasealloy
S	Sybraloy	Kerr

SEM/EDS analyses of all amalgams were conducted at 18 KV accelerating
voltage. A minimum of ten EDS spot analyses were obtained from the
reaction zones of each amalgam system. The x-ray intensities were
corrected using a standard ZAF program and averaged to give the compositions of the reaction zones, using procedures described previously
(Marshall, et al 1977). These compositions were considered to be
representative of the phase mixture in the reaction zone for each
amalgam. Compositions of the alloy pellets and the phases in them
were also determined by EDS in a similar fashion.

X-ray diffraction was used to determine which phases were present in
tne set amalgams as well as the alloy pellets, following procedures
already described (Marshall and Marshall, 1979). These results were
used to separate the compositions of the reaction zones into different phases. In each case γ_1, Cu_6Sn_5 and phases present in the alloy
pellet were assumed to be present in the reaction zone. The weight
percentages of each element in each phase were determined by solving
simultaneous equations. The weight fractions of residual alloy, γ_1,
Cu_6Sn_5 and Cu_3Sn were converted to volume fractions by dividing the
weight fraction of each phase by its density to obtain a volume per
phase. Comparisons were made of the volume fractions of all phases
as well as the ratio of γ_1 to copper-tin phases.

RESULTS AND DISCUSSION

The typical appearance of the reaction zone of blended systems such as D, E and M is shown in Figure 1. The reaction zone around the Cu-rich particle is distinct but the multiphase structure cannot be resolved. The Cu-rich particle of systems P and C contain more Cu, 62 and 53 weight per cent, respectively. The reaction zones also appear somewhat different, as shown in Figures 2 and 3. System S, a single particle amalgam, reacts with the formation of large amounts of Cu_6Sn_5 in the γ_1 matrix, as shown in Figure 4. However, unlike other single particle formulations, there is an apparent reaction zone formed within the circular boundary of the particles. This can be seen as the lighter area surrounding the dark remnants of the original alloy in the large particle in the center of Figure 4. Since this structure is unique among the Cu-rich single particle systems, and contains unresolved phases it was included in this study.

The results of the spot analyses from the reaction zones of all amalgam systems are shown in Table 2. It is clear that the reaction zone compositions varied widely from system to system. The resulting volume fractions are shown in Table 3. Both γ_1 (Ag-Hg) and Cu_6Sn_5 form in all of these systems and other phases are present which vary from system to system, including Cu_3Sn and remnants of the alloy particle. It appears that the ratio of Cu-Sn compounds to γ_1 can vary considerably in the blended systems. Systems C and P had the highest Cu-Sn to γ_1 ratios in their reaction zones, 9.0 and 6.7, respectively. Systems D and E had moderate values, 1.8 and 1.2, while M exhibited a value of 0.9, the lowest ratio of Cu-Sn to γ_1. It is interesting to note that the samples with higher ratios have shown superior clinical performance (Osbourne and Gale, 1979). There is also evidence that the Cu-Sn phases are subject to electrochemical dissolution <u>in vivo</u> (Marshall, et al, 1980). Those samples with higher fractions of Cu-Sn phases may, therefore, be expected to exhibit increased susceptibility to such corrosion. Other properties could also be expected to vary and it seems clear that a substantial increase in understanding of the behavior of amalgams will depend on careful characterization of microstructural variations and their implications on performance.

TABLE 2. Average compositions of reaction zones

Amalgam	Hg	Sn	Ag	Cu
C	11.4+6.4	39.2+5.3	4.1+1.0	45.3+7.8
D	29.0+9.1	31.1+6.1	17.3+4.4	22.6+6.0
E	44.6+3.5	22.9+3.8	13.6+1.7	18.9+1.6
M	38.2+5.8	24.8+4.2	21.5+3.5	15.6+3.9
P	14.8+10.5	41.4+7.7	4.9+2.6	38.8+9.3
S	41.4+10.4	17.9+6.3	14.7+4.6	26.0+5.3

TABLE 3. Approximate volume per cents in reaction zones

Amalgam	γ_1	Cu_6Sn_5	Cu_3Sn	Alloy
C	10	55	35	
D	31	56		13
E	46	54		
M	46	40		14
P	13	66	21	
S	43	16	33	8

System S presents a different characteristic. It is well known that large amounts of Cu_6Sn_5 form in the matrix. In addition, it can be seen from this work that the reaction zones also contain substantial amounts of Cu-Sn phase and these contributions must be taken into account as the various microstructural contributions to properties are considered.

CONCLUSIONS

1. The reaction zones of the systems studied vary considerably in composition and volume fraction of phases present.

2. All the reaction zones contained γ_1 and Cu_6Sn_5.

3. Systems C, P and S also contained Cu_3Sn in amounts between 20 and 35%.

4. Residual alloy was found in the reaction zones of D, M and S with volume fraction of approximately 10%.

5. In future explorations of alloy properties and performance considerations must be given to the variations in reaction zones demonstrated here.

ACKNOWLEDGEMENTS

This work was supported by NIH-NIDR Grants DE 04704 and DE 03637.

REFERENCES

Eames, W. B. and MacNamara, J. F. (1976) Eight high copper amalgam alloys and six conventional alloys compared. Oper. Dent., 1, 98-107.
Mahler, D. B., Terkla, L. B. and Van Eysden, J. (1973) Marginal fracture of amalgam restorations. J. Dent. Res., 52, 823-827.
Mahler, D. B., Adey, J. D. and van Eysden, J. (1975) Quantitative microprobe analysis of amalgam. J. Dent. Res., 54, 218-226.
Marshall, G. W., Marshall, S. J. and Greener, E. H. (1977) SEM/EDX analysis of new dental amalgams, in Scanning Electron Microscopy/1977 (Ed., O. Johari), Vol. 1, pp. 129-136, IITRI, Chicago.
Marshall, G. W., Jackson, B. L. and Marshall, S. J. (1980) Copper-rich and conventional amalgam restorations after clinical use. J. Amer. Dent. Assoc., 100, 43-47.
Marshall, S. J. and Marshall, G. W. (1979) Time dependent phase changes in Cu-rich amalgams. J. Biomed. Mater. Res., 13, 395-406.

Okabe, T., Mitchell, R., Butts, M. B., Bosley, J. R. and Fairhurst, C. W. (1977) Analysis of Asgar-Mahler reaction zone in Dispersalloy amalgam by electron diffraction. J. Dent. Res., 56, 1037-1043.
Osbourne, J. W. and Gale, E. N. (1979) Failure rate of margins of amalgams with a high content of copper. Oper. Dent., 4, 2-8.

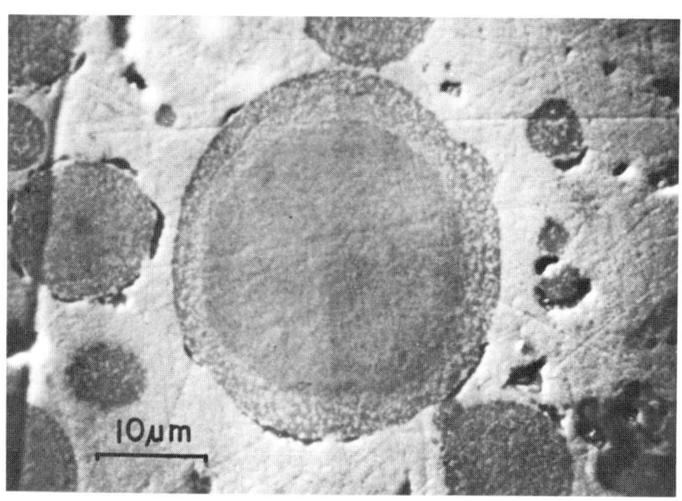

Fig. 1. Typical appearance of reaction zone surrounding Cu-rich particles in blended systems (D, M, E).

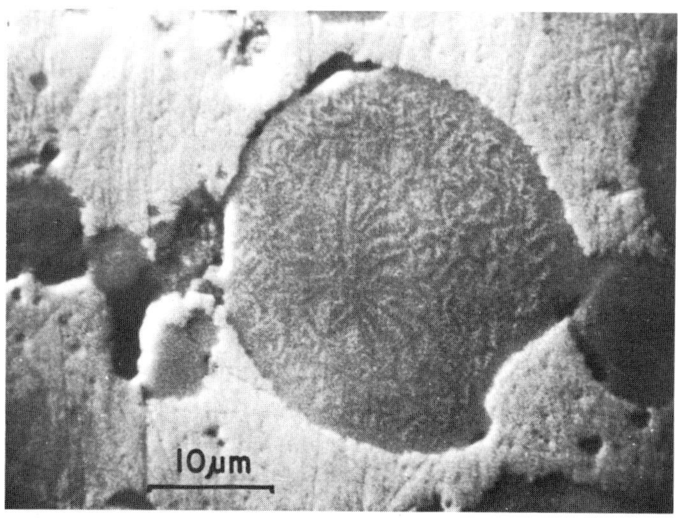

Fig. 2. Dark reaction zone at the periphery of the Cu-rich particles in system P.

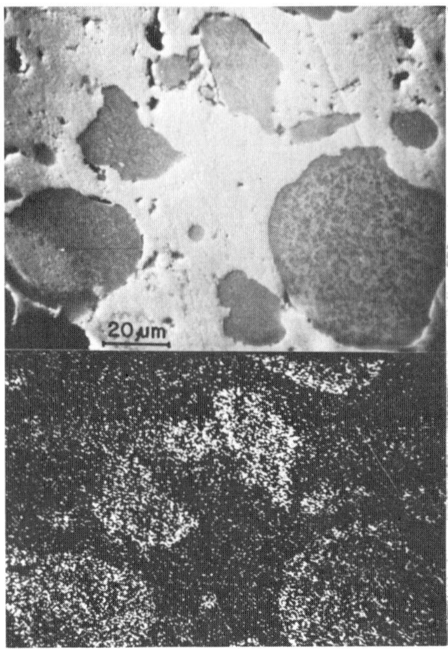

Fig. 3. Characteristics of amalgam system C. (Top) Microstructure showing dark reaction zone surrounding Cu-rich
particles. (Bottom) Sn map demonstrates Cu-Sn phases in
the reaction zones.

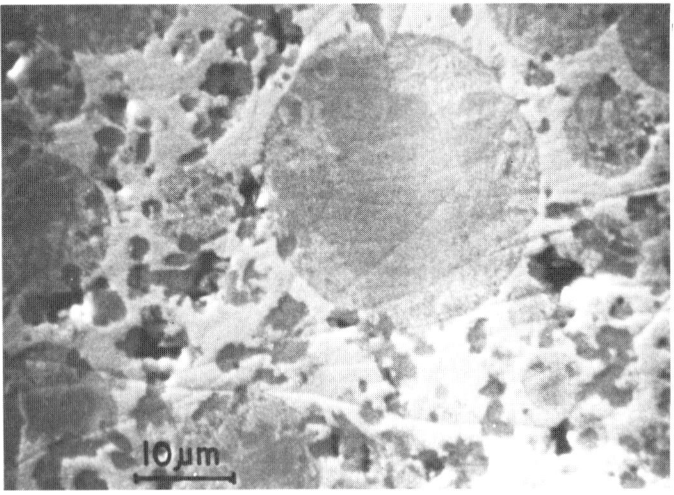

Fig. 4. Microstructure of single particle system S. Original
alloy particles contain darker central region surrounded by
a lighter irregular reaction zone.

Biomaterials 1980
Edited by G. D. Winter, D. F. Gibbons, and H. Plenk, Jr.
© 1982 John Wiley and Sons Ltd.

EXPERIMENTAL CLINICAL RESEARCH ON DENTAL AMALGAM RESTORATIONS

H. Letzel and M.M.A. Vrijhoef

Dental School University of Nijmegen,
Nijmegen, The Netherlands

SUMMARY

In a clinical study the influence of the high copper alloy, the
patient and the operator on the oral behaviour of amalgam restorations
was investigated. In all patients and with all alloys the restorations
can be polished to the same quality of marginal adaptation. The
operator has a significant influence as to this quality. After one
year the influence of the alloy, the patient and the operator on the
marginal fracture are significant. The patient and the alloy have influence on the surface corrosion of the restorations.

INTRODUCTION

Recently, attention has been focused on clinical research in order to
investigate the oral behaviour of amalgam restorations. Up to now
several factors have been identified which influence their behaviour.
The factors are the amalgam alloy (Mahler et al, 1970; Osborne et al,
1978 and Letzel et al, 1978a), the operator (Letzel et al, 1978a and
Mahler & Marantz, 1979), the cavity preparation (Akerboom et al, 1979)
the trituration time (Osborne & Gale, 1974), the condensation
technique (Letzel et al, 1978b), the polishing technique (Leinfelder
et al, 1979) and the patient (Letzel et al, 1978a and Goldberg et al,
1979). This study assesses the influence of the alloy, the patient
and the operator.

MATERIALS AND METHODS

Five hundred and fourty class I and II amalgam restorations were made
by 3 dentists, each dentist placing 180 restorations. Seventy seven
patients participated in the trial, their ages varied between 15 and
44 years. Sixty four patients received one series of 6 restorations,
each made from different amalgam alloys. Thirteen patients received
two such series. In each series the six alloys were randomly distributed. The alloys were I (Indiloy, Shofu Dent. Corp, USA), S (Sybralloy, Sybron-Kerr, USA), D (Dispersalloy, Johnson & Johnson, USA), T
(Tytin, SSWhite-Penwalt, USA), L (Luxalloy, Degussa, Germ.) and A
(A-76, Degussa, Germ.).

341

The last alloy is an experimental ternary alloy mixed with small amounts of conventional alloy (US-patient 4,008,073; USA-tradename will be Amalcap non gamma-2).

The cavity preparation was performed in a conventional way. A rubber-dam was used for all restorations. The cavity walls were varnished with Copalite and deep cavities were first lined with Dycal. All alloys were triturated according to the directions for use provided by the manufacturer. The condensation of the amalgam mix and the over-filling of the cavity was performed mechanically with a Bergendal vibrator. However, in deep cavities the first amalgam portion was condensed by hand. Each series of six restorations was polished in one session, after a minimum time of one day. Immediately after polishing black and white photographs were taken of each restoration (Letzel, 1978a).

After one year, the patients were called back for an examination of the restorations. Again, photographs were taken of each restoration. The size of the occlusal marginal integrity of the restorations - after polishing and after one year - was quantified on the pictures with a 6-point photo rating scale. Each restoration was independent-ly rated 3 times by a trained evaluator. These ratings were averaged. At the one year examination the marginal integrity, corrosion (by means of the discoloration) and roughness of the occlusal surface of the restorations were also quantified clinically with 4-point rating scales by the same trained evaluator (Letzel, 1978b).
The sets of ratings for the 4 criteria (clinical evaluation of margi-nal integrity, corrosion, roughness and photographic evaluation of marginal integrity - after polish and after one year) were analyzed as to differences with 2-way analyses of variance. The first ANOVA analysed for differences between the main effects of operator and alloy, the second between the main effects of patient and alloy. No interactions between main effects were discovered.

RESULTS

At the one year recall all the patients were examined. One restora-tion showed an isthmus fracture and was replaced after the rating procedures. The level of significance of the F-values for the main effects in both ANOVAS are summarized in Table 1. It is apparent that the influence of the operator on the marginal integrity after polis-hing is highly significant ($p \leq 0.001$). After one year the influence of the patient, alloy and operator on marginal integrity obtained both from photographs and clinical evaluations are highly significant ($p \leq 0.001$). The patient and alloy factors have a significant in-fluence on the discoloration and roughness after one year ($p \leq 0.001$). Because of the highly significant influence of the patient on the one year marginal integrity, the mean of the photographic ratings were calculated.

TABLE 1. Level of significance for the F-values calculated
in the two 2 - way ANOVAS for 4 clinical
characteristics

Clinical characteristic	Patient	Factor Alloy	Operator
Marginal integrity (after polish)	-	-	++
Marginal integrity (after 1 year)	++	++	++
Marginal integrity (after 1 year clinically)	++	++	++
Discoloration	++	+	-
Roughness formation	++	++	-

$-$ = $p > 0.05$ $+$ = $0.01 \geq p > 0.001$
$(+)$ = $0.05 \geq p > 0.01$ $++$ = $p \leq 0.001$

The means were divided into classes and listed in a freuqency distribution. The distribution is shown as a histogram in figure 1.

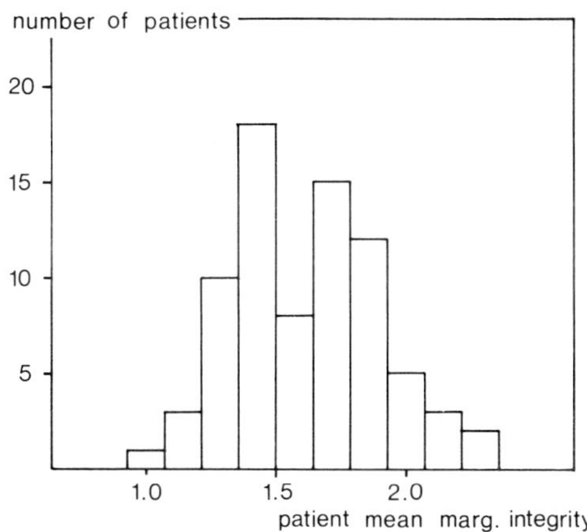

Fig. 1. Histogram for the distribution of patients means
for marginal integrity after one year.

Because of the highly significant influence of the alloy on the one
year marginal integrity, the alloy means were computed both after
polishing and after one year (Table 2). The marginal integrity after
polishing is to be considered as a base line for marginal adaptation,
while that after one year as a cumulative effect of marginal adaptation and marginal fracture. The mean marginal integrity values per
alloy obtained clinically are also listed in table 2.

TABLE 2. Mean values per alloy for marginal integrity, discoloration and roughness

Marginal integrity

	Photographic rating		Clin. rating			
All.	After pol.	One year	One year	All.	Discol.	Roughness
I	1.07	1.29	1.22	T	1.12	1.19
D	1.05	1.45	1.31	L	1.21	1.36
S	1.08	1.53	1.36	D	1.30	1.52
T	1.11	1.66	1.47	A	1.51	1.45
A	1.07	1.68	1.51	S	1.58	1.55
L	1.11	1.92	1.59	I	1.93	1.92
SE	0.03	0.06	0.05		0.05	0.05

SE is standard error of the means of the subsets. Vertical lines indicate homogeneous subsets at the 0.01 level of significance.

The operator means for marginal integrity for the two periods are given in table 3. For discoloration and roughness the mean scale values per alloy are listed in table 2.

TABLE 3. Mean marginal integrity per operator after polish and after one year obtained with pictures of the restorations.

Operator	Mean marginal integrity	
	After polish	After one year
2	1.03 (0.02)	1.45 (0.04)
3	1.07	1.58
1	1.14	1.75

Vertical lines indicate homogeneous subsets at the 0.01 level of significance.
Numbers in parentheses are standard errors of the means.

CONCLUSIONS

The operator has a minor, but significant influence on the marginal adaptation of the polished restorations. Although the operators in this study both standardised their restorative procedures and had a 3 year experience in making restorations for clinical studies, a personal influence on the quality of the marginal adaptation is still noticeable. Since the group of three operators is an incidental sample from the population of general practioners, this group probably is very selective. It is therefore expected that the operator effect is much more substantial for the whole population of general practioners. The alloy and the patient have no influence on the marginal adaptation. All patients can be supplied with high quality restorations, irrespective of the alloy used.

The patient, the operator and the alloy all have a significant influence on the marginal fracture. A patient and operator influence also has been demonstrated by Letzel (1978), Mahler (1978) and Goldberg (1979). No explanation can be given for this phenomenon. Alloy influences have been demonstrated many times. In this study Indiloy exhibited the least marginal fracture, Luxalloy the most. In this respect Luxalloy is comparable to New True Dentalloy (SSW-Penwalt) (Letzel, 1978b).

The factors of patient and alloy have a significant influence on the discoloration of the occlusal surface of the restoration. The operator has no influence on this phenomenon. For discoloration the alloys can be divided into 3 groups. Restorations of D, T and L show no or very little discoloration, those of A and S slightly more. Alloy I gives by far the most discoloration. The color changes vary from alloy to alloy. Restorations of A discolour to light yellow or brown, those of S to light or dark grey and those of I to dark grey or black. In our opinion alloy I is not clinically acceptable as far as its esthetics is concerned.

The patient and the alloy have a significant influence on the disappearance of the original luster of the polished occlusal surface of the restoration. In this respect the 6 alloys also can be divided into 3 groups. Restorations of T show no or very little roughness, those of D, S, A and L somewhat more and those of I the most. Again, the last alloy is clinically unacceptable.

The restorations from the new dental amalgam alloy A-76 have the same marginal adaptation as those from the other tested alloys. With respect to the marginal integrity after one year A-76 is identical to Tytin and Sybralloy. As far as surface corrosion is concerned the amalgam behaves like Sybralloy and Dispersalloy. However, for more definite statements about its clinical behaviour the restorations need to be followed for a longer period.

REFERENCES

Akerboom, H.B.M.; Advokaat, J.G.A.; van Amerongen, W.E.; Borgmeier, P.J. & van Reenen, G.J. (1979): The influence of the preparation on the durability of the amalgam restoration. J. Dent. Res. 58, Special Issue A abstr. 423.
Goldberg, J.; Munster, E.; Spangberg, E.; Sanchez, L. & Lambert, K. (1979): Experimental Design in the Clinical Evaluation of Amalgam Restorations. J. Dent. Res. 58, Special Issue A, abstr. 419.
Leinfelder, K.F.; May, K.N. & Wilder, A.D. (1979): Two year clinical evaluation of pre-carve burnished Amalgam Restorations. J. Dent. Res. 58, Special Issue A, abstr. 426.
Letzel, H.; Aardening, Chr.; Fick, J.M.; van Leusen, J. & Vrijhoef, M.M.A. (1978a): Tarnish, Corrosion, Marginal Fracture and Creep of Amalgam Restorations: A two-year Clinical Study. Operative Dent. 3, 82-91.
Letzel, H.; Aardening, Chr.; Fick, J.M.; van Leusen, J. & Vrijhoef, M.M.A. (1978b): Condensation Technique versus Clinical Behaviour of Amalgam Restorations. J. Dent. Res. 57, Special Issue A, abstr. 497.
Mahler, D.B.; Terkla, L.G.; van Eysden, J. & Reisbick, M.H. (1970): Marginal Fracture vs Mechanical Properties of Amalgam J. Dent. Res. 49, 1452-1457.
Mahler, D.B. & Marantz, R. (1979): The effect of the operator on the clinical performance of Amalgam. J. Amer. Dent. Ass. 99, 38-41.
Osborne, J.W. & Gale, E.N. (1974): A two-, three- and four-year follow-up of a clinical study of the effect of trituration on amalgam restorations. J. Amer. Dent. Ass. 88, 795-797.
Osborne, J.W.; Gale, E.N.; Chew, C.L.; Rhodes, B.F. & Phillips, R.W. (1978): Clinical Performance and Physical Properties of Twelve Amalgam Alloys. J. Dent. Res. 57, 983-988.

Dental implants

Biomaterials 1980
Edited by G. D. Winter, D. F. Gibbons, and H. Plenk, Jr.
© 1982 John Wiley and Sons Ltd.

DESIGN OF A TRANSDUCER FOR MEASURING IN VIVO
FORCES ON ENDOSSEOUS DENTAL IMPLANTS

J. B. Brunski

Center for Biomedical Engineering
Rensselaer Polytechnic Institute,
Troy, N.Y. 12181   USA

SUMMARY

The performance of a dental implant is related to the status of the
tissues which support it. It is suggested that these supporting
tissues can be influenced by the biting forces on the dental implant.
Data have not yet been reported on the in vivo forces which implants
experience in various human and laboratory animals. This hampers
understanding of implant-tissue biomechanics. In the present study
dental implants are themselves strain-gaged and tested as transducers
for measuring axial bite force components. The results point toward
the use of similar transducers for in vivo trials.

INTRODUCTION

The design of a successful endosseous dental implant is a multivari-
able problem. Variables of importance are the implant material,
bacteriologic factors, surgical/clinical methods, and implant-tissue
biomechanics. In regard to biomechanics, an endosseous dental
implant must transmit biting forces to the tissues in which it is
anchored. Finite element computer stress analyses (Norton et al.
1974; Cook et al. 1980; Lavernia et al. 1980) have investigated how
the geometry of an implant, its elastic modulus, and interface tissue
properties influence the stress distribution in tissues around the
implant. In vivo work with animal models (Brunski et al. 1979) has
suggested that the interface tissue response can depend strongly on
the forces on the implant. Interpretation of results from both
theoretical and in vivo studies has been hampered because we lack
quantitative data on the forces which implants experience in the
many different animals (dogs, monkeys, baboons, humans) used for
dental implant research. The present project suggests a method for
the in vivo measurement of forces on dental implants.

DESIGN CRITERIA

An ideal transducer for measuring in vivo bite forces on a dental
implant should have the following characteristics: (1) accuracy in
the expected bite force range (say, 0-1333N); (2) reasonable
precision ($\pm$ 8.8N); (3) durability in the oral cavity; (4) capability
for measurement of three components of a resultant force on an
implant; (5) interchangeability with various implant designs; (6)

348   J.B. Brunski

reliability and negligible hysteresis. Also, the transducer should
be relatively compact so that it does not alter masticatory conditions, and the output from the transducer should be easy to record.
Force transducers used in previous dental studies (Table 1) were not
appropriate for the present work primarily because of size constraints.

TABLE 1.   Transducers used to measure biting forces in
various dental studies not involving implants

1. inductance strain gages   Howell and Manley (1948)
                                     Howell and Brudevold (1950)
                                     Yurkstas and Curby (1953)
2. resistance strain gages   Anderson and Picton (1958)
                                     McNicholas et al. (1975)
                                     Haddad (1976)
                                     Pruim et al. (1978)
3. solid state transducers   Scott and Ash (1966)
4. piezoelectric crystals   Mansour (1974)
                                     Graf et al. (1974)
5. piezoelectric polymer film   Fry (1977)
                                     Cummings et al. (1980)

The approach of the current work was to design a strain-gaged dental
implant that would itself be sensitive to biting forces. A strain-
gage installation that could accomplish this was suggested by a
scheme of Anderson (1948), who measured the three orthogonal components of an unknown resultant force on a cylindrical structural
member (Figure 1). The axial force component is separately measured
by an arrangement of four gages distributed circumferentially around
the cylinder and connected in a full bridge configuration. This
installation gives temperature compensation and insensitivity to
bending and torsional forces (Dally and Riley, 1978).

A method for simultaneous measurement of all three force components
on a dental implant would necessitate twelve strain gages and would
therefore be impractical for the small implants currently used.
However, if a given dental implant had a removable head, then three
separate heads could be strain gaged for separate sensitivity to the
three force components, and attached at selected times when force
readings were desired. Data would consist of separate profiles of
the three force components over different periods of time, from
which conclusions could be drawn about the nature of the average
forces on the implant under study. In the current work a method is
explored for the measurement of only the axial force component on an
endosseous dental implant.

METHODS

Two commercially-available carbon (Pyrolite^{K}) post-type implants
(Figure 2) were used in initial trials. The "head" of this implant
design was approximately cylindrical (diameter ~ 5 mm), and the modulus was nominally 28 GPa (Bockros et al. 1972). These values meant

that the expected bite forces would produce measurable strain values.
Two prototype transducers were fabricated. The strain gage installation on each implant consisted of four strain gages (Micro
Measurements #EA-06-031EC-350), two oriented axially and two oriented transversely for Poisson strain (Figure 3). The gages were
connected in a full bridge configuration for temperature compensation, and sensitivity to bending and torsional loads (Dally and
Riley 1978). Laboratory trials of the transducers were conducted
using a simple axial load applicator and a V/E-20A digital strain
indicator. Static compressive loads of up to 78N were applied along
the long axis of the implant, the apical end of which was held in
epoxy resin. Tests for hysteresis involved cyclic loading and
unloading of the implant.

RESULTS AND DISCUSSION

For the two transducers tested, a linear relationship was observed
between the measured microstrain ($\mu\varepsilon$) and the axial load P. Figure
4 shows the collected data from a total of fifteen load-unload tests
of the two prototype transducers. The open circles are the average
strains, and the error bars show the range of strains recorded at
the indicated applied loads. There was negligible hysteresis observed in these transducer calibration tests. Tests in which
relatively smallforces (< 5N) were applied at 90° to the long axes
of the transducers indicated negligible senstitivity to bending
loads. Tests of temperature compensation, however, showed that the
gage installation was slightly sensitive to temperature ($\pm$ 15$\mu\varepsilon$ for
$\Delta T = \pm 30^{o}C$). The measured strains in transducer tests agreed with
those calculated from the implant's modulus, geometry and the
applied axial load, within experimental error. The range of error
in the measured strains, however, meant that the force which would
be deduced in transducer operation could be off by $\pm$ 15% (Figure 4).

Based on these results, other transducers have been fabricated. In
these cases, a small strain-gaged cylinder of the carbon material
serves as part of a screw-in head portion for a dental implant body
that may be of arbitrary material and shape. Further laboratory and
in vivo trials of these transducers are currently underway.

CONCLUSIONS

A method for measuring in vivo forces on endosseous dental implants
has been presented and discussed. A strain-gaged dental implant has
been designed to measure the axial component of force on the dental
implant. The preliminary results are consistent with the envisaged
use of the removable head of a dental implant as a force transducing
element.

ACKNOWLEDGEMENT

The support of the NIDR through Grant DE05418-01 is gratefully
acknowledged.

<u>REFERENCES</u>

Anderson, A.R. (1948). A three component force recorder. <u>Proc. Soc. Expt'l. Stress Anal.</u>, 5(2), 42-48.

Anderson, D.J. & Picton, D.C.A. (1958) Masticatory stresses in normal and modified occlusion. <u>J. Dent. Res.</u>, 37, 313-317.

Bockros, J.C., La Grange, L.D. & Schoen, G.J. (1972) <u>Chemistry and Physics of Carbon, Vol. 9</u> (Ed. P.L. Walker), p 123, Marcel Dekker, New York.

Brunski, J.B., Moccia, A.F. Jr., Pollack, S.R., Korostoff, E. & Trachtenberg, D.I. (1979) The influence of functional use of endosseous dental implants on the tissue-implant interface. Part I. Histological aspects. <u>J. Dent. Res.</u>, 58(10), 1953-1969.

Cook, S.D., Klawitter, J.J., Weinstein, A.M. & Lavernia, C.J. (1980) The design and evaluation of dental implants with finite element analysis. <u>Finite Elements in Biomechanics</u> (Ed. B.R. Simon), pp 169-178, University of Arizona, Arizona.

Cummings, R.N., Baumeister, H.K. & Proffit, W.R. (1980) Maximum biting force (MBF) measured at rest vertical position of the mandible. Abstract #883, Annual Session of the AADR, <u>J. Dent. Res.</u>, 59, Special Issue A, p 488.

Dally, J.W. & Riley, W.F. (1978) <u>Experimental Stress Analysis</u>, pp 262-264, McGraw-Hill, New York.

Fry, R.W., Baumeister, H. & Proffit, W.R. (1977) Development of an occlusal force transducer utilizing piezoelectric film. <u>J. Dent. Res.</u>, 56, Special Issue B, p B191.

Graf, H., Grassel, H. & Aeberhard, H.J. (1974) A method for measurement of occlusal forces in three directions. <u>Helv. Odont. Scand.</u>, 18, 7-11.

Haddad, W.W. (1976) The functioning dentition. <u>Frontiers of Oral Physiology</u>, 2, 146-183.

Howell, A.H. & Brudevold, F. (1950) Vertical forces used during chewing of food. <u>J. Dent. Res.</u>, 29, 133-136.

Howell, A.H. & Manly, R.S. (1948) An electronic strain gage for measuring oral forces. <u>J. Dent. Res.</u>, 27, 705-712.

Lavernia, C.J., Cook, S.D., Klawitter, J.H., Weinstein, A.M. & Das, S.C. (1980) The effect of implant elastic modulus on the stress distribution surrounding dental implants. <u>Finite Elements in Biomechanics</u> (Ed. B.R. Simon), pp 179-192, Univ. of Arizona, Arizona.

McNicholas, T., Milillo, F. & Eisenstadt, R. (1975) Strain and force determination and distribution in a maxillary and mandibular second molar. <u>Biotelemetry</u>, 2(1-2), 31-32.

Mansour, R.M. (1974) Analysis of occlusal forces in mandibular terminal hinge position and lateral excursive positions. Ph.D. Thesis, Drexel University, Phila. PA.

Norton, R., Knoell, A., Gupta, K. & Grenoble, D. (1974) Biomechanical modeling and structural analysis of a human mandible containing a blade implant. <u>Proc. 5th Int'l. Conf. on Expt'l Stress Analysis</u>, Paper 34, Udine, Italy.

Pruim, G.J., Ten Bosch, J.J. & de Jong, H.J. (1978) Jaw muscle EMG-activity and static loading of the mandible. <u>J. Biomech</u>, 11, 389-395.

Scott, I. & Ash, M.M. Jr. (1966) A six-channel intraoral transmitter for measuring occlusal forces. J. Prosth. Dent., 16(1),
56-61.
Yurkstas, A. & Curby, W.A. (1953) Force analysis of prostehtic
appliances during function. J. Dent. Res., 3, 82-87.

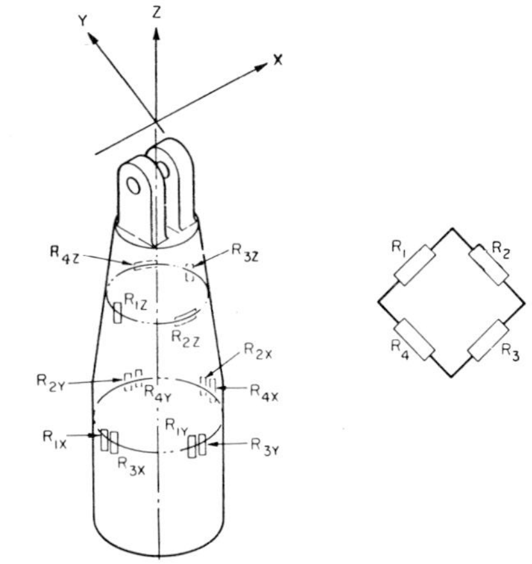

Fig. 1   Strain gage arrangement to measure three
         components of a resultant force on a structural
         member (after Anderson, 1948, "A three-component
         Force Recorder", Proc.SESA 5(2):42-48, by
         permission of the Society for Experimental
         Stress Analysis, Saugatuck Station, CT).

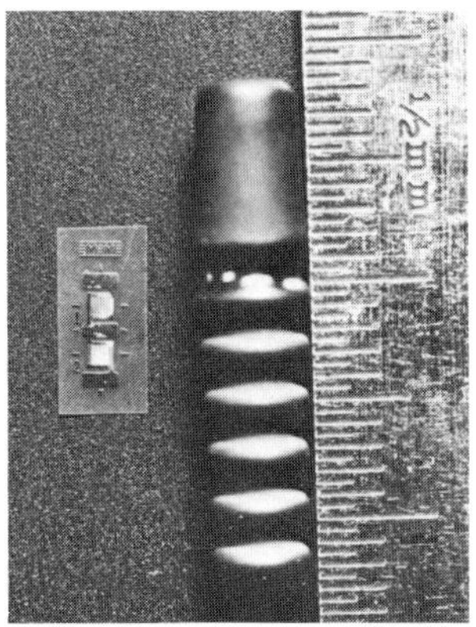

Fig. 2   A Pyrolite[R] carbon dental implant and a
         miniature strain gage.

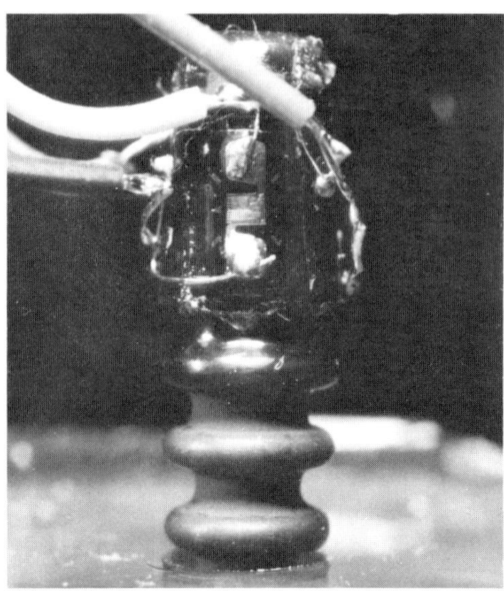

Fig. 3   Carbon implant showing a gage oriented
         for transverse strain (other three gages
         not shown).

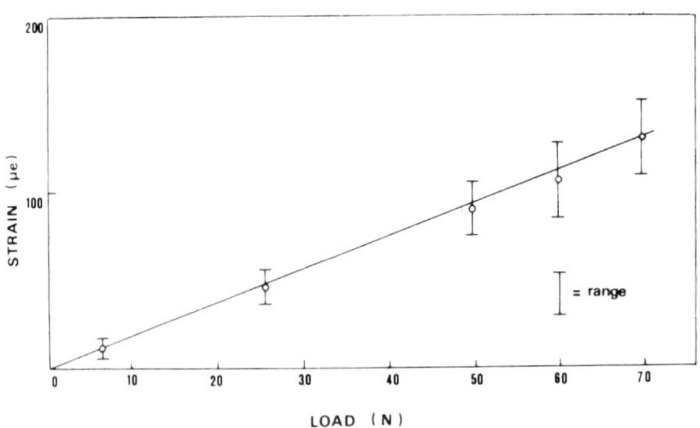

Fig. 4   Calibration curves for two gaged
         implants; results of 15 tests.

Biomaterials 1980
Edited by G. D. Winter, D. F. Gibbons, and H. Plenk, Jr.
© 1982 John Wiley and Sons Ltd.

THE EFFECT OF OCCLUSION ON THE PERFORMANCE
OF POROUS ROOTED TITANIUM DENTAL IMPLANTS

F.A. Young, C.H. Kresch, and C.F. Marcinak

Medical University of South Carolina,
Charleston, SC   29403

INTRODUCTION

Endosteal dental implants of numerous designs have been fabricated
from metals, polymers, and ceramics in order to seek solutions to the
problems associated with substituting for missing natural teeth. Reviews of these attempts have been published by several authors (Linkow
1970, Cranin 1970, DHEW 1974). The use of tissue ingrowth in porous
material to anchor dental implants was suggested at the Engineering
Foundation Conference "Bioceramics" held in 1970 (Young. 1972). Tissue ingrowth into porous titanium alloy specimens was reported at the
same meeting (Hirschorn 1972). Titanium and titanium alloys are
achieving recognition as corrosion resistant and biocompatible materials with properties desirable for the construction of prosthetic
devices (Solar 1979).

Clinical and histological results of the use of porous titanium implants as roots for artificial teeth which were in function but not
in occlusion have been reported by the author (Young 1979 a and b).
The objective of this study was to obtain long term clinical performance data on mandibular implants supporting crowns and bridges in
occlusion against natural opposing dentition. A corollary objective
was to compare the performance of implants supporting crowns and
bridges in occlusion with the clinical results obtained in previous
studies where single tooth implants were in function but not in
occlusion.

MATERIALS AND METHODS

The implant used was fabricated from 6Al-4V titanium alloy powder.
It consisted of a primary endosseous stage containing a solid core
with 0.5mm of spherical powder sintered to the exterior. The porous
titanium coating contained 34 volume per cent porosity. A secondary
stage which was added to the primary stage (root) after a suitable
healing period was fabricated from solid titanium in a slightly
tapered cylindrical form to enhance application of the crowns and
bridges. Crowns and bridges were cast gold restorations which were
placed in functional occlusion using conventional dental techniques.
Bridges were placed using two implants as abutments or using a natural

tooth as a mesial or distal abutment. Twelve Rhesus monkeys are being
used in the study. Implants were placed in healed mandibular premolar
or first molar extraction sites. Evaluations were conducted monthly.
Radiographs were used to assess changes in bone height and density.
Mobility was estimated in millimeters of movement at the crown of the
implant. Pocket depth in millimeters was measured at six locations
around the implant with a graduated periodontal probe. Bleeding was
evaluated on an arbitrary scale of 4 units. The width of keratinized
tissue surrounding the implant was measured in millimeters. Condition
of the gingiva was assessed as good, fair, or poor. Plaque accumulation on the implant was estimated on a scale of 4 units. Where evidence of acute bacterial infection was present, cultures were taken by
aspiration through the buccal surface of the gingiva.

<u>RESULTS</u>

Thirty implants have been placed for this study. Seven implants are in
single unit functional occlusion. Eighteen implants are supporting
bridges. Five of the animals which were implanted for this study were
used in a previous study in which the implants were in function but
were not necessarily in occlusion. The crowns or bridges were placed
on these animals' implants after periods of function up to 29 months,
thus allowing comparison of the same implant in function and in occlusion. Three of the implants were placed in animals whose anatomy
dictated that the abutments were in occlusion; these implants were
therefore in full occlusion for the entire functional period. Three
implants did not receive crowns or bridges because of anatomical difficulties. Figure 1 below summarizes the results of the experiments
as of September 1, 1980. The length of each bar represents the time
period during which the secondary stage (abutment) has been in function. The letter "B" appears at the point in time when the bridge was
placed. The letter "C" appears at the point in time when the crown
was placed. The letter "0" occurs when the implant abutment was
placed in occlusion without an anatomical crown. Open portions of
the time bars represent periods during which the implants functioned
without clinical indications of difficulty. Periods during which implants were observed to display minor clinical symptoms of difficulty
are indicated by hatched portions of the bars. The symptoms were
typically gingivitis, and increased bleeding. Periods during which
the implants experienced severe difficulties are indicated by vertical stripes. Difficulties observed were infection, edema, increased
pocket depth, and bone loss. All implants which exhibited severe
difficulties were removed at the time period indicated by the length
of the bar. The presence of bridges was found, in general to result
in an increase in plaque accumulation which was associated with increased gingivitis. The increased gingivitis did not cause increased
pocket depths or loss of bony support. Four implants were removed.
Two of the implants developed infections immediately after placement
of the abutments. One implant became infected after functioning

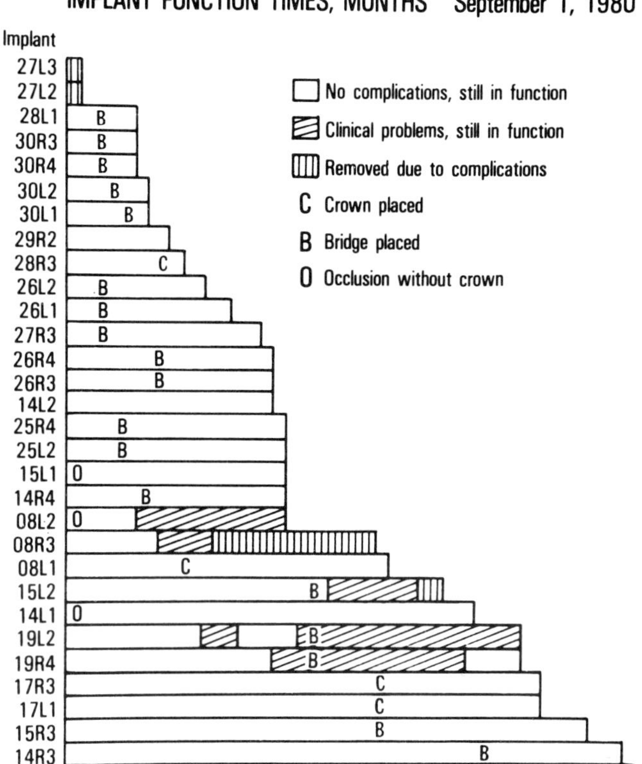

Figure 1. Summary of implant clinical results. The first two numbers
of each implant indicate the animal. Open bars indicate asymptomatic
implants. Hatched bars represent period of minor clinical sympto-
mology. Vertical striped bars represent periods of rapid bone loss,
infection and increasing pocket depth. The total length of the bars
represent time of function. Placement of crown, bridge, or presence
of occlusion is indicated by the letter indicated by the legend.

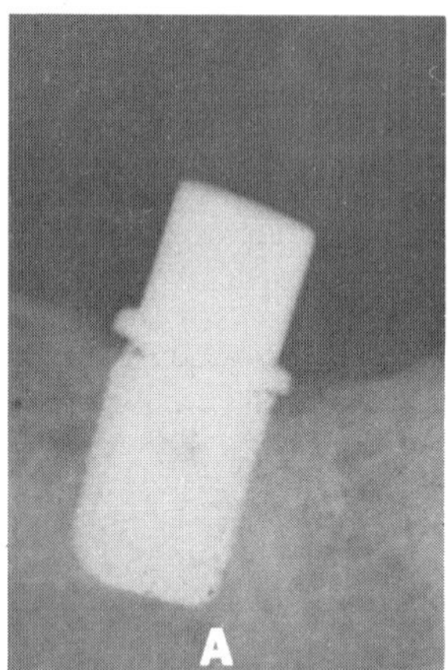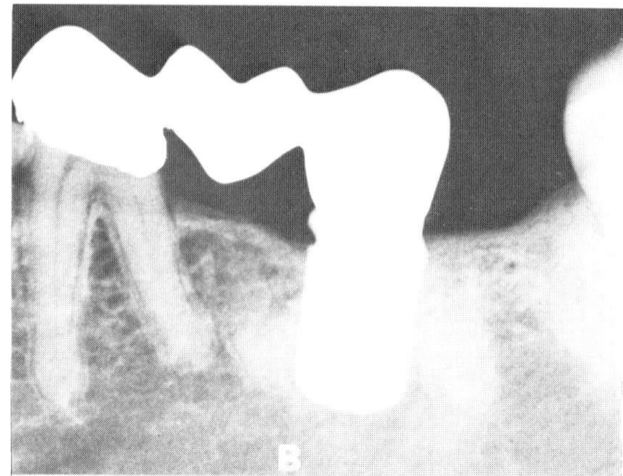

Fig. 2. Radiographs of implant 19L2. (A) Implant after functioning out of occlusion for 18 months. (B) Implant 14 months after bridge has been placed. This implant has been in place for 40 months and has been evaluated as having gingivitis and bleeding.

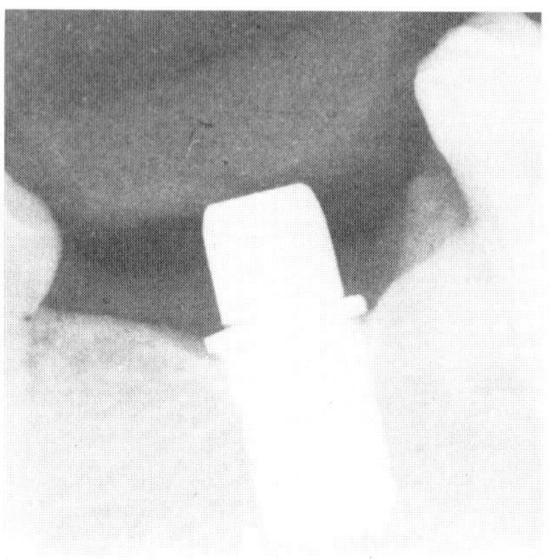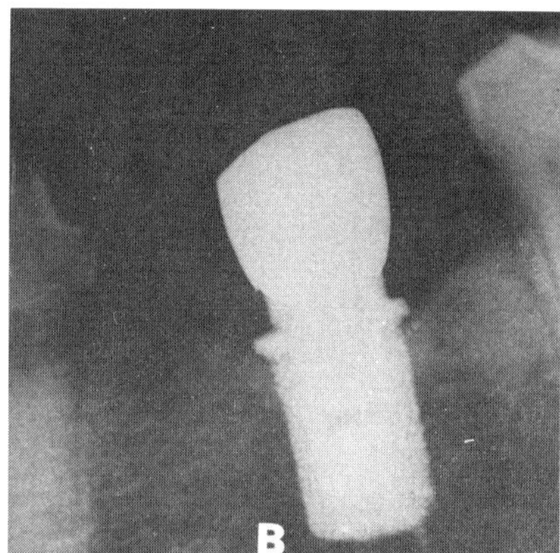

Fig. 3. Radiographs of implant 17L1. (A) Implant after functioning out of occlusion for 27 months. (B) Implant 10 months after crown was placed. This implant displayed no adverse clinical symptoms.

out of occlusion for eight months. Attempts to treat the infection
were unsuccessful, and the implant was removed after a fourteen month
period of complications. No prosthesis was placed on this implant.
One implant became infected after an eight month period of moderate
clinical symptoms following bridge placement. This implant was removed after three months of severe complications. Implant removal
sites healed without complications. Figure 2a illustrates the radiographic appearance of implant 19L2 which has been in function for 18
months. Figure 2b shows the same implant 14 months after the bridge
had been in place. The minor bone loss about the crestal regions of
the implant is typical of the response to these implants. The bone
loss occurs during the first few months of function. This implant
experienced bleeding and gingivitis both before and after placement of
the bridge. Figure 3a illustrates the radiographic appearance of implant 17L1 after 27 months of function. Figure 3b illustrates the
appearance of the implant after the crown has been in place 10 months.
This implant displayed no adverse clinical symptoms. The crestal bone
loss shown occurred during the first few months of function. This implant has functioned asymptomatically for over three years.

The presence of bridges was found to cause increased gingivitis but
did not cause increased pocket depth or loss of bony support. The
increased gingivitis was associated with a higher plaque index. Other
clinical indicators were not found to differ with performance of implants in a previous study which were identical and were in function
but not occlusion.

Monkeys with implants giving a wide range of clinical indicator per
formance were found to have gram positive cocci in blood cultures.
Cultures of the acutely failing implants were positive for beta hemolytic streptococcus and staphylococcus Aureus. The presence of gram
positive cocci in the tissue surrounding these failing implants were
confirmed histologically.

DISCUSSION AND CONCLUSIONS

The increased plaque index and inflammation associated with bridges
were concluded to be the cause of the anatomical design of the
bridges coupled with a lack of hygiene. After the first few bridges
were placed and the increased plaque index was noted, design of the
bridges was modified to leave space under the pontic. Although none
of the implants supporting the redesigned bridges has failed to date,
it is not certain that the design has lowered plaque accumulation or
improved gingival response. It was concluded that no major difference
can be detected in the performance of implants which are in occlusion
versus those only in function for the periods indicated. Although
chronic difficulties were encountered with seven implants, the four
which were removed all failed from infection, rather than the gradual
deterioration of bony support which has characterized solid implants.

While porous rooted implants support the loads of mastication without deleterious chronic changes, their vulnerability to infectious agents may be greater than that of solid implants, a factor which may limit the usefulness of the porous artificial root.

REFERENCES

Cranin, A. (1970) Oral Implantology, Thomas, Springfield.
DHEW publication NIH 74-548 (1974) Dental Biomaterial Research Priorities, U.S. Government Printing Office, Washington.
Hirschorn, J., McBeath, A. & Dustoor, M. (1972) Porous titanium surgical implant materials in Bioceramics-Engineering in Medicine (Eds. Hall, Hulbert, Levine & Young) p. 49-67, Wiley, New York.
Solar, R. (1979) Corrosion resistance of titanium surgical implant alloys. A review in Corrosion and Degradation of Implant Materials (Eds. Syrett & Acharya) p. 259-273. ASTM STP 684, Baltimore.
Young, F. (1972) Ceramic tooth implants in Bioceramics-Engineering in Medicine (Eds. Hall, Hulbert, Levine & Young) p. 281-296, Wiley, New York.
Young, F., Kresch, C. & Spector, M. (1979a) Porous titanium tooth roots: Clinical Evaluation, J. Prosthetic Dentistry, 41, 561-565.
Young, F., Spector, M. & Kresch, C. (1979b) Porous titanium endosseous dental implants in Rhesus monkeys: Microradiography and histological evaluation, J. Biomed. Mater. Res., 13, 843-856.

Biomaterials 1980
Edited by G. D. Winter, D. F. Gibbons, and H. Plenk, Jr.
© 1982 John Wiley and Sons Ltd.

ARTIFICIAL TOOTH ROOTS WITH POROUS POLYMER
COATINGS

M. Spector, C.F. Marcinak, F.A. Young,
J.T. Eldridge and S.L. Harmon

Medical University of South Carolina
Charleston, South Carolina, U.S.A.

SUMMARY

Porous high density polyethylene and porous polysulfone coated artificial tooth roots were implanted in healed mandibular extraction
sites in dogs and Rhesus monkeys. Implants were free-standing in
function, but not in occlusion. Unacceptable performance of canine
implants appeared to be related to resorption of the bone ingrowth
attachment mechanism, perhaps due to overload, mechanical failure.
Failed implants in monkeys were attributed to bacterial infection.

INTRODUCTION

Investigations of the intraosseous application of porous materials
initially proposed that they be employed as surface coatings for the
cement-free fixation of orthopedic implants. Subsequent studies demonstrated that a bone ingrowth attachment vehicle can also serve to
stabilize artificial tooth roots in alveolar bone. Dental implants
with porous metallic (Karagianes, 1976; Young et al., 1979; Weiss and
Rostoker, 1980; Peterson et al., 1980), ceramic (Klawitter et al.,
1977) and polymeric (Peterson et al., 1979) coatings have been evaluated in dogs, swine, and non-human primates. Studies in progress are
attempting to determine the causes of implant failure and to develop
design criteria for porous coated dental implants.

The objective of this study was to determine the efficacy of cylindrical-shaped endosseous dental implants with porous high density
polyethylene (Spector et al., 1976) and porous polysulfone (Spector
et al., 1978) coatings. Investigations were conducted in dogs and
Rhesus monkeys.

MATERIALS AND METHODS

The artificial tooth roots consisted of cylindrical-shaped pure titanium cores coated with either porous high density polyethylene*

*Glasrock Plastics Division of Glasrock Medical Services Corp.

                          M. Spector et al.

(Fig. 1) or porous polysulfone (medical grade)**. These coatings,
fabricated by sintering particles of the plastics, measured approximately 0.8mm in thickness. The porous polyethylene coatings were
40% porous with pore sizes of 120 and 250µm, while the average pore
size of the porous polysulfone material was 200µm. The superior
central aspect of the titanium core of the tooth root was tapped to
accept a supracrestal titanium abutment to be inserted 8 weeks after
the initial submucosal stage (Fig. 2). Thirty-nine porous polyethylene and four porous polysulfone tooth roots were implanted in healed
mandibular premolar extraction sites in 16 dogs. Nine porous polysulfone implants were placed in molar sites in four Rhesus monkeys.
All implants were free-standing and functional but not in occlusion.
Monthly evaluations were conducted to monitor mobility, pocket
depth, width of keratinized tissue around the implant, condition of
the gingiva, plaque accumulation and radiographic appearance of the
artificial tooth roots. Curettage was performed when indicated.

Implants and surrounding bone retrieved at sacrifice or after block
resection were fixed in formalin and embedded in a low viscosity
plastic embedding medium in preparation for sectioning for microradiography and ground section histology. Selected specimens were allocated for decalcification and paraffin processing.

RESULTS

Clinical Observations. Of the 39 polyethylene implants placed in the
dogs for as long as 78 weeks 21 were clinically acceptable with a
mobility of $\leq \frac{1}{2}$ mm. The 18 failures had a mobility greater than $\frac{1}{2}$ mm
and radiographic bone loss. Other clinical signs were unremarkable.
Two implant failures were related to the separation of the porous
coating from the titanium core.

Five of the porous polysulfone implants in monkeys inserted for as
long as 84 weeks were rated clinically successful. The 3 unsuccessful tooth roots exhibited a relatively rapid implant failure mode occurring over a period of a few weeks. The clinical signs which
characterized these failing implants were very different from those
generally seen. Gingival inflammation and swelling were accompanied
by radiographic bone loss which revealed itself as well-demarcated
saucerization around the coronal aspect of the root; mobility measurements remained $\leq \frac{1}{2}$. These features of the acute failure mode were
distinguishable from the more chronic gradual increase in mobility
or radiographic bone loss seen in the polyethylene implant failures
occurring in the dog. Sterile cultures taken by aspiration through
the buccal mucosa were positive for normal oral flora.

**Union Carbide Corporation

The 3 polysulfone failures in the dogs exhibited clinical features
similar to those of the canine polyethylene implants except that 2
of the polysulfone implants did not exhibit mobility. In one case
the coating separated from the core.

<u>Histological Evaluation</u>. Evaluation of 37 polyethylene implants in
dogs revealed 3 characteristic histological profiles (Fig. 3). One
tissue response (Fig. 3, I) included bone ingrowth into the porosity
of the implant with little fibrous tissue seen in the pores. The
crestal bone height was maintained at the level of the superior aspect of the root. Inflammatory infiltrate was confined to the sul-
cular region of the implant. A second histological profile (Fig. 3,
II) displayed bone adaptation to the porous coatings, with a thin
fibrous layer often interposed between the bone and the implant.
Bone ingrowth, if present, was limited to a few pores. Osteoclastic activity along the crestal bone was occasionally evidenced by
a scalloped surface. Associated with this response was densely organized fibrous tissue with spindle shaped cells and occasional inflammatory cell infiltrate extending into the porosity. A third
tissue response (Fig. 3, III) included bone resorption along the
coronal and apical aspects of the porosity, and excessive inflammatory
cell and fibrous infiltrate completely involving the apical porosity.
No difference in tissue response could be correlated with pore size
of the polyethylene implants.

Histological evaluation of the 3 clinically failing polysulfone implants in dogs revealed a tissue response similar to that of the
polyethylene implants in which bone adaptation with no or limited
bone ingrowth was seen (Fig. 3, II). Fibrous tissue predominated in
the porosity and inflammatory cell infiltrate was seen in some pores.

Examination of the 3 primate failures revealed bone ingrowth throughout the apical porosity (Fig. 4). A well demarcated zone of inflammatory reaction and bone loss encompassed from 1/3 to 2/3 of the
coronal aspect of the implants. The crestal surface of the remaining
bone displayed marked osteoclastic activity. These histopathological
changes were consistent with bacterial infection. Brown and Brenn
stains of paraffin sections of the adjacent gingival tissue revealed
the presence of bacteria. Gross destruction of the connective tissue
and inflammatory changes in the gingiva were also consistent with bac-
teria-induced reactions.

<u>DISCUSSION</u>

The histological profiles of the polyethylene implants could be classified as acceptable, potentially problematic, or unacceptable. The
potentially problematic implants were those that displayed histological features that could predispose the implant to failure with

longer implantation time. These features included limited or no bone ingrowth with fibrous tissue and inflammatory cell infiltrate. Nine of 19 polyethylene implants which were rated clinically acceptable displayed histological features which required them to be designated as potentially problematic or unacceptable. These results evidence the inadequacy of clinical measures for rating implant status.

Failure of the polyethylene canine implants appeared to be due to re-sorption of the bone ingrowth attachment mechanism and subsequent re-placement by fibrous tissue and inflammatory cell infiltrate. Im-plants immobile at one examination period was found to exhibit sig-nificant mobility at the next exam (1 month interval) with little im-mediate change in radiographic appearance. Bone loss was noted, how-ever, as the mobility increased. This failure mode is different from periodontal disease type processes which initially involve crestal bone and subsequently progress apically. Rather these observations would seem to be consistent with an overload failure of the bone in-growth attachment mechanism. The high loads applied during canine mastication and the small surface area of the tooth root are factors predisposing to this type of failure mode (Young, 1980).

Failure of the porous polysulfone implants in the monkeys could be related to acute bacterial infections. This failure mode was not observed in canine implants.

Results of the present study suggest that differences in the mode of failure of porous polymer coated dental implants in dogs and monkeys may be species related. Implants in dogs may undergo overload failure of the bone ingrowth attachment mechanism while primate implants may be more susceptible to bacterial infection.

ACKNOWLEDGEMENTS

This work was supported by NIH-NIDR grants DE00067 and DE04414. The authors gratefully acknowledge H. Mercer and N.J. Ballintyn of Glas-rock Plastics and Union Carbide Corporation, respectively, for their assistance in the fabrication of the porous polyethylene and porous polysulfone coated tooth roots.

REFERENCES

Karagianes, M., Westerman, R., Rasmussen, J., and Lodmell, A. (1976) Development and evaluation of porous dental implants in miniature swine. J. Dent. Res., 55, 85.
Klawitter, J., Weinstein, A., Peterson, L., Pennel, B., and McKinney, R. (1977) An evaluation of porous alumina ceramic implants. J. Dent. Res., 56, 768.

Peterson, L., Pennel, B., McKinney, R., Klawitter, J, and Weinstein,
A. (1979) Clinical, radiographic and histological evaluation of porous
rooted polymethylmethacrylate dental implants. J. Dent. Res., 58, 489.
Peterson, L., McKinney, R., Pennel, B., Klawitter, J., and Weinstein,
A. (1980) Clinical, radiographic, and histological evaluation of
porous rooted cobalt-chromium alloy dental implants, J. Dent. Res.,
59, 99.
Spector, M., Flemming, W., Kreutner, A., and Sauer, B. (1976) Bone
growth into porous high-density polyethylene. J. Biomed. Mater. Res.
Symp., No. 7, 595.
Spector, M., Michno, M., Smarook, W., and Kwiatkowski, G. (1978) A
high-modulus polymer for porous orthopedic implants: Biomechanical
compatibility of porous implants. J. Biomed. Mater. Res., 12, 665.
Weiss, M. and Rostoker, W. (1980) Free-standing single tooth replacement by use of an endosseousmetallic dental implant. Trans. 4th Ann.
Mtg. of Soc. for Biomaterials, San Antonio, Texas', U.S., April 29-
May 2, 1978, p. 45.
Young, F., Spector, M., and Kresch, C. (1979) Porous titanium endosseous dental implants in Rhesus monkeys: Microradiography and
histological evaluation. J. Biomed. Mater. Res., 13, 843.
Young, F., Kresch, C., and Spector, M. (1980) Mechanical properties
of the bone-implant interface for porous titanium and polymeric implants in Mechanical Properties of Biomaterials (eds. G. Hastings,
D.F. Williams and G. Winter, J. Wiley and sons, NY) in press.

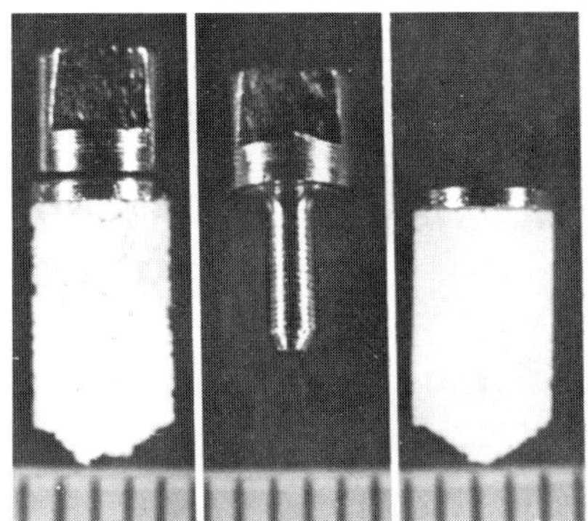

Fig. 1. Porous polyethylene
coated dental implants. Left-
250μm; right-120μm.

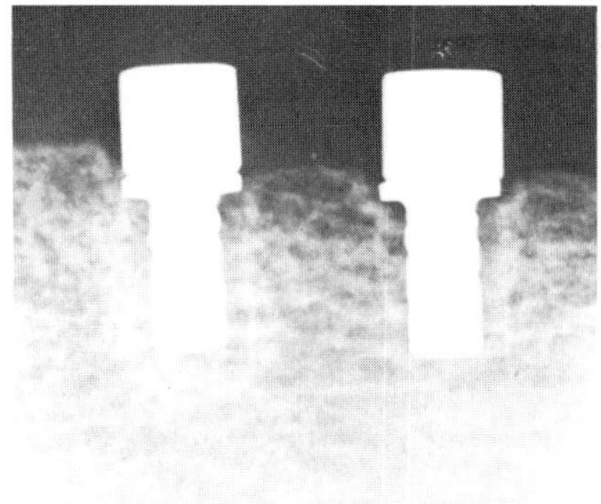

Fig. 2. Radiograph of polyethylene
implants after placement of the
transgingival abutment stage.

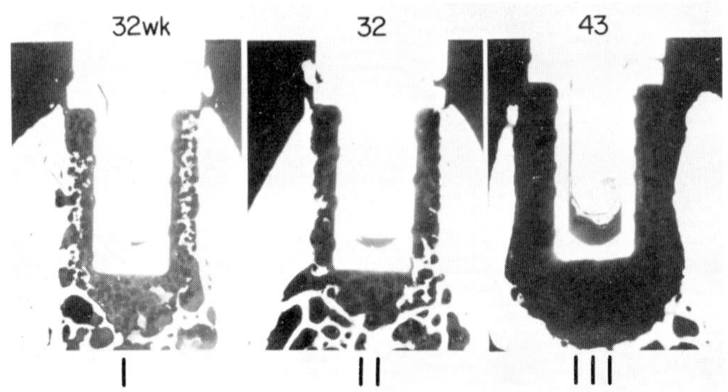

Fig. 3. Microradiographs of acceptable (I), potentially problematic (II), and unacceptable (III) porous polyethylene implants in dogs.

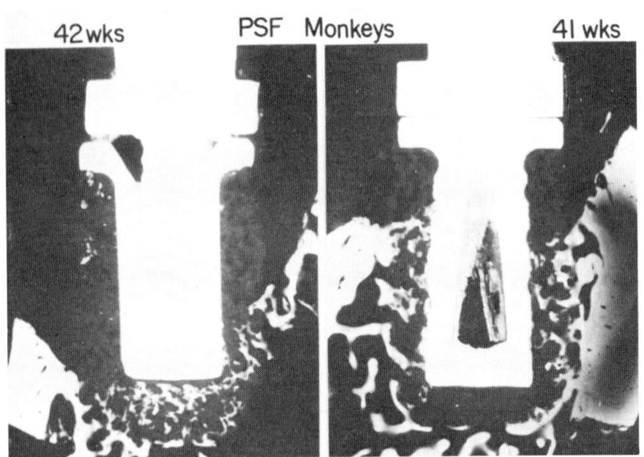

Fig. 4. Microradiographs of two failed porous polysulfone implants in monkeys.

Biomaterials 1980
Edited by G. D. Winter, D. F. Gibbons, and H. Plenk, Jr.
© 1982 John Wiley and Sons Ltd.

LONG TERM OSSEOUS ANCHORAGE OF ENDOSSEOUS DENTAL IMPLANTS MADE OF TANTALUM AND TITANIUM

F.Grundschober*, G.Kellner*, J.Eschberger** and H.Plenk Jr.*

* Bone Research Laboratory and Institute for Histology and Embryology of Vienna University, Austria.
** AUVA Institute for Osteological Research, Vienna, Austria.

SUMMARY:

The anchorage of different designs of endosseous dental implants made of the highly biocompatible metals tantalum and titanium was investigated microscopically using ground sections and corresponding radiomicrographs prepared from the implants removed from human patients together with the surrounding tissue.

4 tantalum "helicoidal screws" and 1 titanium diadontic screw - removed for different reasons after 8 to 12 years of implantation, though still clinically stable under loaded conditions - all showed tight implant-bone contact without an intermediate layer of connective tissue.

Of 3 tantalum needle implants, a single needle and a needle-tripod were loose after 6 weeks and 18 months. The third implant, however, was a stable needle-tripod splinted together with a diadontic needle and exhibited tight tantalum-bone contact 8 years after implantation.

It is concluded that durable skeletal attachment of endosseous dental implants is possible by direct osseous anchorage. The prerequisites for this tissue reaction are highly biocompatible materials and biomechanically suitable designs.

INTRODUCTION

Numerous endosseous dental implants of various designs and manufactured from different materials have been developed during recent years. Both experimental and clinical trials have shown that, apart from the biocompatibility of the material used, several other factors play an important role in the success or failure of such an implant. The geometry of the implant can be regarded as one of the most important factors, since the transmission of forces from implant to the supporting bone structure is largely dependent on this factor.

Dental implants must sustain mainly compression and shearing forces and if these stresses are concentrated in a few regions, they lead to resorption of the alveolar bone. The formation of a connective tissue sheath around the implant indicates micromovements of the implant, which may result in loosening after different periods of time. This connective tissue membrane is regarded by several authors as analogous

365

to the periodontal membrane, which supports the natural teeth (Linkow and Chercheve, 1970). It has not therefore been interpreted as a sign of implant loosening. The majority of clinically successful endosseous dental implants - especially blade-type implants - show this support mechanism.

However, some authors have observed direct bone-to-implant apposition, especially under unloaded conditions. In this study, histological evidence is presented to show that well designed endosseous dental implants made of the highly biocompatible metals tantalum and titanium can lead to direct bony anchorage over a long period of loading in human patients.

MATERIALS AND METHODS

Three types of dental endosseous implants were investigated:
1. Helicoidal screws (n=4) after Heinrich (1971), made of pure tantalum.
2. Diadontic screws (n=1) after Pruin (1974), made of pure titanium.
3. Needle implants (n=3) after Scialom (1962), made of pure tantalum.

All implants were loaded immediately after implantation or a few days later by a superstructure. The reasons for removal can be seen from the results.

The material from patients consisted of the implants removed together with the surrounding tissue. This was fixed in neutral formaline and embedded in methylmethacrylate without decalcification, in some cases after staining with basic fuchsin. Microscopic evaluation using transmitted and polarized light was performed on transverse and longitudinal ground sections and on corresponding radiomicrographs.

RESULTS

1. Tantalum helicoidal screws after Heinrich (1971)

Four implants of this type (Figure 1) were investigated and all were clinically stable under loaded conditions before removal. The first screw was splinted together for 8 years with three other screws, which became loose, breaking the superstructure. The second implant was removed after 10 years due to resorption of the buccal alveolar-bone. The third screw was splinted to an adjacent tooth, which became loose after 8 years, causing the shaft of the implant to break due to overloading. In the case of the fourth screw, removed after 10 years, a metal sensitivity was suspected.

In all four cases histological examination using polarized light and radiomicrographs revealed the presence of lamellar bone tissue between the broad horizontal threads of the screws (Figure 2a). At higher magnification, tight tantalum-to-bone contact without an intermediate layer of connective tissue can be seen at the interface of the implants (Figure 2b). Osteons and osteocytes are found close to the implants.

2. Titanium diadontic screw after Pruin (1974) (Figure 3)

This transdental titanium screw was splinted together with other implants and a natural tooth. After loosening of the transfixed tooth, the
bony anchorage provided the sole support for the implant. When the natural tooth onto which the superstructure was also fixed became loose
after 10 years, this implant had to be removed. In the histological
preparations, tight bone to implant contact can be demonstrated
(Figure 4).

3. Tantalum needle implants after Scialom (1962)

The first implant was found to be loose after 6 weeks and was removed
with a bony sequester. The needle seemed to be in contact with necrotic
bone (Figure 5) but histological examination demonstrated impact damage
to the drilled hole at insertion, bacterial and fungoid inflammation,
and sequestration of bone. The second implant was a needle tripod and
was removed after 18 months because of loosening. Histological examination shows a cleft between implant and bone filled by dense fibrous
connective tissue and local bone resorption (Figure 6).

The third specimen, also a needle tripod splinted to a diadontic pin,
was obtained post mortem 8 years after implantation (Figure 7). A remarkable reduction in the height of the alveolar bone crest did not seem
to have impaired the bone reaction. There was tight tantalum-bone contact around both types of needle implant, but one pin of the tripod
showed encapsulation by fibrous connective tissue (Figure 8).

DISCUSSION

These histological observations demonstrate that a durable skeletal
attachment of endosseous dental implants is possible by direct osseous
anchorage. This bone reaction seems to be directly related to the design
of the implants. All the screw-type implants in this study exhibited
this bone reaction, as did similar dental implants already investigated
(Kellner et al, 1978). Branemark et al, (1977) reported on a two-stage
procedure in which the screw-shaped titanium implant was allowed to
stabilise first without loading. They achieved direct osseous anchorage in both experimental and clinical long-term implantations . Zarb et
al, (1979) and Brunski et al, (1979) observed direct bone contact only
in unloaded bladevent-type dental implants, whereas loaded implants
showed connective tissue encapsulation.

The needle-shaped implants were unsatisfactory as single implants. As
with the blade-type implants, this design makes insertion easier, but
does not seem to provide adequate stabilization.

It can therefore be concluded that the prerequisites for adequate skeletal attachment are not only highly biocompatible materials, but also
biomechanically suitable designs. Additionally, the effects of surgical
trauma, the epithelial seal, local inflammation and implant stabilization through splinting to natural teeth or other implants are also

important in determining whether or not there will be satisfactory anchorage by bone in direct contact with the implant.

REFERENCES

Branemark, P.I., Hansson, B.O., Adell, R., Breine, U., Lindström, J., Hallen, O. & Öhman, A. (1977) Osseointegrated implants in the Treatment of the Edentulous Jaw-Experiences from a 10-year period pp 7-132. Almquist & Wiksell International, Stockholm.
Brunski, J.B., Moccia, A.F., Jr., Pollack S.R., Korostoff, E., & Trachtenberg, D.I. (1979) The influence of functional use of endosseous dental implants of the tissue-implant interface. I. histological aspects. J. Dent. Res. 58, 1953-1969.
Heinrich, B. (1971) Schrauben-Implantate. Quintessenz, 22/9, 1-5.
Kellner, G., Pruin, E.H. & Heinrich, B. (1978) Regeln und Ausnahmen in der enossalen odonto-stomatologischen Implantologie. Quintessenz, 29/2, 11-19.
Linkow, L.I. & Chercheve, R. (1970) Implant histology, in Theories and techniques of oral implantology (Ed. Jones, M.), Vol. 1, pp 132-133, C.V. Mosby Company, Saint Louis.
Pruin, E.H. (1974) Implantationskurs in der Odonto-Stomatologie, pp 98-109. Die Quintessenz, Berlin.
Scialom, J. (1962) Immediate needle implants. Inform. Dent. 44, 1606-1611.
Zarb, G.A., Smith, D.C., Levant, H.C., Fraham, B.S., & Zingg, W. (1979) The effects of cemented and uncemented endosseous implants. J. Prosthet. Dent., 42, 202-210.

FIGURES

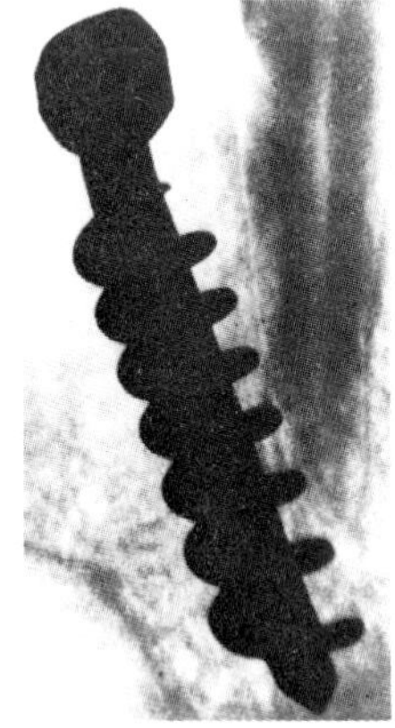

Fig. 1.

Fig. 1. Radiograph of a tantalum helicoidal screw.

Fig. 2a. Radiomicrograph (x9) of a ground section of a tantalum helicoidal screw, 10 years after insertion. The tangentially cut section shows dense lamellar bone tissue between the threads of the screw.

Fig. 2b. Detail (x100) of direct bone-to-tantalum contact.

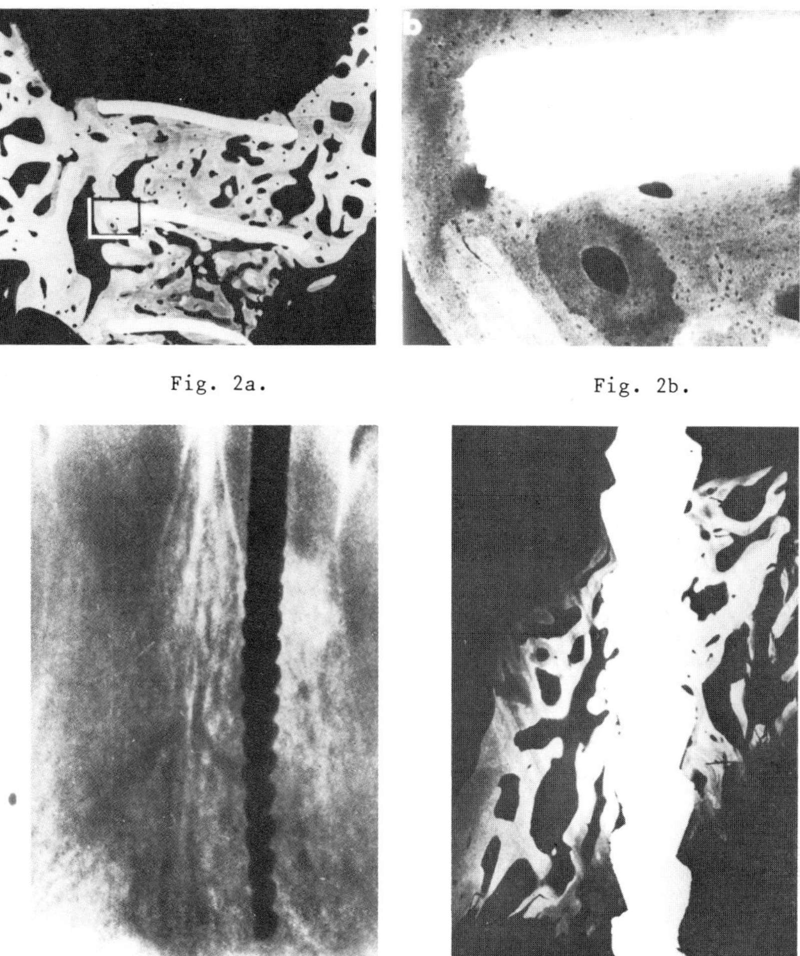

Fig. 2a.   Fig. 2b.

Fig. 3.   Fig. 4.

Fig. 3. Radiograph of a titanium diadontic screw.

Fig. 4. Radiomicrograph (x12) of a longitudinal ground section of a titanium diadontic screw 8 years after insertion. Trabecular bone tissue has tightly enveloped this portion of the broken implant.

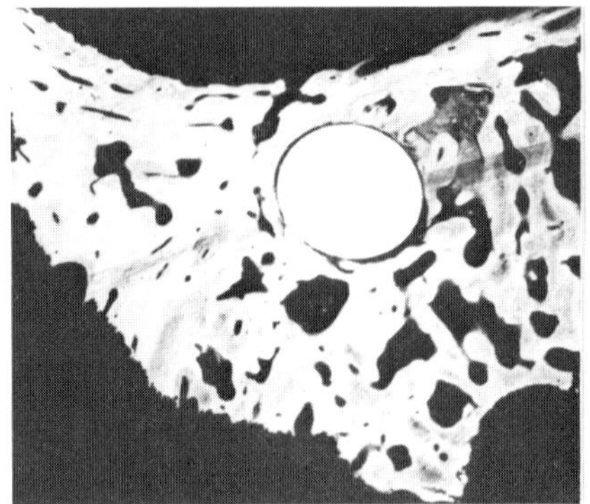
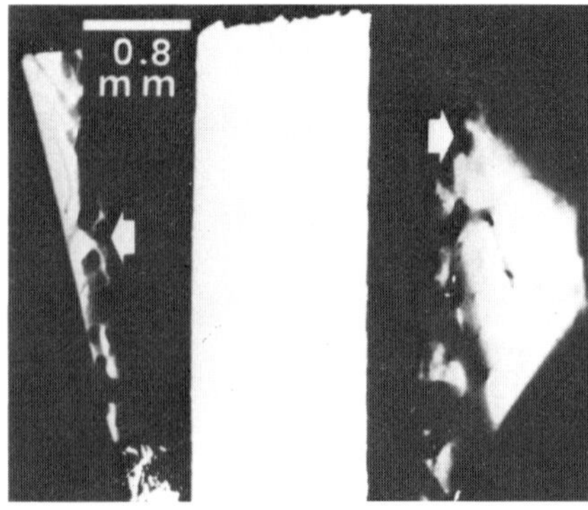

Fig. 5.   Fig. 6.

Fig. 5. Radiomicrograph (x14) of a transverse ground section
of a loose tantalum needle implant 6 weeks after insertion.
The alveolar bone shows close primary contact with the implant, but no reaction due to necrosis.

Fig. 6. Radiomicrograph (x20) of a longitudinal ground section of a loose tantalum needle implant 18 months after
insertion. The adherent bone tissue is separated from the
needle implant by a cleft which contains fibrous connective
tissue. Note lacunar bone resorption on both sides.

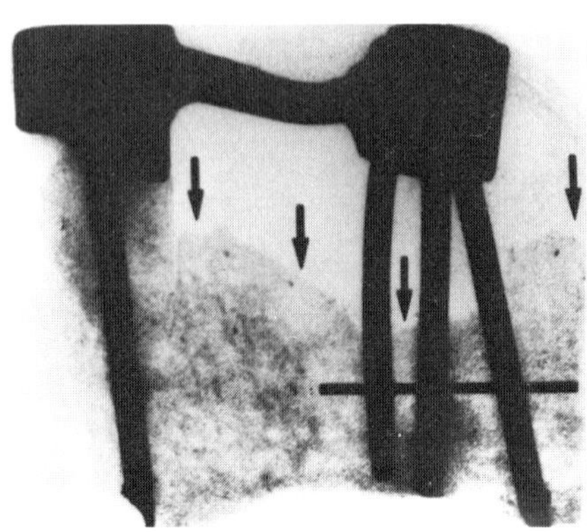
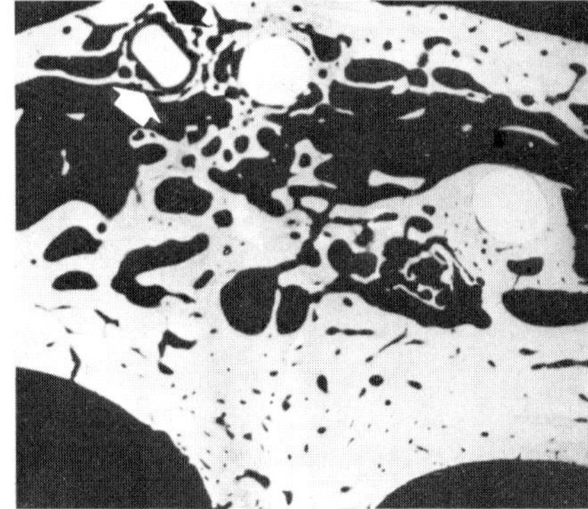

Fig. 7.   Fig. 8.

Fig. 7. Radiograph of a transdental tantalum needle implant
(left) splinted with a tripod needle implant. Note the reduction of the alveolar bone crest. Horizontal line shows
plane of section illustrated in Figure 8.

Fig. 8. Radiomicrograph (x7) of a transverse ground section
of the same tripod needle implant 10 years after insertion.
Two of the needles show tight bone contact; the third needle
was surrounded by fibrous connective tissue (arrow).

Biomaterials 1980
Edited by G. D. Winter, D. F. Gibbons, and H. Plenk, Jr.
© 1982 John Wiley and Sons Ltd.

A CLINICAL STUDY OF AL_2O_3 CERAMIC IMPLANTS FOR THE RECONSTRUCTION OF THE TERMINAL ENDENTULOUS MANDIBLE

P.A. Ehrl and G. Frenkel

Universitätsklinik, 6000 Frankfurt 71, FRG

SUMMARY

Twenty seven Al_2O_3-dental endosteal implants were clinically tested. The mean time of observation was 18.4 month, the longest 3.25 years. One of the implants was lost after three month. Photoelastic analysis was used to demonstrate stress distribution around the implant body. Clinical evaluation consisted of visual observation of the state of the oral mucosa, measurements of the pocket depth and gingival crevicular fluid. A radiological examination showed formation of bone around the implants.

INTRODUCTION

Dense Al_2O_3 ceramic has been in medical use since 1965. It has been used in the following medical applications: substitution of one tooth (Schulte & Heimke 1976, Sandhaus 1969, Mutschelknauss 1970); dental endosteal blade implants (Driskell & Meller 1977, Mutschelknauss & Dörre 1977); orbital floor repair (Iancu-Löbel 1979); canine fossa reconstruction (Geiger et al. 1980); temporo-mandibular-joint prosthesis (Frenkel & Niederdellmann 1977) ans as a hip endoprosthesis (Heimke et al. 1974). An endosteal blade implant described previously (Ehrl & Frenkel 1979) was modified and this report-concerns our clinical experience with the implant in 27 patients.

            P.A. Ehrl and G. Frenkel

MATERIAL AND METHODS

The implants used are made of high density multicristal-
line aluminium oxide ($99.7\%\,Al_2O_3$ + 0.25% MgO). Photoelastic analyses led to an implant design in which
rounded edges reduce stress concentration caused by the
wedge effect (Fig. 1).

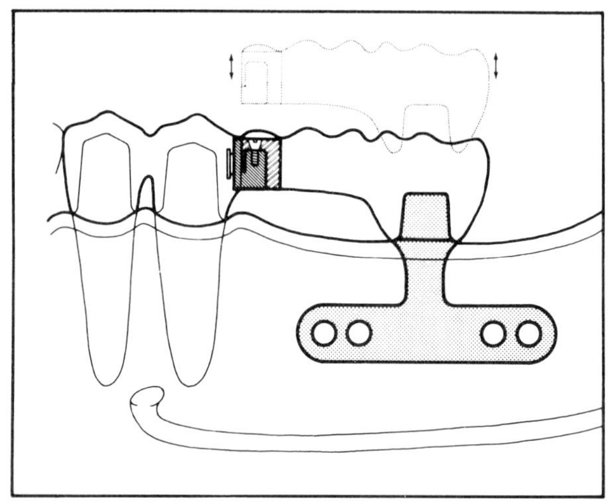

Fig. 1. Diagram of the implant and its position
in the mandible. The crown on the implant and the
attached bridge can be removed by opening a screw
in a precision attachment element.

Twenty seven patients are included in this survey. Observation of the implants was during an average of 18.4
months, the implant incorporated the longest was 40
months old. In each case it was a second class situation,
that is anterior teeth were present which could be attached to the implant by a bridge (Fig. 1).
Immediately after implantation temporary bridges were
placed. Permanent bridges were placed after 6 to 9 months.
Precision attachments were used to allow exact investigation and fabrication of removable prostesis in the event
of implant failure.

Clinical reexamination consisted in questioning the
patients, clinical inspection of the peripheral mucosa

condition and measurement of periimplant pocket depth. The gingival crevicular fluid (GCF) was withdrawn from the sulcus according to the method of Löe and Holm-Pedersen (Löe et al. 1965) and measured with a periometer (Periotron, Harco). These results were also compared with results from natural teeth of the same individual. Apical and orthoradial x-ray pictures of the implant area were taken by standard method.

<u>RESULTS</u>

After surgery the wound usually ached, but the patients discomfort was less than had been expected. In all cases four analgesic pills (Noramidopyrinmethansulfonate 0.5) were given to the patients, only in seven cases did the patient ask for more. Suspected wound infection complaints were stilled by antibiotic treatment in 10 cases. After prosthetic restoration was completed only four patients complained about slight discomfort, and one patient about great discomfort. After correction of occlusal contacts three of these patients had no further complaints. In two cases the attached gingiva had to be widened. In one case inflammation of the tissue could be seen. Surprisingly enough the mean depth of the sulcus of the implant was 1.3 mm which was a better result than that of natural teeth with a mean depth of 1.8 mm (Fig. 2). The average quantity of GCF around implants was 0.037 ul and around natural teeth was 0.038 ul.

The radiographs show that in two thirds of the cases there is a structure similar to a lamina dura around the bone impacted implant. In the other cases no changes of the bone structure in the vicinity of the implant could be found. The formation of a crater around the implanted post could vaguely be interpreted in six cases, in two cases a crater was obvious. There was no correlation between these results and those of the gingival-implant junction.

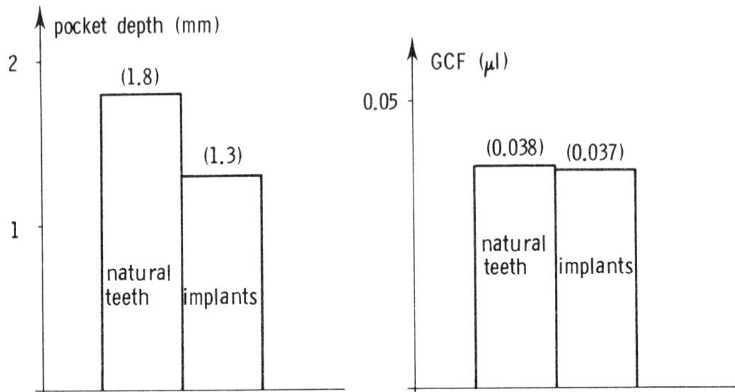

Fig. 2. a) The pocket was deeper in comparable
natural teeth than in the implant. b) The gingival crevicular fluid (GCF) was almost the same
in each group and was slight.

DISCUSSION

Twenty seven implants were not enough to give statistically valid information, yet useful observations were
possible. Firstly all implants but one are still functioning correctly. Concerning the implant that was
finally lost it must be mentioned that the implant was
initially unstable and this could not be compensated
by the temporary reconstruction. The precision of the
fit which should provide a large contact area between
implant and bone is decisive for an inital stable position of the implant and consequently for its life span
(Tetsch 1973). This initial stability can be achieved
for class 2 implants by connecting the implant with
natural teeth.

The ability to maintain a healthy mucosa around the
implant post depends on the ability of the patient to
carry out good plaque control (see Fig. 3 a). The gingival collar must come in contact only with the implant-
material. The danger spots in which plaque will accumu-

late must be easily accessible for the patient when he
cleans his teeth. In five cases it could be shown that
slight peripilary inflammation could be treated with
success by periodontal methods.

The examination of the mucosa by visual inspection,
measurement of the periodontal pockets and GCF measurements indicate that conditions around these ceramic
implants were better then around comparable metal implants (Babbush et al. 1977, Smithloff et al. 1976,
Brinkmann 1978). However, because of the many variables
associated with a clinical investigation of this kind
we do not have enough evidence to draw valid conclusions
comparing the performance of different types of implants.

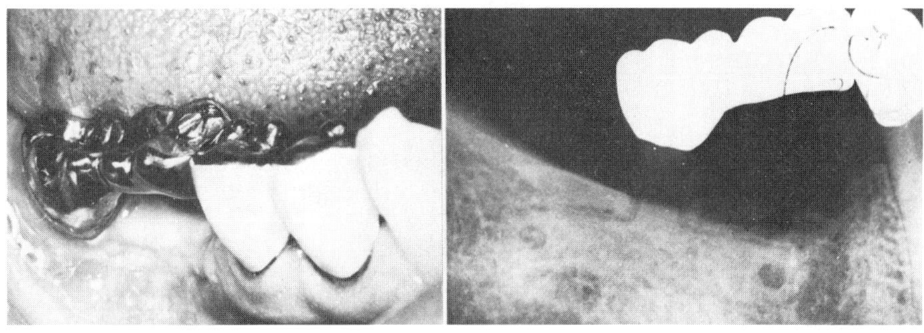

Fig. 3 a). A 30 months old implant. The gingiva
is without irritation and at no point is the
sulcus deeper than 1 mm. Plaque control is easy.
b) The radiograph showing radiolucent zone and
lamina dura around the implant.

The development of a lamina dura like structure around
the implant body, as seen in radiographs, can be interpreted as an adaptation of the bone. We observed that
these structures develop during the function of the implant. In the ideal case the lamina dura on implants
has the same characteristics as on natural teeth (Fig.3b).
At the moment a decision cannot be made about the interpretation of this zone, wether it is a functional adaptation or indicates an inflammatory reaction. We are

unable to explain, as yet, why the development of an
bone crater around the implant post can be seen in a
radiograph and suggests bone absorption does not correspond with clinical epithelial invagination.

REFERENCES

Babbush, C., A. & GREENE, A. H. (1977) Implant dentistry:
A long-term survey & comparative study with foxed
bridgework, J. Oral Implantol., 7, 89-105.
Brinkmann, E. (1978) Parodontalbefunde bei enossalen
Implantaten, Dtsch. zahnärztl Z., 33, 52-53.
Driskell, T.D. & Meller, A. L. (1977) Clinical use of
aluminium oxide endosseous implants, Oral Implantology,
7, 53-76.
Ehrl, P. A. & Frenkel, G. (1979) Vorläufiger Bericht zur
Entwicklung eines Extensionsimplantates. Qintess. zahn.
Lit. I:30, Ref. 6015, 1-7, & II:31, Ref. 6015, 8-18.
Frenkel, G. & Niederdellmann, H. (1977) The possibilities
afforded by the use of dense aluminium oxide ceramics in
the reconstruction of the temperomandibular joint.
Quintess. Internat. 7, 295.
Geiger, S.A. & Pesch, H. J. (1980) Langzeitverhalten von
Aluminiumoxid-Keramik-Implantaten. Dtsch.zahnärztl.Z.35,57.
Heimke, G., Andrian-Werburg, H. v., Krempien, B. & Griss,
P. (1974) Endoprothesen aus Al_2O_3-Keramik, Dtsch. Keram.
Ges. 51, 29.
Iancu-Löbel, R. (1979) Die Versorgung der Orbitabodenfrak-
tur mit Implantaten aus Aluminium-Oxid-Keramik.Med.dent.Diss.
Löe, E. & Holm-Pedersen, P. (1965) Absence and presence of
fluid from normal and inflamed gingivae, Periodontics 3,
171-177.
Mutschelknauss, E. (1970) Enossale Implantation von Por-
zellankörpern, Quintess. zahn. Lit. 21, No. 6, 17-23.
Mutschelknauss, E. & Dörre, E. (1977) Extensions-Implan-
tate aus Aluminium-Oxid-Keramik, Quintess. zahn. Lit. 21,
Ref. 5623, I:7, 1-5 and II:8, 6-10.
-, (1978) Enossale Stiftimplantate aus Aluminium-Oxid-
Keramik, Zahnärztl. Prax. 29, 362-366.
Sandhaus, S. (1969) Nouveaux aspects de l'implantologie -
L'implant CBS, Lausanne.
Schulte, W. & Heimke, G. (1976) Das Tübinger Sofortim-
plantat, Quintess. zahn. Lit., Ref. 5456.
Smithloff, M. & Fritz, M.E. (1976) The use of blade im-
plants in a selected population of partially edentulous
adults. A five-year-report, J. Periodontol., 47, 19-24.
Tetsch, P. (1973) Experimentelle Untersuchungen zur pri-
mären Stabilität von Extensionsimplantaten, Zahnärztl.
Welt Ref. 82, 665-669.

Biomaterials 1980
Edited by G. D. Winter, D. F. Gibbons, and H. Plenk, Jr.
© 1982 John Wiley and Sons Ltd.

HISTOLOGICAL EVALUATION OF CARBON COATED MANDIBULAR CONDYLE REPLACEMENT, 1.5 YEARS IN A DOG

D. Leake*, S. Michieli** and A. Pizzoferrato***

*Dental Research Institute, UCLA
UCLA Schools of Dentistry & Medicine
Los Angeles, California, U.S.A.
**University of Padua
Padova, Italy
Harbor-UCLA Medical Center
Torrance, California, U.S.A.
***Rizzoli Institute
Bologna, Italy

SUMMARY

The purpose of this report is to present the histological
evaluation of a prosthetic mandibular condyle taken from
a dog at sacrifice 18 months after implantation. The
condyle was made of cast Vitallium and coated with ULTI
carbon. There were posts on the medial aspect of the
implant designed to be placed in holes countersunk on the
lateral aspect of the mandible in order to increase stability. Screws were placed through the implant to provide
stability immediately after implantation. The prosthetic
condyle functioned normally allowing an unimpaired range
of motion. Histologically the implant was surrounded by
a layer of fibrous connective tissue. Aside from occasional areas of sclerotic bone adjacent to the screws,
the bone underlying the implant was normal in appearance.

INTRODUCTION

The replacement of the mandibular condyle with an implant
may fail because the implant loosens or because of excessive fibrous connective tissue deposition in the area of
the head of the condyle and of the glenoid fossa. The
heavy connective tissue fibers anchor the condyle and an
ankylosed mandible is the result (Leake, et. al., 1979).
Because carbon has demonstrated exceptional biocompatibility in other implant uses (Haubold, et. al., 1979)
and because earlier studies suggest that carbons may be
used as a component for artificial joints (Shim, 1977),

carbon-coated cast Vitallium implants were prepared as
prostheses to replace the mandibular condyles in mongrel
dogs. This paper reports histological observations on an
implant removed after 1.5 years.

MATERIALS AND METHODS

The prostheses were cast in Vitallium by Ceram-Dent
(Phoenix, Arizona) from models prepared in acrylic in the
Oral and Maxillofacial Laboratory at Harbor-UCLA Medical
Center. The implants were then carbon-coated with ULTI
carbon (CarboMedics, Austin, Texas). They were sterilized
by autoclaving.

Under intravenous barbiturate anesthesia, and using standard surgical techniques, the dogs' right mandibular
condyles were removed through an extra-oral approach. An
air-driven surgical burr was used to section the neck of
the condyle at its base. The implant was carefully positioned and secured. The wound was closed in layers.

The prosthesis was designed with pins on the lingual
aspect to be inserted in holes drilled through the
lateral cortical plate of the ascending ramus of the
mandible. The condylar implants were cast with perforations so that screws could be placed to provide immediate
stabilization. The dogs' mandibles functioned normally
postoperatively. Altogether 4 dogs have been operated
upon. At one and one-half years, a dog was sacrificed
and the mandible was resected en bloc with the glenoid
fossa. The implant was found to be firmly attached to
the mandible and the tissue surrounding the implant
appeared perfectly normal. The specimen was fixed in
ten percent formalin. After embedding in acrylic, blocks
were cut as shown in Figure 1. Multiple sections were
prepared from each block and stained in a variety of ways.

RESULTS

The hole where a pin was inserted in the bone is surrounded by a thin connective tissue layer (Fig. 2). A
thick layer of connective tissue is interposed between
the underlying bone (the lateral aspect of the ascending
ramus) and the implant. There is no evidence of inflammatory cells or of any other abnormality. A section
through the bone below the level of the pin at the inferior border of the plate reveals very well-defined Haversian systems and a connective tissue capsule surrounding

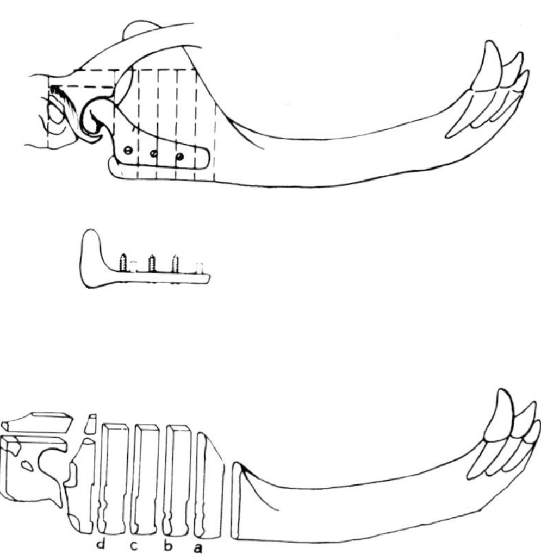

Fig. 1. A drawing of the mandibular condylar
prosthesis. There are pins to be countersunk
through the lateral cortical plate and 7 mm
screws to be placed for immediate stabilization.
Histologic sections were prepared from each of
the blocks labeled (a) through (f).

the pin (Fig. 3). Examination of a section of the mandible where a screw was placed shows that the neck of the
screw is surrounded by a fibrous connective tissue capsule. Deeper into the bone, around the screws, the
fibrous tissue capsule is thinner. In the deepest portion, the screw has not elicited any visible fibrous
tissue reaction. The bony trabeculae surrounding the
screw are sclerotic, and Haversian systems are absent.
The hypermineralized state of the trabeculae is consistent with decreased vascularity secondary to the
presence of the screw. Normal bone is much better
vascularized in nearby areas. (Fig. 4)

The bone below the implant does not show atrophy or
sclerosis although there are a few, small, newly formed
spicules that jet out from the bony border (Fig. 5).

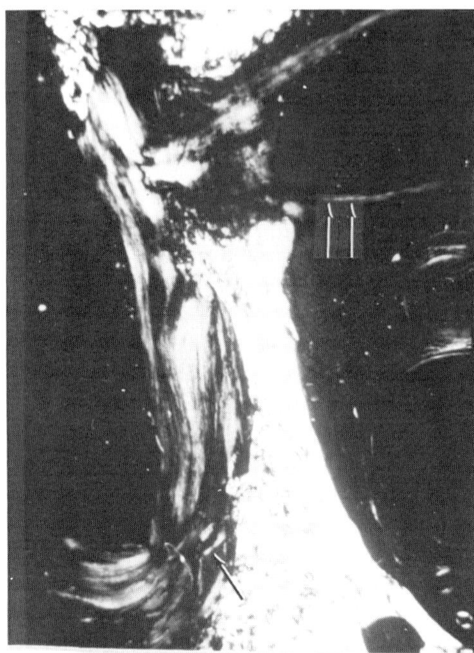

Fig. 2. Paragon
stain. 2.5x. Single
arrow denotes the
connective tissue
surrounding the im-
plant. Double arrow
indicates the area
of the pin.

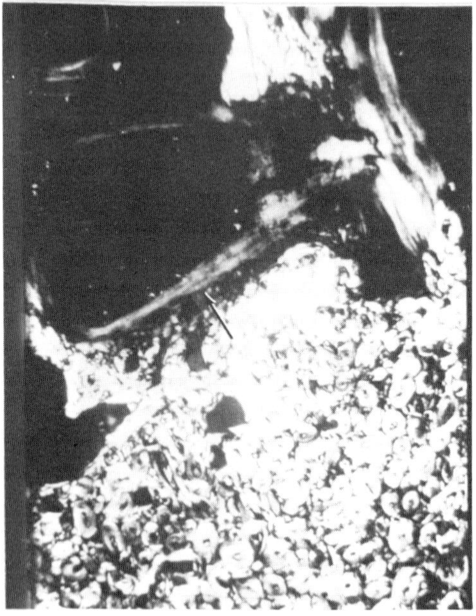

Fig. 3. Paragon
stain. 2.5x. The
area where a pin was
embedded in bone.
The arrow indicates
the thin connective
tissue capsule
around the pin.

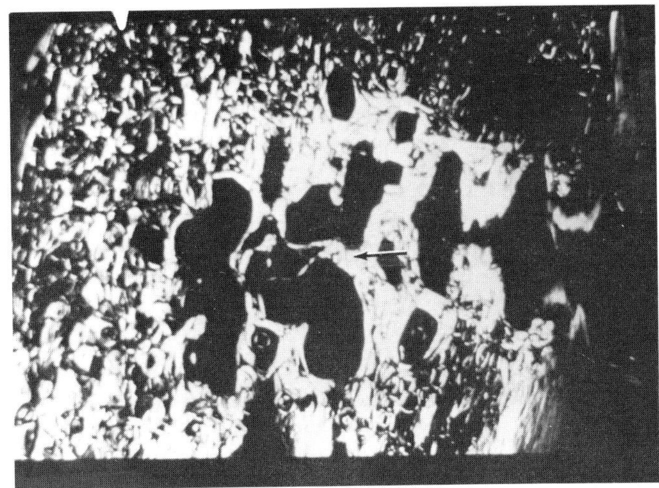

Fig. 4. Paragon stain with polarized light.
2.5x. The area occupied by a screw. The
spaces occupied by the screw threads can be
seen (arrow).

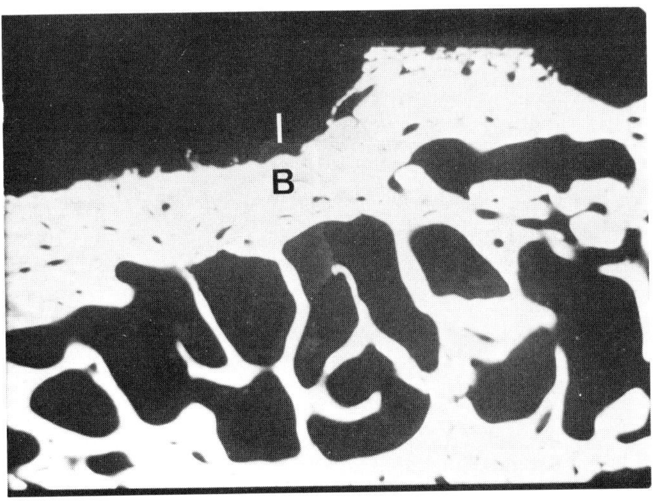

Fig. 5. Radiomicrograph. 2.5x. Healthy appear-
ing bone underlying the implant (B - bone;
I - implant).

DISCUSSION

The ULTI carbon-coated Vitallium implant did not cause
bony atrophy nor did any new bone formation occur below
the implant. Between the prosthetic implant and the
underlying bone, a thin layer of fibrous connective
tissue is interposed. This connective tissue discontin-
uously surrounds both the pins and the screws. In a few
areas surrounding the screws, there are moderate elements
of osteosclerosis. This dense bone firmly holds the
implant's posts and screws.

A new fibrous capsule was formed, partially fastened to
the temporal bone, serving as an articular capsule. This
capsule does not impede the movement of the condyle.
Additionally, this capsule is partially covered by a
synovial tissue, probably originating from synovial
remnants left behind at the time of surgery.

ACKNOWLEDGEMENTS

The collegial support and cooperation of Jack Bokros and
Axel Haubold of CarboMedics is gratefully acknowledged.

Dr. Michieli died January 27, 1980 at home in Vescovana,
Italy.

REFERENCES

Haubold, A., Shim, H. & Bokros, J. (1979). Developments
in carbon prosthetics. Biomat., Med. Dev., Art. Org., 7,
263-269.
Leake, D., Schwartz, H., Michieli, S., Habal, M. &
Freeman, S. (1979). Status of selected biomaterials for
oral and maxillofacial surgery. Biomat. Med. Dev., Art.
Org., 7, 213-227.
Shim, H. (1977). The wear of titanium, titanium alloy,
and UHMW polyethylene caused by LTI carbon and Stellite
21. J Bioeng., 1, 223-229.

PART 2

CARDIOVASCULAR APPLICATIONS OF BIOMATERIALS

Protein interaction with implants

Biomaterials 1980
Edited by G. D. Winter, D. F. Gibbons, and H. Plenk, Jr.
© 1982 John Wiley and Sons Ltd.

SURFACE ENRICHMENT OF PLASMA PROTEINS ON
POLYHYDROXYETHYLMETHACRYLATE-ETHYLMETHACRYLATE POLYMERS

T. A. Horbett

Department of Chemical Engineering, BF-10
University of Washington
Seattle, Washington 98195

SUMMARY

Plasma protein adsorption is an important initial event in the
response of tissue to foreign materials. In this study, the amounts
of fibrinogen, immunoglobulin G, albumin, and hemoglobin adsorbed
from plasma to a series of HEMA-EMA copolymers varying in hydrophilicity was measured. The adsorption of each protein varied in a
characteristic way with copolymer composition, probably reflecting
a different affinity of the proteins for the various copolymers.
Surface enrichment of the proteins, calculated as the ratio of the
surface and bulk fraction of each protein, also varied with copolymer
composition, and indicated substantial differences in the composition
of the surface and bulk phases.

INTRODUCTION

Plasma protein adsorption to implanted materials is an important
initial event in the response of tissue to foreign materials (Salzman,
1972; Brück, 1977; Baier, 1977). Most biological interactions with
materials occur after protein adsorption has occurred, so that the
material does not react directly with tissue but instead through the
adsorbed protein/material interface (Baier and Dutton, 1969; Vroman
and Adams, 1969). The nature of this interface has therefore been
explored in some detail in recent years, using both physicochemical
(Morrissey and Stromberg, 1974; Nyilas et al, 1974; McMillin et al,
1974) and biochemical approaches (Lyman et al, 1974; Vroman et al,
1975; Limber and Mason, 1975; Lee et al, 1974).

In previous studies in my laboratory, the affinity of fibrinogen and
hemoglobin for polymers was found to depend on both the nature of the
proteins and the properties of the surface (Horbett et al, 1977;
Weathersby et al, 1976). These studies indicated that the composition of the adsorbed protein layer varies systematically with surface
hydrophilicity. To confirm these results, this study of the adsorption of pre-labelled proteins from plasma to the hydroxyethylmeth-
acrylate-ethylmethacrylate copolymer series was undertaken.

383

T. A. Horbett

MATERIALS AND METHODS

Plasma was prepared from citrated bovine blood. Fibrinogen was
prepared from plasma by a method developed in my laboratory
(Weathersby et al, 1977b) and was found to be 95% or more clottable.
Bovine immunoglobulin G (electrophoretically homogeneous) and hemoglobin (2x crystallized) were obtained from Miles Laboratories, Inc.
Bovine albumin ("crystalline") was obtained from Nutritional Biochemicals Corporation. The buffer used in this study was 0.01 M sodium
citrate, 0.01 M sodium phosphate, 0.12 M NaCl, 0.02% sodium azide,
pH 7.4 ("CPBSz").

Hydroxyethylmethacrylate and ethylmethacrylate polymers were radiation
grafted to polyethylene, using techniques for synthesis and characterization described previously (Weathersby et al, 1977c). The
polymers were stored dry, and were rehydrated in buffer overnight
before use.

Iodine-125 radiolabelled proteins were usually prepared with the ICl
method of MacFarlane (1955) as modified by Helmkamp et al (1960),
using 1-4 fold molar excess of ICl over protein. In one study,
iodinated hemoglobin was prepared with the solid state lactoperoxidase
method (David and Reisfeld, 1974). The ^{125}I labelled proteins were
subjected to sodium dodecylsulfate polyacrylamide gel electrophoresis
(Weber and Osborn, 1969). The molecular weight of the subunit of the
^{125}I proteins were identical to the native proteins. The ^{125}I
proteins also retained their native subunit molecular weights after
exposure to plasma at 37°C for two hours.

Analysis of plasma to obtain the concentration of individual proteins
was done with the following methods: Fibrinogen was analyzed by re-
dissolution of the thrombus induced clot (Ratnoff and Menzie, 1950);
immunoglobulin G was determined by quantitative radial immuno-
diffusion; albumin was measured by bromoscrescol dye binding (Doumas
et al, 1971); and hemoglobin was determined by tetramethylbenzidine
binding (Standefer and Vanderjagt, 1977).

In all adsorption experiments, the surfaces were first immersed in
37°C buffer; an equal volume of plasma (at 37°) was added, and after
the desired time, the adsorption was terminated by a dilution-
displacement rinsing technique with buffer. In this rinsing technique, buffer is run through the equilibration tube at about 400
ml/min for approximately 0.5 minute, using a two-hole stopper fitted
with glass tubes, one for entrance and one for exit of buffer.

To measure adsorption of single proteins from the plasma, the pure
I-125 labelled form of the desired protein was added in small volume
and amounts at high specific activity to the plasma, resulting in
plasma specific activities in the range of 100-2000 cpm/µg. The
amounts adsorbed in µg/cm^2 were calculated from the radioactivity
retained by the film, using the specific activity of the plasma pool
and the planar surface area of the film. Duplicate adsorption

measurements were made. Surface enrichment was calculated from the absolute adsorption data as described in the text.

<u>RESULTS</u>

The adsorption of I-125 labelled proteins from plasma to a series of copolymers was measured after two hours of equilibrium at 37°C. Fibrinogen, immunoglobulin G, albumin, and hemoglobin adsorption were measured in separate experiments, but in each set of experiments, the same plasma and polymer preparations were used. The pHEMA-pEMA copolymers studied were radiation grafted to polyethylene. Four sets of such experiments were done, each with different plasma and copolymer preparations, using freshly iodinated proteins. Each of the iodinated proteins was made from a highly purified protein preparation. The iodinated proteins appear to retain their high purity and are stable in plasma, when examined by SDS polyacrylamide gel electrophoresis.

The results of the adsorption experiments are summarized in Figure 1.

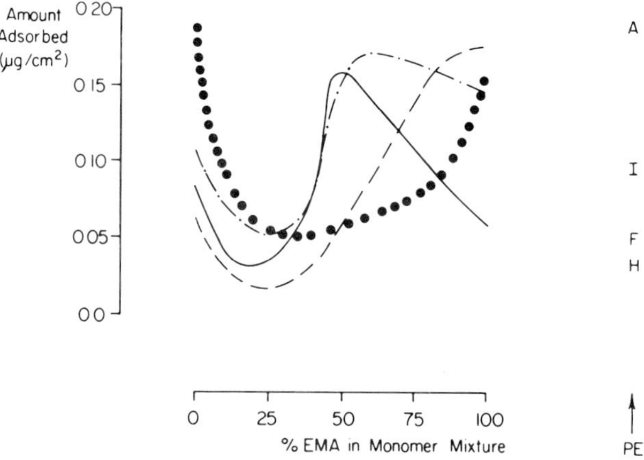

Fig. 1. Adsorption of plasma proteins to HEMA-EMA/PE. Fibrinogen (solid line), immunoglobulin G (—·), albumin (•), and hemoglobin (— —) average adsorption curves are plotted. Data for PE are also shown to the right (F = fibrinogen, I = immunoglobulin G, A = albumin, H = hemoglobin).

The ordinate is the amount of each protein adsorbed, in micrograms per square centimeter, while the abscissa is the per cent EMA in the monomer solution used to make polymer. Two of the polymers were made with either 100% EMA or 100% HEMA in the monomer solution, while the rest were made with various ratios of these monomers. For convenience, each polymer will be identified by the per cent EMA in the

monomer solution used in its preparation. The difference between 100
and the per cent EMA is the per cent HEMA used in the monomer
solution. The curves shown were obtained by drawing a line connecting
the average adsorption data for each protein. The standard deviations have been deleted for the sake of clarity.

The adsorption of each of the proteins varies among the polymers,
resulting in a specific shape to the plots of adsorption versus % EMA
for each protein. Thus, fibrinogen adsorption is maximal at 50% EMA
and is five times lower at 20% EMA. Hemoglobin is also minimal at
20% EMA, but does not reach a maximum until 100% EMA. Albumin
adsorption is minimal over a wide range of intermediate composition
polymers and is much higher to the pHEMA or pEMA. Immunoglobulin G
adsorption is maximal between 50 and 100% EMA, but is much less in
the 0-50% EMA range.

Thus, the absolute plasma adsorption of the four proteins studied
varies markedly in the pHEMA-pEMA copolymer series. The variance
appears to be due to intrinsic differences in the relative or competitive affinity of the plasma proteins for each of the surfaces. The
affinity differences cause variable degrees of preferential adsorption of each protein to each surface. However, absolute adsorption
figures do not provide much insight into how different the composition of the adsorbed protein mixture is from the bulk phase nor
how the surface composition varies with polymer.

To better elucidate surface protein compositional variations in this
copolymer series, I calculated an estimate of the surface enrichment
of each protein on each surface. The fractional amount of each
protein in the adsorbed phase was calculated by dividing its absolute
adsorption by the total adsorption of all four proteins measured. The
fractional amount of each protein in the bulk phase was similarly
calculated. The ratio of the surface fraction to the bulk fraction
provides an estimate of the surface enrichment. Essentially, this
parameter reflects the excess (or deficit) fraction of a particular
protein in the adsorbed layer relative to the fraction expected if
all proteins were present in the same ratio as in the bulk phase.

The next four figures summarize the surface enrichment calculations
for each of the four proteins on each of the polymers studied. The
data are based on the average absolute adsorption values obtained
from the four sets of experiments represented in Figure 1. The error
estimates represented by the bars (one standard error long) include
contributions from all the variables used to calculate the enrichment,
and were calculated with standard formulas for propagation of errors
(Bevington, 1969).

The enrichment data for fibrinogen shown in Figure 2 displays a similar
shape to the absolute adsorption data, with a maximum at 50% EMA.
The values range between 0.8 and 3.4. The adsorbed layer is thus
enriched in fibrinogen over the bulk phase by a factor of 3.4 on 50%
EMA, while it is only 80% as rich in fibrinogen as the bulk phase on

the 20% EMA surface.

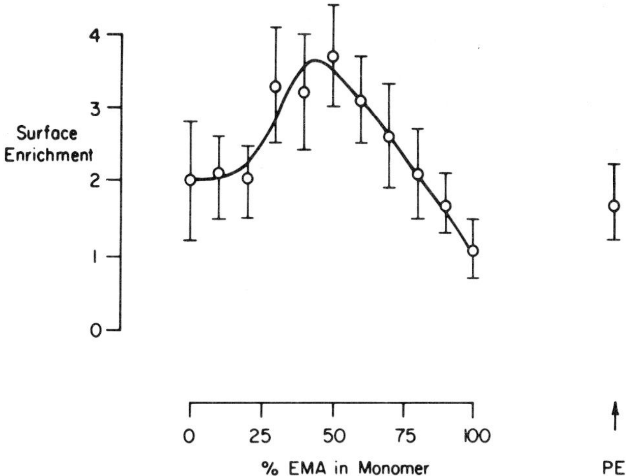

Fig. 2.   Surface enrichment of fibrinogen on HEMA-EMA/PE.

Figure 3 shows the enrichment for immunoglobulin G, which ranges
between 0.8 and 1.5.   There is less variation in the surface enrichment of immunoglobulin G than in the absolute adsorption data, and
the variation with polymer composition is quite different than the
adsorption data.   The differences between the adsorption and enrichment data stem from the fact that the enrichment calculations depends
on the variation in adsorption of all the proteins, since the fraction
of the proteins of interest relative to the total is calculated.   Thus,
variations in immunoglobulin G adsorption which are paralleled by
similar variations in the adsorption of other proteins will result in
little variation in surface enrichment, as observed.

The surface enrichment of albumin shown in Figure 4 varies between
0.3 and 0.8.   Since enrichment values less than 1 mean that the
protein is present on the surface in lesser amounts than in the bulk
phase, albumin can be said to be non-preferentially adsorbed to all
the polymers.

Hemoglobin surface enrichment (shown in Figure 5) is very much higher
than the other proteins studied, due to the high affinity of this
protein for surfaces, as I have previously reported (Horbett et al,
1977).

To summarize, the composition of the surface phase differs markedly
from that of the bulk phase, and the degree of difference depends on
the copolymer.   The enrichment figures for fibrinogen support the

                    T. A. Horbett

idea that this protein is important in the protein layer on some
surfaces does not seem to justify the idea that this protein somehow
dominates the layer, since each of the other proteins is also present
in concentrations approximating the bulk phase values.

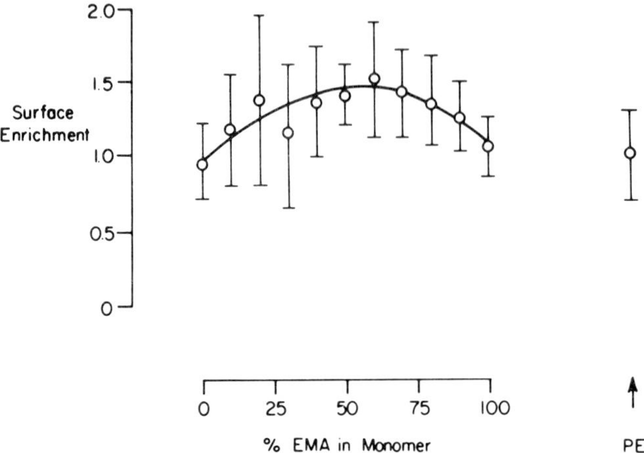

Fig. 3.   Surface enrichment of immunoglobulin G on HEMA-EMA/
PE.

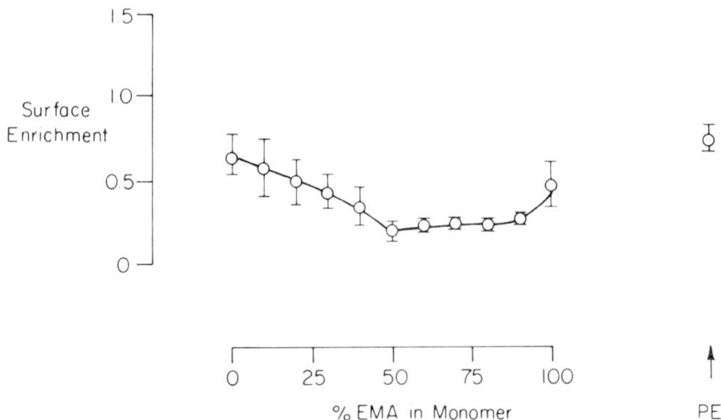

Fig. 4.   Surface enrichment of albumin on HEMA-EMA/PE.

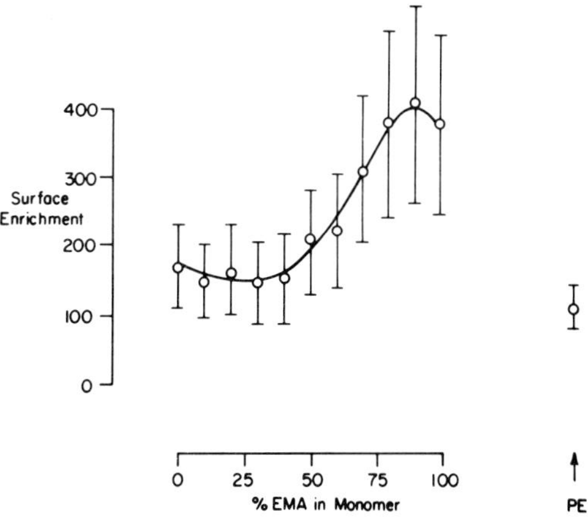

Fig. 5. Surface enrichment of hemoglobin on HEMA-EMA/PE.

DISCUSSION

The adsorption of proteins from plasma to surfaces is a competitive
process in which all of the plasma proteins participate to some
degree. All proteins appear to be surface active, so that the
adsorption process is driven by the spontaneous tendency towards
surface adsorption of each of the proteins in the plasma. Both mass
action (due to bulk phase concentration differences) and intrinsic
differences in the affinity or rate of adsorption among the proteins
influence the adsorption process. Thus, the adsorbed protein layer
that forms on a polymer surface is a mixture reflecting the final
result of the interplay of these various competitive factors. Since
the surface phase is much more highly concentrated than the bulk
phase and, in addition, may preferentially adsorb some proteins more
than others, an opportunity for much more intense interaction than
usual is provided for reactions of these proteins both with one
another and, in the in vivo setting, with cells. It is generally
thought that such interactions are important in the processes mediating in vivo tissue response to implants and also influence
cellular processes necessary for existence in culture (e.g., adhesion,
growth, motility, etc.).

The results of this study clearly illustrate both the competitive and
selective nature of the plasma adsorption process. Thus, for example,
while all of the surfaces adsorb at least some of each of the four
proteins studied, the relative amounts of each of the proteins in the
adsorbed layer vary greatly. The surface enrichment is much greater
for some of the proteins (especially hemoglobin) than others. For
each protein, a different pattern of enrichment among the various
polymers was observed. These differences undoubtedly originate in
both intrinsic differences in affinity of the proteins for each

surface, as well as variations in the affinity of each protein for the
series of surfaces studied. It appears that the composition of the
protein layer which adsorbs to polymers from plasma is neither constant nor directly reflective of the bulk phase composition. Such
variations in the adsorbed layer probably constitute an important
mechanism whereby polymer properties can influence cellular responses
via their influence on the adsorbed protein layer.

The systematic variations in the adsorption of fibrinogen, immunoglobulin G, albumin, and hemoglobin from plasma to the pHEMA-pEMA
copolymer series reveal that the composition of the adsorbed protein
layer is dependent on the surface chemical properties of polymers.
Some of the proteins in plasma can elicit strong responses from
various cells, especially when the proteins are concentrated at interfaces. The ability of polymers to fractionate the plasma proteins
and concentrate them at their surface therefore is probably a key
determinant in the complex processes which occur when polymers are
implanted _in vivo_ or used as supports for cells _in vitro_. Further
delineation of the role of specific plasma proteins in specific
cellular reactions with polymers and the way in which the organization
of the adsorbed layer affects accessibility and reactivity of cells
for such proteins is clearly needed.

ACKNOWLEDGEMENTS

The financial support of the National Heart, Lung, and Blood Institute
grant number 19419, is gratefully acknowledged.

REFERENCES

Baier, R.E. (1977) The organization of blood components near interfaces. Ann. N.Y. Acad. Sci., 283, 17.
Baier, R.E. & Dutton, R.C. (1969) Initial events in interactions of
blood with a foreign surface. J. Biomed. Mater. Res., 3, 191.
Bevington, P.R. (1969) Data Reduction and Error Analysis for the
Physical Sciences. McGraw Hill, New York.
Brück, S.D. (1977) Interactions of synthetic and natural surfaces with
blood in the physiological environment. J. Biomed. Mater. Res. Symp.,
8, 1.
David, G.S. & Reisfeld, R.A. (1974) Protein iodination with solid
state lactoperoxidase. Biochemistry, 13, 1014.
Doumas, B.T., Watson, W.A. & Biggs, H.G. (1971) Albumin standards and
the measurement of serum albumin with bromoscrescol green. Clin.
Chim. Acta, 31, 87.
Helmkamp, R.W., Goodland, R.L., Bale, W.F., Spar, I.L. & Mutschler,
L.E. (1960) High specific activity iodination of γ-globulin with
iodine-131 monochloride. Cancer Res., 20, 1495.
Horbett, T.A., Weathersby, P.K. & Hoffman, A.S. (1977) The preferential adsorption of hemoglobin to polyethylene. J. Bioengineering, 1,
61.
Lee, R.G., Adamson, C. & Kim, S.W. (1974) Competitive adsorption of
plasma proteins onto polymer surfaces. Thromb. Res., 4, 485.

Limber, G.K. & Mason, R.G. (1975) Studies of proteins elutable from cuprophane exposed to human plasma. Thromb. Res., 6, 421.

Lyman, D.J., Metcalf, L.C., Albo, D., Richards, K.F. & Lamb, J. (1974) The effect of chemical structure and surface properties of synthetic polymers on the coagulation of blood III. In vivo adsorption of proteins on polymer surfaces. Trans. Amer. Soc. Artif. Int. Organs, 20, 474.

MacFarlane, A. (1958) Efficient trace-labelling of proteins with iodine. Nature, 182, 53.

McMillin, C.R., Saito, H., Ratnoff, O.D. & Walton, A.G. (1974) A circular dichroism technique for the study of adsorbed protein structure. J. Clin. Invest., 54, 1312.

Morrissey, B.W. & Stromberg, R.R. (1974) The conformation of adsorbed blood proteins by infrared bound fraction measurements. J. Coll. Interf. Sci., 46, 152.

Nyilas, E., Chieu, T.-H. & Herzberger, G.A. (1974) Thermodynamics of native protein/foreign surface interaction I. Calorimetry of the human γ globulin/glass system. Trans. Amer. Soc. Artif. Int. Organs, 20, 480.

Ratnoff, O.D. & Menzie, C. (1950) A new method for the determination of fibrinogen in small samples of plasma. J. Lab. Clin. Med., 37, 316.

Salzman, E.W. (1972) The events that lead to thrombosis. Bull. N.Y. Acad. Med., 48, 225.

Standefer, J.C. & Vanderjagt, D. (1977) Use of tetramethylbenzidine in plasma hemoglobin assay. Clin. Chem., 23, 749.

Vroman, L. & Adams, A.L. (1969) Identification of rapid changes at plasma-solid interfaces. J. Biomed. Mater. Res., 3, 43.

Vroman, L., Adams, A.L., Klings, M., & Fischer, G. (1975) Fibrinogen, globulins, albumin and plasma at interfaces. Adv. Chem. Ser., 145, 255.

Weathersby, P.K., Horbett, T.A. & Hoffman, A.S. (1976) A new method for analysis of the adsorbed plasma protein layer on biomaterial surfaces. Trans. Amer. Soc. Artif. Int. Organs, 22, 242.

Weathersby, P.K., Horbett, T.A. & Hoffman, A.S. (1977a) Fibrinogen adsorption to surfaces of varying hydrophilicity. J. Bioengineering, 1, 395.

Weathersby, P.K., Horbett, T.A. & Hoffman, A.S. (1977b) Solution stability of bovine fibrinogen. Thromb. Res., 10, 245.

Weathersby, P.K., Horbett, T.A. & Hoffman, A.S. (1977c) Surface analysis of methacrylate graft copolymers varying in hydrophilicity. J. Bioengineering, 1, 381.

Weber, K. & Osborn, M. (1969) The reliability of molecular weight determinations by dodecyl sulfate polyacrylamide gel electrophoresis. J. Biol. Chem., 274, 4406.

Biomaterials 1980
Edited by G. D. Winter, D. F. Gibbons, and H. Plenk, Jr.
© 1982 John Wiley and Sons Ltd.

ADSORPTION/DESORPTION STUDIES OF PLASMA PROTEINS ON
POLYMER SURFACES

A. Baszkin

Physico-Chimie des Surfaces et des Membranes, CNRS,
45 rue des Saints-Pères, 75270 Paris cedex 06, France

D.J. Lyman

Department of Materials Science and Engineering
BME Center for Polymer Implants, The University of Utah,
Salt Lake City, Utah 84112, USA

SUMMARY

Adsorption of bovine albumin, γ-globulin, fibrinogen and of the
mixtures of proteins onto several polymer films was studied using
the radioiodinated proteins (^{125}I). After adsorption the proteinated
polymer films were desorbed in bovine plasma.

Surface energetics measurements of the studied polymers by means of
various pure liquids allowed the calculation of polar (I_p) and
dispersive (W_A^d) components of the polymer-protein solution free
energy of adhesion. Results from these measurements and from
adsorption/desorption studies show that the non-dispersive-dispersive
force balance at the polymer-protein solution interface, expressed
by the I_p/W_A^d ratio, is an important factor for binding of proteins
on polymer surfaces. In terms of selectivity of adsorption, studies
of protein mixtures (the mixture contained the main blood proteins)
showed that albumin preferentially adsorbs on the copolyurethane
samples.

INTRODUCTION

Polymers exposed to whole blood adsorb proteins on their surfaces
(Lyman & al, 1974). It is interesting to note that platelets do not
adhere to albumin coated surfaces, whereas γ-globulin and fibrinogen
coatings cause platelet adhesion and realease of platelet constituents (Lyman & al, 1975 ; Lyman & al, 1974 ; Packham & al, 1969).
It was proposed (Kim & Lee, 1979) that platelet adhesion is mediated
via bridges between transferase enzymes on a cell membrane and glycoproteins in the adsorbed layer. γ-globulin and fibrinogen contain
oligosaccharide chains and thus may induce platelet adhesion and
aggregation while albumin which has no oligosaccharide chains fails
to cause a glycosyl transferase reaction. This provides a favorable
argument for the idea that a less thrombogenic surface should preferentially adsorb albumin in vivo.

In this study we have attempted to apply the surface energetics treatment to explain the difference in adsorption of the three main plasma proteins to four polymers of different chemical nature and hydrophobicity.

MATERIALS AND METHODS

Polymers. Fluorinated ethylene-propylene copolymer (Teflon FEP 10 mil films E.I. du Pont), polydimethyl siloxane (10 mil medical grade Silastic Rubber film, Dow Corning) and two segmented copolyurethanes based on polypropylene glycol (molecular weight 700 and 1000) were used. The synthesis of these copolyurethanes and the casting method to obtain 5 mil films was already described (Lyman & al, 1971). The polymers were cleaned according to the procedure proposed by Baszkin & Lyman (1980).

Proteins. Albumin, bovine crystalline (FRV) and γ-globulin bovine (FRII) were from Nutritional Biochemicals and were used as received. Two different bovine fibrinogens were used. FRI from Nutritional Biochemicals and highly purified bovine fibrinogen from IMCO, Sweden (coagulability $98.1 \pm 0.003\%$). Some of the fibrinogen from Nutritional Biochemicals was purified using the method of Weathersby & al (1977). Iodination of proteins with ^{125}I was performed according to the method of Marchelonis (1969).

Bovine plasma. The plasma obtained from citrated fresh bovine blood by high speed centrifugation.

Contact angle measurements. The following liquids (Aldrich Chemical, analytical reagent grades) were used : formamide (γ_1 = 58.2 dyn/cm) ; methylene iodide (γ_1 = 50.8 dyn/cm) ; ethylene glycol (γ_1 = 48.3 dyn/cm) ; and 1-bromo-naphtalene (γ_1 = 72.8 dyn/cm). Advancing contact angles were measured by a sessile drop method using a Contact Angle Goniometer (Rame Hart Inc.). An average of at least six measurements were taken for each liquid and polymer.

Adsorption/desorption from the solutions containing one protein. Adsorption measurements were made using protein solution in phosphate buffer (Na = 0.05 M ; pH = 7.5) (35 mg/100 ml sol). The films were placed in the solutions for 180 min. It was experimentally found that this time of adsorption gave the plateau value. Films were then rinsed with 300 ml of distilled water (flow rate of 11/min). The proteinated films, after having their radioactivity counted, were transfered to bovine plasma for desorption experiments. All adsorption/desorption experiments were carried out at 23°C and the disintegrations were counted in γ-vials on a Beckman Biogamma Counter (Beckman Instruments).

Adsorption from the solutions containing mixture of proteins. Adsorption measurements were performed from two phosphate buffer solutions (Na = 0.05 M ; pH = 7.5), one containing 0.7 mg/ml and the other 1.4 mg/ml of a mixture of proteins of the following composition:

albumin 55%, γ-globulin 11%, β-globulin 15.5%, α-globulin 14% and fibrinogen 6.5%. The adsorption/desorption experiments were conducted as above.

RESULTS

TABLE 1. γ_S^d for polymers and I_p, W_A^d for polymer-protein solution systems.

Polymer	γ_S^d erg/cm^2	I_p erg/cm^2	W_A^d erg/cm^2	I_p/W_A^d
FEP	16	20.3	37.4	0.54
SR	23.1	34.2	44.9	0.76
PU-700	32.6	46.8	53.3	0.89
PU-1000	34.6	52.0	54.9	0.95

γ_S^d is the dispersion force contribution to the surface free energy of the solid.
W_A^d is the dispersion component of the solid-liquid work of adhesion.
I_p is the polar component of the solid-liquid work of adhesion.

TABLE 2. Protein concentration on polymer surfaces after adsorption (180 min) and after desorption (330 min).

Polymer	after adsorption (plateau values)	after desorption (plateau values)	desorption/ adsorption ratio
	Albumin (mg/m^2)		
FEP	8.6	2.3	0.27
SR	9.2	3.3	0.37
PU-700	12.3	4.9	0.40
PU-1000	23.5	10.8	0.46
	γ-globulin (mg/m^2)		
FEP	8.0		
SR	18	6	0.33
PU-700	25	10	0.40
PU-1000	50	24	0.48
	Fibrinogen (mg/m^2)		
FEP	23	6	0.26
SR	33	9	0.28
PU-700	63	41	0.65
PU-1000	145	82	0.57

Table 1 summarizes the thermodynamic parameters related to the
interactions of proteins solutions. The details of the calculated
values are given by Baszkin & Lyman (1980).

The results of adsorption/desorption measurements from solutions
containing one protein are shown in Table 2. It should be noted that
SR surface is rough compared to FEP and copolyurethanes and so the
real concentrations per sq. m. for SR are probably much lower.
Fibrinogen used for these measurements was purified according to
Weatherby & al (1977). Similar results were obtained with the
fibrinogen from IMCO (Sweden).

TABLE 3. Adsorption (mg/m^2) of albumin from protein
mixtures (adsorption time : 180 min, plateau values).

Polymer	albumin concentration 0.39 mg/ml	albumin concentration O.78 mg/ml
FEP	1.7	2.4
SR	4.0	4.1
PU-700	5.3	6.3
PU-1000	15.5	14.4

The reproductibility of the surface concentration measurement was
about ± 15%.

DISCUSSION

The analysis of adsorption results from the solutions containing
only one protein reveals that the degree of coverage depends on both
the nature of protein and the polymer. The contact angle measurements of protein coated surface made by Lee & al (1973) show that
water and glycerol contact angles on albuminated FEP are much higher
than for other polymers. This would support the microscopic observation of the partial coverage of albuminated hydrophobic surfaces
made by Eberhart & al (1978). However, the results may also be interpreted as an easier stripping of albumin molecules from the FEP
surfaces by a liquid drop as suggested by Van der Scheer & Smolders
(1978). Our results from the desorption of albuminated surfaces in
bovine plasma (Table 2) suggest this later argument e.g. for FEP
surfaces the desorption/adsorption ratio is smaller than for the
copolyurethanes. That is, for the FEP, the fraction of irreversibly
attached proteins is smaller than for other polymers.

The reason for the difference in binding of proteins to hydrophobic
surfaces may be due to differences in their polar/non polar force
relationship. Analysing the data of Table 1, it can be seen that the
polar/non polar force relationship, i.e. the I_p/W_A^d ratio for the
copolyurethanes, on which adsorption is high, approaches 1.

It is worthwile to note that when adsorption of albumin takes place
from the mixture of proteins, the adsorbed amounts are less that for
the solution containing only albumin. For the four studied polymers
these amounts represent for FEP 23%, for SR 43%, for PU-700 43%, and
for PU-1000 65% of albumin adsorbed from the solution containing
albumin only. These results show that PU-1000 preferentially adsorbs
albumin from the protein mixture solution and confirm the previous
findings from ex vivo experiments (Lyman & al, 1974). Although the
actual percentages of adsorbed albumin determined in the ex vivo
experiments differ from the above results, these differences may
result from both flow effects and differences in albumin concentrations being 50-100 times lower than in blood.

In conclusion, it appears that a more equal balance of non-disper-
sive/dispersive forces on the polymer surface is a factor in
controlling the optimal interaction of protein with the polymer
surface.

REFERENCES

Baszkin, A. & Lyman, D.J. (1980) The interactions of plasma proteins
with polymers. I. Relationship between polymer surface energy and
protein adsorption/desorption. J. Biomed. Mater. Res., 14, 393-403.
Eberhart, R.C., Wissinger, J., White, W. & Wilkow, M. (1978) Polymer
pretreatment with albumin decreases the area of subsequent fibrinogen coverage. Transaction of the 10th Annual International Bio-
materials Symposium, San Antonio, p.136.
Kim, S.W. & Lee, E.S. (1979) The role of adsorbed proteins in plate-
let adhesion onto polymer surfaces. J. Polymer Sci. Polymer
Symposium, 66, 429-441.
Lee, R.G., Adamson, C., Kim, S.W. & Lyman, D.J. (1973) Determination
of the surface energy of proteinated polymer surfaces. Thrombosis
Res., 3, 87-90.
Lyman, D.J., Kwan-Gett, C., Zwart, H.M.J., Bland, A., Eastwood, N.,
Dawai, J. & Kolff, W.J. (1971) The development and implantation of
R polyurethane hemispherical artificial heart. Trans. Amer. Soc.
Artf. Int. Organs, 17, 456-463.
Lyman, D.J., Metcalf, L.C., Albo, D.J., Richards, K.F. & Lamb, J.
(1974) The effect of chemical structure and surface properties of
synthetic polymers in the coagulation of blood. In vivo adsorption
of proteins on polymer surfaces. Trans. Amer. Soc. Artf. Int.
Organs, 20, 474-478.
Lyman, D.J., Knutson, K. McNeill, B. & Shibatani, K. (1975) Effect
of chemical structure and surface proterties of synthetic polymers
on the coagulation of blood. Relation between polymer morphology
and protein adsorption. Trans. Amer. Soc. Artf. Int. Organs, 21,
49-53.
Marchalonis, J.J. (1969) An enzymic method for the trace iodination
of immunoglobulins and other proteins. Biochem. J., 113, 299-305.

     A. Baszkin and D.J. Lyman

Packham, M.A., Evans, G., Glynn, M.P. & Mustard, J.F. (1969) The effect of plasma proteins on the interaction of platelets with glass surfaces. J. Lab. Clin. Med., 73, 683-691.
Van der Scheer, A. & Smolders, C.A. (1978) Dynamic aspects of contact angle measurements on adsorbed protein layers. J. Colloid Interface Sci., 63, 7-15.
Weathersby, P.W., Horbett, T.A. & Hoffman, A.S. (1977) Solution stability of bovine fibrinogen. Thrombosis Res., 10, 245-252.

Biomaterials 1980
Edited by G. D. Winter, D. F. Gibbons, and H. Plenk, Jr.
© 1982 John Wiley and Sons Ltd.

STRIKING DIFFERENCES OBSERVED IN THE EFFECT OF AMPHIPATHIC POLYELECTROLYTES ON CONTACT AND OTHER CLOTTING FACTORS

M.C. Boffa[*], J.P. Farges[**], B. Dreyer[**], B. Conche[*],
C. Pusineri[***] and G. Vantard[**]

[*]   Centre National de Transfusion Sanguine, 6 rue
     A. Cabanel F. 75015 Paris
[**] Rhône-Poulenc Research Centre, 13 Quai Jules Guesde
     F. 94400 Vitry-sur-Seine
[***] Rhône-Poulenc Research Centre, F. 69190 Saint-Fons

SUMMARY

Modification of contact phase proteins and other plasma clotting
factors are studied in the presence of positive and negative charges
provided by amphipathic polyelectrolytes or by polyanions and poly-
cations derived from copolymerization of acrylonitrile at different
surface/plasma ratios.

Both global clotting assays and specific one stage assays for
factors V, VII, IX, XI and XII have been performed ; prekallikrein
and Xa levels have been determined with specific chromogenic substrates and high molecular weight kininogen (HMWK) with the guinea-
pig ileum method.

Two types of responses of clotting factors are obtained. Negatively
charged polymers activate the contact phase through the HMWK –
prekallikrein system with insignificant modifications of factor XI
and XII activities. The measurement of HMWK level appears to be more
sensitive than prekallikrein assay. Positively charged polymers
develop an anticoagulant, surface-dependent effect observed in a
global cephalin clotting time and prothrombin time.

Among clotting factors, factor V activity is the most affected by
contact with charged polymers. In conclusion, this systematic
analysis on well-characterized polymers shows that both HMWK and
factor V activity could be used as sensitive tools for biomaterial
screening.

INTRODUCTION

The present work is a part of a larger study including other research
teams (Pusineri et al., 1980 ; Sultan et al. 1980) designed to screen
biomaterials based upon such criteria as plasma clotting factors,
platelet behaviour and protein deposition. This paper reports the
effects of physico-chemical characteristics, especially ionic charges,
of specifically defined biomaterials on the clotting process, with
special emphasis on the contact phase. The clotting protein modifications have been studied in presence of positive and negative charges

provided by amphipathic polyelectrolytes or by polyanions and poly-
cations derived from copolymerization of acrylonitrile at different
surface/plasma volume ratios.

MATERIALS

All materials tested in this work derive from amphipathic polyelectrolytes ; they are statistical copolymers which have been polymerized with monomers of acrylonitrile including either pyridinium or
sulfonic groups as fixed ionic sites.

Two types of materials have been studied :

(1) Precipitated powders of an amphipathic polycation (P.A.C.) and
of an amphipathic polyanion (P.A.A.). The former is a polyelectrolyte
with 0.95 mEq/g of pyridinium groups, the latter a polyelectrolyte
with 0.6 mEq/g of sulfonic groups. The exchangeable counter ions are
respectively iodide and sodium. These powders have high specific surfaces but in the case of such highly porous materials, there are numerous pores unaccessible to plasma proteins.

(2) Ground powder of polyelectrolyte complexes (P.E.C.s) formed by
ionic association of a polyanion and a polycation. For this study
they were synthesized from the same P.A.C. (see above) and from a
similar polyanion (P.A.A. above) but richer in sulfonic groups
(1.33 mEq/g instead of 0.6).

Two P.E.C.s have been formed : anionic and cationic, - 0.8 mEq/g and
+ 0.8 mEq/g respectively. Powders of these P.E.C.s have been obtained
by thin grinding which yields powders with limited specific surfaces.
The particles obtained are very compact and wall surfaces must be
accessible to blood components.

The surface/plasma volume ratios for amphipathic polymers and P.E.C.s
were chosen according to the porosity of the materials and the accessibility of ionic sites to plasma, after a precise determination of
their specific surface (B.E.T. method) and of their ionic surface
concentration (adsorption of ionic dyes).

METHODS

Incubation of the materials. The materials were swollen for 24 hours
in buffered isotonic solution (pH : 7.3, 94.10^{-3}M.NaCl, $1.63\ 10^{-3}$M.
$CaCl_2$, $0.5\ 10^{-3}$M.$MgCl_2$, 2.10^{-3}M.KCl, 38.10^{-3}M.NaCOOCH$_3$) at room temperature.

After centrifugation, the materials were suspended and stirred at
37° C in human platelet-poor plasma (from a pool of 10 donors) at
different polymer surface/plasma volume ratios.

Control tests were identical but were performed without polymer
present. After different incubation times, an aliquot of the suspension was centrifuged (5 min - 3000 g) and the plasma obtained immediately frozen in 0.3 ml fractions at - 80° C.

<u>Clotting assays</u>. Clotting assays were performed at 37° C in an electro-magnetic water bath with the incubated plasmas : thrombin time was measured using 0.1 ml plasma + 0.1 ml thrombin solution (2 U/ml). Prothrombin time was measured using 0.1 ml plasma + 0.2 ml thromboplastin Stago/0.025 M $CaCl_2$ (1 : 1). Recalcification time was performed in polystyrene tubes in the presence of phospholipids (human brain cephalin - Bell and Alton) using 0.1 ml plasma + 0.2 ml 0.025 M.$CaCl_2$/cephalin (1 : 1). Specific one-stage assays were performed with congenital deficient plasmas (VIII, XI, XII) or with plasmas specifically deprived of one factor (II, V, VII + X, IX).

<u>Prekallikrein and factor Xa assays</u> were performed on chromogenic substrates using chromozym P.K. Pentapharm Basel and S.2222 Kabi respectively. Prekallikrein was measured in presence of celite eluates (Soulier and Gozin, 1979).

<u>High molecular weight (H.M.W.) kininogen assay</u> was performed by detection of kinin activity on isolated guinea-pig ileum with reference to a bradydinin scale (12 939 R.P.). Kinin activity, liberated from the H.M.W. kininogen remaining after incubation, was revealed, in presence of O-phenanthroline chloride, by adjunction of kallikrein. The latter was obtained from prekallikrein (semi-purified by DEA E52 chromatography) from whole plasma which was activated by enzyme agarose-trypsin (Miles Laboratories).

RESULTS

1. <u>Effect on the contact phase proteins</u>. The activities of factor XII and factor XI are unaffected by contact with the P.E.C.s, whatever the charge is ; only a slight decrease is observed with the largest surfaces (Table 1).

TABLE 1. Factor XII and factor XI activities in plasmas
after 60 min incubation with charged polymers

	P.E.C. - 0.8 mEq/g					P.E.C. + 0.8 mEq/g		
$S.cm^2/ml$	5	10	25	50	75	5	25	75
Factor XII	100	100	100	100	85	100	100	90
Factor XI	90	90	100	100	80	95	100	95

100 % = Plasma incubated without any material

P.E.C. = Polyelectrolyte complex

S = Polymer surface in contact with plasma

P.P.K. activity and H.M.W.K. level progressively decrease when the surface of the polymer increases. The level of H.M.W.K. is more affected by negative charges than P.P.K. activity since a 50 % decrease in P.P.K. activity corresponds to a complete disappearance of H.M.W.K. (fig. 1 and Table 2).

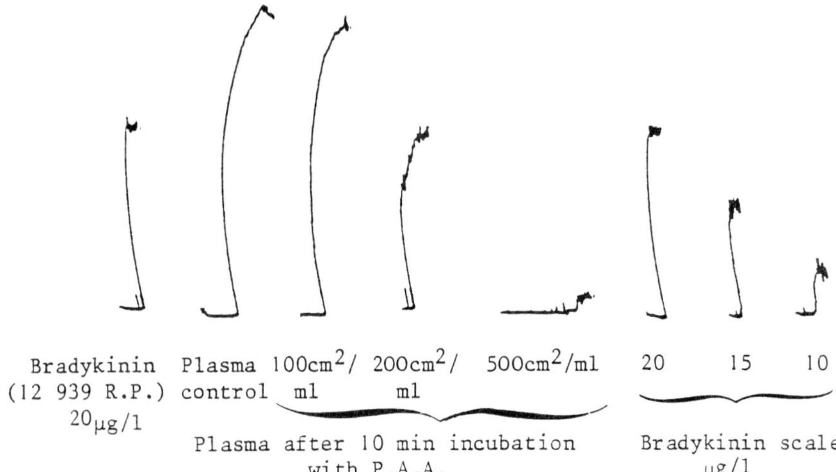

Bradykinin   Plasma 100cm^2/ 200cm^2/   500cm^2/ml   20   15   10
(12 939 R.P.) control   ml   ml
  20μg/l
                  Plasma after 10 min incubation   Bradykinin scale
                        with P.A.A.   μg/l

Fig. 1. Effect of different surface of amphipathic polyanion (P.A.A.) on kinin response of guinea-pig ileum.

TABLE 2. Kallikrein-kinin system : Prekallikrein and kinin
          activity of plasmas incubated with negatively
          charged polymers

	P.A.A.					
	P.P.K.			H.M.W.K.		
Incubat. S.cm^2/ml	10 min	30 min	60 min	10 min	30 min	60 min
100				104	97	
150	80	81	88	51	53	53
200	86	84	84	57	54	52
250	63	60	59	0	2	
500	64	72	69	6	4	
1 000	16	12	12	7	5	
2 500	14	14	14	0		

100 % = Plasma incubated without any material

P.A.A. = Amphipathic polyanion ; P.P.K. = prekallikrein ;
H.M.W.K. = high molecular weight kininogen
S = Polymer surface in contact with plasma

P.E.C. - 0.8 mEq/g

| Incubat. | P.P.K. | | | H.M.W.K. | | |
$S.cm^2/ml$	10 min	30 min	60 min	10 min	30 min	60 min
5	91	102	93	100	87	100
10	89	98	102	100	93	100
25	85	94	93	80	60	74
50	78	70	76	54	61	29
75	50	46	48	5	0	0

100 % = Plasma incubated without any material

P.E.C. = polyelectrolyte complex ; P.P.K. : prekallikrein ;
H.M.W.K. = high molecular weight kininogen

On the contrary no effect on both P.P.K. and H.M.W.K. level is observed in the case of positively charged polymers (Table 3).

TABLE 3. Kallikrein-kinin system : Prekallikrein and
          kinin activity of plasmas incubated with posi-
          tively charged polymers

P.A.C. + 0.95 mEq/g

| Incubat. | P.P.K. | | | H.M.W.K. | | |
$S.cm^2/ml$	10 min	30 min	60 min	10 min	30 min	60 min
250	87	96	116	–	100	95
1 000	96	94	96	–	–	97
2 000	95	96	96	–	100	–

P.E.C. + 0.8 mEq/g

| Incubat. | P.P.K. | | | H.M.W.K. | | |
$S.cm^2/ml$	10 min	30 min	60 min	10 min	30 min	60 min
5	89	91	94	–	93	103
25	92	92	92	–	90	100
75	87	87	85	–	93	100

100 % = Plasma incubated without any material

P.A.C. = Amphipathic polycation ; P.E.C. = polyelectrolyte complex ;
P.P.K. = prekallikrein ; H.M.W.K. = high molecular weight kininogen

2. <u>Effect on prothrombinase formation</u>. Thrombin formation is not modified by any polymer ; on the contrary, plasma recalcification time
in presence of phospholipids or thromboplastin shows distinctly different behaviours according to the charges of the polymers (fig. 2
and 3). For negative charges a surface-related shortening is observed at 10 min incubation, followed by a delay in clot formation after
1 hour incubation. For positive charges no modification is observed
in the case of P.E.C. + 0.8 mEq/g while an anticoagulant effect develops in plasma incubated with P.A.C.. In the case of this latter
materials, it has been possible to study the effect on plasma clotting with larger polymer surface/plasma volume ratios.

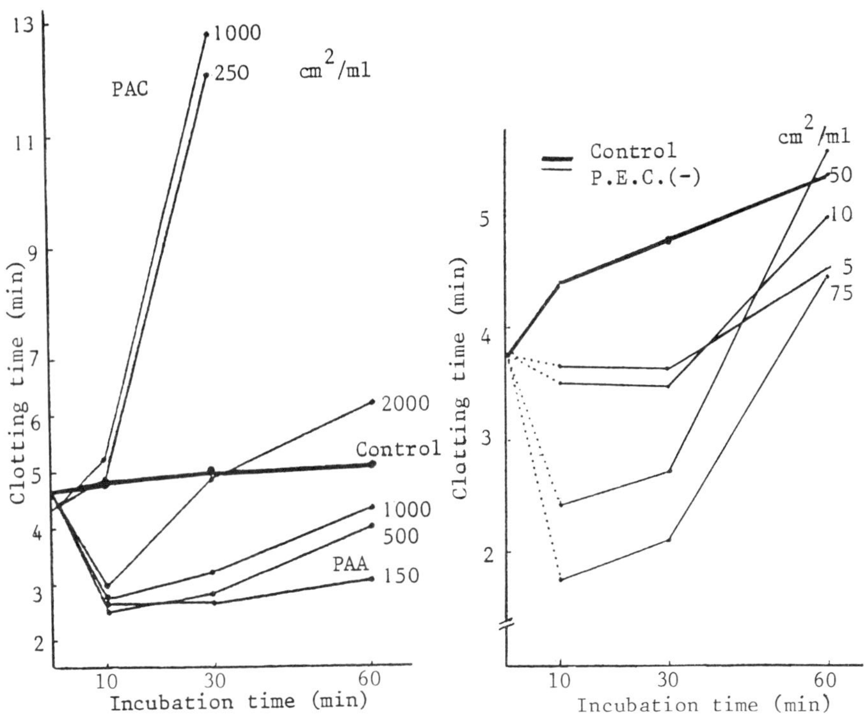

(for legend, see next page)

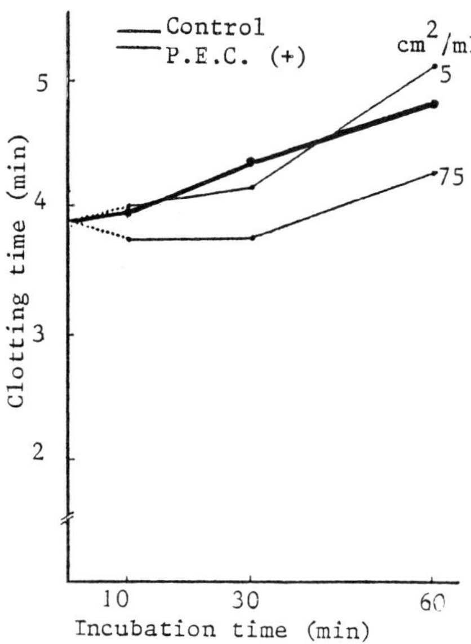

Fig. 2. Recalcification time of plasma incubated with
charged polymers (amphipathic polyanion P.A.A. and polycation P.A.C. ; polyelectrolyte complexes - 0.8 mEq/g and
+ 0.8 mEq/g) in the presence of phospholipids.

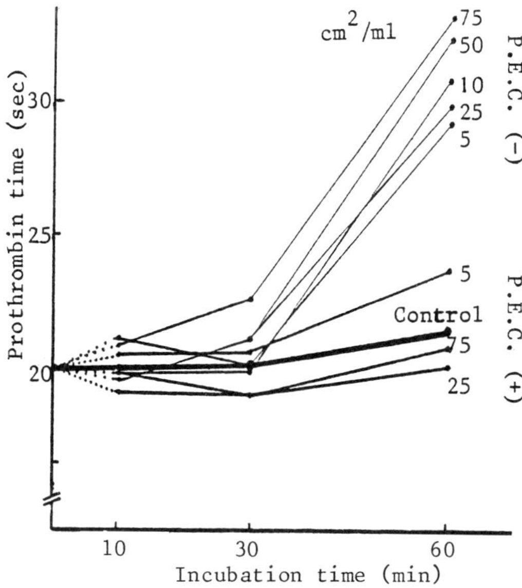

Fig. 3. Prothrombin time of plasmas incubated with polyelectrolyte complexes + 0.8 mEq/g and - 0.8 mEq/g

It has not been possible to explain the negative charge-induced
shortening of recalcification time by the presence of an activated
factor (Table 4).

TABLE 4. Are there activated factors in plasma incubated
with amphipathic polyanions (10 min 37° C) ?

Surface cm^2/ml	XII	XI	IX	Xa	IIa	VII
	Assay without activator			on S.2222	on Fb	
500	–	–	70 %	$<$ 1 %	$>$3h	150 %
1000	87 %	70 %	65 %	$<$ 1 %	$>$3h	90 %

Fb : Fibrinogen

The decrease in factor V activity – already suspected on prothrombin
time (see fig. 3) – appears to be time and surface dependent and more
important in the case of P.E.C. – 0.8 mEq/g than in the case of
P.E.C. + 0.8 mEq/g (fig. 4).

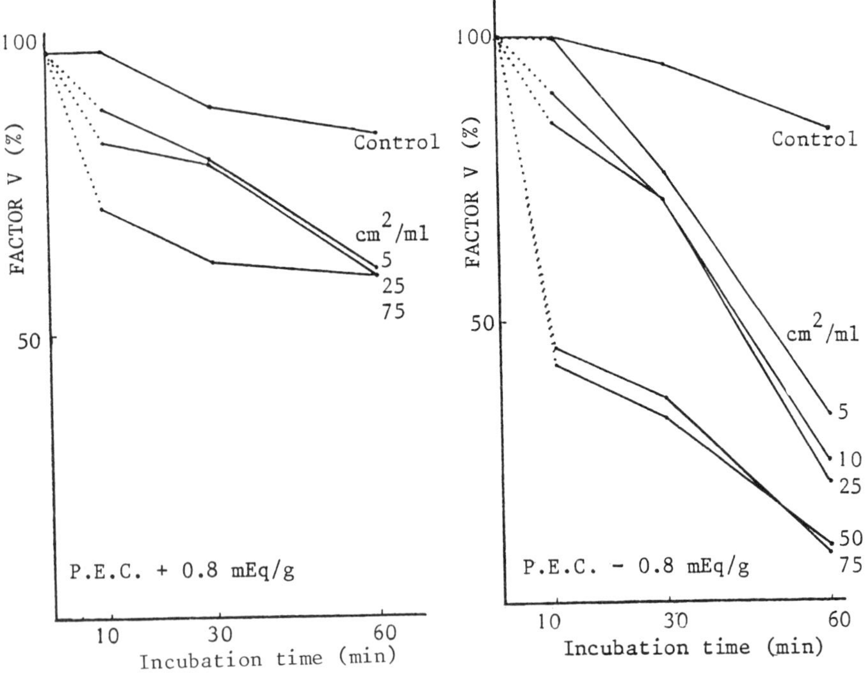

Fig. 4. Evolution of factor V activity in plasma incubated
with polyelectrolyte complexes (P.E.C.) + 0.8 mEq/g and
– 0.8 mEq/g.

DISCUSSION

Only few data on the effect of specifically charged polymers on plasma clotting factors are presently available. Our study shows that negatively charged polymers activate the coagulation process through the kallikrein-kinin system ; surprisingly no striking effect has been observed on factor XI and factor XII activities.

It should be noted that materials are amphipathic ; thus, results might partially arise from cooperative effect between ionic and hydrophobic interactions.

The measurement of H.M.W. kininogen level appears to be more sensitive than prekallikrein assay that has been reported as a good tool for biomaterial screening (Becker et al., 1979).

Among clotting factors, plasma factor V activity is the most affected by contact with charged polymers ; for equivalent surfaces a more pronounced effect of negatively charged polymers is observed. Thus the presence of negative charges on the polymer emphasizes the decrease in factor V activity reported by Fuhge et al. (1979). However, inactivation of clotting factor V appears not sufficient to be used as the only screening clotting test for development of blood compatible biomaterials. Emphasis has to be given to more thorough studies, especially concerning the mechanism of contact activation since the kallikrein-kinin system seems to be very sensitive to contact with polymer surfaces. Additional studies with these materials concerning platelet behaviour (Sultan et al. 1980) have shown that platelet adhesion decreases with the increase of negative charges on the polymer surface. Therefore, an exhaustive approach should include both plasma proteins and cellular behaviour at interfaces. Such a systematic study using well-characterized polymers could allow the development of a precise screening for biomaterials and offer an interesting tool for a better understanding of the coagulation process.

REFERENCES

Becker, U., Fuhge, P., Heimburger, N. & Fischer, P. (1979) Evaluation of the blood compatibility of biomaterials by plasma kallikrein derived from contact activation. Communication to the VIIth International Congress of Thrombosis and Haemostasis, London (G.B.), July 18th, Abstract N° 0554 p. 235.
Fuhge, P., Becker, U. & Heimburger, N. (1979) Inactivation of Clotting factor V - a simple in vitro test for screening biomaterials. Communication to the 6th Annual Meeting of the European Society for Artificial Organs, Geneva (Switzerland), September 29-30th and October 1st ; Abstract p.9.
Pusineri, C., Farges, J.P., Brash, J.L. & Schmitt, A. (1980) Hydrophobic and amphipathic ionic interfaces : physico-chemical characterization, adsorption of plasma proteins. Communication to the 1st World Biomaterials Congress, April 8-12th, Baden (Austria).
Soulier, J.P. & Gozin, D. (1979) Assay of Fletcher factor (plasma prekallikrein) using an artificial clotting reagent and a modified chromogenic substrate. Thromb. Haemostas. 42, 538-547.

Sultan, Y., Maisonneuve, P. & Pusineri, C. (1980) Characterization
of artificial surfaces by protein adsorption and platelet adherence.
Communication to the 1st World Biomaterial Congress, April 8-12th,
Baden (Austria).

Biomaterials 1980
Edited by G. D. Winter, D. F. Gibbons, and H. Plenk, Jr.
© 1982 John Wiley and Sons Ltd.

PHYSICAL STUDIES OF IMPLANT SURFACES

B. Ivarsson, U. Jönsson, I. Lundström and D. McQueen.

Laboratory of Applied Physics,
Linköping Institute of Technology,
581 83 Linköping, Sweden.

SUMMARY

We use ellipsometry in the study of implant materials to obtain information about the initial adsorption of human serum fibrinogen (HFIB) and human serum albumin (HSA) onto the implant surface. The ellipsometric measurements are combined with measurements of Galvani potential and electrode impedance to learn more about the implant-protein solution interface. We present a short description of the experimental techniques used, focusing mainly on ellipsometry. Model experiments on protein adsorption from electrolytes on titanium, aluminum and gold are described. Correlations between protein adsorption as measured using ellipsometry and changes in the electrical properties of the metal-electrolyte interface are demonstrated. The possibility of using a small organic molecule as a probe for the packing of proteins on the surfaces is also discussed.

INTRODUCTION

It is of interest to study the surface properties of implant materials to better understand their behavior in contact with body fluids and tissues. However, there are few direct methods for such studies on a molecular level. We have chosen to use and compare ellipsometric, Galvani potential and capacitance measurements to study the attachment of molecules to implant surfaces, and which mechanisms of attachment are most important. In the initial phase of our study we have studied the adsorption of polypeptides on substrates of aluminum, titanium and gold. These measurements are reported here.

MATERIALS AND METHODS

The three polypeptides used were the following: a) Human serum fibrinogen (HFIB), more than 90 % clottable, lyophilized, Grade L. b) Human serum albumin (HSA), more than 97 % pure, lyophilized. c) Tripeptide Bz-Phe-Val-Arg-pNA (S-2160). They were all obtained from AB Kabi, Stockholm. The buffer used was in all cases Hanks's physiological phosphate buffer, pH 7.4. All protein solutions were made within half an hour before each measurement.

The three substrates, aluminum, titanium and gold, were made by evaporating films onto glass slides masked with copper foil to give well defined geometrical sample areas.

In the experiments for comparison between the three metals the starting concentrations of the proteins were chosen to be 5 % and 100 % of
the normal human blood concentration (BC) for HFIB, and 0.4 % and 50 %
BC for HSA. The simultaneous Galvani potential and ellipsometry experiments were done on gold with HSA 10 % and 50 % BC followed by HFIB
100 % BC. The simultaneous capacitance and ellipsometry experiments
were done on gold with HSA 0.4 % and 0.8 % BC followed by HFIB 5 % and
10 % BC. The simultaneous capacitance and ellipsometry experiments on
gold using S-2160, 90 μM, as a probe were done on HSA 0.1 % and 0.2 %
BC. After initial S-2160 adsorption the adsorbed molecules were rinsed
away by 400 ml buffer followed by two HSA injections. After the HSA
adsorption the HSA solution was rinsed away similarly and S-2160 injected again.

Ellipsometry. We used a Rudolph Research ellipsometer type 43603.
Since the measurements were all carried out in the liquid phase, special attention was paid to maintaining constant temperature in all
parts of the system. Protein solutions were temperature equilibrated
before being injected into the ellipsometer sample volume, which was
carefully thermostated (24°C). These extensive precautions were necessary because it was found that even the slightest thermal instability greatly disturbed the ellipsometric measurements.

In ellipsometry one measures two quantities tan ψ and Δ, where tan ψ
is the amplitude ratio between the reflection coefficients for light
polarized parallel to and perpendicular to the plane of incidence, and
Δ is the corresponding difference in phase shifts of the light. These
quantities are related to the properties of the sample surface through
the refractive indices of the various layers, and their respective
thicknesses. We have used a model in which there is a thick metal base
and oxide layer, a protein layer, and buffer. Refractive indices were
measured for the metal base and oxide layer and the buffer. The final
refractive index of the protein film was measured to be about 1.5.

The model assumed for the calculation of the protein film thickness
is that of a homogeneous film of constant refractive index (1.5) with
discrete boundaries treated in the Drude equations (Azzam and Bashara,
1977). Since the adsorbed molecule will show some refractive index
distribution normal to the surface, the relative values of the calculated film thicknesses on the different surfaces may be compared assuming that the refractive index distribution does not change markedly
from one surface to another (Fenstermaker et al, 1974).

Current understanding of ellipsometric measurements indicates that the
ellipsometric signal is proportional to the amount adsorbed (Bootsma
and Meyer, 1969). According to these authors an incomplete monolayer
having only a fraction of the possible sites occupied (coverage θ < 1)
behaves like a continuous film (constant index of refraction) of
effective thickness $\theta \cdot dm$, where dm is the diameter of the molecules.
The calculated film thickness from the Drude model (d(A)) may be
described as this effective thickness.

Galvani potential. By coupling the metal-solution interface under
study with a non polarizable interface it is possible to equate chang-
es in cell potential (metal|electrolyte|polarizable electrode) with
changes in the Galvani potential ΔE (the inner potential) across the
interface under examination (Bockris, 1977). The Galvani potential is
made up of contributions from the charges which give the outer potential difference $\Delta\psi$, and from the dipole layers which give the surface
potential difference $\Delta\chi$ at the metal-solution interface ($\Delta E = \Delta\psi + \Delta\chi$).
The measurable Galvani potential changes thus yield information on the
distribution of charges and orientation of dipoles which make up the
structure of the electrified interface.

Since adsorbed proteins may contain both charge and dipole moments,
and the protein adsorption probably displaces water dipoles and ions,
it is natural to detect protein layers on metal surfaces using changes
in the Galvani potential.

In practice one uses a reference electrode (saturated calomel electrode
(SCE), platinum, etc.) and measures voltage differences between the
reference and test electrodes using a high impedance (more than 10^{14}
ohms) millivoltmeter.

Electrode capacitance. The capacitance of a clean electrode in an
electrolyte is mainly determined by the double layer capacitance which
for a strong electrolyte is determined by the amount of adsorbed water
molecules and ions and the extension of this double layer in the
electrolyte (Bockris, 1977). In reality the capacitance is influenced
by oxide layers, surface structure etc. When proteins adsorb onto the
electrode this double layer is disturbed, due to the displacement process mentioned above, at the sites on the surface where the protein
makes close contact to the electrode. Since the double layer has a
large specific capacitance while the protein molecules generally represent a small capacitance the total capacitance of an electrode
drops on the adsorption of the protein. The capacitance and the Galvani potential are related, but are expected to give complementary information about protein adsorption. In practice the capacitance can
be measured by a lock-in amplifier. We used a measurement frequency
of 1 kHz and an amplitude of 10 mV.

RESULTS

We have used the above methods to study HFIB and HSA adsorption on
different metal surfaces and applied in different sequences. This gives
an indication of relative binding energies for the two proteins to the
three metals.

Figure 1 shows simultaneous ellipsometric and Galvani potential measurements immediately after the gold electrode's immersion in Hanks's
solution. The potential isotherm indicates an adsorption of some potential determining species. The ellipsometric and potential data for
adsorption of high concentrations of HSA and HFIB correlate well. Also,
HFIB can adsorb on a surface which is already covered with HSA,
according to these results.

Figure 2 shows simultaneous ellipsometric and capacitance measurements
on gold after the capacitance has stabilized in the buffer. For this
experiment lower concentrations of HSA and HFIB were used. Again we
note a good correlation of the two measurement techniques for the first
protein adsorbed. However, the HFIB adsorption is not detectable by
capacitance measurements but by the ellipsometric technique. The
complementary data obtained from both methods are discussed below.

We have carried out a large number of measurements of this type in order to discover characteristics of the binding of these two proteins.
The results of these measurements are summarized in figure 3. In figure 3a the curves show what happens when HSA is adsorbed on HFIB covered surfaces, and figure 3b shows the corresponding results for HFIB
on HSA covered surfaces. We note that HSA has little or no effect on a
HFIB covered surface, but HFIB increases the effective thicknesses
of HSA covered surfaces. This can be indicative of stronger binding
forces or energies for HFIB than for HSA. We further notice that the
film thicknesses increase from aluminum to titanium to gold. Aluminum
and titanium have oxide films, but gold does not. However, the stabilized Galvani potentials of titanium and gold in Hanks's solution are
almost equal (about +150 mV and +200 mV relative SCE, respectively),
while the potential for aluminum is large and negative (about -700 mV
relative SCE). These data suggest a correlation between effective
film thickness and Galvani potential. We also found two types of gold-
structures, Au_1 and Au_2, with different protein adsorption properties.

The effective film thickness is dependent on both the size of the in-
divudual protein molecules (dm) and their coverage (θ). Thus it is of
interest to test how tightly packed the protein layers are. Figure 4
illustrates how we have used the small tripeptide S-2160 for this purpose. S-2160 was adsorbed onto the gold surface, and then rinsed off.
HSA was then adsorbed irreversibly onto the surface in two stages
according to the sequence described in figure 4. Finally S-2160 was
admitted to the sample chamber again, and adsorbed. Due to the change
in capacitance on the adsorption a probable interpretation of this result is that S-2160 fits into gaps between the HSA molecules, thus introducing new contact points between organic molecules and the electrode surface.

DISCUSSION

The effective thickness of the protein film was calculated assuming a
constant refractive index of the film during adsorption. The refractive indices of fibrinogen and albumin during adsorption have been measured (Cuyper, 1976) on hydrophilic and hydrophobic chromium and silicon. For fibrinogen on hydrophilic chromium both the analyzer and
polarizer stabilized simultaneously after 10 minutes. Cuyper's interpretation of this stability was that the refractive index did not
change much during the adsorption. The refractive index of fibrinogen
($10\mu g/ml$) was 1.4 and the corresponding film thickness 120 Å. For albumin adsorption ($10\mu g/ml$) on hydrophilic·chromium a stable refractive
index at 1.55 was reached after about 7 minutes giving a film thickness
of about 15 Å.

In our measurements on both HFIB and HSA the analyzer change is less
than 10 % of the polarizer change and both are stable simultaneously
also indicating a constant refractive index. In our model a decrease
in the refractive index from 1.5 to 1.4 will nearly double our effective film thickness, which exemplifies the relation between refractive
index and film thickness. We feel that the agreement in these results
between Cuyper and us indicates that we have selected reasonable values for the refractive index parameter in the model. Our results thus
show how ellipsometry combined with suitable proteins can be applied
to biometals as a screening method for prediction of biocompatibility.
According to Vroman et al (1971) and Kim et al (1974) a fibrinogen
film is believed to be required for platelet adhesion on a foreign
surface while a precoating of these surfaces with albumin is known to
reduce this adhesion suggesting that an albumin film may prevent fibrinogen adsorption on the surfaces. Our ellipsometric findings for
fibrinogen (figure 3a) indicate a decreasing ability for platelet adhesion and thrombosis for the series gold to titanium to aluminum.
Furthermore an albumin film was found to reduce fibrinogen adsorption
(figure 3b) but not to prevent it. The latter result is in accordance
with that of Vroman et al (1971) and Fenstermaker et al (1974) for
silicon surfaces.

Conformational information from capacitance measurements is shown in
figure 2. We feel that the difference between ellipsometric and capacitance data is caused by the fact that upon protein adsorption the
number of contact points to the electrode ($\sim\theta$) is not changed. Thus
the double layer capacitance will not change, even if the effective
protein layer thickness ($\sim\theta \cdot dm$) is increased.

The capacitance change upon adsorption of S-2160 on an incompletely
preadsorbed albumin film (figure 4) has consequently been interpreted by us as an increase in coverage (θ) of organic material which also
increases the effective film thickness.

<u>REFERENCES</u>

Azzam, R.M.A. & Bashara, N.M. (1977) Reflection and transmission by an
ambient-film-substrate system, in Ellipsometry and Polarized Light
(Eds., Azzam & Bashara), pp 283-288. North-Holland Publ., Amsterdam.
Bockris, J.O'M. & Reddy, A.K.N. (1977) The potential difference across
electrified interfaces, in Modern Electrochemistry (Eds., Bockris &
Reddy), pp 644-761. Plenum Press, New York.
Bootsma, G.A. & Meyer, F. (1969) Ellipsometry in the submonolayer re-
gion. Surface Sci. 14, 52-76.
Cuyper, P.A. (1976) Dynamic ellipsometry, biochemical and biomedical
applications, PhD Thesis. Rijks Universiteit, Limburg, Maastricht,
The Netherlands, pp 113-146.
Fenstermaker, C.A., Grant, W.H., Morrissey, B.W., Smith, L.A. & Strom-
berg, R.R. (1974) Interaction of plasma proteins with surfaces,
N.B.S.I.R. 74-470 Nat. Bur. of Standards, Washington.
Kim, S.W., Lee, R.G., Oster, H., Coleman, D., Andrade, J.D., Lentz,
D.J. & Olsen, D. (1974) Platelet adhesion to polymer surfaces. Trans.
Amer. Soc. Artif. Int. Organs, 20, 449-455.
Vroman, L., Adams, A.L. & Klings, M. (1971) Interactions among human
blood proteins at interfaces. Federation Proceedings, 30, 1494-1502.

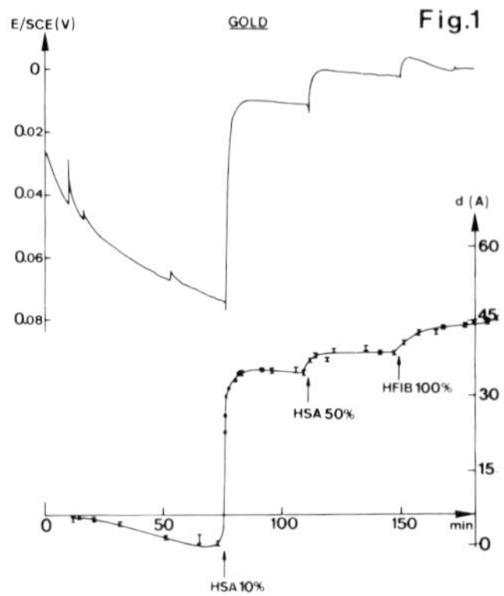

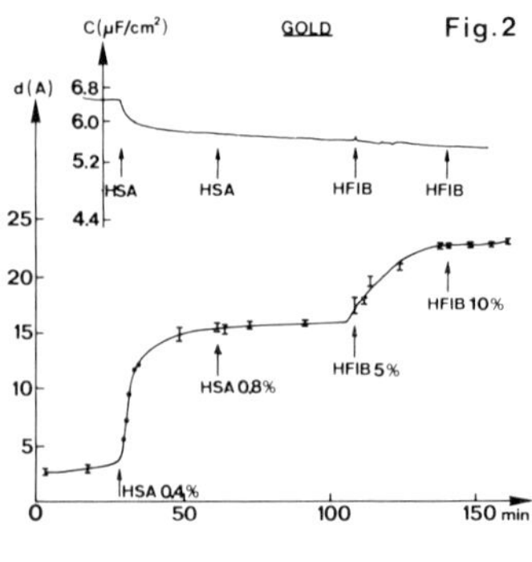

Fig. 1. Sample data for adsorption of HSA and HFIB on gold as
measured using Galvani potential and ellipsometry.

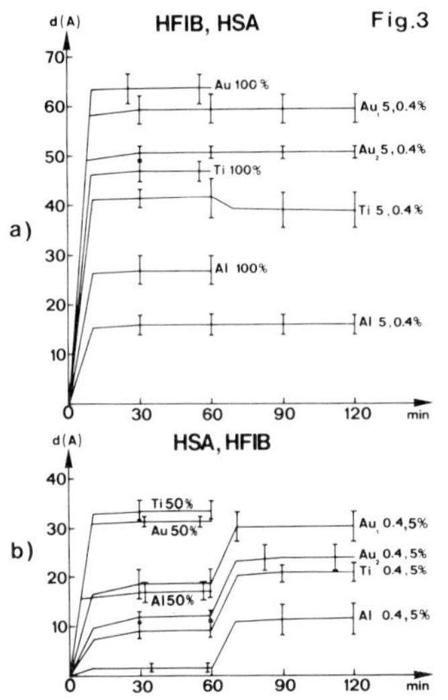

Fig. 2. Sample data for adsorption of HSA and HFIB on gold as
measured using capacitance and
ellipsometry.

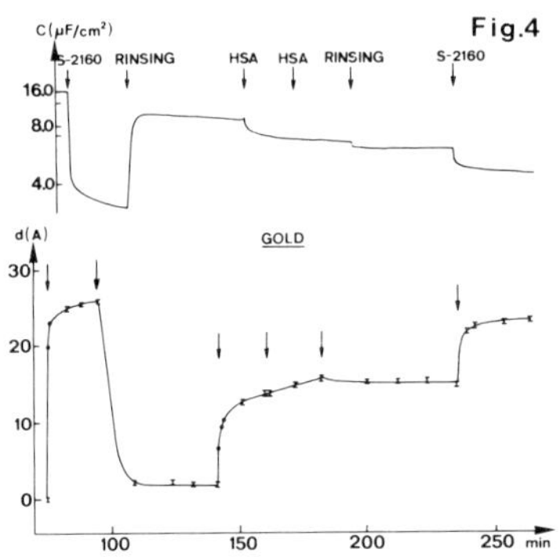

Fig. 3. Summary of ellipsometer data on adsorption of HSA and
HFIB on aluminum, titanium and two classes of gold. The first
protein is injected at the starting point and after 30 minutes. The second protein is added after 60 and 90 minutes,
respectively. The concentration of the first injection of
each protein is shown. For the following injection of the proteins the concentration is nearly doubled.

Fig. 4. Sample data from capacitance and ellipsometer measurements showing the use of S-2160 as a probe for testing protein packing. For experimental procedure see methods. Arrows
on lower curve describe the same sequence followed in the
upper curve. (Note that the time sequence in the upper curve
was somewhat distorted in the photographic reduction).

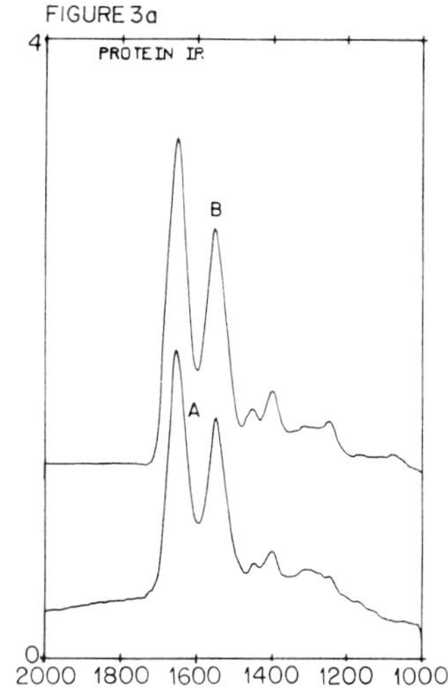

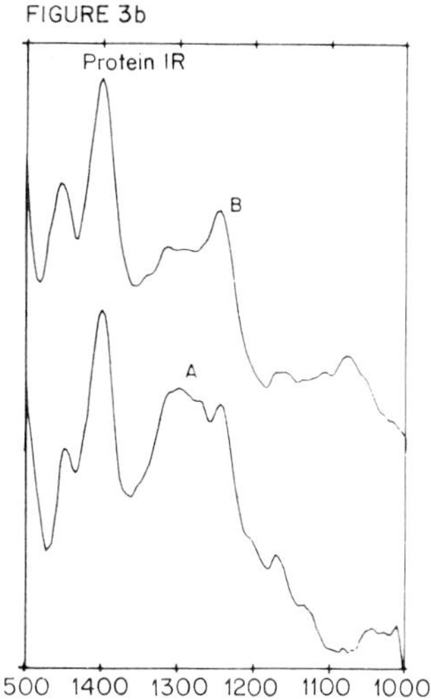

Fig. 3a. Spectrum of (A) albumin (B) fibrinogen adsorbed onto germanium after water subtraction. 3b. Scale expansion of albumin (A) and fibrinogen (B) spectra to illustrate detail. Note that bands in the neighborhood of 1250 cm^{-1} are quite different between the two proteins.

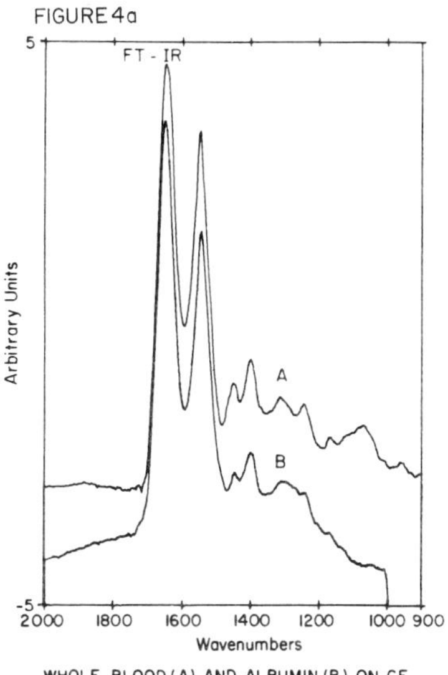

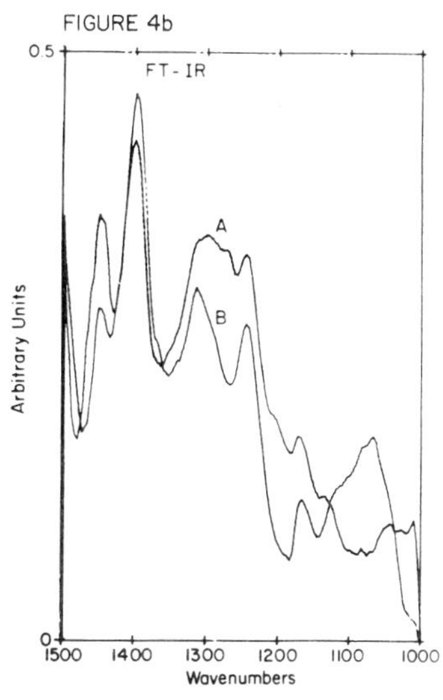

Fig. 4a. Spectra of whole blood (A) and albumin (B) adsorbed onto germanium after water subtraction. 4b. Scale expansion to illustrate differences. Carbohydrate band at 1084 cm^{-1} in whole blood is lacking in albumin (A) spectrum.

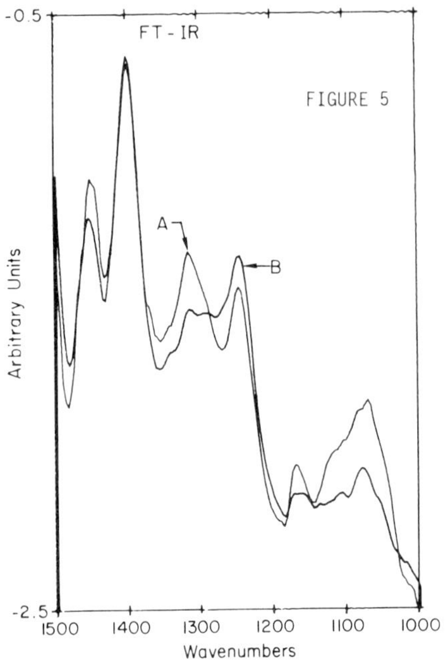

Fig. 5. Scale expanded comparison of whole blood (A) and fibrinogen (B) on germanium. Note differences in 1250 cm^{-1} region and 1084 cm^{-1} (carbohydrate) region.

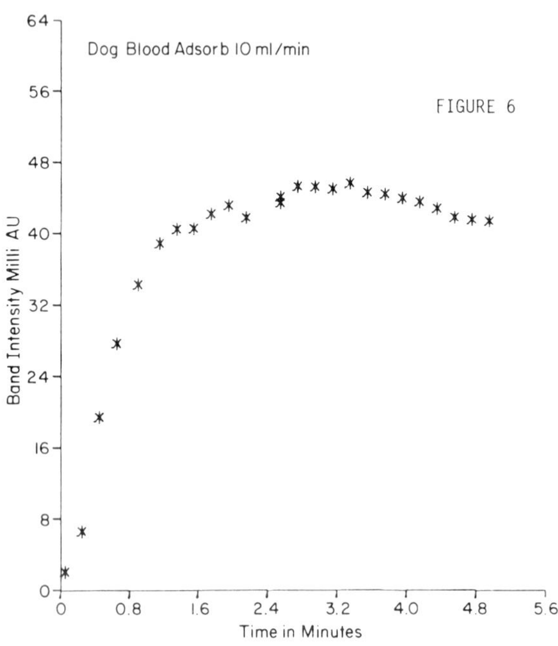

Fig. 6. Plot of Amide 11 (1550 cm^{-1}) band intensity versus time. Whole dog blood adsorbing on germanium.

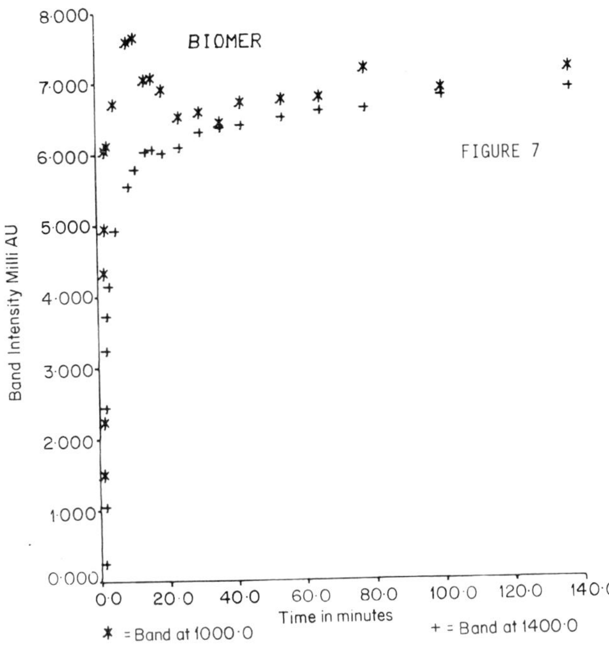

Fig.7. Plot of 1400 cm^{-1} band and 1084 cm^{-1} bands, normalized to roughly same intensity. Note that 1084 cm^{-1} band reaches max.intensity at about 10 min. then falls. This is significant since total proteins as indicated by 1400 cm^{-1} band continued to increase throughout. Whole dog blood adsorbing on Biomer[R].

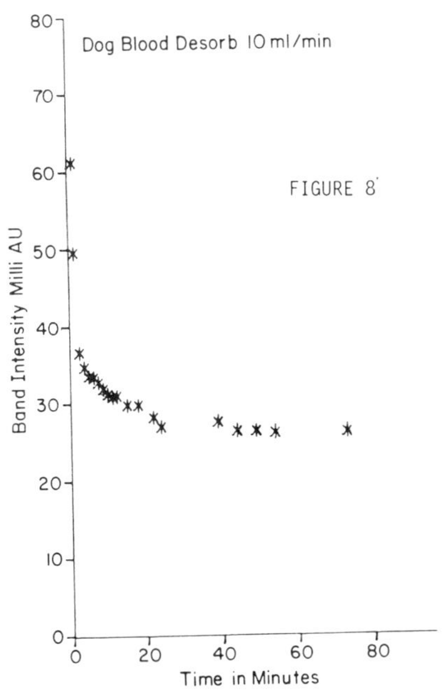

Fig. 8. Typical desorption plot. Amide II intensity plotted versus time. Whole dog blood desorbing from Biomer[R].

Biomaterials 1980
Edited by G. D. Winter, D. F. Gibbons, and H. Plenk, Jr.
© 1982 John Wiley and Sons Ltd.

FTIR-ATR SPECTROSCOPIC ANALYSIS OF
POLYURETHANE-SILICONE BLOODCONTACT SURFACES

R. Kellner and G. Gidaly

Institute of Analytical Chemistry
Technical University, A-1060 Vienna, Getreidemarkt 9

F. Unger

Surgical Clinic I, University Innsbruck
A-6020 Innsbruck, Anichstraße 35

SUMMARY

The application of infrared-attenuated total reflectance (IR-ATR)
spectrometry as a method for the analysis of polymer bloodcontact
surfaces is described. The sensivity and information depth of this
method of 0,4 - 1,6 μm makes a quantitative analysis of polymer
mixtures in the surface area possible. For polyurethane-silicone
bloodcontact materials (Avcothane-51) an index of chemical blood-
compatibility has been formed which can be used as quality control
in the development of new models of the artificial heart. Of more
general importance to the problem is the investigation of protein
adsorption on polymer surfaces, which can be done by Fourier
transform spectrometry on a molecular basis. Experiments to correlate reversibility of protein adsorption and bloodcompatibility of
the respective polymer surfaces have been done.

INTRODUCTION

Organic polymers like polyetherurethanes, siloxanes or polyurethane-
silicone mixtures are widely used as basic materials for artificial
organs in the cardiovascular system. A good blood compatibility of
their blood contact surfaces is of outmost importance in that it
dictates the success or failure of a polymer for cardiovascular
applications.

The problem of blood compatibility being mainly a problem of surface
chemistry and hydrodynamic aspects (Baier and Dutton, 1969,
Nyilas, 1976) can be analyzed by Infrared Attenuated Total Reflectance (IR-ATR) Spectrometry (Kellner, 1979, Nyilas and Ward, 1977).
This technique may be used to measure the chemical composition of
the blood contact surface itself and also the effect of different
materials on the adsorption of blood proteins.

423

IR-ATR-spectroscopy can contribute to both ways on a molecular
basis since the information depth of the method can be adjusted to
the submicrometer range (0,4 - 1,6 µm) and since the method can be
used for the analysis of solid and liquid (aqueous) materials.

RESULTS AND DISCUSSIONS

A. The Effect of the Chemical Composition on the Blood Compatibility for a Polyurethane-silicone-material (Avcothane-51). It has
been shown experimentally that the air facing side (AFS) of Avco-
thane-51 has a very good bloodcompatibility whereas the substrate
facing side (SFS) is usually thrombogeneous (Nyilas and Ward, 1977).
The reason for this is an enrichment of the siloxane component at the
SFS due to the influence of a diffusion process. This enrichment can
be controlled by the IR-ATR spectra of the respective surfaces
(Fig. 1). In a special design of the artificial heart, the AFS, however, cannot be used as blood contact surface (Unger, 1975).

By substituting steel as mandril material by epolene which can be
pentrated by the solvent and by a careful optimization of the
dipping and drying process an acceptable bloodcompatibility could be
reached also for SFS's. A strict control of the surface composition
of these samples is however necessary and the following procedure
based on IR-ATR spectroscopy has been successfully applied. The
IR-ATR spectrum of the sample to be tested is evaluated quantitatively
by measuring the absorbance values at 770 cm^{-1} (polyurethane band),
800 cm^{-1} (siloxane band) and 1850 cm^{-1} (background) and by forming
the ratio $R = \dfrac{E_{770} - E_{1850}}{E_{800} - E_{1850}}$ (Fig. 2).

The AFS of an intraaortic balloon pump with a very good blood compatibility was used as a standard and R_{ST} was determined to be 2,08
with new (unscratched) KRS-5 crystals. A baseline slope can be corrected by introduction of a term E_C in the following equation and
also be calculated for the standard condition.

$$R_{ST} = \frac{E_{770} - E_{1850} + E_C}{E_{800} - E_{1850} + E_C} = 2,08.$$

E_C has than to be used in the equation for R_S of the test sample. An
"Index of Chemical Blood Compatibility" is formed
($I_{CBC} = R_S/R_{ST} \cdot 100$ [%]) and it was found that I_{CBC} can be used as
quality control in the development of new ways for producing Avcothane membranes for artificial hearts. Indices $\geq$ 80 % point to good
bloodcompatibility, samples with indices $\leq$ 65 % are thrombogenic
(Kellner and Unger, 1977).

B. FTIR-ATR Spectroscopic Analysis of Adsorbed Protein Films on
Polymers after Blood Contact. The study of the protein adsorption
on an implanted polymer seems to be of a more general importance
than the study of the surface composition of the polymer alone.
FTIR-ATR-spectrometry has enabled us to register the IR-spectra of
polymer films on Avcothane-51 and on Avcomat-610 (a pure polyetherurethane) by subtraction of the strongly absorbing background
(fig. 3, fig. 4). From the striking band intensity differences in the
spectra shown in Fig. 4 a and b, representing samples of one min. and
seven hrs exposure time respectively, we can conclude that the nature
of the adsorbed proteins must be a function of the exposure time
and/or the actual state of the blood contact surface. Glycoproteins
with their γ-C-O around 1060 cm^{-1} are adsorbed on Avcomat-610 at a
greater rate than other plasma proteins at the begin of the exposure.

The adsorption of proteins on the polymer samples under investigation
may be reversible or at least partially irreversible. The latter would
point to a denaturation of the adsorbed proteins by strong interaction
with the polymer surface. In order to investigate this effect for
Avcomat 610 one segment of each explanted shunt was rinsed with
distilled water, then stored in a 0,9 % NaCl solution for up to
12 hours and finally analyzed by FTIR-ATR spectroscopy. Fig. 5 shows
the IR-spectra of the same samples as in fig. 4, also after complete
compensation of the polyurethane band (x). No amide bands are detected.
The conclusion is that the proteins have been desorbed from the polymer surface, because only weak interactions exist, what is in agreement with the clinical observation that Avcomat 610 is non thrombogenic.

REFERENCES

Baier, R.E. & Dutton, R.C. (1969) Initial Events in Interactions of
Blood with a Foreign Surface. J.Biomed.Mater Res 3, 191.
Kellner, R. (1979) Infrared Spectroscopy of Biocontact Polymers,
Proceedings of the Euroanalysis III conference, 1978, Applied Science
publ., London.
Kellner, R. & Unger, F. (1977) IR-spektroskopische Charakterisierung
der Blutverträglichkeit von Polyurethan-Silicon-Copolymeren, Z.Anal.
Chem. 283, 349.
Nyilas, E. (1976) Development of antithrombogenic artificial materials:
Theory and practice, in: Blood vessels p. 165, Springer-Verlag,
Heidelberg.

Nyilas, E. & Wards, R.S.Jr. (1977) Development of blood compatible
elastomers V: Surface structure and blood compatibility of Avcothane
elastomers, J. Biomed. Mater. Res. Symposium 8, 69.
Unger, F. (1975) Konstruktion eines künstlichen Herzens: Ellipsoid-
herz, Österreichische Patentanmeldung 1495/75.

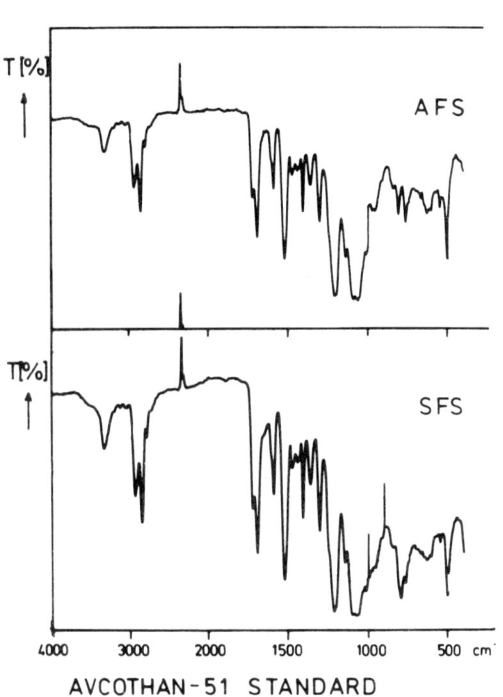

Fig. 1: IR-ATR spectra of the air facing side (AFS)
and the substrate facing side (SFS) of Avcothane-51

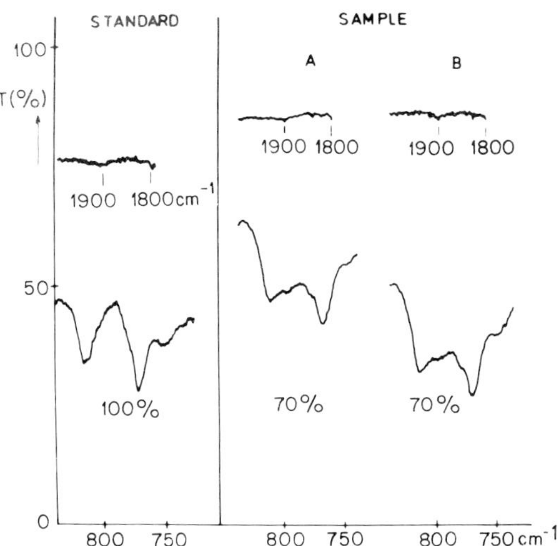

Fig. 2.
Quantitative evaluation of the IR-ATR spectra of Avcothane-51

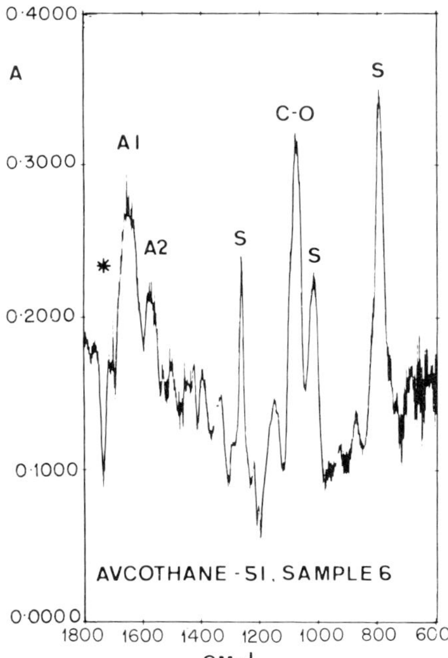

Fig. 3.
FTIR-ATR spectrum of Avcothane-51 minus spectrum of the polyurethane component.

* = compensated polyurethane band.
A1, A2 = protein amide 1 & 2 band.
S = siloxane bands.
C-O = glycoprotein band

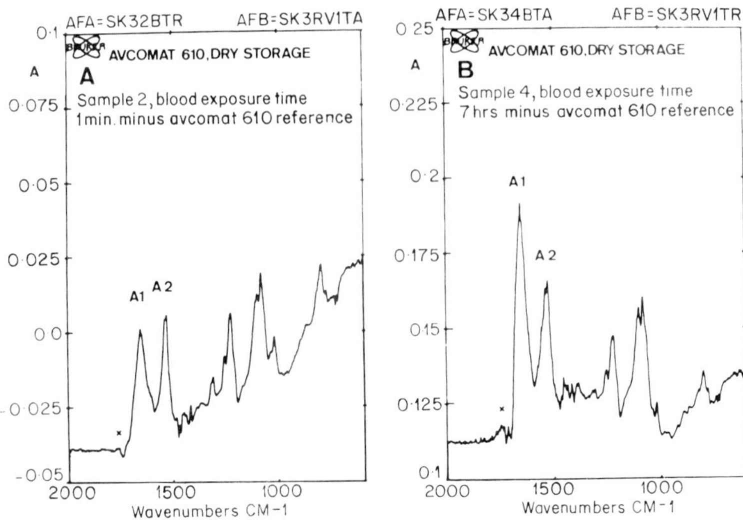

Fig.4:FTIR-ATR spectra of protein layers on Avcomat 610 samples, background compensated at 1730 cm^{-1}, A)blood-exposure time 1 min., B)blood exposure time 7 hrs

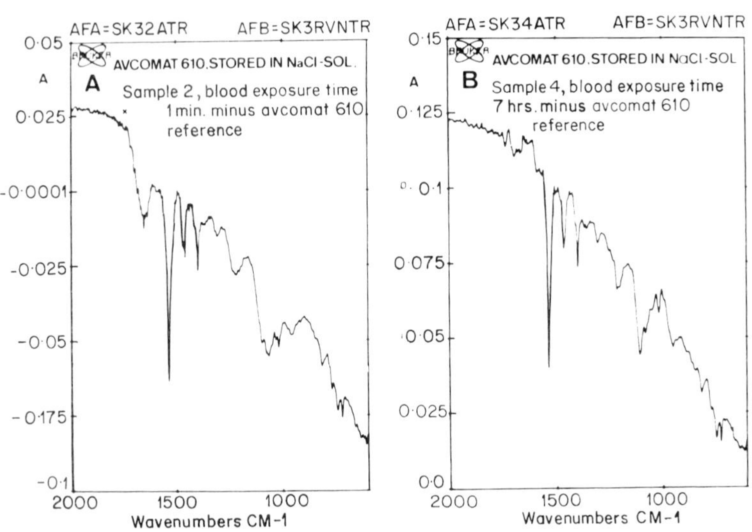

Fig.5:As in fig. 4, but aliquote samples after storage in aqueous NaCl-solution (0,9%), no protein bands detectable

Platelet interaction and thromboresistance

Biomaterials 1980
Edited by G. D. Winter, D. F. Gibbons, and H. Plenk, Jr.
© 1982 John Wiley and Sons Ltd.

DEVELOPMENT OF A NEW 'IN VITRO' TEST SYSTEM FOR MEASURING PLATELET INTERACTIONS WITH BIOMATERIALS

J. Olijslager[*], C.H.N. Veenhof[**], T. Beugeling[*] and J. Feijen[*]

[*] Twente University of Technology, Department of Chemical Technology, Enschede, The Netherlands.
[**] Department of Internal Medicine, 'Binnengasthuis', University of Amsterdam, Amsterdam, The Netherlands.

SUMMARY

An in vitro test system for measuring initial platelet adhesion on materials is described. In this system a test material mounted in one flow cell is directly compared with a reference material in a second cell. In this way both materials are tested under the same experimental conditions (flow, hematology). Freshly drawn canine blood is anticoagulated with heparin (3 IU ml^{-1}) and applied in the test system for 5 min under continuous flow (2 ml min^{-1} per cell). The results show a very good reproducibility and accordingly statistically significant differences are obtained with only a few experiments. A direct correlation is found between the number of adhering platelets and platelet morphology, but no correlation is found between these two phenomena and aggregate formation on material surfaces.

INTRODUCTION

In the past decade initial platelet adhesion on biomaterials has been extensively studied, because it is one of the first steps in thrombus formation. A number of factors influence platelet adhesion and thrombus formation on materials during the contact with blood. These factors are the surface properties of the materials, blood composition, flow conditions, and temperature. Various well defined test systems have been developed to study the adhesion process as a function of these factors. Well known examples are a number of flow cells (Lyman, 1968; Friedman, 1971; Grabowski, 1976), the spinning disc (Turitto, 1972), the Couette type (Feuerstein, 1975), and the stagnation point apparatus (Nyilas, 1975). If the platelet adhesion process is not diffusion controlled, such a system can also be used to differentiate between materials. A disadvantage of the systems mentioned before is, however, that a single test cell is used and that only one material is tested at a time. In the test system described in this article, two materials each placed in separate flow cells and connected to the same blood supply, are compared simultaneously.

Because flow rates and blood composition are equal in these cells, only a few experimental runs are required to obtain statistically significant differences in platelet adhesion. The principle of this test system has been described before (Beugeling, 1976). In this paper an improved design of the test system is described. The results of initial platelet adhesion for a number of materials in contact with heparinized canine blood is given.

METHODS

The schematic drawing of the initial platelet adhesion test system is given in Figure 1. The components used are successively a 3-way

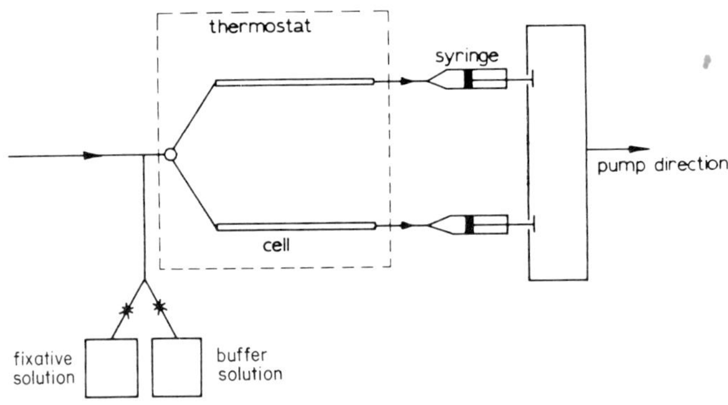

Fig. 1 Schematic set up for measuring initial platelet adhesion.

stopcock, 15 centimeters of silicone rubber tubing, a Y-connector, two test cells, two 3-way stopcocks, and two 60 ml syringes. The test cells consist of a silicone rubber gasket with in- and outflow tubing (manufactured by Talas, Ommen, The Netherlands), two pieces of test material (coated or mounted on glass plates), and two perspex plates. In this way a flow channel is created of 5 x 30 mm cross section and a length of 50 mm with smoothly curved in- and outflow sections. The cells are placed in a vertical position in a water bath (38°C). The cells are primed with a previously degassed buffer solution (0.15 M NaCl, 0.01 M NaH_2PO_4, pH 7.4). Blood (23.5 ml) is collected by venapuncture from anaesthetized mongrel dogs. The syringe contained 1.5 ml of a heparin solution (Thromboliquine; from porcine intestine, Organon Teknika BV, Oss, The Netherlands) yielding a final heparin concentration of 3 IU ml^{-1}. Immediately after venapuncture the syringe is placed into an electrically thermostated housing, carefully rocked, and connected to the first 3-way stopcock. After 5 min of blood flow (2 ml min^{-1} in each cell), the 3-way stopcock is turned to allow the buffer solution to displace the blood. The whole system is immediately turned upside down to facilitate the removal of blood by the action of gravity. After 5 min the flow is increased to 20 ml min^{-1} in each cell for 1.5 min, and then stopped. After 5 min a 2% glutardialdehyde buffer solution is introduced into the cells for fixation of the adhering blood cells. After fixation overnight the surfaces are dehydrated using a series of ethanol-water mixtures, and dried. In each cell three samples are cut from either side. These samples are sputter coated with a gold layer and are then studied by scanning electron microscopy (SEM).

On each sample 10 surface areas are studied to count the adhering platelets; these areas are located at fixed distances on a straight line perpendicular to the flow direction. When more then half of the number of platelets present in a surface area are incorporated in aggregates, this is recorded as an 'aggregated surface area'. Generally a magnification of 2000 x is used, which results in a surface area for counting of 2500 μ^2. The average platelet adhesion number for a material is obtained from counts on 60 different surfaces of 2500 μ^2. The platelet adhesion ratio is calculated by dividing the average platelet adhesion number on the test material by the corresponding number on the reference material. The mean platelet adhesion ratio is calculated by averaging over the number (n) of experiments. The aggregation ratio is the number of 'aggregated surface areas' in the test cell divided by the corresponding number in the reference cell. The mean aggregation ratio is obtained by averaging over the number of experiments. The statistical significance of the determined ratios is calculated by testing the null-hypothesis using the two sided Student distribution (Diem, 1972).

<u>MATERIALS</u>

The following materials were used for testing. Silicone rubber sheeting (SR$_E$; 120 μ, Edwards Laboratories Santa Ana, California, U.S.A.), silicone rubber medical sheeting (SR$_D$; 120 μ, Dow Corning Corporation, Medical Products, Midland, Michigan, U.S.A.), cuprophane (Cup; 18 μ, cellophane PT 150, Enka Glanzstoff AG, Bemberg W-Germany), cellulose acetate (CA; TV 20, Fabelta SA, Tubize, Belgium), poly(vinyl chloride) (PVC, applied for blood bags, Draka Plastics, Enkhuizen, The Netherlands), and glass (Glass, glass plates used for thin layer chromatography art. 5715, Merck, Darmstadt, W-Germany). Cup films contain additives which are removed by soaking in double distilled water (changed often) for 24 hours. Because Cup also swells in water the films are mounted in the test cell in a wet state. Ca films are prepared by casting a solution of CA in acetone (2%, w/w) on glass plates. Residual acetone is removed in a vacuum oven at room temperature.

SR$_D$ and SR$_E$ surfaces are also modified by grafting a low molecular weight polyelectrolyte (PLE) with heparinoid activity onto these surfaces using gamma radiation (Sederel, 1979). An albuminated surface is obtained by displacing the priming solution in <u>one</u> cell, which is equiped with SR$_D$ sheeting, by <u>a</u> dog albumin solution (4 g L^{-1}, 38 C; fraction V, no A9263, Sigma® Chemical Co., St. Louis, USA). After 2 h adsorption, this solution is again displaced by buffer, and blood flow is initiated within ten min. From previous experiments it is known that under these conditions the plateau value for albumin adsorption is reached within 2 hours.

All solutions used have a pH of 7.4, and are previously degassed at room temperature for ten minutes at a pressure of 20 mm Hg. This procedure proved to be very succesfull in avoiding the formation of air bubbles onto the polymer surfaces.

RESULTS

The mean platelet adhesion ratio and the mean aggregation ratio for combinations of materials are presented in Table 1. Cup is usually

Material	n	Mean adhesion ratio	Signifi- cance level (P)	Mean aggregation ratio	Signifi- cance level (P)
SR_E/Cup	3	0.46	0.03	–	–
SR_D/Cup	16	0.83	0.001	4	0.001
PVC/Cup	2	0.91	0.08	0.5	–
CA/Cup	7	0.94	0.52	0.02	0.001
Glass/Cup	3	0.70	0.03	2	0.56
SR_E-PLE/SR_E	1	0.36	–	1	–
SR_D-PLE/SR_D	4	0.38	0.001	3	0.50
SR_D-DA/SR_D	4	1.26	0.005	0.05	0.001

Table 1 Mean Platelet adhesion- and aggregation ratio

taken as the reference material. But when the surface properties of materials are modified, e.g. by grafting or by adsorption of proteins, the untreated material is used as a reference. Except for CA/Cup and PVC/Cup all mean platelet adhesion ratios are statistically signifi- cant different from unity at a 5% level. The values for the mean aggregation ratios undicate that there is no relationship between ad- hesion and aggregate formation on materials. This is illustrated in Figure 2 for the system CA/Cup. These materials show equal platelet

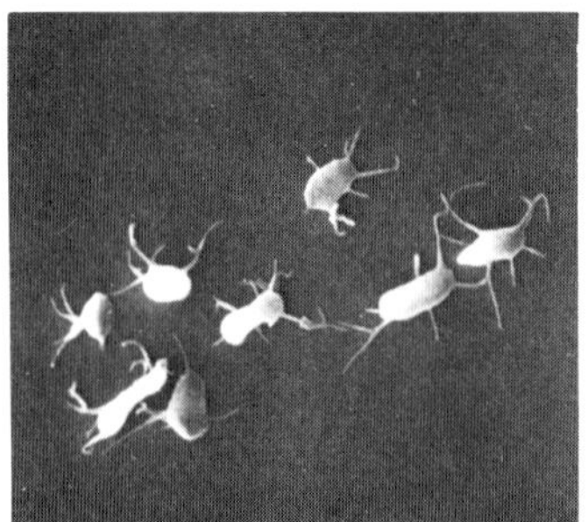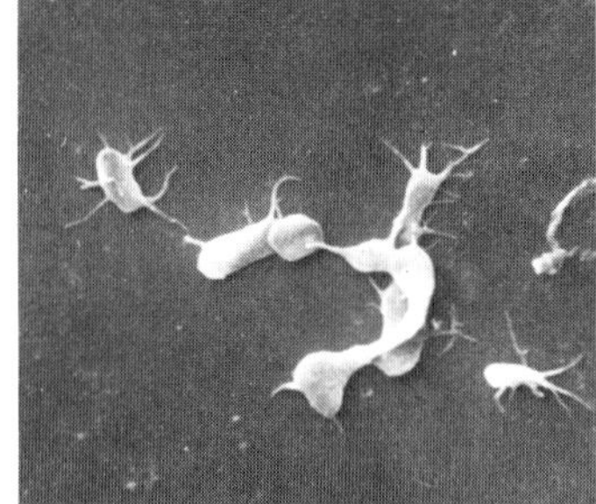

Fig. 2 Comparison of aggregate formation on CA (left) and Cup.

adhesion numbers but aggregate formation is almost exclusively found
on Cup. The shapes of the individual platelets on different materials
also differ. They can be long or round with many, few, or no pseudopodia. Typical examples are given in Figure 3.

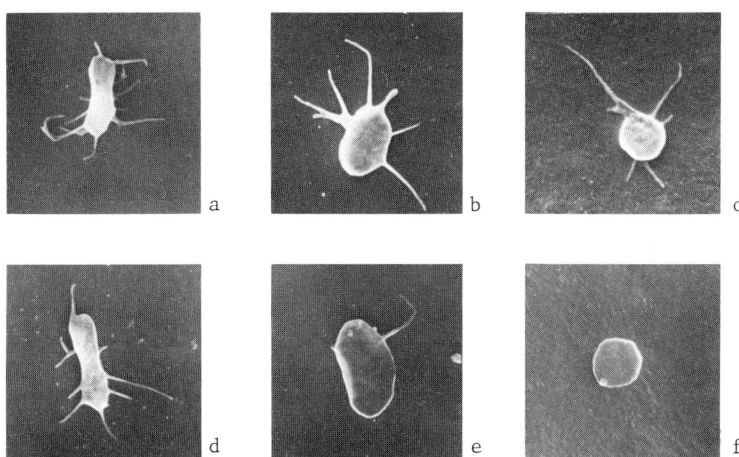

Fig. 3 Typical examples of the shapes of platelets on CA (a),
PVC (b), SR_E (c), Cup (d), Glass (e), and SR_E-PLE (f).

DISCUSSION

With the system described, differentiation between materials with
respect to initial platelet adhesion can be obtained. Because of the
good reproducability of the method only a few experiments are required to obtain statistically significant results. Platelet adhesion
for different positions in the cell do not show differences, which
implies that during the blood material contact, sufficient platelets
are available for adhesion. The measured differences in platelet adhesion numbers must therefore be attributed to differences in affinity of platelets for different materials.

In addition to the measurements of initial platelet adhesion numbers,
the test also provides insight into platelet aggregate formation. No
relationship is found between adhesion and aggregate formation on
materials, however, platelets found on different test materials exhibit differences in pseudopod formation. In general, adhering platelets
with many pseupopods are found on materials with high platelet adhesion numbers. In our opinion the amount of platelet aggregates found
on material surfaces might be a better indication for eventual thrombus formation than the number of adhering platelets.

It was expected that both the silicone rubber modified with DA and
that with PLE would show a significant decrease in platelet numbers
as compared to the untreated material (Wicher, 1978; Beugeling, 1976).
The decrease was only found with the PLE grafted surface. The DA
treated surface showed an increased platelet adhesion number, which

might be due to the presence of 4% of α_2 macro globulines in the albumin.

In conclusion, the system described can be used as a fast screening method for materials with respect to initial platelet adhesion and aggregate formation on the surface. Furthermore there is no relationship between aggregate formation and the number of platelets on the surface.

ACKNOWLEDGEMENT

We like to thank the members of the team of the animal facility in Muiderberg for their assistance during the experiments, and mr. M.A. de Jongh for his valuable support during the work with the scanning electron microscope.

REFERENCES

Beugeling, T., Feijen,J., Tijhuis, A.H.J., Froehling, P.E., de Jongh, M.A., Looze-van Iperen, M., and Bantjes, A. (1976). Reduced Platelet Adhesion onto Polymer Surfaces Coated With a Synthetic Heparinoid Polyelectrolyte - Investigations on Blood-Surface Interactions With the Aid of a Flow System. in Proceedings European Society for Artificial Organs 3 (ed. E.S. Bücherl), pp. 76-82, Westkreuz, Berlin.
Diem, K., and Leutner, C. (1972), Scientific Tables. 7th ed., Ciba-Geigy Limited, Basel.
Feuerstein, I.A., Brophy, J.M., and Brash, J.L. (1975). Platelet transport and adhesion to reconstituted collagen and artificial surfaces, Trans. Amer. Soc. Artif. Int. Organs 21, 427-435.
Friedman, L.I., and Leonard, E.F. (1971), Platelet adhesion to artificial surfaces: consequences of flow, exposure time, blood condition, and surface nature. Federation Proceedings 30, 1641-1646.
Grabowski, E.F., Herther, K.K., and Didisheim, P. (1976). Human vs. dog platelet adhesion to Cuprophane under controlled condition of whole blood flow. J. Lab. Clin. Med 88, 368-374.
Lyman, D.J., Brash, J.L., Chaikin, S.W., Klein, K.G., and Carini, M., (1968), The effect of chemical structure and surface properties of synthetic polymers on the coagulation of blood. II Protein and platelet interaction with polymer surfaces. Trans. Am. Soc. Artif. Int. Organs 14, 250-255.
Nyilas, E., Morton, W.A., Lederman, D.M., Chiu, T.H., and Cumming, R.D. (1975). Interdependence of hemodynamic and surface parameters in thrombosis. Trans Amer. Soc. Artif. Int. Organs 21, 55-70.
Sederel, L.C. Olijslager, J., de Koning, H.W.M., van der Does, L., Beugeling, T. Feijen, J. and Bantjes, A., (1979). Non-thrombogenic surfaces by radiation-induced grafting and crosslinking of a synthetic polyelectrolyte: Preparation and in vitro studies, to be published in the Proceedings of the COMAC Workshop on New Aspects in Anticoagulant Therapy during Extracorporeal Circulation, Lindhurst, United Kingdom.
Turitto, V.T., and Leonard, E.F. (1972). Platelet adhesion to a spinning disc. Trans Amer. Soc. Artif. Int. Organs 18, 348-354.
Whicher, S.J., and Brash, J.L. (1978). Platelet foreign surface interactions: Release of granule constituents from adherent platelets, J. Biomed. Mat. Res. 12, 181-201.

Biomaterials 1980
Edited by G. D. Winter, D. F. Gibbons, and H. Plenk, Jr.
© 1982 John Wiley and Sons Ltd.

BLOOD COMPATIBILITY OF POLYMERS: AN IN VITRO METHOD OF ASSESSMENT

S. K. Bowry, J.M. Courtney, C.R.M. Prentice* and J.P. Paul

Bioengineering Unit, University of Strathclyde, Glasgow
*Royal Infirmary, Glasgow

SUMMARY

Research in the area of biomaterials is limited by the lack of acceptable biocompatibility test methods which characterise the properties of biomaterials.
This paper presents a new in vitro method for the assessment of the blood compatibility of polymers.

It is believed that the rate of platelet aggregation and thrombus formation
depends on the type of material which the blood contacts. The method
involves rotation of citrated platelet-rich plasma in loops in different materials
under test, and the observation of the time of appearance of the "snowstorm"
after recalcification of the plasma. The snowstorm of small platelet aggregates
is the first of the aggregation parameters observed towards the formation of a
thrombus. The method is based on Chandler's (1958) original concept of
studying in vitro thrombi.

Preliminary experiments showed that the method is capable of differentiating
materials in terms of their thrombogenicity: PVC from two different sources
was tested and one was significantly less thrombogenic than the other. Also,
when two different types of silicone rubbers and natural rubber were compared,
there was little difference between the silicone rubbers, but both were superior
to the natural rubber. The results are in agreement with the PTT (partial
thromboplastin time) test, which is another method of assessing blood
compatibility. Further, scanning electron microscopy studies were carried out
to compare in vitro and in vivo thrombi.

INTRODUCTION

In recent years development of blood-contacting devices has stimulated research
into problems of the compatibility of blood with the foreign surfaces used. Ideal
materials should not activate clotting factors, cause platelet aggregation, or
cause local damage to the surrounding tissues. The main limitation in the
development of implantable artificial organs and devices has been the thrombotic
problems associated with these materials. Despite several advances, no

synthetic material has been produced that is totally free from a thrombogenic
response, to match the normal endothelium which has the unique property of
being totally compatible with blood.

Blood compatibility may be defined as the ability of an artificial surface to
prevent activation of platelets or the intrinsic mechanism of blood coagulation
(Mason et al 1974).   Protein denaturation, haemolysis, thrombo-embolism and
loss of leukocytic function are further consequences of protein adsorption at the
blood-material interface.   Further, blood compatibility covers certain dynamic
factors inherent in an implantable system.   Device manifold cross-sections, for
example, cause changes in blood flow which may lead to cavitation or emergence
from solution of dissolved blood gases.

The Report of the Task Force on Biomaterials (Galletti et al 1978), states that the
major roadblock to the development of materials to handle blood is the lack of
an operational definition of blood compatibility.   Consensus on such a definition
will not be forthcoming until there is at least a provisional agreement among
scientists on test and evaluation methods which quantitatively define the blood
compatibility of materials, and which characterise the surface and bulk
properties of biomaterials in physical-chemical terms.   The Report lists three
main problem areas in biomaterials research: a) definition of materials (b)
definition of blood and (c) definition of the test system.   In this study we have
directed our attention to the last of these problems.

Chandler (1958) devised a technique to produce an _in vitro_ thrombus, its histological structure resembling a thrombus formed _in vivo._   Since then this method
has been used to study platelet aggregation and plug information (Silver, 1970),
the effect of anticoagulant drugs on platelet aggregation (Cunningham et al 1965)
the acceleration of thrombus formation by certain fatty acids (Connor, 1961)
and in the prevention of platelet adhesion and aggregation by a glutaraldehyde
stabilised heparin surface (Olsson et al 1977).   In our project we have used the
Chandler's loop to develop a new method for evaluating the blood compatibility
of polymers used in surgery.   Since it has been shown that platelet adhesion
and aggregation is dependent on the type of material with which the blood
comes into contact, (Feijen, 1976), and as Chandler's method has been used
to study adhesion and aggregation phenomena, it is reasonable to deduce that,
for different materials, the rate of platelet aggregation would be directly proportional to the compatibility with blood of the material of which the loop is
composed.   If this method could show a difference between materials already in
use for blood-contact purposes according to their known thrombogenicity, then
new materials could be tested for blood compatibility.

The general aims of this project were, first, the development of a new technique
of assessing the blood compatibility of polymers, and second, the assessment of
candidate polymers for their thrombogenicity using the rotating loop method and
the comparison of results with another blood compatibility method.   The materials
were investigated in two groups: in the first group, two types of polyvinyl-

chloride were compared and, in the second group, silicone rubber from two
different sources and natural rubber were compared.

MATERIALS AND METHOD

(a)   The "tube method" of Lee and White (1913) was employed as a preliminary
screening test for all blood donors to check that clotting times were within the
normal range.
(b)   Partial throboplastin time test (PTT).   This was performed as described by
Biggs (1976) by using a commercial PTT reagent (BCL London).   The test is
normally carried out in test tubes coated with the material under test, but as
tubing was used for the rotating loop test, small pieces of the tubing were
clamped at the bottom and used for the PTT test.   For glass, the test was
carried out in new test tubes measuring 3 in x 3/8th in.
(c)   The rotating loop test.   (Chandler tube, 1958).

(i)   The test is a closed loop system made from the material under test.   These
tubes are used to measure the time taken for platelet aggregation and thrombus
to occur after insertion and recalcification of citrated platelet-rich plasma
(PRP).

The test involves rotating a tube of the material under consideration with human
citrated PRP, and, after the addition of calcium observing the time of
appearance of the following events for tests of platelet function (Fig. 1):

       1.   first particles
       2.   "snowstorm"
       3.   aggregates
       4.   plug
       5.   thrombus

The time of appearance of the snowstorm after recalcification was taken as the
end point, since the rate of formation of thrombus depends on the rate of
formation of the snowstorm.   The snowstorm is the first stage in the formation
of a thrombus due to the sudden appearance of many small particles which
increase rapidly in size.

(ii)   The rig consisted of the loop on a blackend aluminium disc rotated at
12-15 rpm at an angle of 80° from the horizontal to simulate flow conditions.
A digital stopwatch was mounted below the disc to observe the time appearance
of the snowstorm.   (Fig. 2).   Nine volumes of blood were mixed with one
volume of trisodium citrate (3.8%) solution and centrifuged at 150g for 3
minutes to obtain PRP.   All glassware was siliconized with dimethyldichloro-
silane in acetone.

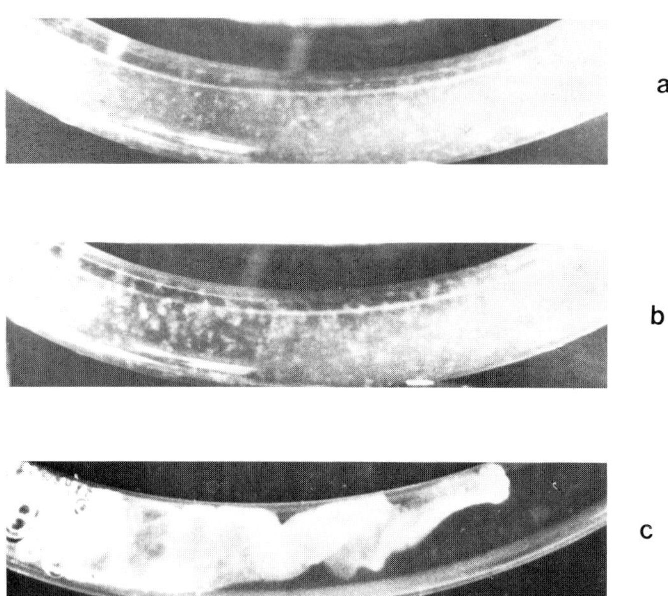

Fig. 1. Events leading to the formation of an <u>in vitro</u> thrombus a) first particles (b) "snowstorm" c) thrombus.

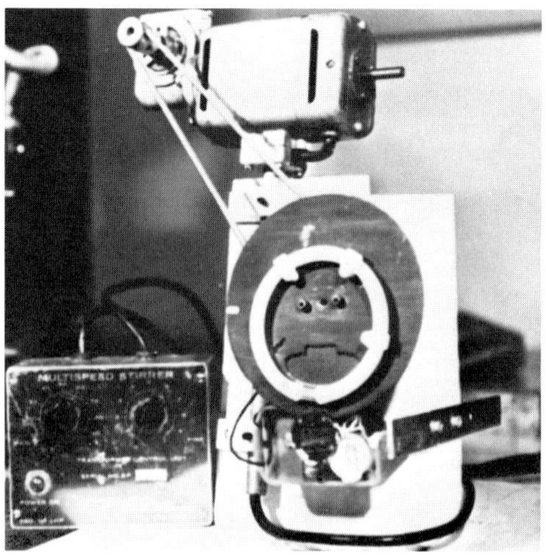

Fig. 2. The experimental rig.

(iii)   25 cm length pieces of tubing of all materials investigated were used. The materials were studied in two groups.   In one group, PVC from arterial extracorporeal sets (LE 611) made by Sorin Biomedica (13040 Saluggia, Italy) was compared with blood tubing, grade VN714/4 supplied by Avon Medicals. In the second group silicone rubber from Dow Corning (Medical grade tubing, lot HO59592) and medical grade tubing supplied by Silicone Altimex Ltd. (Nottingham, England) were compared with tubes extruded from purified, untreated natural rubber latex (from Malaysian Rubber Producers' Research Association).   For transparent materials such as PVC, the two ends of the tube were brought together and joined firmly by an external plastic collar to form a circle.   For opaque materials e.g. natural and silicone rubbers a small standard piece of transparent PVC was inserted in the material to enable the snowstorm to be observed.   The two ends of the PVC window were tapered with abrasive paper so that a minimal lip was exposed to the blood.   While the insertion of the window may itself induce thrombus formation, it must be remembered that this is essentially an in vitro test method; for instance, an air-blood interface is present.   However, the irregularities were minimised and standardised.

(iv)   0.1 ml of buffered physiological saline solution (0.15M sodium chloride buffered with 0.05M imidazole buffer, pH 7.4), was run into the tubing followed by 1 ml of PRP and the loop rotated for 30 seconds.   After this mixing period, 0.1 ml of 0.25M calcium chloride solution was added, the stop-watch started simultaneously and the loop rotated at 12 rpm.   The time of appearance of the snowstorm was recorded by a photographic method.

(v)   It is often difficult to ascertain the exact time of appearance of the snow-storm.   The post-snowstorm period can last for several seconds and can often be erroneously regarded as the endpoint.   Further, as it was hoped to assess loops of opaque materials, the insertion of a transparent window allows only about one second to observe the plasma.   Hence another method, preferably one which allowed the aggregation events to be recorded, was required.

On the principle that protein solutions opalescent to visible light are clear in infrared, high speed infrared photography was first used in an attempt to solve the problem of detecting the snowstorm.   However, as infrared film has to be loaded and unloaded in the dark and filters have to be used, Ektachrome film, ED136, ASA200 for colour slides was tried and found to give results far superior than those from infrared photography.   Best results were obtained at f5.6 and shutter speed of 1/25th of a second using a vivitar close-up lens (35 - 105 mm).   To measure the start of the snowstorm, the frames were exposed once every three seconds.

RESULTS

(a)   The partial thromboplastin times are given in (Fig. 3).   Mean values are based on a minimum of three tests for each material.   Figure 3 shows that the

Biomedica PVC differs from the Avon PVC, but the test does not differentiate
the silicone rubber varieties.   However, making no assumptions on the distribution characteristics of the PTT values a Rank Sum Test was performed using
the data on the PVCs and SRs.   The PTTs are significantly different at the
0.025 – 0.05 level.   This must be considered as an approximate level of
significance.

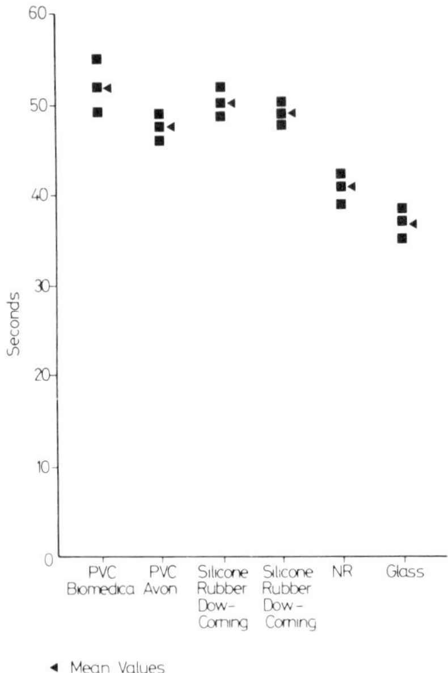

Fig. 3   The PTT Test

(b)   Rotating loop test.   In group one (polyvinylchlorides), 1 ml of plasma
from the same donor was used for the two types of PVC, and in group two
(silicone rubbers and natural rubber), 0.5 ml of plasma from the same donor
was used for each of the three materials, thus minimising variation in samples.
Also, as the time of standing of plasma may change platelet function, the first
test run was alternated between materials in each group.   Platelet count for
all plasma samples was between 225,000 – 450,000 per cubic microlitre.

Fig. 4 gives the time of appearance of the snowstorm after recalcification for
the two types of PVC.   A statistical test of significance, the t-test for paired
samples (correlated data), was applied.   The difference between the two
PVCs is significant at the 5% level; the calculated value of t is 2.885 while
the p value from the table is 2.306.

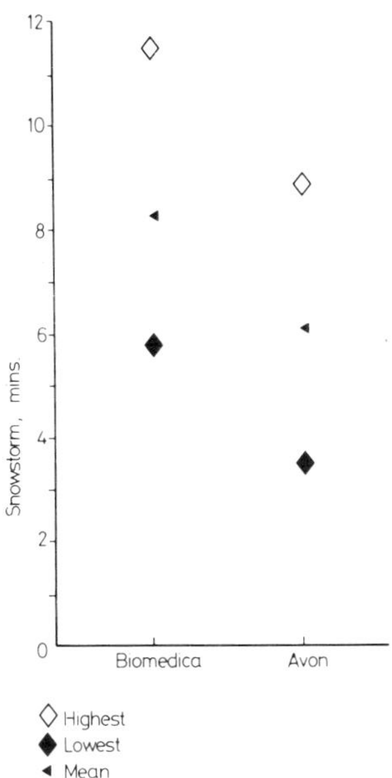

Fig. 4.   Rotating loop test on the PVC's

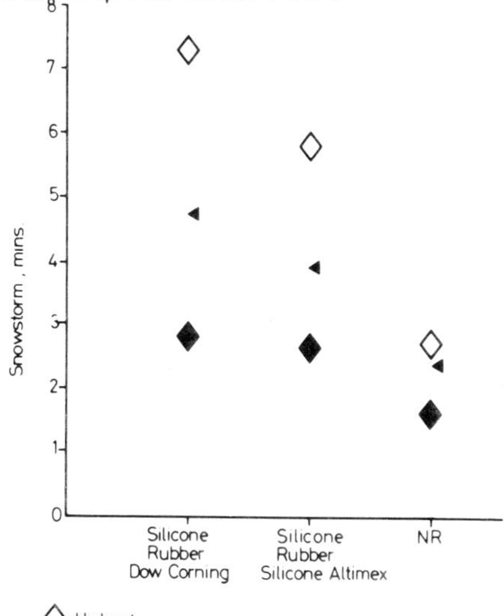

Fig. 5.   Rotating loop test on silicone rubbers and natural rubber

Fig. 5 gives the time of appearance of the snowstorm for materials in group two.   As the number of tests was small, no test of significance was carried out. However, the difference between the two types of silicone rubbers is small while the NR is different from the silicone rubbers.   The method thus detects differences between different materials.   The results of experiments in both groups are in agreement with those obtained from the PTT test.

(c)   Factors influencing platelet aggregation. (i)   Effect of time of mixing of saline with PRP.   It was found that if the period of mixing prior to calcium addition was increased from the standard 30 second period, the rate of platelet aggregation became longer compared to the 30 second control.   Spontaneous aggregation occurred when mixing was allowed for longer periods, even in the absence of calcium ions.   In these cases large aggregates or plugs were not formed after calcium addition.   Silver (1970) made similar observations.

(ii) Time of standing of normal PRP.   The appearance of normal platelet aggregation depended on the time of standing of PRP at room temperature after venipuncture before the tests were carried out.   Abnormal aggregation was observed before 12 minutes and after 30 minutes of standing PRP after veni- puncture.   Silver (1970) reported similar observations although he obtained abnormal parameters before 24 min. and after one hour, and refers to this as the "fade-in" and "fade-out" phenomena.   Thus, it is important, as far as possible, to conduct the tests between the two time intervals.

(d)   Scanning electron microscopy .   The thrombus formed by the rotating loop method is   (Figure   6a)   in many ways, similar to an in vivo thrombus.   In particular, the common features were platelet adhesion and aggregation and formation of a plug which is trapped in a network of fibrin to form the thrombus.

DISCUSSION

Platelet count of PRP.   It was observed that, in general, the appearance of the aggregation parameters was prolonged when the platelet count was decreased. However, no absolute relationship between platelet count and the time of appearance of the snowstorm could be determined.

The tests done on two different types of PVC show that the rotating loop method is capable of differentiating polymeric materials in terms of their thrombo- genicity.   The results from the rotating loop test are supported by results from the other blood compatibility method (PTT test).   Biomedica PVC is signi- ficantly less thrombogenic than the Avon PVC.   The silicone rubbers were found less thrombogenic than NR.   Very little difference was detected between Dow Corning silicone rubber and that supplied by Silicone-Altimex Ltd; these two rubbers have the same formulation, verified by Silicone-Altimex Ltd after the experiments were complete.

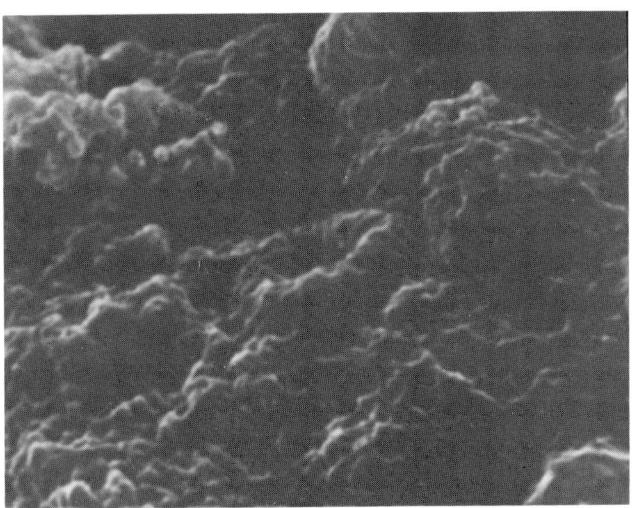

Fig. 6   SEM of thrombus formed with whole blood

The SEM studies showed that the thrombus formed in the rotating loop is, in many ways similar to the formation of an <u>in vivo</u> thrombus.   The morphology of the <u>in vitro</u> thrombus (in Fig. 6) shows platelet aggregates and the fibrin network deposited over the blood contents.

Hence, although the objectives of the project have been satisfactorily fulfilled, and that the method has the potential of being adopted as a test of blood compatibility, further refinements of the method need to be done to obtain quantitative results if the method is to become acceptable.   In particular, the spontaneous aggregation and the fade-in and fade-out phenomena observed need to be understood and defined.   Studies on the rotating loop method using platelets labelled with ^{111}Indium are being carried out.

ACKNOWLEDGEMENT

We are grateful to Avon Medicals, Birmingham, England, Malaysian Rubber Producers' Research Association and Silicone-Altimex Ltd., Stapleford, Nottingham, England for the provision of materials.

REFERENCES

Biggs, R. (1976) <u>Human blood coagulation, Haemostasis and Thrombosis</u> 2nd Edition, Blackwell Scientific Publications, Oxford.

Chandler, A. B. (1958) Lb. Investigation Vol. 7
Connor, W. E. (1961) J. Clin. Invest. 41, 1199 - 1205
Cunningham, G.M., McNicol, G.P. & Douglas, A. S. (1965) The Lancet April 1965.
Feijen, J. (1976) In Artificial Organs, (Ed. R.M. Kenedi et al) pp 235
Galletti, P.M., Brash, J.L., Keller, K.H., LaFarge, G., Mason, R.G., Pierce, W.S. & Reynolds, J.A. (1978) Biomaterials Task Force Report Artificial Organs, Vol. 2, 189 - 201
Lee, R. I. & White, P. D. (1913) Am. J. of Med. Sci. 145: 495 -
Olsson, P., Lagergren, H., Larsson, R. & Radegran, K. (1977) Thrombos Haemostase 37, 274 -
Silver, M.J. (1970) Am. J. of Physiology Vol. 218, 384 -
Mason, R. G., Shermer, R. W. & Zucker, W.H. (1974) An in vitro test system for estimation of B.C. of Biomaterials J. Biomed. Mater. Res. Vol.18 341 - 356.

ROLE OF MICROPHASE SEPARATED STRUCTURE IN INTERACTION
BETWEEN POLYMER AND PLATELET

T.Okano*, M.Shimada**, I.Shinohara**, K.Kataoka*
T.Akaike* and Y.Sakurai*

*Institute of Medical Engineering, Tokyo Women's Medical
College, Shinjuku-ku, Tokyo 162, JAPAN
**Department of Polymer Chemistry, Waseda University,
Shinjuku-ku, 162, JAPAN

SUMMARY

ABA type block copolymers composed of 2-hydroxyethyl methacrylate(HEMA),
a hydrophilic monomer, and styrene(St), a hydrophobic monomer were
synthesized in order to elucidate the effect of hydrophilic and hydrophobic microdomains in interaction of the polymer with blood platelets.
Platelet adhesion and deformation on teh block polymer surface with or
without protein precoating were studied by microsphere column method
comparing with homogeneous surfaces of PHEMA and PSt, It was found
that orientation and distribution of adsorbed protein regulated by
the microstructure of hydrophilic and hydrophobic sites played an
important role in interaction between polymers and platelets.

INTRODUCTION

Platelet adhesion plays a major role in the <u>in vivo</u> initiation of
thrombus formation on a foreign surface. In order to design antithrombogenic polymers, therefore, it is important to clarify the
influence of adsorbed proteins on interaction between polymer and
platelet (Sakurai, et al., 1980)

We have been studying the interaction between polymer and blood, so
as to elucidate the effect of the hydrophilic and hydrophobic microphase separation of copolymers. It was found that a 2-hydroxyethyl
methacrylate(HEMA)-styrene block copolymer, having a microphase
separated structure, exhibited excellent antithrombogenic properties
due to the inhibition of platelet adhesion and aggregation (Okano,
et al., 1979a). Measurement of the adsorbed blood proteins on the
copolymer surface showed that serum albumin was adsorbed on the
hydrophilic domain, while γ-globulin and fibrinogen were selectively
adsorbed on the hydrophobic domains (Okano, et al., 1978a)

In this paper, the interaction of platelets with the HEMA-styrene
block copolymer surface with or without preadsorped blood proteins
was investigated by the microsphere column beads method (Kataoka,

445

et al., 1978). From these results, the effect of adsorbed protein,
on the block copolymer surface, on platelet adhesion was discussed in
comparison with the case of homopolymer surfaces.

EXPERIMENTAL

<u>Material</u>: Fig.1 shows the structure formula of ABA type block co-
polymer composed of HEMA(A) and styrene(B), synthesized from teleche-
lic ologomers by the method described in a previous paper (Okano,
et al., 1978b). This block copolymer containing 0.608 mole fraction
of HEMA exhibits alternate lamellae, as shown in Fig.2.

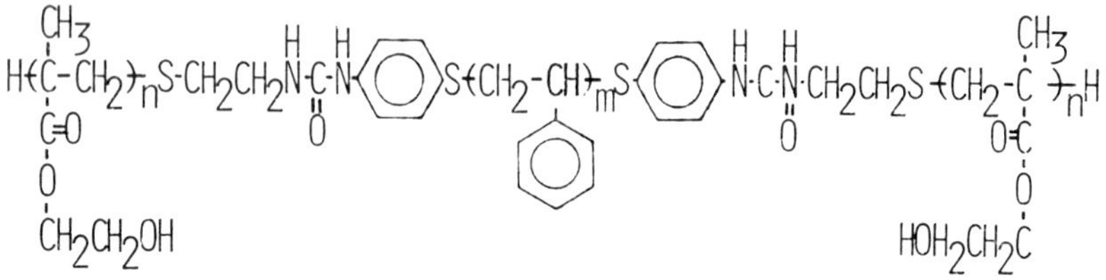

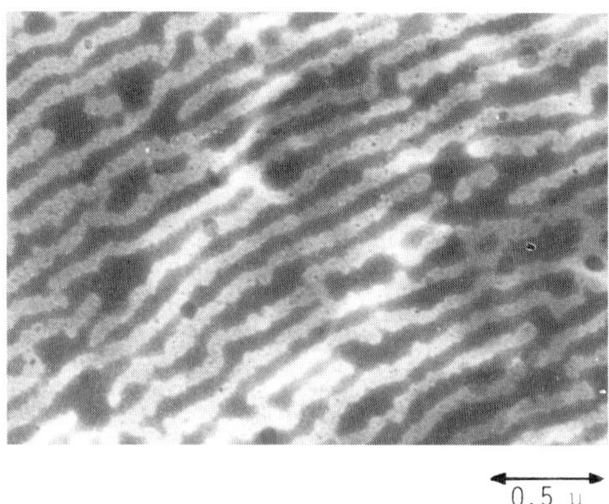

Fig.1 Chemical structure of HEMA-St ABA type block
copolymer

Fig.2 Electron micrograph of HEMA-St ABA type block
copolymer film cast from DMF at 40°C stained with osmium
tetroxide (HEMA mole fraction 0.608)

<u>Analysis of Platelet Adhesion and Deformation</u>: Glass beads (40-60 mesh) precoated with polymer samples with or without preadsorped proteins were packed into a column (i.d. 3 mm, length 10 cm) of poly(vinyl chloride) through which fresh canine blood collected from the jugular vein was pumped at 1.2 ml/min for 1 min. Eluted blood is collected and examined by counting retention of platelets on the column according to the method of Brecher and Cronkite (Brecher, et al., 1950). After blood perfusion, the beads were rinsed with the saline solution, then treated with glutaraldehyde and freeze-dried. The morphology of adhered platelets was observed by scanning electron microscopy.

<u>RESULTS AND DISCUSSION</u>

<u>Effect of Adsorbed Proteins on Platelet Adhesion</u>: The number of adhered platelets on the block copolymer surface with or without precoating of proteins was examined and compared with the homopolymer surface systems. These results are shown in Fig.3. The block copolymer, which has a hydrophilic-hydrophobic microphase separated structure of alternate lamellae, showed less platelet adhesion as

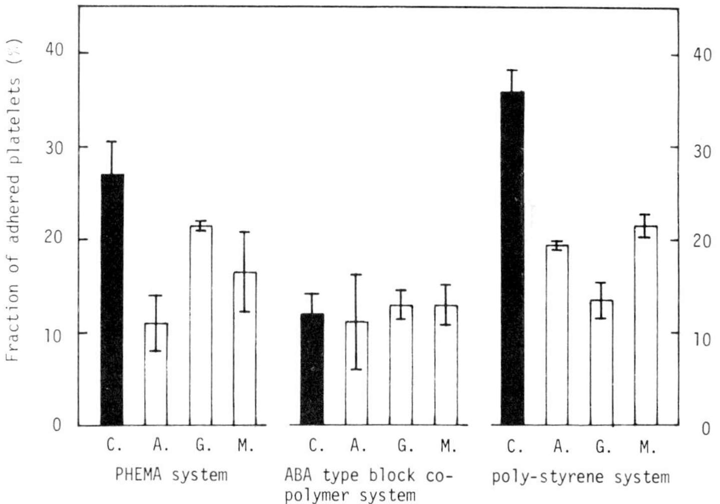

Fig.3 Fraction of adhered platelets on blood protein precoated surfaces C.; control, A.; albumin precoated, G.; γ-globulin precoated, M.; albumin-γ-globulin micture precoated, % = (number of adhered platelets)/(number of whole blooc platelets) x 100 ± s.e.m.

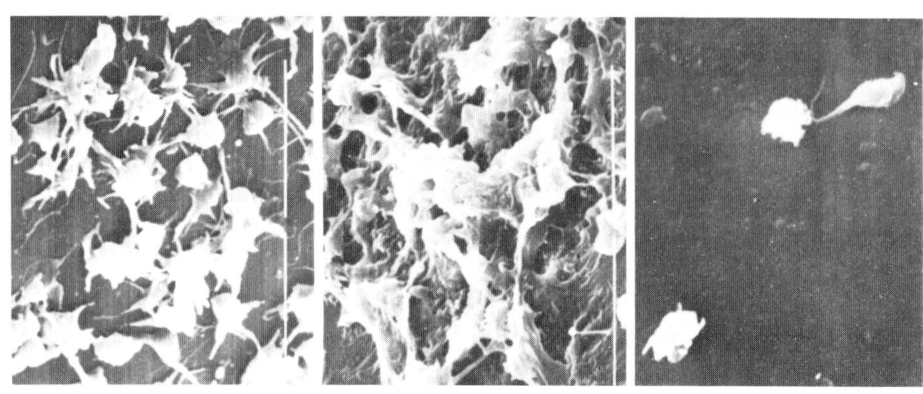

PHEMA   Poly-Styrene   ABA type block copolymer

Fig.4   Influence of polymer surfaces on platelets adhesion
(protein non-coated system, canine whole blood, X 4,700)

compared with the hydrophilic or the hydrophobic homopolymers. In the
block copolymer system, the number of adhered platelets was constant
and independent of albumin and/or γ-globulin precoating. In the homopolymer systems, however, the number of adhered platelets was decreased
when precoated by proteins. The PHEMA surface precoated with albumin
and the polystryrene surface precoated with γ-globulin, however, also
showed reduced platlet adhesion.

Effect of Adsorbed Proteins on Morphology of the Adhered Platelet:
Remarkable differences in the morphology of the adhered platelet on
the surfaces of the block copolymer, PHEMA and polystyrene were
observed as shown in Fig.4. In the case of polystyrene surface, the
adhered platelets exhibited many speudopods and were aggregated.
In the case of PHEMA surface, adhesion and aggregation of platelets
was also observed. On the contrary, only isolated adhered platelets
were observed, without aggregation, on the surface of the block copolymer. In this case, the morphology of the adhered platelets
showed less pseudopodia.

On surfaces precoated with serum albumin, the morphologies of the
adhered platelets were similar to the block copolymer.

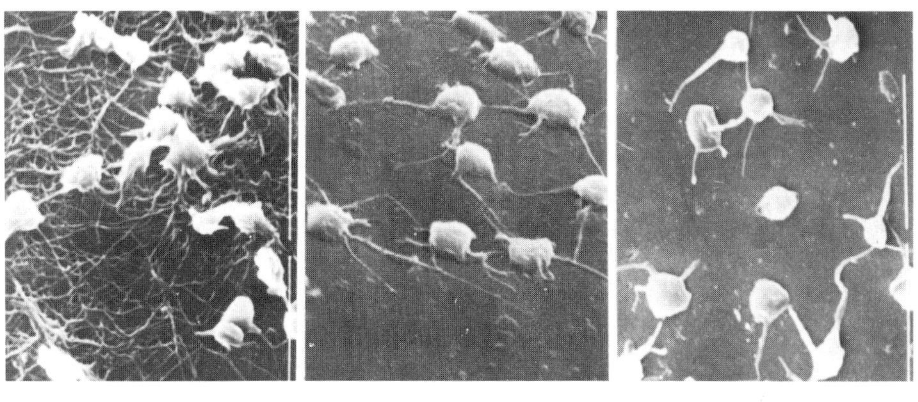

PHEMA   Poly-Styrene   ABA type block copolymer

Fig.5   Influence of polymer surfaces on platelet adhesion
(γ-globulin precoated system, canine whole blood, X 4,700)

On the surfaces precoated with γ-globulin, the morphology of adhered
platelet on PHEMA differed from that on polystyrene, as shown in Fig.5.
That is, platelets adhered moderately without aggregation on the
γ-globulin precoated hydrophobic surface of polystyrene, whereas,
the adhered platelets on the γ-globulin precoated hydrophilic surface
of HPEMA exhibited spreading and many pseudopodia. This difference is
considered to be due to the different orientation of adsorbed γ-globulin
on the hydrophilic and the hydrophobic surface. The γ-globulin molecule
has an anisotropic structure, i.e., the Fc segment of γ-globulin is
more hydrophobic, the Fab segment more hydrophilic (Van Oss, et al.,
1975). Our experimental results on the conformational change of adsorbed
γ-globulin (Sakurai, et al., 1980) and wettability of γ-globulin solution
on the hydrophilic and hydrophobic surfaces (Okano, et al., 1979) also
suggested that γ-globulins were adsorbed onto the hydrophobic surface
with their Fc segment, but adsorbed onto the hydrophilic surface with
their Fab segment. These data suggest that the deformation of the
adhered platelets was large on the γ-globulin precoated PHEMA surface
because of specific reaction of platelet Fc receptor with the Fc
segment which is exposed to liquid phase. On the surface of the
γ-globulin precoated block copolymer, the adhered platelets were
observed to be round, similar to the hydrophobic surface system.

<u>Role of Hydrophilic and Hydrophobic Microdomains in Polymer-Platelet
Interaction</u>: In contrast to the homopolymers, the block copolymer
surface, with or without protein precoating (albumin or γ-globulin),
exhibited the remarkable inhibition not only of platelet attachment
but also of platelet deformation and aggregation. That is, the
organized structure of adsorbed proteins, formed on the block copolymer surface with hydrophilic and hydrophobic microdomains, plays
an important role in antithrombogenecity.

<u>REFERENCES</u>

Brecher, G., Cronkite, E.P., Morphology and Enumeration of Human
Blood Platelets (1950) <u>J.Appl.Physiol.</u>, 3, 365-377
Kataoka, K., Tsuruta, T., Akaike, T., Sakurai, Y. (1978) Effect of
charge and molecular structure of polyion complexes on the morphology
of adherent blood platelets, <u>Makromol.Chem.</u>, <u>179</u>, 1121-1124
Okano, T., Nishiyama, S., Shinohara, I., Akaike, T., Sakurai, Y.,
(1978a) Interaction between plasma protein and microphase separated
structure of copolymers, <u>Polymer J.</u>, <u>10</u>, 223-228
Okano, T., Katayama, M., Shinohara, I., (1978) The influence of
hydrophilic and hydrophobic domains on water wettability of 2-hydroxy-
ethyl methacrylate-styrene copolymer, <u>J.Appl.Polymer Sci.</u>, <u>22</u>, 369-377
Okano, T., Nishiyama, S., Shinohara, I., Akaike, T., Sakurai, Y.,
Kataoka, K., Tsuruta, T., (1979a) Role of microphase separated structure
in the interaction of polymer with blood, <u>ACS Polymer Preprints, 20,</u>
571-574
Okano, T., Nishiyama, S., Shinohara, I., Akaike, T., Sakurai, Y.,
(1979b) Influence of hydrophilic-hydrophobic type of microphase
separated structure on interfacial behaviour between polymer and blood
proteins, <u>Kobunshi Ronbunshu</u>, <u>36</u>, 209-216
Sakurai, Y., Akaike, T., Kataoka, K., Okano, T., (1980) Interfacial
Phenomenon in Biomaterials Chemistry, <u>Biomedical Polymer, Polymeric
Materils and Pharmaceuticals for Biomedical Use</u>, pp 335-379,
Academic Press
Van Oss, S.J., Gillman, C.F., Newman, A.W., (1975) <u>Phagocytic
Engulfment and Cell Adhesiveness as Cellular Surface Phenomena</u>, Marcel
Dekker, New York

Biomaterials 1980
Edited by G. D. Winter, D. F. Gibbons, and H. Plenk, Jr.
© 1982 John Wiley and Sons Ltd.

THROMBOGENESIS: AN IONIC/STERIC PHENOMENA

S. A. Barenberg, J. M. Anderson, and K. A. Mauritz

University of Michigan
Ann Arbor, Michigan 48109

SUMMARY

A differential empirical epitaxial model has been derived which correlates and interrelates the ultrastructure morphology, surface charge,
surface chemistry, and surface molecular motions of a model semi-crystalline hydrophobic triblock copolymer to thrombogenesis. This paper
addresses the aspects of: 1. ultrastructure order vs. disorder, 2. primary and secondary molecular motions, 3. surface and side chain chemistry, 4. thrombogenesis, and 5. the derived epitaxial model. This model
can be extrapolated to predict the relative thrombogenic responses of
various crystalline and semi-crystalline hydrophobic aliphatic polymer
substrates.

INTRODUCTION

In defining and correlating the surface properties of crystalline and
semi-crystalline polymeric prosthetic materials to thrombogenesis, the
surface free energy, surface charge, ultrastructure morphology, surface
chemistry, surface molecular motions, surface topography, critical surface tension, electrical conductivity and water content have evolved as
important factors (Vroman 1977). It is apparent from the above that a
complex interrelationship exists between the surface properties of a
prosthetic material and thrombogenesis. It is the intent of this paper
to present a semi empirical epitaxial/thrombogenic model which correlates and interrelates the ultrastructure morphology, surface molecular
motions, and ionic and steric order of a model triblock copolymer to
thrombogenesis.

The precept with which we will be presenting is that morphologically
ordered polymeric systems, of given side chain chemistry can sequester
ions, which can subsequently serve as an ionic array/template for protein epitaxial crystallization. Additionally, we will be addressing
the effect of side chain motion of the substrate on the epitactic process based, in part, on our previous work (Barenberg 1979). A comprehensive review of polymer epitactic processes is given by (Mauritz 1978).

The polymeric system used in this study was a semi-crystalline hydrophobic triblock copolymer synthesized and characterized in our laboratories
(Barenberg 1976). The salient aspects of this triblock copolymer are:

1. the ultrastructure morphology of the copolymer (long range order vs. no order) can be controlled through solution casting from selected solvents, 2. the onset of secondary side chain motion occurs between 12 - 25°C, 3. the side chain motion can be restricted by casting the copolymer from a nonpreferential solvent, 4. the pendant side chain groups are projecting normal to the helical backbone, and 5. the copolymer can be extracorporeally evaluated with strict control of morphology and molecular motion.

METHODS

The polymer used in this study was a triblock copolymer, $A_x B_y A_x$, of poly[(γ-benzyl-L-glutamate)(acrylonitrile/butadiene)(γ-benzyl-L-glutamate)], (PBLG)(ATBN)(PBLG), (Barenberg 1976).

Solutions (0.1% & 1.0% w/v) of the copolymer were prepared from dioxane and chloroform. The dioxane and chloroform systems being preferential and nonpreferential solvent systems, respectively.

The dynamic mechanical measurements were done using an inverted torsion (braid) pendulum (Armeniades 1968).

Morphological and electron diffraction studies were done on thin films of the copolymer as cast onto carbon coated glass slides. The thin films were vapor stained with osmium tetroxide.

Conventional and scannign transmission electron microscopy was done on a J.E.O.L. 100C electron microscope. The scanning electron microscopy was done on a J.E.O.L.U3.

The animals used in the extracorporeal (Schultz 1977) studies were conditioned male dogs. Access to the animals' circulatory system was via a chronic shunt surgically implanted into the neck. The shunt was anastomosed to the carotid artery and jugular vein. Blood flow through the shunt was 1 liter/minute.

Twenty-four hours prior to the experiment the platelets were labeled with ^{51}Cr and human ^{125}I labeled fibrinogen were injected into the dog. No anticoagulants were used prior and/or during the experiment. The morphological studies were done on unlabeled dogs.

Experiments were carried out for periods of 5, 10, and 60 minutes at a shear rate of 150 sec^{-1}.

At the completion of the test the exposed shafts (not used in the counting studies) were placed in buffered glutaraldehyde. The shafts were postfixed and critically point dried (Barenberg 1979). The critically point dried coatings were removed, embedded in Spurr (via propylene oxide) and ultramicrotomed. The unstained (osmocated) thin sections were carbon coated and examined by conventional and scanning transmission electron microscopy.

RESULTS

The copolymer morphology as cast from dioxane exhibited a lamellar morphology, figure 1, with the ATBN midblock layers being on the order of 15 nm thick while the alternating PBLG layers were on the order of 50 nm thick. The copolymer morphology as cast from chloroform exhibited a homogeneous morphology with the ATBN midblock domains being on the order of 15 nm.

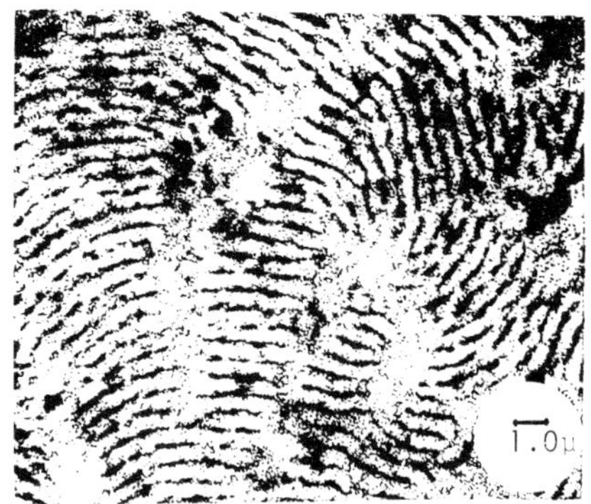

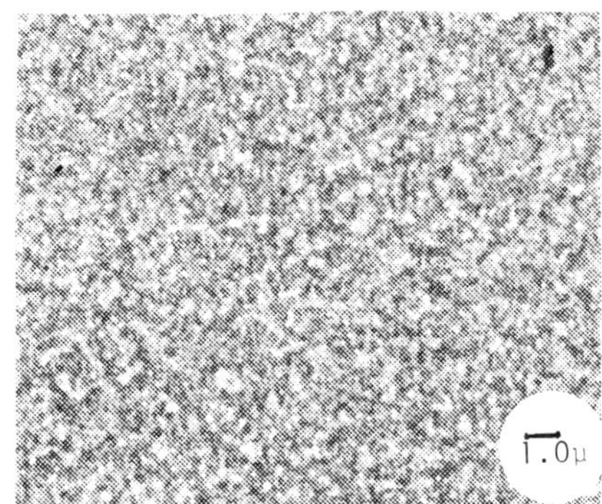

Figure 1, dioxane cast copolymer.   Figure 2, chloroform cast co-
                                                       polymer

Reproduced by permission of A.S.A.I.O.

The electron diffraction patterns of the above films indicated that the PBLG segment of the copolymer was α-helical.

The dielectric and dynamic mechanical measurements (Barenberg in press) of the copolymer as cast from dioxane and chloroform revealed a dispersion maxima at 298°K and a split dispersion at 298°K and 315°K, respectively. The 298°K dispersion maxima has been ascribed (Fukuzawa 1974) to the onset of motion of the PBLG side chains. The onset of molecular motion of the PBLG backbone occurs at 408°K (McKinnon 1968). Therefore the only molecular motion occurring in the copolymers over the physiological temperature range affecting hemocompatibility are those that can be ascribed to the onset of side chain motion of PBLG. The single dispersion maxima for the dioxane cast copolymer infers unrestricted side chain motion, whereas the split maxima, chloroform cast, infers restricted side chain motion. This change then infers that at physiological temperatures, in conjunction with the morphological results, the motion of the side chains in the dioxane cast copolymer are unrestricted and occur in an ordered steric array, whereas in the chloroform cast copolymer the side chain motion is restricted in a disordered array. This type of side chain motion has been previously postulated (Merrill 1977) and demonstrated (Barenberg 1979) to influence the initial sorption of the plasma protein(s) and subsequent interaction with blood. These interaction effects in conjunction with the results of the extracorporeal experiments will be discussed below.

When the copolymers were exposed to canine blood for 60 minutes,figures
3 and 4, the dioxane cast copolymer exhibited a large thrombus,whereas
the chloroform cast copolymer exhibited a limited thrombus.

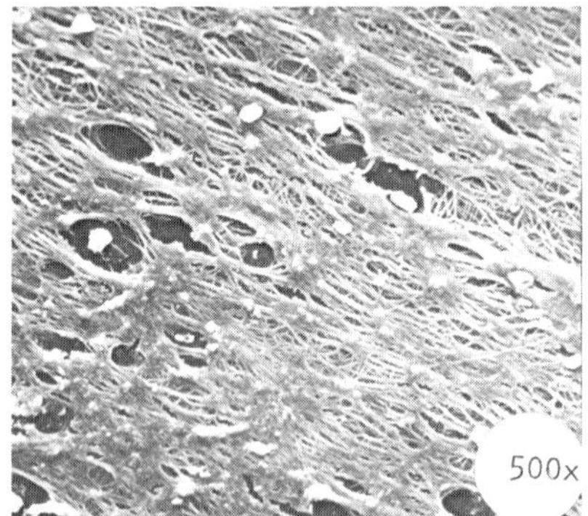

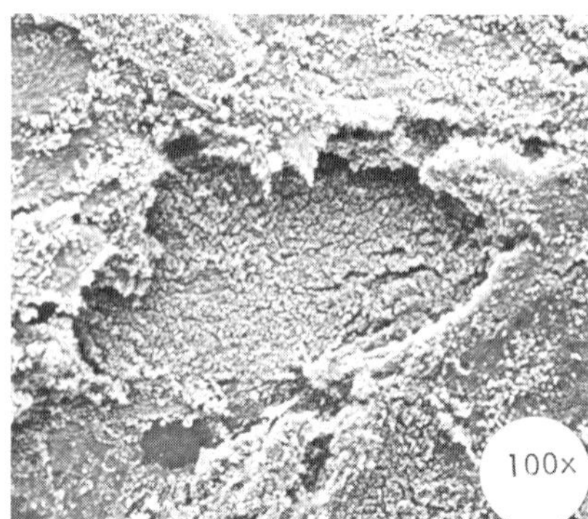

Figure 3,dioxane cast copolymer   Figure 4,chloroform cast copolymer
exposed to canine blood 60 minutes   exposed to canine blood 60 minutes
Reproduced by permission of A.S.A.I.O.

These series of experiments were replicated using different dogs and
different substrate shafts, i.e. stainless steel and polypropylene,
with consistent reproducibility.

The above exposed copolymers were ultramicrotomed in cross section and
examined by transmission electron microscopy (Barenber 1980). The
dioxane cast copolymer exhibited a tightly bound 10 nm osmophilic interfacial layer, whereas the chloroform cast copolymer exhibited a loosely
bound 50 nm interfacial layer.

DISCUSSION

The epitaxial model takes into account the differences between the two
types of secondary molecular motions observed, the ultrastructural
differences between the ordered phase separated and the disordered
phase mixed morphologies of the block copolymers, the electronegativity
of the side chain carbonyl oxygens, the ionic clustering effects due
to the above electronegativity and the surface chemistry of the copolymers. The model does not take into account any effects due to stream-
ing potential and/or local surface pH differences (Helmus 1980); two
very important areas which need to be addressed.

The model is divided into four parts: 1. the definition of the surface
to be interfaced with blood, 2. the mode of the plasma protein(s)
and/or electrolyte adsorption, 3. relaxation motion of the blood inter-
facing side chain groups, and 4. protein denaturation and/or liquid
crystalline order.

The first aspect of the model is the definition of that surface which
is to be interfaced with blood. The dioxane cast copolymeric surface,

figure 5, represents a dynamic quasiordered hydrophobic array.Whereas
the chloroform cast copolymeric surface represents a disordered array.

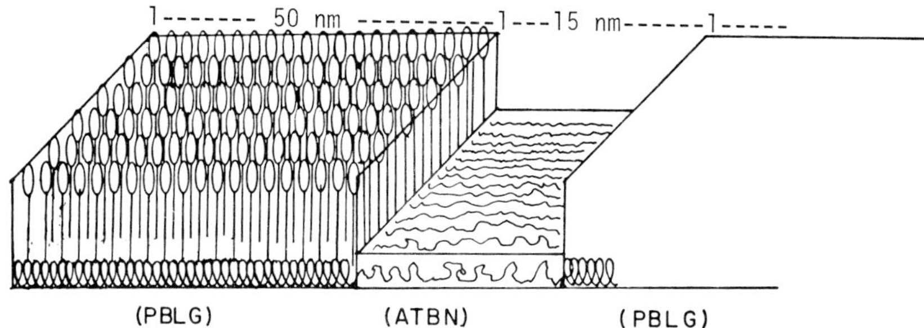

Figure 5, Schematic representation of the dioxane cast copolymeric
surface.

The second aspect of the model incorporates the two concurrent types
of adsorption occurring at the surface: (1) that of the plasma
protein(s) and (2) that of either ions and/or polyelectrolytes. The
sorption of the protein(s) occurs, in part, by a two step process. The
proteins, figure 6, would initially hydrophobically bond to the exposed
phenyl groups in a metastable state and (2) the proteins in the metastable state would then surface diffuse to a lower free energy state
located in the potential trough between the benzyl ester side chains.

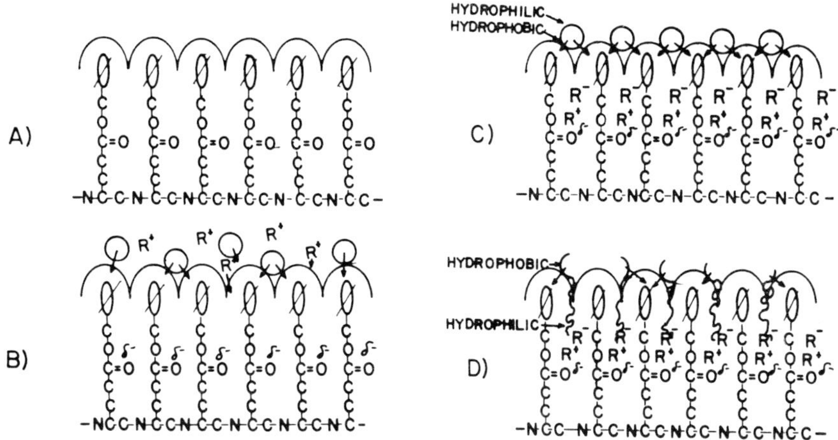

Figure 6, Schematic representation of the adsorption process;A. definition of the surface,B. initial mode of adsorption, C. ion sequestering
and development of an ordered surface, and D. denaturation.

These proteins would then align in an ordered fashion with the hydrophilic portion of the sorbed protein being exposed to the blood interface, this being the case for the dioxane cast copolymer. In the case
where there is not an ordered array, as in the chloroform cast copolymer, the sorbed protein would not sorb in an ordered array nor form an
ordered type of surface, i.e. liquid crystalline. The third aspect of
the model takes into account the relaxational motion of the side chains
and the electronegativity of the carbonyl oxygen. In that the side
chain mobility of the solution interface may facilitate ionic diffusion
to the proximity of the electronegative oxygen, figure 6c and 6d.

In the vicinity of these oxygens,the electrostatic potential energy of
cations will be most favourable. As a result of this, one might envision coordinations of a number of carbonyl groups with these cations,
figure 7. Additionally, since the macromolecular side chains are in an
ordered packing mode, one might hypothesize that (assuming that the
sodium ions are reasonably immobilized) a relatively ordered subsurface
cationic array.

It is then at this step that the differences between the effects of
surface chemistry and secondary molecular motions as dictated by morph-
logical order can be observed on thrombogenesis. In the case of the
sterically ordered substrate, in conjunction with the subsurface
cationic array, the sorbed protein(s) can assume a liquid crystalline
(and/or paracrystalline) and subsequently be subjected to further per-
tubations. Whereas, in the case of the disordered substrate the sorbed
proteins can not assume a paracrystalline state and subsequently will
not, per se, be subjected to any further conformational changes.

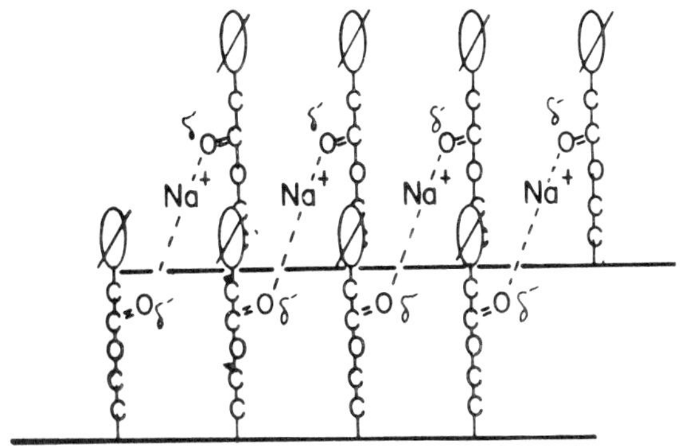

Figure 7, Schematic representation of sequestered ions forming a
cationic array.

The initial evidence for this model can be observed in figure 1,2,3,& 4.
When the ordered copolymer was exposed to canine blood a difference in
the initial adsorption of the protein(s) could be observed. In the case
of the dioxane cast copolymer a tightly bound layer was observed,whereas
a loosely bound layer was observed for the chloroform cast copolymer.
These initial differences are felt to be the mediating/chemotactic factors responsible for the resultant thrombogenic responses. It is presumed, a priori, that the tightly bound and loosely bound layers are a
result of the epitaxial (ionic and steric) and non epitaxial aspects of
the above model, respectively.Recently Filisko (Filisko), in his microcalorimetry studies, observed an exothermic heat of adsorption for protein adsorption on a series of inorganic and organic hydrated substrates,
rather than endothermic heats. Additionally, Nyilas (Nyilas 1977) also
observed similar calorimetric results in his hydrated adsorption studies. The exothermic results have been interpreted in two ways: 1. the
exotherm being indicative of surface ordering (Filisko) and 2. the exotherm being indicative of initial bonding followed by denaturation
and/or conformational changes (Nyilas 1977). Both Filisko and Nyilas in
this studies in the dehydrated state did observe endotherms. The endotherms being indicative of denaturation. It can be assumed, a priori,
from their studies the observed differences between the exothermic and
endothermic heats can be attributed, in part, to the presence of the
buffer which may have been substrate sequestered and served as an ionic
template for protein adsorption. In order to further substantiate the
above observations and hypothesis, high resolution electron microscopy,
x-ray dispersion mapping, and microcalorimetry of the above copolymers
is currently underway in our laboratories. Additionally, angular resolved ESCA studies of the homo and block copolymers are underway in
Dr. Ratner's laboratory.

Therefore in summary it appears that the interaction between the immediate substrate surface and hydrophobic groupings will contribute to the
overall adsorption process. However, the dynamic state of the side
chains would present a dynamic "liquid" steric template rather than the
conventional "solid" steric template, with an ill defined periodic potential energy profile, in the near interfacial region. Whether or not
this dynamic template would serve to induce an orientational influence
on incoming sections of proteins has yet to be proven. However, the
electrostatic force field of the substrate ions will be strong,long
range and not suffer a drastic attentuation. Therefore, given the assum-
tions of surface order and ionic distribution, an epitaxial adsorption
orientation mechanism may appear credible as the initial nucleation
event in thrombogenesis on biomaterials having microstructural crystallinity.

<u>REFERENCES</u>

Armeniades, C.D., Kuriyama,I.,Roe,J.M.,and Baer,E.,(1968) Mechanical
behaviour of poly(ethylene terphthalate) at cryogenic temperatures,in
<u>Cryogenic Properties of Polymers</u> (Eds. Serafini and Koenig),pp 155 -
170. Dekker, New York

Barenberg,S.A.,(1976) The Structure and Properties of Selected Plastic Peptides, Ph.D. Dissertation, Case Western Reserve

Barenberg,S.A.,Schultz,J.S.,Anderson,J.M., and Geil,P.H.,(1980) Hemocompatibility: Macromolecular motions and order of the polymer interface, Trans. Amer. Soc. Artif. Int. Organs,25, 159 - 162.

Barenberg,S.A., Anderson,J.M., and Geil,P.H., (in press) Structure and Properties of two plastic peptide triblock,ABA, copolymers of poly(γ - benzyl-L-glutamate), A,and poly(butadiene/acrylonitrile),B,Int.J.Biol. Macromol.

Filisko,F.E., Malladi,D., and Barenberg,S.A., (in preparation) Isothermal Enthalpy Studies of Plasma Protein Adsorption on Synthetic Surfaces, Adv. Chem. Series

Fukuzawa,T., and Uematsu,Il, (1974) Viscoelastic Properties of poly(γ - benzyl-L-glutamate), Polymer J., 6, 431-437.

Helmus,M.N., (1980), The Effect of Surface Charge on Arterial Thrombosis Ph.D. Dissertation, Case Western Reserve University

Mauritz,K.A., Baer,E., and Hopfinger,A.J., (1978) The Epitaxial Crystallization of Macromolecules, J.Polym.Sci.Macromol.Rev.13, 1 - 61

Merrill,E.W.,(1977), The Behaviour of Blood at their Surfaces,Annals, N.Y.Acad. Sci., 283, 6 - 16

McKinnon,A. and Tobolosky,A., (1968) Structure and Properties of poly (γ-benzyl-L-glutamate) cast from Dimethylformamide,J.Phys.Chem., 72, 1157 - 1161

Nyilas,E.,Chiu,T-H.,and Turcotte,L.R., (1977) Study of the Interaction of Plasma Proteins with Prosthetic Surfaces IV. N.I.H. Annual Report NIH-N01-HV-3-2917-4

Schultz,J.S.,Goddard,J.D.,Ciarkowski,A.A.,Penner,J.A.,and Lindenauer, S.M. (1977) An Ex Vivo Method for the evaluation of Biomaterials in Contact with Blood, Annals N.Y. Acad. Sci., 283, 494 - 523

Vroman,L.,and Leonard,E., Eds. (1977) The Behaviour of Blood and Its Components at Interfaces, Annals N.Y.Acad.Sci., 283

ACKNOWLEDGEMENTS

This work was supported by an N.I.H. grant 5 R01 HL 23288-02

The authors wish to thank L.J.C.R. in the preparation of this manuscript.

Biomaterials 1980
Edited by G. D. Winter, D. F. Gibbons, and H. Plenk, Jr.
© 1982 John Wiley and Sons Ltd.

POLYURETHANE – POLYDIMETHYLSILOXANE MIXTURES WITH IMPROVED
THROMBORESISTANCE, THEIR CHEMICAL AND BIOLOGICAL PROPERTIES

W. Lemm and E. S. Bücherl

Chirurgische Klinik und Poliklinik, Klinikum Charlottenburg
der Freien Universität Berlin, Spandauer Damm 130,
D-1000 Berlin 19

SUMMARY

Although some polyurethanes have proved a satisfactory antithrombogenicity, the thrombus formation on a polyurethane surface can be reduced
by addition of small quantities of a polydimethylsiloxane (PDMS). The
exact ratio of both components has to be established. The two incompatible polymers were dissolved separately and finally mixed that the polyurethane contains 2, 3, 4, 5 and 10 % PDMS. The different PDMS-con-
tent of the glass facing and the air facing surface were analyzed by
IR-ATR-spectroscopy and protein adsorption tests. Two in vitro blood
compatibility tests were performed: material-thrombelastography, Nosé-
blood-chamber-test. The improved biological properties must be paid by
a loss of mechanical strength.

INTRODUCTION

Within past years there has been considerable utilization of some segmented polyetherurethane materials for biomedical applications like
flexible tubing, heart assist pumps and the artificial heart (Mirko-
vitch et al, 1962;Kantrowitz, 1968; Pierce et al, 1969). One reason for
this choice is their high mechanical strength when compared with other
elastomeric polymers; this is achieved without the inclusion of additives. In addition thus exhibit a sufficient resistance against biodegradation together with a reasonable blood compatibility. Different
procedures have been proposed to reduce the thrombogenicity on polyurethane surfaces, for example heparinization (Grode et al, 1969), car-
bonization (Taylor et al, 1971), albuminization (Imai et al, 1970) or a
bioelectric treatment (Sharp et al, 1966 & 1968). Avcothane 51 is described as a polyether-urethane crosslinked with segments of polydimethylsiloxane. The silicone additive is covalently bound (Nyilas, 1971;
Sung & Hu, 1979 a, b). However the blood compatibility of a polyurethane can also be improved by a simple addition of small quantities of
a polydimethylsiloxane-prepolymer, which vulcanizes at room temperature
in the presence of a humid atmosphere. In this case a mixture of the
polymers is obtained. The silicone additive is not covalently bound but
its polymer chains are crosslinked to each other.

MATERIALS AND METHODS

Normally mixtures of the polymers are not compatible, their solutions
have a tendency to separate. If both polymers dissolved in suitable
solvents and at optimal concentrations, however, mixtures of the two
polymer solutions are homogenous, stable and can be stored. The optimal preparation of the polyurethane-silicone mixtures requires a 5 %
solution of the polyetherurethane (Pellethane 2363-80A) in N,N-di-
methylacetamide and a 1 % solution of polydimethylsiloxane in tetrahydrofuran. Both solvents must be anhydrous otherwise the silicone
prepolymer will vulcanize. The polymer solutions were mixed so that
the polyurethane contained 2, 3, 4, 5 and 10 % silicone.

To obtain films of a constant quality, the solutions were poured onto
polished glass and dried for 24 hours at $70^{\circ}C$. Under these conditions
and concentrations the polymers phase separate. Simultaneously the
PDMS-component crosslinks as a result of the moisture in the air.
Consequently the polymer distribution in a cast film differs from
that in solution.

Surface characterization by IR-ATR-spectroscopy. Both surfaces, the
air-facing and the glass-facing, differ in their content of PDMS.
Because the infrared spectra of the polymers differ, IR-ATR-spectroscopy can be used to analyse the surface composition (Harrick, 1967;
Wesley, 1966) of polyurethane-silicone-mixtures as well as that of
the polyurethane-polydimethylsiloxane-block-copolymer (Avcothane 51).
Nylas (1977) proposed to control and characterize the blood contact-
ing surface of intra-aortic-balloons made of Avcothane 51 by an IR-ATR
Index. He compared the IR-absorption at $770\ cm^{-1}$ which represents the
aromatic ring of the polyurethane with the IR-absorption at $800\ cm^{-1}$

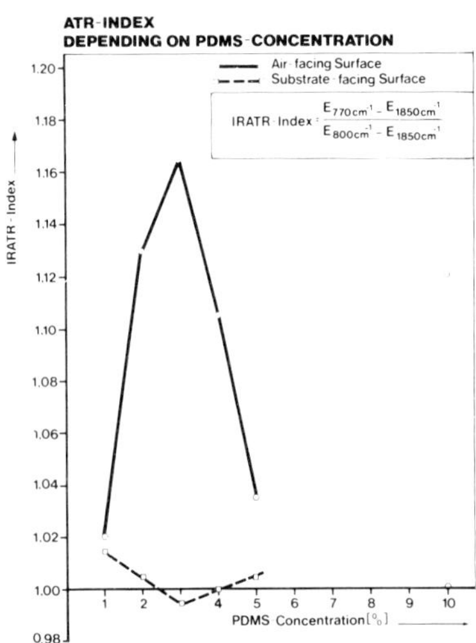

Fig.1. IR-ATR-Index on films of polyurethane-PDMS-mixtures depending on PDMS-concentration.

which can be related to the Si-O-oscillation of the PDMS-component
(Kellner & Unger,1977). This method was utilized for the polyurethane
silicone-mixtures. Figure 1 shows the ATR-index of polyurethane films
with increasing content of silicone. The air-facing surface has a distinct maximum at a PDMS-concentration of 3 %, whereas the glass-facing
surface varies only slightly around 1.00. The air-dried surface thus
has a lower concentration of silicone than the glass-facing surface.

Competitive protein adsorption. Each polymer also differs significantly in its affinity for the blood protein albumin. Therefore competitive protein adsorption tests on the air-dried and glass-dried surfaces
were also performed. Polyurethanes generally show a preferential adsorption for albumin (Unger et al.1976; Lemm et al.1977 & 1978).
Therefore the proteins albumin and fibrinogen can be used to indicate
the surface molecular composition. Films of the different polymer
compositions were exposed to synthetic protein solutions which contained both proteins in their physiological concentrations (4,5 g/100 ml
albumin; 0,3 g/100 ml fibrinogen) until the surfaces of specimens had
reached equilibrium. The protein solutions contained I(125)-albumin
and I(131)-fibrinogen to identify and to quantify the adsorbed protein
layer. Protein adsorption numbers were defined as the ratio of albumin
to fibrinogen. In figure 2 the results are shown. The pure polyurethane adsorbs 16 times more albumin than fibrinogen. With increasing content of PDMS the protein adsorption ratio decreased. The dottet line
represents the glass-facing surfaces. At identical PDMS concentrations
the protein adsorption numbers of the glass-dried surfaces are always
smaller than of the air-dried surfaces. This indicates a lower silicone content at the air-dried surface.

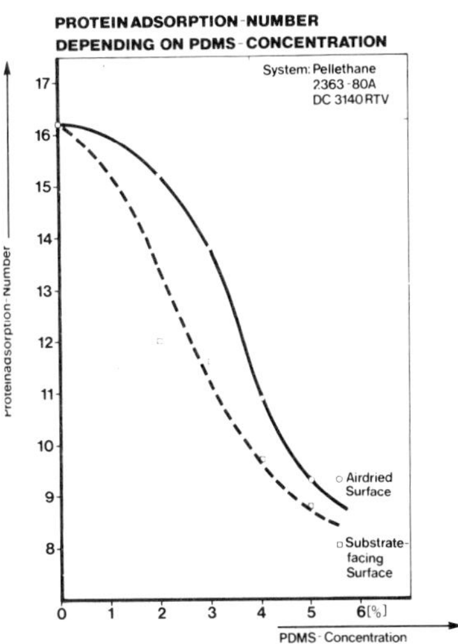

Fig. 2. Protein adsorption on films of
polyurethane-silicone mixtures.

<u>In vitro blood compatibility.</u> Two <u>in vitro</u> blood compatibility tests
with native blood were performed: the material-thrombelastography
(MTEG) (Affeld et al. 1974; Lemm et al. 1979) and the blood chamber
test (Nosé et al. 1973). The MTEG is a modification of clinical
thrombelastography and a quick and sensitive method to test the throm
bogenic properties of biomaterials. Fig. 3 shows the relationship

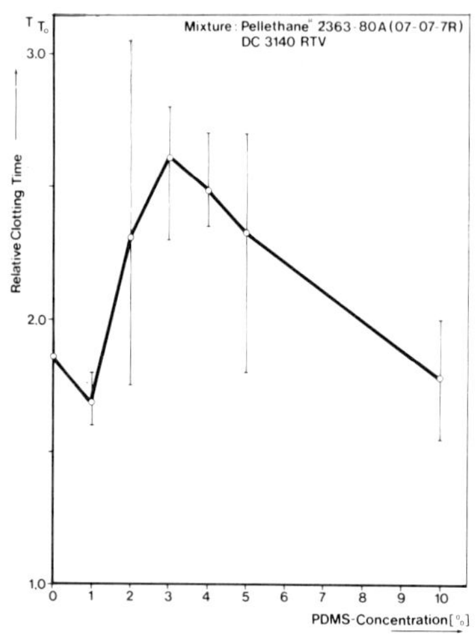

Fig. 3. Relative clotting time depending on PDMS-concentration (MTEG-test)

between the relative clotting time as criterion for antithrombogenicity and the concentration of PDMS. The optimal thromboresistance was
obtained with a mixture which contained 3 % silicone additive and
coincides within the IR-ATR-analysis.

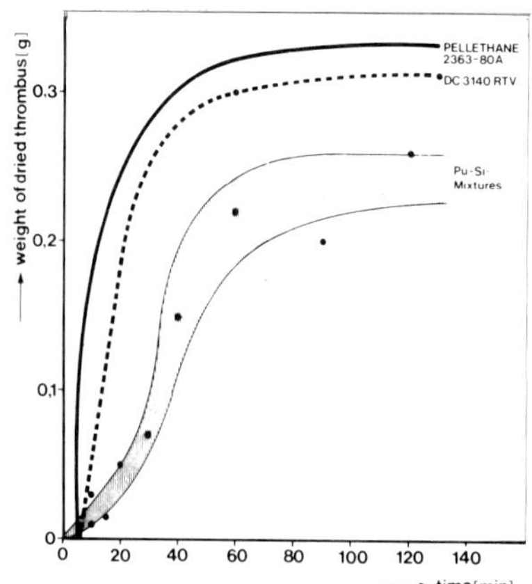

Fig. 4. Nosé-blood-chamber-test with
polyurethane-PDMS-mixtures.

Figure 4 shows the results of the Nosé blood chamber test. A high
weight of dried thrombus indicates a bad blood compatibility. No
distinct maximum was found which could be related to one of the polyurethane-PDMS mixtures, as it could be done with the MTEG-test. But
all results obtained with the polymer mixtures exceed those of the
pure polymers.

<u>Mechanical strength.</u> The improved thromboresistance of the materials
is compensated by a loss of mechanical strength. Ten specimens of each
polymer composition were tested in a tensile test machine. Both the
tensile strength and the elongation at break were measured and compared with the pure polyurethane (Fig. 5). The addition of 3 % PDMS,
the composition which exhibited the optimal blood compatibility, reduces the elongation at break by more than 3 % and the tensile strength
by 35 % compared with the pure polyurethane. Therefore these polymer
mixtures should not be recommended for highly stressed applications
for example the diaphragms of blood pumps. These mixtures could be
used however as coatings.

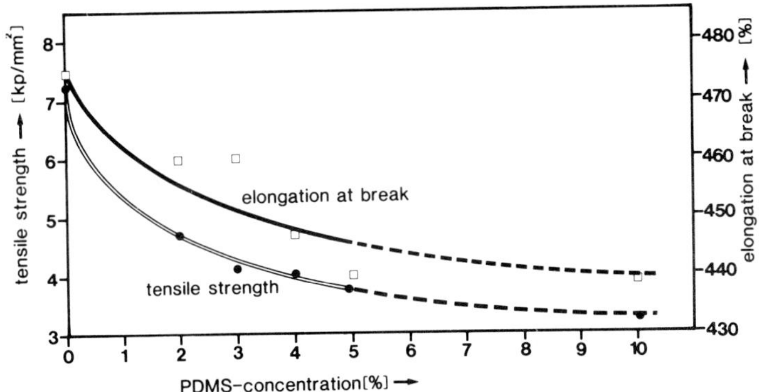

Fig. 5. Mechanical properties of polyurethane-
PDMS mixtures.

CONCLUSION

The <u>in vitro</u> blood compatibility of polyurethanes can be improved by
small additions of PDMS. Because of the loss of mechanical properties
these polyurethane-PDMS mixtures could be used as coatings. So far
the investigations were limited to physical and biological <u>in vitro</u>
tests. For <u>in vivo</u> evaluation catheters and polyurethane tubes will be
coated. The polyurethane which is coated with a polyurethane-PDMS
mixture will change the surface composition in as yet unknown manner.
The IR-ATR-method can be used to evaluate and optimize such a coating
process and hopefully produce a more antithrombogenic surface.

REFERENCES

Affeld, K., Beyer, J., Müller, R., Bücherl, E.S. (1974) A new method for an in vitro test of blood contact materials. Proc. Europ. Soc. Artif. Organs (ESAO) I, 26 - 28.

Grode, G., Falb, R. and Anderson, S. (1969) Development of materials for use in circulatory assist devices. Proc. Artif. Heart Progr. Conf. 19 - 24.

Harrick, N.J. (1967) Internal reflection spectroscopy. New York Interscience. Publ.

Imai, Y., Bally, K., Nosé, Y. (1970) New elastic materials for the artificial heart. Trans. Am. Soc. Artif. Int. Organs XXI, 17 - 18.

Kellner, R., Unger, F. (1977) IR-Spektroskopische Charakterisierung der Blutverträglichkeit von Polyurethan-Silikon-Copolymeren. Z.Anal. Chem. 283, 349 - 354.

Kantrowitz, A. (1968) Trans. ASAIO, XIV, 344.

Lemm, W., Unger, V., Große-Siestrup, Ch., Olsen, D.B., Bücherl, E.S. (1977) Blood compatibility tests of biomaterials on the basis of the protein-adsorption-hypothesis. Proc. ESAO IV, 168 - 171.

Lemm, W., Unger, V., Große-Siestrup, Ch., Kaiser, M., Bücherl, E.S. (1978) A comparing evaluation of three blood compatibility tests for biomaterials. Proc. ESAO V, 29 - 32.

Lemm, W., Affeld, K., Bücherl, E.S. (1979) Die modifizierte Thrombelastografie, ein geeigneter in-vitro-Blutverträglichkeitstest für Biomaterialien. Biomed. Techn.,24, 297 - 298.

Mirkowitch, V., Akutsu, T., Kolff, W.J. (1962) Trans.ASAIO,VIII, 79-81.

Nosé, Y., Kambic, H. (1973) Development of blood and tissue compatible materials. 1st Annual Report, Cleveland Clinic Foundation.

Nyilas, E. (1971) US-Patent 3562352.

Nyilas, E., Ward, R.S. (1977) Development of blood compatible elastomers. Surface structure and blood compatibility of Avcothane elastomers. J. Biomed. Mater. Res. Symposium 88, 69 - 74.

Pierce, W.S., Turner, M.S., Boretos, J.W., Nolan, S.P., Morrow, A.G. (1969) Surgery, 66, 1034.

Sharp, W.V., Gardner, D.L., Andresen, G.J. (1966) A bioelectric polyurethane elastomer for intravascular replacement. Trans. ASAIO, XII, 179 -182.

Sharp, W.V., Gardner, D.L., Andresen, G.J., Wright, J. (1968) Electrolour: A new vascular interface. Trans. ASAIO XIV, 73.

Sung, C.S., Hu, S.B. (1979) Application of Auger spectroscopy for surface chemical analysis of Avcothane. Journ. of Biomed. Mat. Res. 13, 45 - 52.

Sung, C.S., Hu, S.B. (1979) ESCA Studies of surface chemical composition of segmented polyurethanes. Journ. of Biomed. Mat. Res. 13, 161 - 169.

Taylor, B.C., Sharp, W.V., Wright, J.I., Ewing, K.L., Wilson, C.L.(1971) The importance of zeta potential, ultrastructure, and electrical conductivity to the in-vitro performance of polyurethane-carbon black vascular prostheses. Trans. ASAIO XVII, 22 - 27.

Unger, V., Lemm, W., Bücherl, E.S. (1976) Kinetics of albumin and fibrinogen adsorption on biomaterials. Proc. ESAO III, 48 - 51.

Wesley, W.M. and Hecht, H.G. (1966) Reflectance spectroscopy. New York Interscience Publ.

Biomaterials 1980
Edited by G. D. Winter, D. F. Gibbons, and H. Plenk, Jr.
© 1982 John Wiley and Sons Ltd.

NEW HEPARIN-LIKE INSOLUBLE MATERIALS

C. Fougnot, J. Jozefonvicz and M. Jozefowicz

Laboratoire de Recherches sur les Macromolécules
Université Paris-Nord
Centre Scientifique et Polytechnique
Avenue J.B. Clément - 93430 Villetaneuse - FRANCE

SUMMARY

Insoluble anticoagulant materials were prepared by reacting different α-amino acids with crosslinked chlorosulfonated polystyrene - These insoluble materials possess high antithrombic activities when suspended in plasma - These activities are heparin-like i.e. these materials act as catalysts of the antithrombin III-thrombin reaction.

INTRODUCTION

The precise mechanism by which heparin exerts its anticoagulant effect remain a matter of some controversy (Rosenberg and Damus, 1973)(Rosenberg, 1977) (Machovich, 1975)(Smith and Craft, 1976) (Sturzebecher and Markwardt, 1977)(Machovich et al., 1975). Indeed, it is generally assumed that the three dimensional structure of the mucopolysaccharide is an essential requirement for binding of antithrombin III or thrombin and thereby inhibiting the action of the coagulation mechanism. We postulated that synthetic macromolecules might possess a three dimensional array of charged groups which are similar to those of heparin. In order to check whether this assumption is valid, we prepared insoluble materials by reacting different α-amino acids with crosslinked chlorosulfonated polystyrene. Sulfonate and sulfonate amino acid sulfamide polystyrene derivatives were synthesized to determine whether specific chemical groups linked to the polymer backbone in a statistical manner are able to endow these macromolecules with high heparin-like activity. The structures of these polymers are given in Fig. 1.

MATERIALS AND METHODS

<u>Preparation of polystyrene derivatives</u>. The samples were synthesized by methods similar to those previously described (Fougnot et al., 1980). They were characterized with regard to their chemical composition by elemental analysis and acidic potentiometric titration. Polymer samples were washed and, then, crushed for various times and products of two different grain sizes were obtained. The particle average diameter of the first one (type A) was 10 microns while that

C. Fougnot, J. Jozefonvicz and M. Jozefowicz

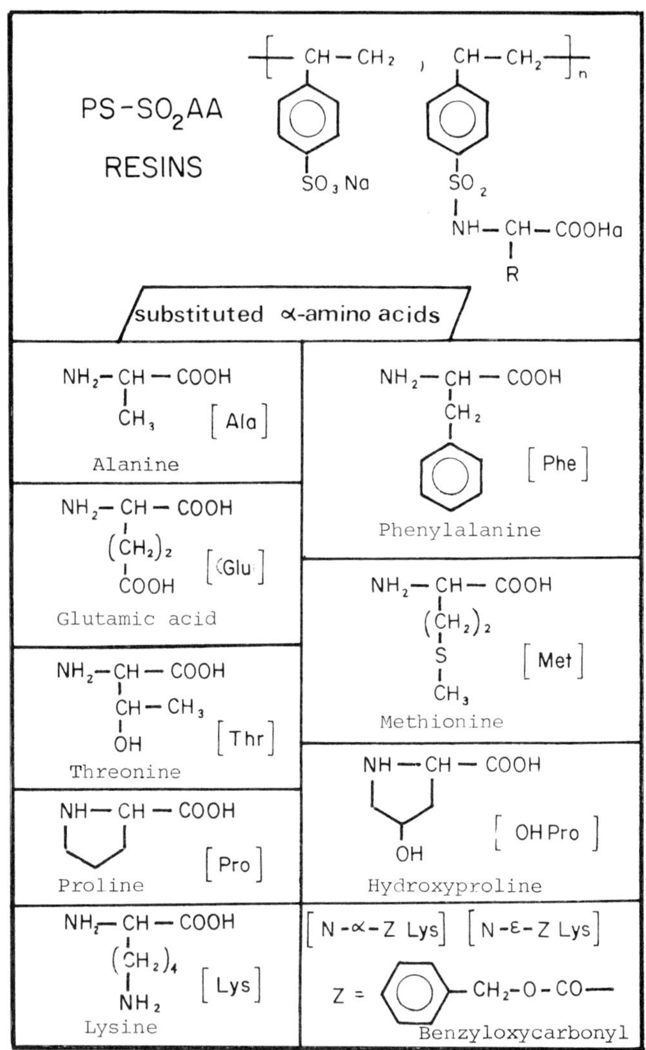

Fig. 1. Heparin-like derivatives of crosslinked polystyrene.

of the second one (type B) was smaller than one micron. Grain size
distribution of the former was determined by use of the quantitative
microscope Technic Analyzer System.

<u>Coagulation assays</u>. Polymer samples were suspended in Michaelis
buffer modified by addition of 1 g/l of an emulsifying agent (Lensex
TA 01-NP 40 Shell).
Platelet poor plasma (PPP) was incubated with each polymer suspension
in glass tubes ; then clotting times were determined at 37°C by
visual observation.
Reagents were : thrombin "Roche" 50 NIH/mg, polybrene and polylysine
"Sigma", antithrombin III, "Kabi" and reptilase "Stago".

<u>RESULTS AND DISCUSSION</u>

<u>Anticoagulant activity of resins</u>. The anticoagulant activity of all
resins (type A) has been determined by measuring the thrombin clotting times of platelet poor plasma incubated with various amounts of
suspended resins. Figure 2   shows the results obtained with several
PS-SO$_2$Pro resins containing various contents of prolin sulfamide
groups. All these resins possess an high antithrombic activity which
increases as the number of -SO$_2$Pro groups increases.
For each resin, thrombin times can be expressed in terms of the
amount of thrombin inactivated by a given amount of the resin
(Figure 3). Similar results have been obtained for each α-amino
acid investigated.
All these data can be normalized by plotting the percent of total
thrombin inactivated versus the amount of polymer utilized (Fig. 4).
The level of resin is expressed as a percentage of the theoretical
quantity needed for total inactivation of thrombin. This latter parameter is obtained by extrapolating the linear portion of the curve
to 100 % inactivation of enzyme. Thus, a virtually linear relationship exists between the amount of thrombin neutralized for all concentrations of enzyme added and the level of polymer employed for
all quantities of resin used. Given these results, the antithrombic
activity, "a", of a given resin can be defined as the reverse of the
resin amount expressed in milliequivalent of total substituting
groups able to inactivate 1 NIH unit of thrombin.
The antithrombic activity of the resins is neutralized by the usual
inhibitors of heparin i.e. polybrene and polylysine. Moreover, the
reptilase times performed on PPP suspensions or the thrombin and
reptilase times performed on fibrinogen suspensions of any resins
were equal to control assays. This suggests that the antithrombic
activities of the resins are heparin-like i.e. require the presence
of a plasma cofactor which does not exist in fibrinogen solution. We
thought it likely that this substance would prove to be antithrombin III.

<u>Catalytic effect of resins on the reaction of the antithrombin III
and thrombin</u>. In order to substantiate this hypothesis, a kinetic
study of the catalytic effect of the PS-SO$_2$Glu resin (type B) on the
reaction of the antithrombin III and thrombin in solution was performed. This catalytic effect was compared with the one obtained with

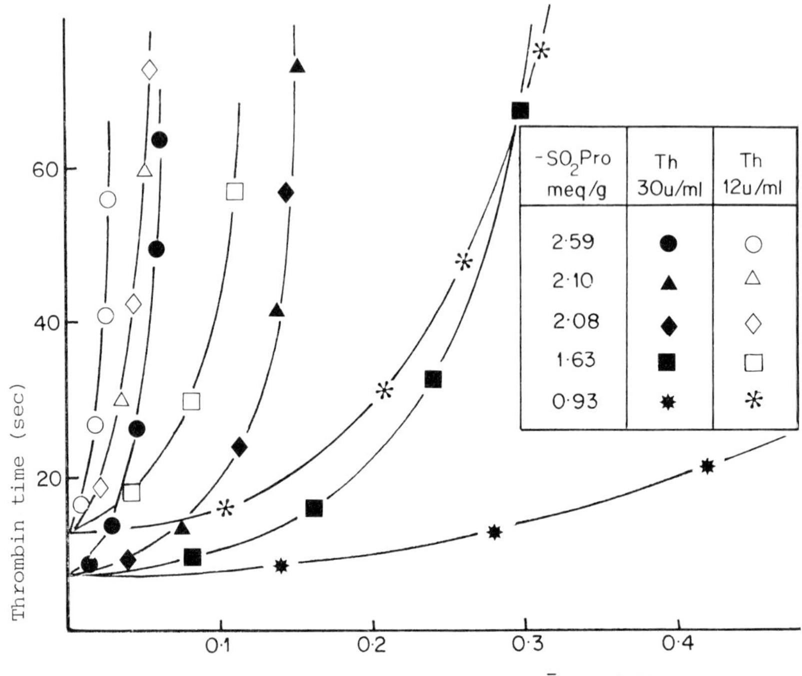

Fig. 2. Influence of the concentration of polymer suspensions on thrombin time for five polymers PS - SO$_2$ - Pro containing various ratios of sulfonate (-SO$_3^-$ meq/g) and prolin sulfamide (-SO$_2$ - Pro meq/g) groups. Two initial concentrations of thrombin were used : 30 U/ml and 12 U/ml). Each curve shows the plot obtained for one polymer its concentration being expressed in milliequivalent of -SO$_3^-$ per ml of polymer suspension.
Clotting system : 0.1 ml of polymer suspension (various contents) was incubated with 0.2 ml of platelet poor plasma for 30 minutes at 37°C. Then, 0.1 ml of thrombin of increasing concentrations was added and the clotting time (sec) was measured. Control times were performed with buffer included emulsifier instead of polymer suspension.

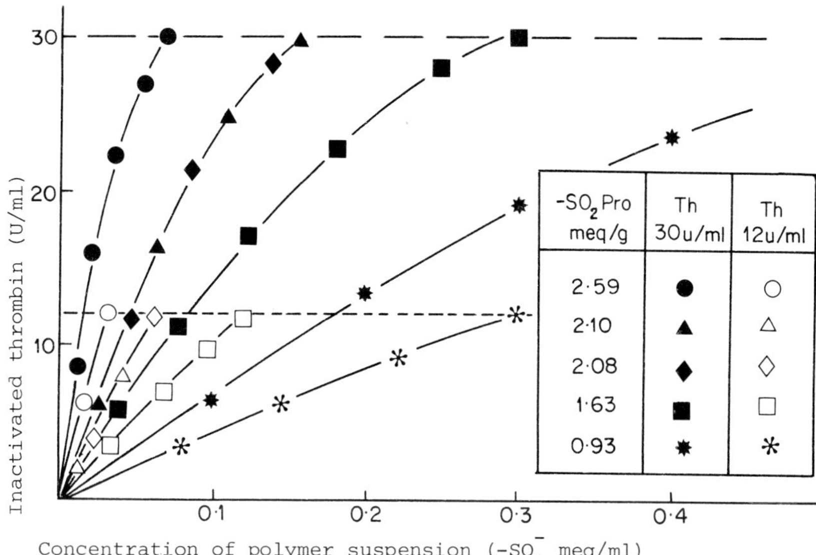

Concentration of polymer suspension ($-SO_3^-$ meq/ml)

Fig. 3. Influence of the concentration of polymer suspensions on thrombin inactivation for the five polymers $PS - SO_2 - Pro$. The conditions and symbols are identical to those expressed in the legend of the figure 2.

soluble heparin. In both cases, the kinetics of the catalyzed reaction was compared with that of uncatalyzed reaction between antithrombin III and thrombin performed under the same conditions.
Fig. 5 depicts the variations in the reciprocal residual thrombin concentration for various antithrombin III concentrations versus incubation time. In the presence of heparin or $PS - SO_2$ Glu resin, the reciprocal of residual thrombin concentration is a linear function of the incubation time ; in both cases, the velocity of the thrombin neutralization is second order in thrombin as published elsewhere (10) in the case of heparin. In contrast, when there is no catalyst, the reaction is bimolecular.
On the other hand, the rate constant appears to be linearly dependent on antithrombin III concentration when the reaction is catalyzed by $PS - SO_2$ Glu resin and independent of antithrombin III concentration in the case of heparin in the concentration ranges studied.
These results suggest that the antithrombic effect of the resins is heparin-like i.e. that the catalytic action of the resin follows the

                C. Fougnot, J. Jozefonvicz and M. Jozefowicz

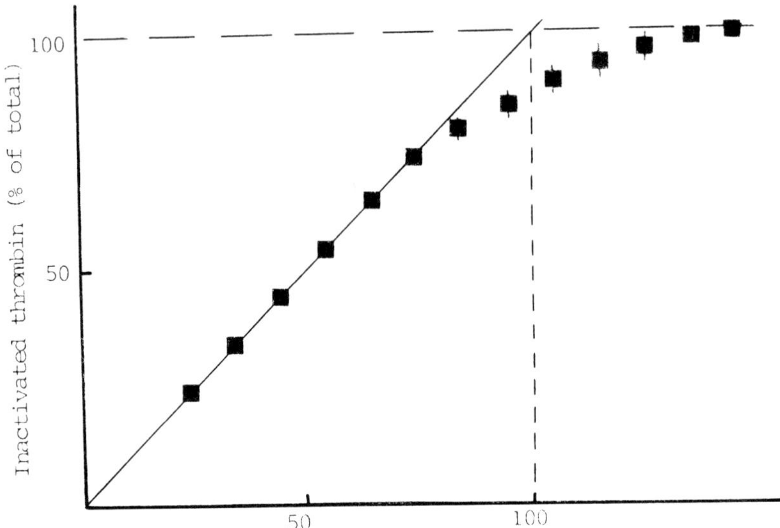

Fig. 4. General relation between the concentration of
suspended polymer and the thrombin inactivation.

same mechanism as that described elsewhere for heparin (Jordan et al,
1979). It is noticeable that the specific heparin-like activity of
these samples (type B) is 2 IU/mg, much higher than that of the
heparin copolymers previously described (Labarre et al., 1977).
Moreover, the differences in the antithrombin III concentration
necessary to reach the same rate constant value indicate that the
resin-antithrombin III complexes are less stable than the corresponding heparin-antithrombin III complexes. Thus, the formation of the
latter interaction product requires lower concentration of antithrombin III than the former one.
The anticoagulant activities of the resins (type A), as previously
defined, are strongly dependent upon the content of amino acid sulfamide groups and sulfonate groups. Given these observations, we wonde-
red whether the heparin-like properties of our polymers are due to a
cooperative or additive effect of the two types of substituents. The
following relation can be postulated :

$$a(C_{SO_3^-} + C_{AA}) = a_{SO_3^-}\, C_{SO_3^-} + a_{AA}\, C_{AA}$$

where "a" is the anticoagulant potency of the resin expressed as the
reverse of the resin amount able to inactivate 1 NIH unit of thrombin. The parameters $C_{SO_3^-}$ and C_{AA} represent the sulfonate and amino

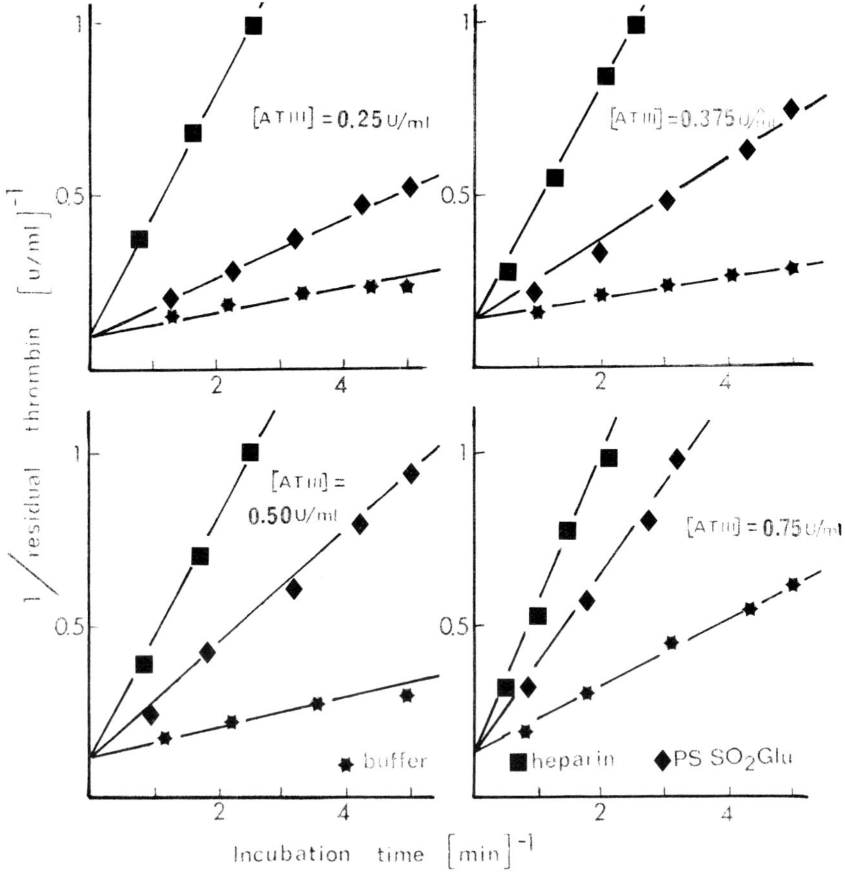

Fig. 5. Kinetics of the inactivation of thrombin by antithrombin III with or without catalyst. Clotting system :
0.1 ml of polymer suspension (0.4 mg/ml) or 0.1 ml of
heparin solution (0.8 u/ml) or 0.1 ml of Michaelis buffer
was incubated with 0.1 ml of thrombin (20 u/ml) and 0.01 ml
of antithrombin III solution of increasing concentration
for various times at 37°C. Then, 0.1 ml of polylysine
solution (5.6 mg/ml) was added and incubated for 1 min..
Then, 0.2 ml of platelet poor plasma was added and the clotting time was measured.
A standard titration curve was utilized to determine the
level of residual enzyme. To obtain this curve 0.1 ml of
Michaelis buffer (or polymer suspension or heparin solution)
was incubated with 0.1 ml of thrombin solution of increasing concentration for various times at 37°C. 0.1 ml of
polylysine solution (5.6 mg/ml) was added and incubated for
1 min.. Then, 0.2 ml of PPP was added and the clotting time
was measured.

acid sulfamide groups content in a given resin. "$a_{SO_3^-}$" and "a_{AA}" are anticoagulant activity coefficients of the sulfonate and amino acid sulfamide groups respectively, expressed in the same unit as "a". The value of "$a_{SO_3^-}$" and "a_{AA}" are given in table I.

TABLE 1.   Activity coefficient of each type of substituent[1]

Substituent	Activity coefficient (meq^{-1} NIH Th unit)
$-SO_3^-$	$\simeq 60$
$-SO_2NH$ But	O
$-SO_2Glu$	$\simeq 370$
$-SO_2Ala$	$60 < a_{AA} < 80$
$-SO_2Phe$	$60 < a_{AA} < 80$
$-SO_2OH$ Pro	$120 < a_{AA} < 150$
$-SO_2$ Pro	$120 < a_{AA} < 150$
$-SO_2Met$	$120 < a_{AA} < 150$
$-SO_2Thr$	$120 < a_{AA} < 150$
$-SO_2\ \alpha$ Z Lys	$120 < a_{AA} < 150$
$-SO_2\ \varepsilon$ Z Lys	$120 < a_{AA} < 150$

[1] For 1 NIH unit of thrombin.

CONCLUSION

In summary, we have obtained resins with significant heparin-like activity by binding sulfonate and/or α-amino acid sulfamide groups onto crosslinked polystyrene. These results suggest that the isolated functional groups borne by the polysaccharide chain of heparin, rather than the secondary or tertiary structure of this mucopolysaccharide, are responsible for its interaction with antithrombin III or thrombin. Moreover, the configuration of the substitutes bound to the crosslinked polystyrene backbone mimics, in some respect, the active sites of heparin.

REFERENCES

Fougnot, C., Jozefonvicz, J., Samama, M. & Bara, L. (1980) New heparin-like insoluble materials : part I, Ann. Biomed. Eng., (in press).
Jordan, R., Beeler, D. & Rosenberg, R.D. (1979) Fractionation of low molecular weight heparin species and their interaction with antithrombin. J. Biol. Chem., 254, 2902-2913.

Labarre, D., Jozefowicz, M. & Boffa, M.C. (1977) Properties of heparin-poly(methylmethacrylate) copolymers. II. J. Biomed. Mater. Res., 11, 283-295.

Machovich, R.B. (1975) Mechanism of action of heparin through thombin on blood coagulation. Biochem. Biophys. Acta, 412, 12-17.

Machovich, R.B., Blasko, G. & Palos, L.A. (1975) Action of heparin on thrombin-antithrombin reaction. Biochem. Biophys. Acta, 379, 193-200.

Rosenberg, R.D. & Damus, P.S. (1973) The purification and mechanism of action of human antithrombin-heparin cofactor. J. Biol. Chem., 248, 6490-6505.

Rosenberg, R.D. (1977) Chemistry of the hemostatic mechanism and its relationship to the action of heparin. Fed. Proc., 36, 10-18.

Smith, G.F. & Craft, T.J. (1976) Heparin reacts stoichiometrically with thrombin during thrombin inhibition in human plasma. Biochem. Biophys. Res. Commun., 71, 738-745.

Sturzebecher, J. & Markwardt, F. (1977) Role of heparin in the inactivation of thrombin, factor X_a, and plasmin by antithrombin III. Thrombos. Res., 11, 835-846.

SYNTHESIS AND PROPERTIES OF COVALENTLY BOUND HEPARIN
SURFACES

D. Labarre[*], J. Lindon[°], M. Silane[°], D. Brier-Russell[°],
M. Jozefowicz[*], E. Merrill[+], and E. Salzman[°].

[*]Laboratoire de Recherches sur les Macromolécules, associé
au CNRS, C.S.P., 93430 Villetaneuse (France)
[°]Beth Israel Hospital, Harvard Medical School, Boston (MA)
02215 (USA)
[+]Department of Chemical Engineering, M.I.T, Cambridge (MA)
02139 (USA)

SUMMARY

Different methods of covalent binding of heparin onto surfaces in
order to obtain longterm anticoagulant materials have been published.
The heparin-like activity of most of these materials was poor or
could not be detected. We described previously the preparation and
the solid state anticoagulant properties of a Heparin-Poly (Methyl
Methacrylate) copolymer. A modification of this method is used to
obtain Poly(Methyl Acrylate) beads bearing heparin onto their surface. The "heparin-beads" possess a solid state heparin-like, non
elutable activity, related to antithrombin III (AT) reversible binding and activation against thrombin. These beads have a reduced
activity towards platelets when pretreated with AT or platelet free
plasma. This activity increases again when pretreated with AT
depleted plasma. The differences of heparin-like activity observed
between the covalent heparinized materials may be related to differences in the ability of AT and thrombin to form the suitable
complexes with bound heparin, as a result of the different pathways
used to heparinize the materials.

INTRODUCTION

Different methods of covalent binding of heparin onto surfaces in
order to obtain long-term anticoagulant materials have been
previously published (Halpern & Shibakawa 1968, Merrill et al 1970,
Hoffman et al 1972, Chawla & Chang 1975). Provided that any released
heparin was not taken into account, the insoluble heparin-like
activity of most of these materials was poor or could not be
detected. This lack of activity was commonly explained in terms of
inaccessibility of the active sites of heparin for proteins such as
AT and thrombin.
We described previously the preparation (Labarre et al 1974) and the
anticoagulant properties (Labarre et al 1977) of a copolymer

475

Heparin-Poly(Methyl Methacrylate) (HEP-PMMA). Furthermore, we
demonstrated that these properties were mainly due to a binding of
antithrombin to the insolubilized heparin and to the activation of
this antiprotease (BOFFA et al 1979).
With this technique it was possible to produce solid state anticoagulant materials, we use it in this study to bind heparin onto
the surface of an already formed material - Poly(Methyl Acrylate)
(PMA) beads. This material has been already studied and modified
(Lindon et al 1978, Dincer 1977) and the bead form appeared to be
very convenient to evaluate the compatibility of surfaces with
blood platelets.

MATERIALS AND METHODS

Principle of the method of binding of heparin. As already described
(Labarre et al 1974), the addition of cerium IV ions to an aqueous
nitric solution of heparin was able to generate heparin radicals
which could initiate the polymerization of acrylic monomers such as
alkyl methacrylates or alkyl acrylates. These copolymers were
probably biblock copolymers (Boffa et al 1979), the acrylic block
having grown on one end of the heparin block. If methyl acrylate
(MA) swollen PMA crosslinked beads were brought in contact with
heparin radicals, it could be possible to initiate the polymerization of MA from the interface to the interior of the beads. Heparin,
which was insoluble in MA, could not penetrate into the beads ; so
it would stay on the surface, only bound through one end. If cross-
linking agents were added to MA, it would be possible to synthezise
a Heparin-PMA network interpenetrating with the original crosslinked
PMA network.

Typical procedure of preparation. The PMA beads, crosslinked by
about 4 % divinylbenzene, were prepared by the Rohm and Haas Co.,
Philadelphia, PA, (Lot J.F.-4967, Methyl Ester of Amberlite IRC 94,
average diameter 0.2 mm). These beads were first washed with a 0.5 M
solution of sulfuric acid in methanol to get rid of surfactant which
was used during bead polymerization, then extensively with methanol
and dried under vacuum. In a typical experiment, 10 g of these beads
were poured into 5 ml of a mixture (9/1 v/v) of MA and 1,4 butane-
diol diacrylate (BDA) previously treated to remove stabilizing
agents. The swelling process was very fast and no monomer remained
in the flask after 10 minutes. During the same time, 0.2 g of
heparin (sodium salt, pig intestinal mucosa, obtained from
Schwarz/Mann, Orangeburg NY, lot ZZ 1825, activity = 187 USP U/mg),
used as supplied, were dissolved under nitrogen bubbling in 10 ml of
a 0.2 M aqueous solution of nitric acid at 40°C. Then 1 ml of a
0.2 M solution of cerium IV salt - $(NH_4)_2Ce(NO_3)_6$ supplied by GFS
Chemical Co., Columbus, Ohio - in 0.2 M nitric acid, was added under
vigorous stirring and immediatly after this the swollen PMA beads
were added. After 30 minutes at 40°C, the reaction medium was
neutralized by addition of a 0.5 M sodium hydroxide solution and the
beads filtered on a sintered glass funnel. Then the beads were
extensively washed with a (3 M sodium chloride, 0.1 M sodium
citrate, 5 % methanol) aqueous solution. Finally the beads were kept

in 0.15 M sodium chloride in the refrigerator. Just before any test,
the beads (Heparin beads) were washed again in order to be sure that
no more unbound adsorbed heparin was present.

Heparin content of the beads. In order to evaluate the heparin content of the beads, ^{14}C labelled heparin was prepared, purified and
characterized as described by Dincer (1977). Samples of heparin
beads were prepared as above with varying the concentrations of the
reagents, using the labelled heparin. The radioactivity of these
samples was measured with a Packard liquid scintillation counter.
Aquasol (New England Nuclear Corporation) was used as the counting
scintillation cocktail.

Biological activity of the beads. Heparin-like activity was measured
using a chromogenic substrate assay to determine thrombin inactivation. Small quantities (≈0.2 ml) of beads were incubated with normal
or de-antithrombinated plasma for 5 min. at 37°C. Thrombin was then
added to the bead/plasma mixture and incubated for 15 sec, and the
remaining thrombin activity was measured. Thrombin inactivation, in
excess of that which occurred in the absence of antithrombin, was a
measure of heparin-like activity of the beads.
The binding of AT III by beads was determined as follows :
small (0.8 x 5.0 cm ; vol. ≃ 2 ml) columns of beads were maintained
at 37°C and exposed to 4 ml of plasma. The columns were rinsed with
10 ml of a buffered saline solution (0.15 M NaCl, 0.05 M Trisma
base ; pH 7.4) and then eluted with 3 ml of a (1 M NaCl, 0.05 M
Trisma base ; pH 8.0) solution. AT III levels in the 1 M NaCl
eluates were determined by radioimmuno assay. Platelet reactivity
was assayed as previously described (Lindon et al, 1978) by pumping
citrated whole blood at 37°C through 2 ml bead columns and measuring
the number of platelets and the presence of released platelet
constituents in the effluent blood fractions.

RESULTS

The heparin radicals created by reaction of cerium IV on heparin,
initiated the polymerization of the monomers inside the beads,
starting from the surface, as described in the following scheme :
(Figure 1). The heparin content of the heparin-beads, as determined
by the level of radioactivity, depended upon the initial concentrations of cerium IV and heparin in the reaction medium (Figure 2). A
side polymerization reaction could occur if the suspension of the
beads was not stirred vigorously enough, with high concentration of
heparin and high swelling ratios of the beads : under these conditions, some monomer diffused outside the beads and polymerized.
Proliferating surface beads and copolymer flakes could result in
this side reaction. The samples containing proliferating surfaces
beads were discarded and the copolymer flakes were eliminated by
successive decantations under slow stirring. When observed by
scanning electron microscopy (10,000 X), the surface of the beads
was "smooth".
The biological activities of a given sample of heparin-beads
depended upon the presence of AT : (Table I). The heparin-like

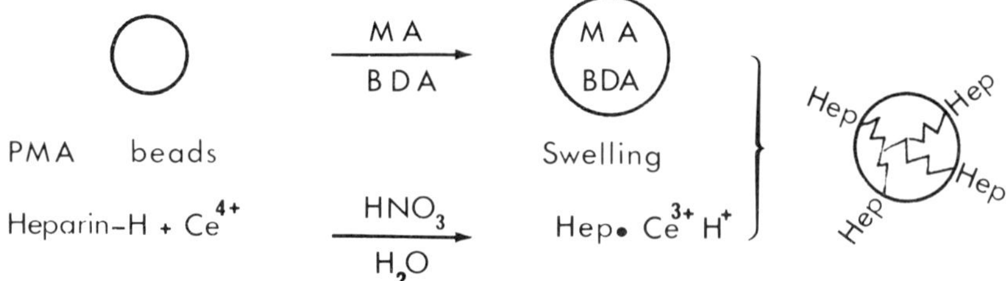

Fig. 1. Scheme of the reactions of binding.
MA = Methyl Acrylate, BDA = 1-4-Butanediol Diacrylate.

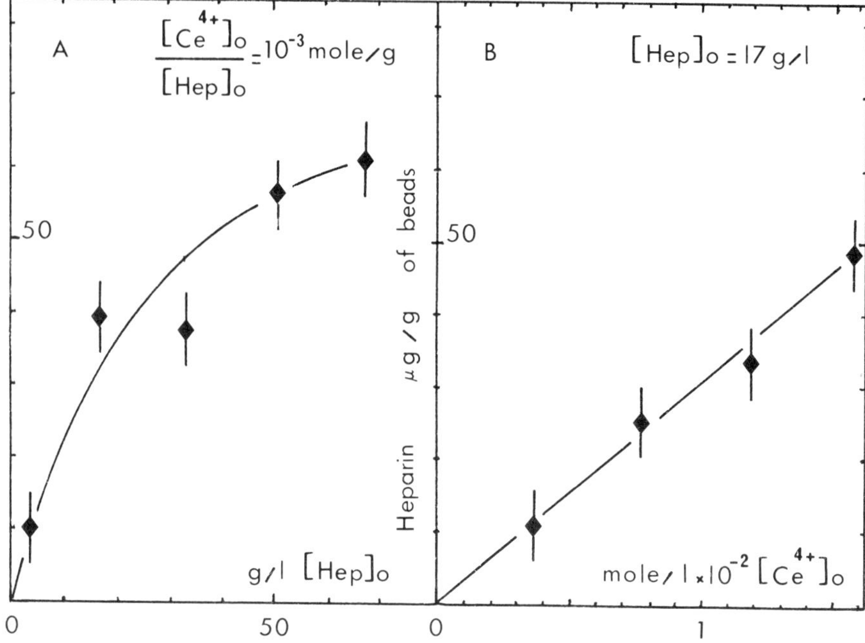

Fig. 2. Amount of bound heparin on the beads as functions of the
initial concentrations of : A - cerium IV salt, B-heparin, in the
reaction medium.

activity was measurable, it was not an elutable one but a solid-
state activity. AT could be bound to the surface and its activation
against thrombin accelerated in presence of the beads. Furthermore,
the blood platelets were less activated by this surface than by the
original one, and this passivation depended upon the presence of AT
in contact with the beads.

Table 1 : Heparin-like activity and platelet reactivity
of a typical sample of "heparin-beads".

Sample	Heparin-like Activity		AT
	Surface	Eluted	binding
	Hep Unit/ml of beads		µg/g of beads
PMA	0.00	0.00	0.12
Hep-PMA	0.035	0.00	1.6

	Platelet Recovery Index[1]			
Pretreatment[2]	None	PPP	PPP-AT	AT
Hep-PMA	0.68	0.80	0.44	0.90

(1) Platelet Recovery Index was determined by measuring
the number of platelets in the column fractions and
was expressed as a percentage of the platelet count in
the whole blood prior to column exposure (Lindon et al
1978).
(2) Prior to whole blood exposure, the "heparin-beads"
were pretreated either by saline, or by platelet poor
plasma (PPP), or by AT depleted plasma (PPP-AT), or by
purified AT.

DISCUSSION

The results of the activities of these beads on which heparin is
covalently bound demonstrate that heparin can be still active when
bound to a surface. It is noticeable that, when using this technique, the binding of heparin likely occurs only through one end of
the macromolecule which was cleaved during its oxidation by cerium
IV ions (Boffa et al 1979). Antithrombin can bind to the surface,
and complex formation between thrombin and AT is accelerated by
heparin on the surface. This behaviour presumes that the bound
heparin active site is accessible enough to allow this accelerated
complex formation (Rosenberg et al 1978).
If a heparin-like activity is a necessary requirement for a surface
designed to be in contact with blood (antithrombogenicity), the
binding technique should allow the heparin molecule a sufficient
mobility in order that it can utilize its catalytic activity. This
requirement has few chances to be satisfied if the reactive groups
of the surface to be heparinized could react with more than one end
of heparin, or if the chemical activation of heparin was able to
produce intramolecular reactions of heparin. This could explain why

covalently-bound-heparin surfaces previously described did not
possess noticeable heparin-like activity.
Heparinization of the surface increases compatibility with blood
platelets tremendously. This result is in agreement with the results
obtained by Dincer (1977). A pretreatment with plasma or purified AT
decreases the reactivity of the heparinized surface towards
platelets and a pretreatment with AT-depleted plasma increases it,
in agreement with previous results (Lindon et al 1978).
From these results concerning the antithrombogenicity and platelets
passivation of such heparinized surfaces, it can be expected to
obtain long-term anticoagulant biomaterials by use of such techniques of covalent binding of heparin through one end.

ACKNOWLEDGMENT

The helpful advice of Doctor A. Dincer is gratefully acknowledged.

REFERENCES

Boffa, M.C., Labarre D., Jozefowicz, M., & Boffa, G.A. (1979).
Interactions between human plasma proteins and heparin-poly(methyl
methacrylate) copolymers, Thromb. Haemost., 6, 346-356.
Chawla, A.S. & Chang, T.M.S. (1975). A new method for the prepara-
tion of nonthrombogenic surface by radiation grafting of heparin.
Preparation and in vitro studies, Polym. Sci. Technol, 7, 147-157.
Dincer, A. (1977). Covalent coupling of heparin to synthetic polymer
surfaces, Ph. D. Thesis, M.I.T.
Halpern, B.D. & Shibakawa, P. (1968). Heparin covalently bonded to
polymer surface, Adv. Chem. Serv., 87, 197-205.
Hoffman, A.S., Schmer, G., Harris, C., & Kraft., W.G. (1972).
Covalent binding of biomolecules to radiation-grafted hydrogels on
inert polymer surfaces, Trans. Amer. Soc. Artif. Int. Organs, 18,
10-18.
Labarre, D., Boffa, M.C., & Jozefowicz, M. (1974). Preparation and
properties of heparin-poly(methyl methacrylate) copolymers,
J. Polym. Sci. Symp., 47, 131-137.
Labarre, D., Jozefowicz, M., and Boffa, M.C. (1977). Properties of
heparin-poly(methyl methacrylate) copolymers, J. Biomed. Mater.
Res., 11, 283-295.
Lindon, J., Rodvien, R., Brier, D., Greenberg, R., Merrill, E., &
Salzman, E. (1978). In vitro assessment of interaction of blood
with model surfaces, J. Lab. Clin. Med., 92, 904-915.
Merrill, E.W., Salzman E.W., Wong, P.S.L., Ashford, T.P., Brown,
A.H. & Austen, W.G. (1970). Polyvinyl alcohol-heparin hydrogel "G",
J. Appl. Physiol., 29, 723-730.
Rosenberg, R.D. Armand, G., and Lam, L. (1978). Structure-function
relationships of heparin species, Proc. Natl. Acad. Sci. USA, 75,
3065-3069.

IN VIVO COMPARISON OF POLY(VINYL CHLORIDE) AND SILICONE
RUBBER TUBING WITH AND WITHOUT THE PRESENCE OF HEPARIN

J. Olijslager[*], J. Feijen[*] and Ch.R.H. Wildevuur[**]

[*] Twente University of Technology, Department of Chemical
Technology, Enschede, The Netherlands.
[**] State University of Groningen, Department of Experimental
Surgery, Groningen, The Netherlands.

SUMMARY

Poly(vinyl chloride) (PVC) and silicone rubber (SR) tubing were
compared in an in vivo test system with and without systemic heparinization. 5 Meters of tubing were interconnected in a veno-venous
shunt in anaesthetized dogs, and a flow of 400 ml/min was maintained.
Though no significant hematological differences were observed,
microscopic study of the surfaces revealed an important phenomenon.
SR with heparinization showed a regular coverage with platelets. In
the absence of heparin, the SR surface was covered with platelet
aggregates, fibrin and clots. The PVC surfaces, however, were
covered with a thin platelet mass and did not show any sign of clot
or fibrin formation. No differences between the use or absence of
heparin were observed. Apparently the platelets adhere on the PVC
surfaces in such a way, that fibrin formation is prevented.

INTRODUCTION

In the early contact between blood and the surface of a foreign
material protein adsorption, blood platelet deposition, and activation of the intrinsic coagulation are known to take place (Salzman,
1972; Bruck, 1977). After 10 or 30 min of blood-material contact
thrombus formation will occur (Ihlenfeld, 1978). Lately several
investigators have studied this thrombus formation, especially the
influence of flow upon the rate of thrombus growth (Schultz et al,
1976; Ruckenstein et al, 1977; Ihlenfeld et al 1978) proved that
thrombus formation is also a material dependent phenomenon. Blood
parameters like platelet number and reactivity, fibrinogen concentration, and heparinization play an important role (Salzman, 1972;
Feijen, 1979). Although significant improvements have been made
towards non-thrombogenic surfaces, all known biomaterials show the
above described process to some extent.

Development of biomaterials for long term use requires test models
which measure biocompatibility for longer time intervals. Well known
in vivo test models are the vena cava ring test and the renal embolus
test (Bruck, 1977). These have been tried extensively in the past ten
years, but are very laborious. Recently more simple in vivo test

481

models have been developed to study blood material interactions, using pieces of tubing in an arterial-venous shunt system (Ihlenfeld et al 1978; Ihlenfeld and Cooper,1979; Lindon et al,1979).

In this article we describe an _in vivo_ veno-venous shunt model, in which commercial available tubing material is tested to study thrombus formation with and without heparinization.

MATERIALS AND METHODS

Healthy mongrel dogs (20 - 30 kg), previously screened for normal haemotalogy, were anaesthetized, intubated and artificially ventilated. Each animal was used for one experiment. Heparin, when administered, was given in an initial dose of 300 IU per kg BW. The effect of heparinization was monitored by the activated clotting time (ACT, Hemochron ® system, International Technidyne Co., Metuchen, New Jersey, U.S.A.). After termination of the extra corporeal circulation (ECC), in cases of heparinization, protamine chloride was administered in a dose which is necessary to neutralize 150 IU of heparin per kg BW.

Cannulation was performed in the following sequence. In the left femoral artery a Deseret ® E-Z catheter (Deseret Pharmaceutical Co., Sandy, Utah, U.S.A.) was inserted for arterial pressure measurement and blood sampling. The right jugular vein was cannulated with a long cannula (Portex ® , 5 mm, Hythe, Kent, England), and the right femoral vein was cannulated with a short cannula (USCI ® , no 14, 15 cm, C.R. Bard Inc., Massachusets, U.S.A.). After priming with a prewarmed sterile saline solution, 5 meters of a medical grade tubing (I.D. 8 mm) was interconnected between these venous cannulas by means of connectors (Polystan ® $\frac{1}{4}$' x $\frac{1}{4}$' straight, Harlev, Denmark). A roller pump (Dreissen, Hellevoetsluis, The Netherlands) set just occlusive, was calibrated to maintain a blood flow of 400 ml min^{-1} from jugular to femoral vein. The temperature of the main part of the tubing was kept constant in a water bath at 38°C. ECC was performed for 2 h. Blood samples were taken during ECC and up to the 14th post experimental day as folows: 0', 5', 15', 30', 60', 90', 120', 180', 240' (taken from the arterial line), 1, 2, 5, 6, 7 and the 14th day (taken by venapuncture). These samples were analyzed for: Hematocrit, total hemoglobin, plasma hemoglobin, erythrocyte, leucocyte and platelet count, and platelet aggregability (maximal optical density loss, ADP induced). Directly after termination of ECC, 200 of the 250 ml of blood present in the tubing was first given back to the animal, whereafter the cannulas were taken out. The tubing was immediately flushed with a phosphate buffered saline solution (0.01 M NaH$_2$PO$_4$, 0.15 M NaCl, pH 7.4) for 10 min at a flow rate of 400 ml min^{-1}. Then at fixed places pieces of tubing were excised and put overnight into a 2% glutaraldehyde solution. Preparations for scanning electron microscope (SEM) studies are described in this book (Olijslager, 1980).

Two different tubing materials were compared: Poly(vinyl chloride) (PVC, 8 x 12 mm, shore °65, Raumedic ® , Rehau, W-Germany) and silicone rubber (SR, 8 x 12 mm shore °55, Raumedic ®). Four series were performed:

I   Silicone rubber with heparinization   n=3
II   Silicone rubber without heparinization   n=5
III Poly(vinyl chloride) without heparinization   n=4
IV   Poly(vinyl chloride) with heparinization   n=1

Series IV was a concluding experiment to control whether the surface
behaviour found on PVC in series III was influenced by heparin
administration.

RESULTS

The hematological results do not show large changes, expecially
during ECC. In Figs. 1 and 2 platelet count and aggregability is
given as a function of time. During ECC a small but continuous
decrease is measured, particular the aggregability, indicating

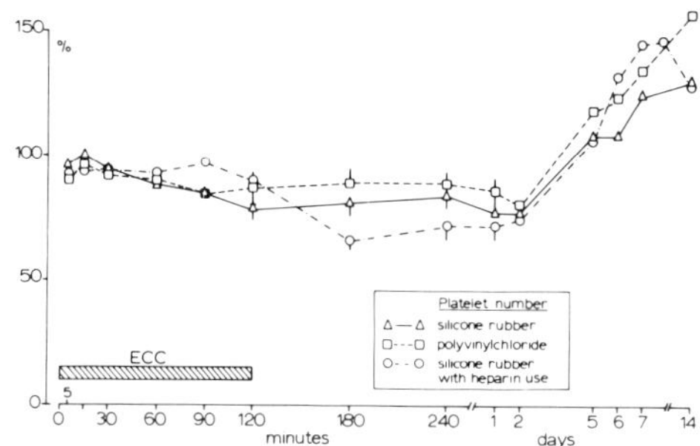

Fig. 1 Platelet numbers for different ECC as a function of
time.

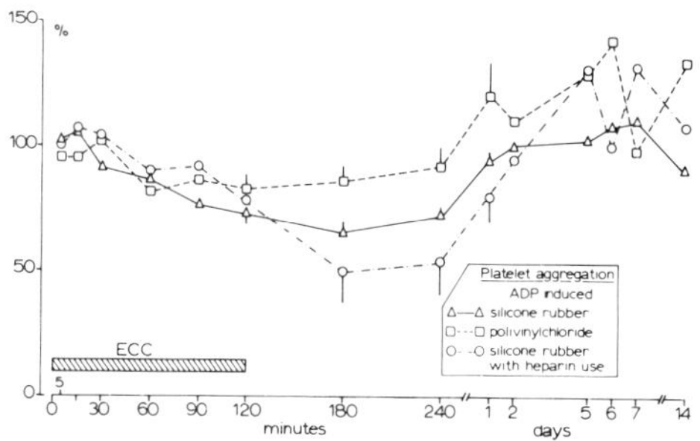

Fig. 2 Platelet aggregability for different ECC as a function of time.

that platelets are affected. The PVC material (series III) seems to
affect platelets somewhat less then silicone rubber (series II).
However when heparin is used in the SR group (series I), a sharp drop
in both platelet count and aggregability is seen at the 180' sample.
In a separate investigation in this laboratory (Velders et al, 1979)
it has been shown that this phenomenon must be attributed to the
excess of protamine given at the end of ECC to neutralize heparin.
It is not possible to differentiate between the series on the second
post experimental day and thereafter.

After flushing with buffer, at the end of ECC, macroscopic examination showed that with heparinization, the SR and the PVC tubings
were free of clot formation. Without heparinization the SR tubing
became largely covered with loosely bound clots. The PVC tubings
showed no clot formation except for the regions in and near the
cannulas and the connectors. The surfaces were further studied in
the SEM, and typical observations are shown in figures 3-8. When
heparin is administered SR tubing is covered with a monocellular
layer of platelets after 2 h of perfusion (Fig. 3). These platelets
show pseudopodia, but no aggregates were observed (Fig. 4). A maximum
surface concentration of 55 platelets per 1000 μ^2 is attained in
this case. When no heparin is administered, the SR surface shows
single platelets and aggregates (Fig. 5), but also fibrin networks
in red- and white (only platelets) thrombi (Fig. 6). The general
picture seen on the PVC tubings, with and without heparinization,
is that of monocellular platelet masses without any detectable fibrin
formation (Fig. 7). The blood platelets lost their integrity, and
only occasionally it is possible to recognize individual platelets
(Fig. 8).

DISCUSSION

Because systemic heparinization during ECC has several drawbacks,
it is important to study the effects of heparin during blood-material
interactions. Minimal heparinization (Gotch and Keen et al,1977) or
even a complete avoidance of heparin (Rottembourg et al, 1979)
received therefore increasing attention. Absence of heparin does not
inevitably result in severe clotting problems. For instance, cardiopulmonary bypass on baboons with or without systemic heparinization
did not show differences with respect to oxygenator performance or
hematological results (Fletcher et al, 1978).

Using our test system we found distinct differences between the
appearance of the SR surface when heparinized or non-heparinized
animals were used. When no heparin is administered, eventually thrombin has been generated as can be seen in the formation of fibrin
threads on the SR surface (Fig. 6). Also thrombi and clots were present,
With heparinization only single adherent platelets were seen.

In the absence of heparin, a monocellular platelet mass was observed
on the PVC surface. No fibrin could be detected and therefore we
assume that no thrombi or clots have been attached to the surfaces
(Fig. 7). The PVC surface becomes passive towards fibrin and thrombus
formation during the two hours of perfusion. The use of heparin did
not change the appearance of the PVC surface.

Ihlenfeld and Cooper (1979) also carried out experiments with PVC
tubing, used as an arterial-venous shunt in dogs. After 2 h of circulation the PVC surface showed the presence of single adherent
platelets (15 per 1000 μ^2). It was found that during the circulation
an intermediate state with thrombus formation existed, but these were
ripped of the surface by high shear forces. After 2 h the surface
became passive for thrombus formation. Under our conditions (low
shear) we have no proof of thrombus formation during the ECC and after
2 h perfusion the surface concentration is over 150 platelets per 1000 μ^2.

We conclude that the presence or absence of heparin has a very distinct effect on the appearance of the SR surface after 2 h ECC, but not on the PVC surface. After 2 h ECC without heparinization there was no thrombus formation on PVC surfaces. Absence of fibrin on the surface suggest that during ECC no thrombi attached to the surface. Using this test model, the most useful results are obtained by SEM study. Hematological data reveal slight differences only.

REFERENCES

Bruck, S.D. (1977). Interactions of synthetic and natural surfaces with blood in the physiological environment, J. Biomed. Mater. Res. Symposium 8, 1-21.

Feijen, J. (1979). Blood-foreign surface contact phenomena, in: Proceedings of the Third International Conference on Plastics in Medicine and Surgery, Enschede, The Netherlands, June 21-22, 28.1-10

Fletcher, J.R., MacKee, A., Anderson, R., & Watson, L., (1978). Baboon venoarterial cardiopulmonary bypass without anticoagulants, Trans. Am. Soc. Artif. Intern. Organs 24, 315-319.

Gotch, F.A. & Keen, M.L. (1977). Precise control of minimal heparinization for high bleeding risk hemodialysis, Trans. Am. Soc. Artif. Intern. Organs 23, 168-176.

Ihlenfeld, J.V., Mathis, T.R., Barberm, T.A., Mosher, D.F., Riddle, L.M. Hart, A.P., Updike, S.J., & Cooper, S.L. (1978). Transient in vivo thrombus deposition onto polymeric biomaterials: Role of plasma fibronectin, Trans. Amer. Soc. Artif. Intern. Organs 24, 727-735.

Ihlenfeld, J.V., & Cooper, S.L. (1979). Transient in vivo protein adsorption onto polymeric biomaterials, J. Biomed. Mater. Res. 13, 577-591.

Lindon, J.N., Collins, R.E.C., Coe. N.P., Jagoda, A., Brier-Russell, D., Merrill, E.W., & Salzman, E.W. (1980). In vivo assessment in sheep of thromboresistant materials by determination of platelet survival, Circulation Research 46, 84-90.

Olijslager, J., Veenhof, C.H.N., Beugeling, T., & Feijen, J., (1980). Development of a new in vitro test system for measuring platelet interactions with biomaterials, in Proceedings of the First World Biomaterial Congress, (Eds. Winter, Gibbons & Plenk), Wiley, Chichester (in press).

Rottembourg, J., Bouayed. F., Durande, J.P., El Shahat, Y., & Guimont, M.C., (1979). No heparin for routine hemodialysis sessions in patients with high bleeding risk, in Proceedings European Soc. Artif. Organs 6 (Ed. E.S. Bücherl), Published by ESAO-Congress Secretariat, Geneva, 121-125.

Ruckenstein, E., Marmur, A., & Gill, W.N., (1977). Growth kinetics of platelet thrombi, J. Theor. Biol. 66, 147-168.

Salzman, E.W. (1972), Surface effects in hemostasis and thrombosis, in The chemistry of Biosurfaces 2 (Ed. M. Hair), Dekker, New York, 489-522.

Schultz, J.S., Ciarkowski, A., Goddard, J.D., Lindenauer, S.M., & Penner, J.A., (1976), Kinetics of thrombus formations, Trans. Amer. Soc. Artif. Intern. Organs 21, 269-277.

Velders, A.J., van den Dungen, J.J.A.M. Westerhof, N.J.W., & Wildevuur, Ch.R.H., (1979), Platelet damage by protamine administration: Protection by reducing protamine or by prostacyclin (PGI2) treatment, Proceedings European Soc. Artif. Organs 6, (Ed. E.S. Bücherl), Published by ESAO-Congress Secretariat, Geneva, pp. 194-197.

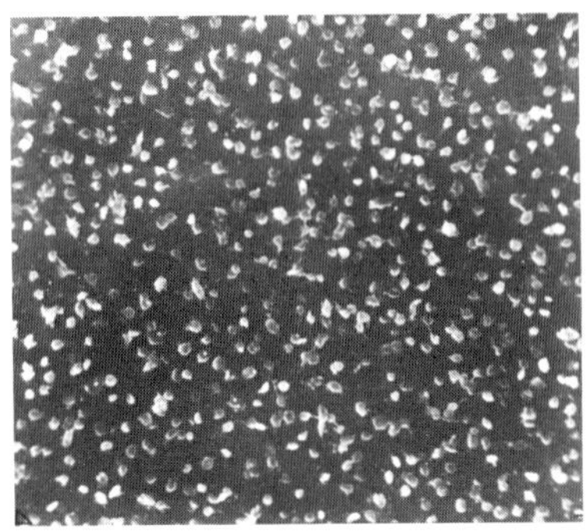

Fig. 3 Platelets on SR surface
with systemic heparinization
(500 x)

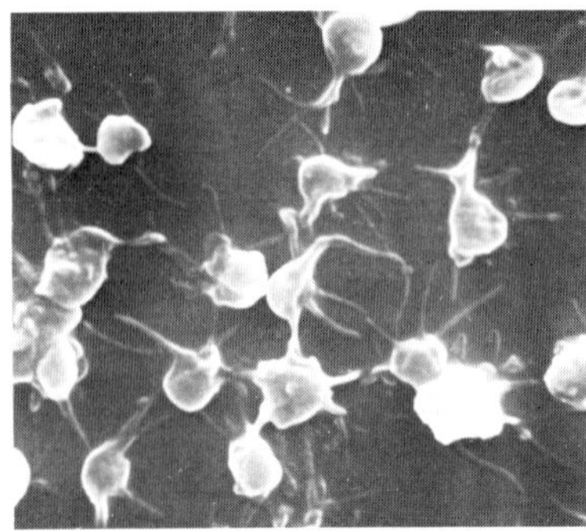

Fig. 4 Enlargment of 3; platelets
are single and show pseudopodia
(2000 x)

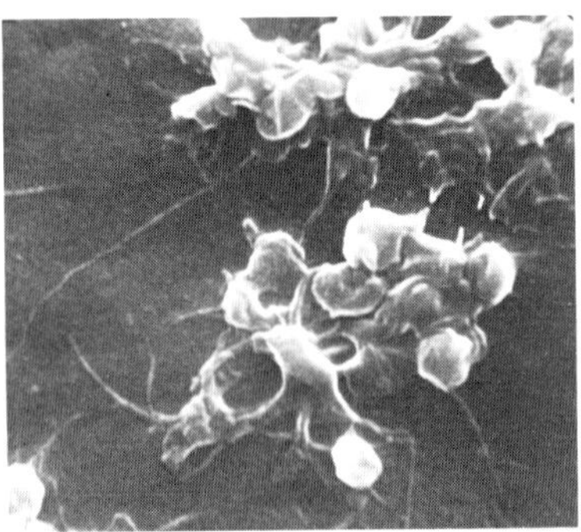

Fig. 5 Platelet aggregates on
SR without systemic heparinization (2000 x)

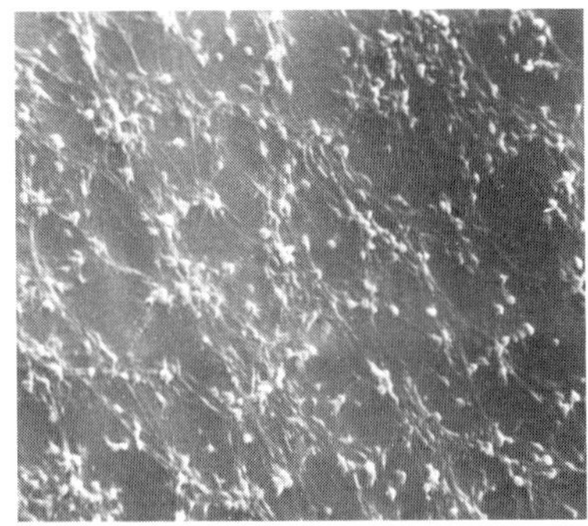

Fig. 6 As Fig. 5; fibrin platelet
networks (500 x)

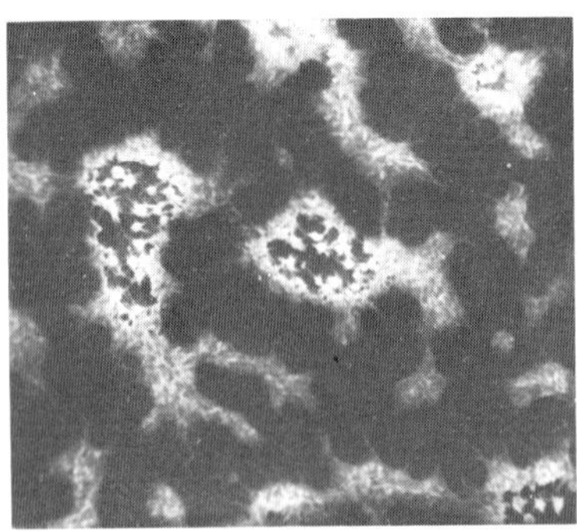

Fig. 7 Platelet masses on PVC
(500 x)

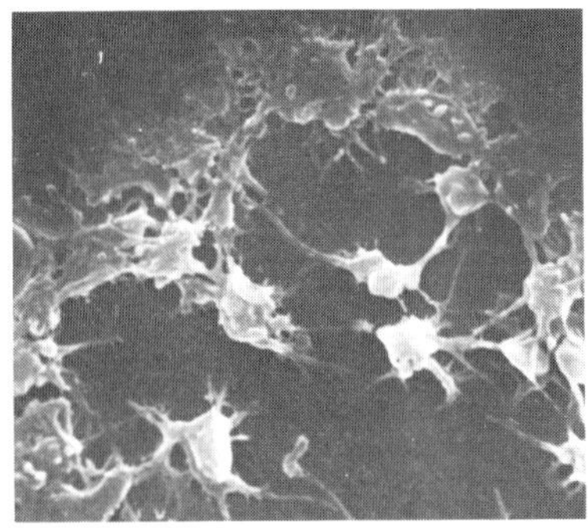

Fig. 8 Enlargment of 7; platelet
masses do not shown fibrin formation (2000 x)

Blood cell interaction

Biomaterials 1980
Edited by G. D. Winter, D. F. Gibbons, and H. Plenk, Jr.
© 1982 John Wiley and Sons Ltd.

A THERMODYNAMIC MODEL FOR THE ASSESSMENT OF LEUKOCYTE AND
PLATELET ADHESION

W. Zingg[1,2], A.W. Neumann[2], C.J. van Oss[3], D.R. Absolom[1,2,3],
O.S. Hum[2] and D.W. Francis[2]

1. Research Institute, The Hospital for Sick Children

2. Institute of Biomedical Engineering and Department of
    Mechanical Engineering, University of Toronto

3. and Immunochemistry Laboratory, Department of Micro-
    biology, State University of New York, Buffalo, N.Y.

<u>SUMMARY</u>

Adhesion of leukocytes and platelets to solid substrates of different
surface tensions and hence different wettability is studied from a
thermodynamic point of view. A simple thermodynamic model predicts
that cellular adhesion should increase with increasing surface tension of the solid substrate if the surface tension of suspending liquid
medium is less than that of the cells. If the surface tension of the
suspending medium is higher than that of the cells, the opposite behaviour is predicted. These predictions are substantiated by adhesion
experiments using granulocytes and platelets.

<u>INTRODUCTION</u>

The explanation of biological observations through physico-chemical
theory is an important aspect of theoretical biology. Such an explanation, rather than empirically obtained data, may also be of practical
value, because it allows logical manipulation of a biological system
and, within well-defined limits, even the prediction of events within
the biological system.

We compare the adhesion of granulocytes and platelets with a simple
thermodynamic model which considers the cells as inert particles.
Adhesion to the solid substrate is then governed by the free energy of
adhesion.

$$\Delta F^{adh} = \gamma_{PS} - \gamma_{PL} - \gamma_{SL} \quad \text{(negative } \Delta F^{adh} \text{ promotes cell adhesion)}$$

γ_{PS} : interfacial tension particle/solid.

γ_{PL} : interfacial tension particle/liquid.

γ_{SL} : interfacial tension solid/liquid.

For a given particle with surface tension γ_{PV}, suspended in a liquid of surface tension γ_{LV}, and interacting with a solid substrate of surface tension γ_{SV}, the quantities γ_{PS}, γ_{PL} and γ_{SL} can be calculated by means of an equation of state approach (Neumann, et al., 1974). The relative magnitude of γ_{LV} and γ_{PV} are decisive. For $\gamma_{LV} > \gamma_{PV}$, the thermodynamic model predicts that adhesion decreases with increasing γ_{SV}, when γ_{SV} is above 30 ergs/cm^2, (Neumann et al., 1974) whereas adhesion increases with increasing γ_{SV}, when $\gamma_{LV} < \gamma_{PV}$. At low values of γ_{SV}, ΔF^{adh} is not very sensitive to changes in γ_{SV}. Such a theoretical prediction of platelet adhesion has been recently published (Neumann et al., 1980).

METHODS

In adhesion experiments with granulocytes the surface tension of the buffer solution was adjusted by adding varying amounts of dimethyl-sulfoxide (DMSO). The thermodynamic predictions were confirmed qualitatively (Fig. 1). The experiments were performed by allowing the granulocytes or platelets to contact the various polymer substrates for 30 min at 21°C (Absolom et al., 1979, 1980a; Neumann et al., 1979). Thereafter the substrates were washed, stained and the number of cells adhering per unit area of substrate was determined.

RESULTS AND DISCUSSION

This method of investigation also provides a novel means for the determination of the surface tension of cells: for the case $\gamma_{LV} = \gamma_{PV}$, ΔF^{adh} becomes independent of γ_{SV}, so that cellular adhesion is independent of γ_{SV} (Fig. 1). The surface tension of granulocytes determined in this way (69.0 ergs/cm^2) was found to agree well with the values obtained from contact angle measurements (via the equation of state approach) on cell layers (Fig. 2). This method is restricted to (those types) of cells which have a propensity for adhesion (Neumann et al., 1979). The effect of the electrostatic interaction between the adhering cells and the substrate cannot be disregarded. However the contribution of these forces to cell adhesion over the range of polymers investigated appears to be constant. This could be shown since when the cells are suspended in a low ionic strength medium ($\mu \approx 0$) containing a chelating agent e.g. Na$_2$EDTA to eliminate the effect of multivalent cationic bridging between the cells and substrate and in which $\gamma_{LV} = \gamma_{PV}$ (made possible through the incorporation of a certain amount of DMSO) cell adhesion virtually disappears (Absolom et al., 1980a)

In platelet adhesion studies, it has not been possible to observe the decrease in the number of platelets adhering to the substrate as γ_{SV} increases (Fig. 3). In view of the marked fragility of platelets it has not been possible to vary the surface tension of the suspending

buffer through the incorporation of surface active additives
(Neumann et al., 1980). Furthermore in those cases where platelets
are suspended in a buffer containing protein (e.g. Tyrodes plus
albumin) there is an inherent difficulty in determining the surface
tension of the buffer (Absolom et al., 1980b). In terms of the thermodynamic model, this implies that γ_{PV} is greater than γ_{LV} under all
circumstances. This may be due to the secretion of proteins by the
platelets which reduces γ_{LV} . Measurements of the surface tension of
the platelet supernatant (γ_{LV} = 63 ergs/cm^2) have confirmed that γ_{LV}
is below the surface tension of platelets ($\gamma_{PV} \approx$ 70 ergs/cm^2). These
measurements were obtained by means of a recently developed photographic contact angle method, in which the contact angle which the
10 $\mu\ell$ sessile drop of platelet supernatant makes with a smooth polymer surface e.g. low density polyethylene, is determined within 2
seconds of deposition (Sherman et al., 1979). In contrast measurements on the supernatant of granulocytes indicate very little, if any,
protein exudation during the experimental period. In both cases the
respective supernatants where obtained by aspiration after centrifugation of the cell suspensions for appropriate times and g forces.
The cell suspensions were allowed to remain standing at 21°C for the
duration of the experimental period prior to centrifugation (Absolom
et al., 1979).

The description of cell adhesion in terms of the Helmholtz Free Energy
of Adhesion (ΔF^{adh}) provides a useful analytical tool to differentiate
between normal and pathological granulocytes which differ in their
surface tensions (Fig. 4). The pathological granulocytes which have
been studied most extensively are obtained from patients with persistent idiopathic juvenile periodontal disease (Absolom et al., 1980a).
The differences in the surface tensions of normal and pathological
granulocytes have been correlated with abnormal adhesion and phagocytic properties (Absolom et al., 1980a; Cianciola et al., 1979).

We have previously documented that a maximum or a minimum exist for
ΔF^{adh} over a range of γ_{SV} for each value of γ_{LV} (Neumann et al., 1980).
Kinetic studies of platelet adhesion as a function of contact time show
an initial linear increase in the number of platelets adhering per unit
area; the slope of these curves depends, however, on γ_{SV} (Fig. 5). After
contact times of approximately 1 to 2 hrs, platelet adhesion ceases at
a level which is again a function of γ_{SV} . A plot of this equilibrium
or saturation amount of adhering platelets against γ_{SV} reveals a levell-
ing off at low values of γ_{SV} as is predicted by the thermodynamic
model (Neumann et al., 1980) (Fig. 6). The observed kinetics of platelet adhesion is in qualitative disagreement with simple transport ideas
combined with a Derajaguin, Landau, Verwey and Overbeek (DLVO) theory
type of activation barrier for platelet adhesion.

Recent work on protein adhesion suggests that the thermodynamic approach-
may have an even wider range of applicability than expected so far.

Considering protein molecules as particles (which adhere to polymers
in a manner similar to cells) it is now possible to obtain a hitherto
inaccessible property of proteins: the intrinsic surface tension of
protein molecules. The protein adsorption studies reveal patterns
very similar to those shown for cells in Fig. 1. Different serum
protein species have unique and characteristic slopes and surface
tensions (van Oss et al., 1980). The method employed is analogous to
that already described for cell surface tension determinations
(Absolom et al., 1979, Absolom et al., 1980a).

REFERENCES

Absolom, D.R., Neumann, A.W., Zingg, W. & van Oss C.J. (1979)
Thermodynamic Studies of Cellular Adhesion.
Trans. Am. Soc. Artif. Intern. Organs, 25, 152-156.

Absolom, D.R., van Oss, C.J., Genco, R.J., Francis, D.W. & Neumann, A.W.
(1980a).
Surface Thermodynamics of Normal and Pathological Human Granulocytes.
Cell Biophysics 2, In press.

Absolom, D.R., van Oss, C.J., Zingg, W. & Neumann, A.W. (1980b).
Determination of Surface Tensions of Proteins II. Surface Tension of
Serum Albumin, Altered at the Protein-Air Interface.
Abstract #109
Second Chemical Congress of the North American Continent, Las Vegas,
August, 1980.

Cianciola, L.J., Genco, R.J., Patters, M.R., McKenna, J. & van Oss, C.J.
(1977)
Defective Chemotaxis and Phagocytosis of Polymorphonuclear Phagocytes
of Patients with Periodontal Disease.
Nature 265, 445-447.

Neumann, A.W., Good, R.J., Hope, C.J. & Sejpal, M. (1974)
An Equation-of-State Approach to Determine Surface Tensions of Low-
Energy Solids from Contact Angles.
J. Coll. Interface Sci. 49,

Neumann, A.W., Hum, O.S., Francis, D.W., Zingg, W. & van Oss, C.J.
(1980)
Kinetic and Thermodynamic Aspects of Platelet Adhesion from Suspension
to Various Substrates.
J. Biomed. Mater. Res. 14: 499-509, 1980.

Sherman, J.A.
The Critical Closing and Critical Opening Phenomena in Canine Heart.
Ph.D. Dissertation, University of Toronto, 1979. pg. 88.

van Oss, C.J., Absolom, D.R., Zingg, W. & Neumann, A.W. (1980)
Determination of the Surface Tension of Proteins. I. Surface Tension
of Native Serum Proteins in Aqueous Media.
Abstract #108
Second Chemical Congress of the North American Continent, Las Vegas,
August, 1980.

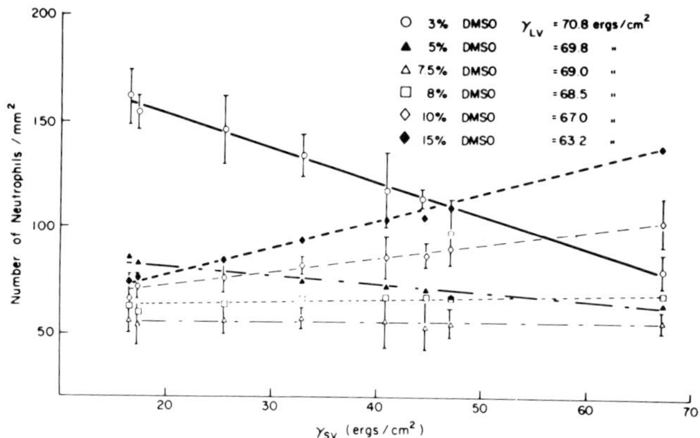

Fig.1   Granulocyte Adhesion as a Function of Substrate Surface Tension (γ_{SV}) for Various Liquid Surface Tensions (γ_{LV})

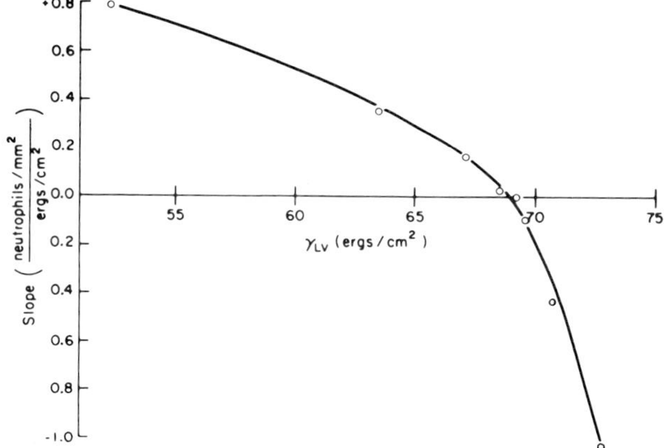

Fig.2   Determination of Cell Surface Tension from Adhesion Studies.   Slope = 0 when $\gamma_{LV} = \gamma_{PV}$

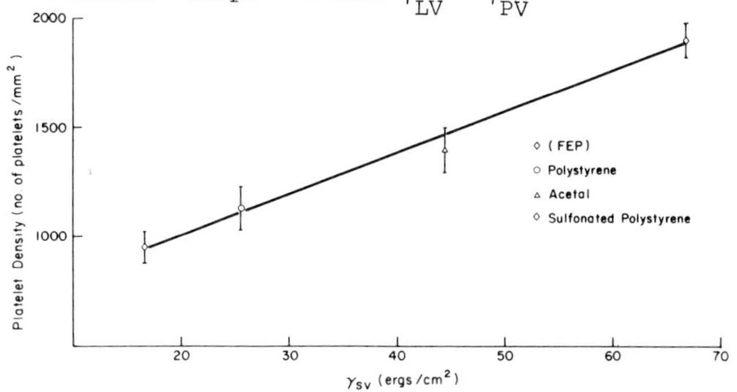

Fig.3   Platelet Adhesion as a Function of Substrate Surface Tension (γ_{SV}).   In the case of platelets γ_{LV} is always < γ_{PV}

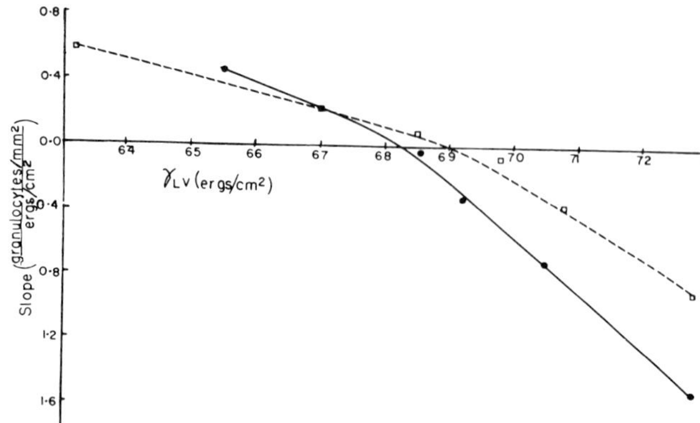

Fig.4   Use of the Thermodynamic Approach to Describe Surface Tension
Difference Between Normal (□) and Pathological Granulocytes (●)

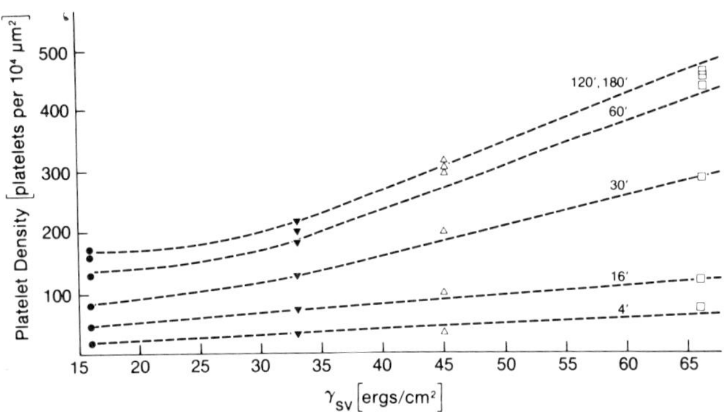

Fig.5   Kinetics of Platelet Adhesion to Various Solid Substrates:
● TEFLON FEP, △ Acetal, ▼ Low density polyethylene,
■ Sulphonated polystyrene

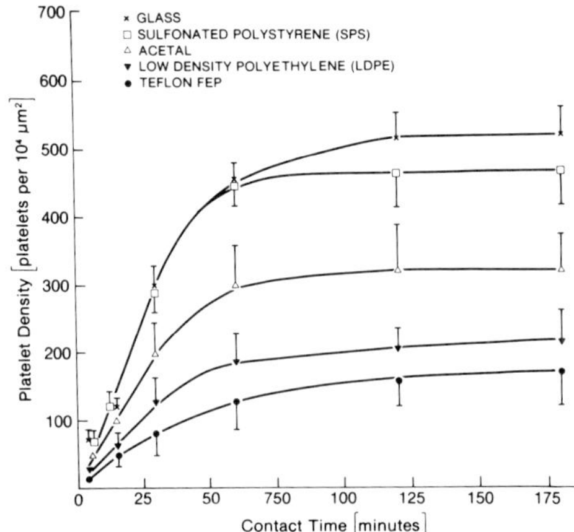

Fig.6   Platelet Adhesion as a Function of Substrate Surface Tension
(γ_{SV}) for Various Contact Times

Biomaterials 1980
Edited by G. D. Winter, D. F. Gibbons, and H. Plenk, Jr.
© 1982 John Wiley and Sons Ltd.

ESTIMATION OF CELL ADHESION ON POLYMER SURFACES
BY THE USE OF "COLUMN-METHOD"

K. Kataoka*, T. Okano*, T. Akaike*, Y. Sakurai*,
M. Maeda**, T. Nishimura**, Y. Nitadori**, T. Tsuruta**,
A. Shimada***, and I. Shinohara***

*Institute of Medical Engineering, Tokyo Women's Medical
College, Shinjuku-ku, Tokyo 162, JAPAN
**Department of Synthetic Chemistry, University of Tokyo,
Bunkyo-ku, Tokyo 113, JAPAN
***Department of Polymer Chemistry, Waseda University,
Shinjuku-ku, Tokyo 162, JAPAN

SUMMARY

Adhesion behavior of rat mesenteric lymph-node lymphocytes was investigated using the "column method". Lymphocytes attached on a γ-
globulin-coated poly(2-hydroxyethyl methacrylate) (γ-G-PHEMA) surface
were found to undergo significant flattening and elongation, in
contrast with moderate shape change of lymphocytes attached on a γ-
globulin-coated poly(styrene) (γ-G-PSt) surface. We consider that
the difference in orientation of adsorbed γ-G molecules (i.e. γ-G adsorb on PHEMA and PSt with its Fab part and Fc part, respectively.)
may be responsible for this difference in lymphocytes morphology. In
another series of experiments, adhesion of rat platelets on poly-
styrene/polyamine comb type copolymers (SA copolymers) was investigated. Shape changes of attached platelets can be controlled from
"negligible" to "marked" by varying the mode of "microphase separation
" of SA copolymer surfaces. Platelets adhesivity can also be controlled by coating SA copolymer surfaces with plasma protein (albumin
and γ-globulin). We assume that the "microphase separated" structure
of SA copolymer may regulate the adhesion and shape change of platelet
through its effect on a redistribution of glycoproteins present at the
plasma membrane of platelets.

INTRODUCTION

Our primary purpose is to control the species, amounts, morphologies,
and functions of adhered cells by designing the physical and chemical
structures of materials on which cells adhere.

After the initial contact with and attachment of the cells to surface,
there is a general reorganization of the microtubules and microfilaments that comprise the cell's cytoskeleton. Morphological and
functional changes, such as pseudopod formation and release reactions
of lysosomal enzymes, of adhered cells may be triggered by these reorganization processes. Prior to this reorganization of microtubules

493

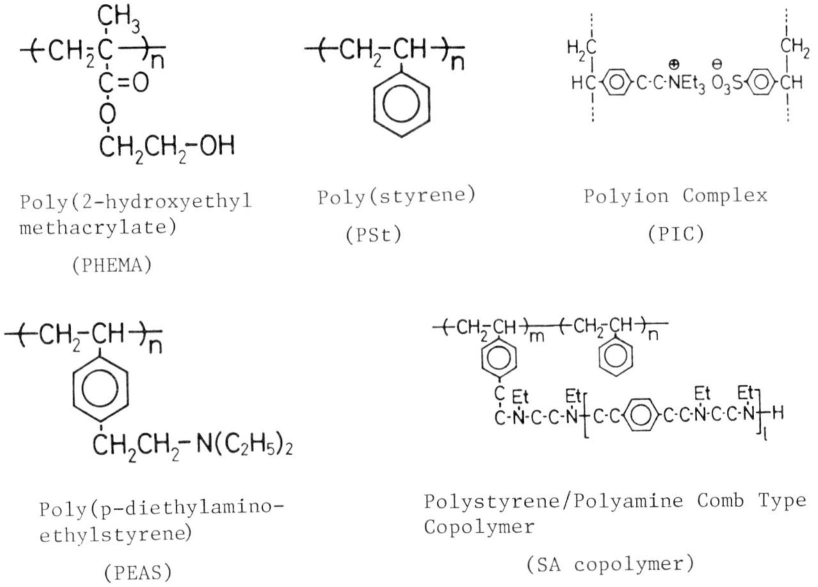

Poly(2-hydroxyethyl
methacrylate)

(PHEMA)

Poly(styrene)

(PSt)

Polyion Complex

(PIC)

Poly(p-diethylamino-
ethylstyrene)

(PEAS)

Polystyrene/Polyamine Comb Type
Copolymer

(SA copolymer)

Fig. 1. Structural formulas of polymers examined.

and microfilaments, redistribution (clustering$\longrightarrow$patching$\longrightarrow$capping)
of the protein molecules of the cell membrane take place. Therefore,
to control cell adhesion, the physicochemical and morphological parameters of the material's surface should control the redistribution of
membrane proteins. We named this concept "capping control".

In this paper, we discuss two important parameters which are considered to affect the capping of cell membrane proteins. First, the
effect of proteins adsorbed on material's surface, and second, the
effect of the material microstructure on cell adhesion.

MATERIALS AND METHODS

The structural formulas of polymers examined are shown in Fig. 1.
Preparation of these polymers and their coating on glass beads (40-60
mesh) are described elsewhere (Kataoka et al, 1980; Nishimura et al,
1980). 0.2M phosphate buffer solutions containing rat albumin (0.09
g/dl) and rat γ-globulin (0.032 g/dl) were used for the precoating of
the beads.

Cell Suspensions. Platelets and mesenteric lymph-node lymphocytes
were obtained from inbred male Wister rats, and suspended in Hank's
Balanced Salt Solution (HBSS), pH 7.2.

The Column Method (Kataoka et al, 1980). A single cell suspension was
passed through the column by use of an infusion pump. When indicated,
cells were incubated in the column for a definite time. The number

of cells in the eluted suspension was determined by a hemacytometer
and phase contrast microscopy. The morphology of the cells adhered
the beads' surface was observed by scanning electron microscope (SEM).

RESULTS AND DISCUSSION

Effect of Adsorbed γ-Globulin Molecules on Lymphocyte Adhesion. We
have previously investigated the adhesion of canine peripheral lymphocytes on various polymer surfaces (Kataoka et al, 1980). In most
cases, lymphocyte adhesion was suppressed when the surface was precoated with autologous serum. However on a PHEMA surface, lymphocyte
adhesion was enhanced by serum-precoating. Among the many components
of serum, we considered γ-globulin molecules to be responsible for
this exceptional phenomenon because of their amphiphilic nature. The
γ-globulin molecule is reported to contain two regions, namely, the
hydrophilic Fab part and the hydrophobic Fc part (Van Oss et al, 1975).
Therefore, it is plausible that adsorbed γ-globulin molecules may assume different orientations depending upon the hydrophobicity of materials; γ-globulin molecules adsorb on hydrophilic surface, like
PHEMA, with their Fab parts, and adsorb on hydrophobic surface, like
PSt, with their Fc parts. The results obtained from circular dichroism and wettability measurements of adsorbed γ-globulin layer also
suggest such orientations (Sakurai et al, 1980).

To confirm this oriented adsorption of γ-globulin molecules, rat
mesenteric lymphocytes were incubated on a γ-globulin-coated PHEMA
surface (γ-G-PHEMA) and on a γ-globulin-coated PSt surface (γ-G-PSt).
Table 1 presents the distribution of adhered cell morphology when
graded by degree of flattening and extent of elongation. In contrast
with lymphocytes on γ-G-PSt, significant flattening and elongation
were observed for lymphocytes adhered on γ-G-PHEMA. Such elongated
shape changes are similar to those observed with Fc receptor-bearing
lymphocytes adhered on immune-complex precoated surfaces (Alexander
and Henkart, 1976).

In the light of these findings, the steep rise of canine lymphocyte
adhesion on serum-coated PHEMA and the significant distortion of rat
lymphocytes adhered on γ-G-PHEMA may be caused by a binding of Fc receptor-bearing lymphocytes to Fc parts of adsorbed γ-globulin molecules.

"Capping Control" of Adhered Cells. The adhesion behavior of rat
platelets on PSt/polyamine comb type copolymers (SA copolymers) was
examined to clarify the role of "microphase separated" structure of
materials on cell adhesion. Fig. 2a shows transmission electron
micrographs of the "microphase separated" structure of SA copolymer
surfaces. The size of the polyamine domain (observed as dispersed
phase) seems to increase with increasing the polyamine content. Morphologies and amounts of adhered platelets on SA surfaces are summarized in Fig. 2b and Table 2, respectively. Since the SA copolymers
have cell-adhesive polyamine domains, almost 80 % of platelets were
adhered on SA copolymer surfaces without protein-coating.

TABLE 1. Distribution of adhered lymphocyte morphology
(% of total adhered cells)[1].

a) γ-G-PSt

		Degree of flattening		
		none	intermediate	marked
Extent of elongation	none	3(20)	23(36)	13(2)
	intermediate	0(3)	18(15)	0(0)
	marked	0(2)	9(7)	34(15)

b) γ-G-PHEMA

		Degree of flattening		
		none	intermediate	marked
Extent of elongation	none	0(44)	0(12)	0(6)
	intermediate	0(13)	0(5)	0(5)
	marked	0(0)	0(11)	100(37)

[1]Incubation time: 10 min. A minimum of 200 cells were
scored. The criteria used to score lymphocytes was according to (Alexander and Henkart, 1976). Values obtained
for γ-G-uncoated polymer surfaces are given in parenthesis.

TABLE 2. % of adhered platelets on SA copolymers with or
without protein coating[1].

Protein precoating	Substrate					
	Glass	PSt	SA9	SA15	SA25	PEAS
none	83± 8	83± 8	75±13	85± 7	77± 9	86± 6
Alb	78±10	76±15	22±13	77±13	44±20	86± 8
γ-G	55±11	53±20	50±23	34± 8	51±14	76± 8

[1]Each value is the mean ± standard deviation of four column
runs each using platelets prepared from a different rat.
Platelet density: 3×10^4 cells/mm^3. Flow rate: 0.2 ml/min.
Contact time: 4 min.

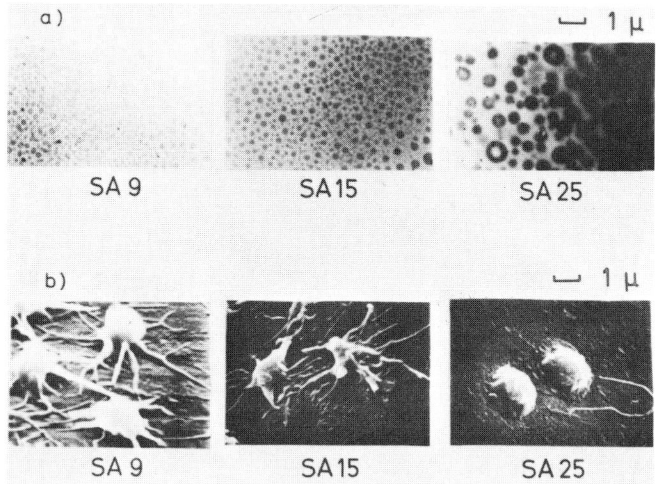

Fig. 2. Microphase separated structures of SA copolymers
(SAx; x=polyamine content, wt%) and the morphology of the
adhered platelets. a) TEM photographs of the surface of
SAx (Nishimura et al, 1980). Polyamine domains are
observed as black dispersed phase. b) SEM photographs of
the adhered rat platelets on SAx without protein-coating.

The morphology of the adhered platelets, however, changed strikingly
with a change in the polyamine contents of the SA copolymers. Particularly, on SA25, platelets attached with hardly any pseudopod formation. This result suggests that reorganization of microtubules and
microfilaments, and therefore, capping of membrane proteins was prevented by SA25 surface.

Table 2 also summarizes the results of platelet adhesion on protein
coated surfaces. γ-Globulin(γ-G)-coated surfaces, except γ-G-coated
PEAS, were found to retain not more than 60 % of applied platelets,
and platelet adhesion seems to be minimum on γ-G-coated SA15.

On albumin(Alb)-coated surfaces, platelet adhesion didn't correlate
with the polyamine content of the polymers. A significant decrease in
platelet adhesion was observed on Alb-coated SA9 ($P<0.02$) and Alb-
coated SA25 ($P<0.05$). Also, essentially no pseudopod formation nor
spreading was observed with the platelets attached on these two surfaces. We have previously reported that cationic polymers enhance
the adsorption and the conformational change (evaluated by α-helix
content) of albumin, compared with neutral polymers including PSt (
Akaike et al, 1979). Since SA copolymer surfaces are separated to two
distinct microphase of weakly cationic polyamine (observed as "islands
") and neutral PSt (observed as "sea"), the "microphase separated"
albumin layer, in terms of adsorbed amounts and conformation, could be
formed on SA copolymer surfaces, corresponding to their "microphase
separated" structure.

As a possible mechanism, we assume that the "microphase separated" albumin layer thus formed may prevent the adhesion and shape change of platelets through its regulating effect on a redistribution (clustering⟶patching⟶capping) of glycoproteins present at the plasma membrane of platelets. However, negligible decrease in plate- let adhesion on Alb-coated SA15 suggests that the formation of "microphase separated" structure alone may be insufficient to account for the decrease in platelet adhesion on Alb-coated SA9 and Alb-coated SA25, and that the differences in their mode of "microphase sepa- ration", in terms of size, shape, and distribution, should also be taken into account, as is the case with platelet adhesion on PHEMA/PSt block copolymer (Okano et al, 1980).

In conclusion, our results establish that shapes and adhesiveness of platelets can be controlled in a wide range by using a series of SA copolymers with or without protein-coating. Blood cell separator com- posed of the column packed with SA copolymer-coated glass beads is now developed in our laboratories.

ACKNOWLEDGEMENTS

Financial support given by the Ministry of Science and Technology, Japan (Special Project Research, Bio-separator) is acknowledged.

REFERENCES

Akaike, T., Sakurai, Y., Kosuge, K., Senba, Y., Kuwana, K., Miyata, S. , Kataoka, K., and Tsuruta, T. (1979) Study on the interaction be- tween plasma proteins and polyion complex by circular dichroism and ultraviolet spectroscopy. Kobunshi Ronbunshu, 36, 217-222.
Alexander, E., and Henkart, P. (1976) The adherence of human Fc re- ceptor-bearing lymphocytes to antigen-antibody complexes II. Morpho- logic alternations induced by the substrate. J. Exp. Med., 143, 329- 347.
Kataoka, K., Maeda, M., Nishimura, T., Nitadori, Y., Tsuruta, T., Akaike, T., and Sakurai, Y. (1980) Estimation of cell adhesion on polymer surfaces with the use of column-method. J. Biomed. Mater. Res., in press.
Nishimura, T., Maeda, M., Nitadori, Y., and Tsuruta, T. (1980) Poly- styrene-polyamine comb-type graft copolymer, synthesis and microphase structure. Makromol. Chem., Rapid Commun., 1, 573-577.
Okano, T., Nishiyama, S., Shinohara, I., Akaike, T., Sakurai, Y., Kataoka, K., and Tsuruta, T. (1979) Role of microphase separated structure on the interfacial interaction of polymer with blood. ACS Polym. Prep., 20, 571-574.
Sakurai, Y., Akaike, T., Kataoka, K., and Okano, T. (1980) Inter- facial phenomenon in biomaterials chemistry. in ACS Advances in Chem- istry Series, American Chemical Society, Washington, D. C., in press.
Van Oss, C. J., Gillman, C. F., and Neumann, A. W. (1975) Phagocytic Engulfment and Cell Adhesiveness as Cellular Surface Phenomena, Marcel Dekker, N. Y.

Biomaterials 1980
Edited by G. D. Winter, D. F. Gibbons, and H. Plenk, Jr.
© 1982 John Wiley and Sons Ltd.

THE BEHAVIOR OF BLOOD COMPONENTS FOLLOWING CONTACT
WITH AN ALL CARBON SURFACED MEMBRANE OXYGENATOR

R. Debski, H. Borovetz, L. Mitchell, B. Griffith,
A. Haubold* and R. Hardesty

Department of Surgery, University of Pittsburgh
School of Medicine, Pittsburgh, Pennsylvania, USA

*Carbomedics, Inc., San Diego, California, USA

SUMMARY

ULTI carbon can be successfully applied to the components of a membrane oxygenator. While the ULTI carbon does not significantly impair O_2 permeability, it does demonstrate less cellular damage and protein denaturation manifested by 1) maintenance of red cell structure and quantity, 2) mean increased numbers of white blood cells, 3) less mean initial thrombocytopenia with rapid return to baseline levels, and 4) less mean depression in serum fibrinogen levels. This correlates with previous experiments showing noticable reduction in the attachment of cellular debris and minimal fibrin formation when the ULTI surface is compared to the uncoated surface during arteriovenous perfusion in dogs.

INTRODUCTION

A variety of vacuum processes have been investigated in an effort to produce carbon coatings at room temperature without suspension in a fluidized bed. These coatings have generally been called vacuum-vapor-deposited carbons. Using a hybrid low pressure process, a new isotropic carbon coating can now be deposited from a gaseous precursor at ambient temperatures using a proprietary catalyst. This new coating is called ultra low temperature isotropic (ULTI) carbon and can be applied to devices having a certain degree of flexibility.

This ULTI carbon has been successfully applied to the microchannels, membranes and connectors of a membrane oxygenator. In this study, the effect of the ULTI carbon on blood components is defined. Red blood cell, white blood cell, platelet and protein morphology and function were evaluated in blood samples from animals undergoing bypass with the membrane oxygenator. Results for the ULTI carbon surface were compared to data obtained when the surface was not coated.

MATERIALS

The oxygenator employs the mass exchange process of blood flowing

through etched microchannels with one side permeable to gas (Hung
et al., 1977). Each channel is semi-circular in shape, 230 $\pm$
20µm wide and 110 $\pm$ 10µmm etched onto a copper sheet, 12 in.
long, 5 in. wide and 0.016 in. thick and is plated with a layer of
nickel one micron thick. To optimize the use of the plate, both
sides are completely etched with parallel channels (a total of 1130
channels per stainless steel plate). The membrane (Gelman Instrument, Co.) is fabricated from polyvinyl chloride (PVC) acrylonitrile
cast on a woven polyester cloth and made hydrophobic by treatment
with a silicone fluid. The membrane has a typical sheet thickness
of 50-100 microns. The nominal pore size is 0.2 microns (40-50%
porosity).

In preparation for coating with the ULTI carbon, the microchannels,
membranes, connectors and polytetrafluoroethylene graft material are
agitated in filtered, deionized water, rinsed with ethyl alcohol and
dried in a lint-free environment (Borovetz et al., 1980). These components are mounted inside the coating apparatus. The entire system
is evacuated to a pressure of less than 5 X 10^{-7} torr and an adherent
layer of ULTI carbon is applied. The thickness of the carbon coating
is monitored optically and deposition is terminated when the pre-
selected thickness is achieved. A membrane is placed flush with each
surface of a plate and sandwiched in a rigid epoxy-coated porous foam
encased in a 1 in. thick Lexan plate. Prior to introduction of blood
into the unit, saline is pumped through the etched microchannels by a
roller pump to eliminate air bubbles from the system.

METHODS

Arteriovenous perfusion was established in 16 (18-22 kg) dogs: 8 dogs
in which the circuit components (inlet/outlet connectors, microchannels, microporous membranes, polytetrafluoroethylene graft material)
were coated with ULTI carbon and 8 dogs in which the components remained uncoated. Phenobarbitol (35mg/kg) anesthesia was used and the dogs
were ventilated with a Harvard ventilator. The dogs were heparinized
with a bolus (2mg/kg) of beef lung heparin. Supplemental heparin was
given to maintain the activated coagulation time between 5 and 7 minutes. The carotid artery was attached directly to the inlet connector
of the oxygenator. Venous outflow was collected by interposition of a
segment of 4 mm polytetrafluoroethylene (PTFE) conduit from the outlet
to a femoral vein (end-to-side).

Flow was monitored on the arterial side with an electromagnetic probe
and regulated at 10% of cardiac output (estimated at 100 cc/kg) with a
gate clamp. Central venous pressure and arterial pressure were monitored continuously. Blood samples were taken prior to bypass and at
15 min., 30 min., 1 hour, 2, 3, 4, 5 and 6 hour intervals and assayed
using the laboratory tests shown in Table 1.

TABLE 1. Laboratory tests and methods performed on blood
          samples.

Test   Method

Red Blood Count   Coulter
White Blood Count   Coulter
Platelet Count   Coulter
WBC Differential   Slide
RBC Morphology   Slide
Hematocrit   Centrifuge
Osmotic Fragility   Hypotonic Phosphate
Plasma Hgb   Tetramethylbenzidine/H_2O_2
Platelet Aggregation   ADP Induction
Fibrinogen   Thrombin/Folin's Reagent

RESULTS

The effect of the ULTI carbon surface on red blood cells, white blood
cells, platelets, and fibrinogen was evaluated and compared to data
from the uncoated surface. Data are expressed as a percent deviation
from baseline. Mean and standard deviations were calculated and are
plotted versus time for the ULTI and uncoated groups.

Red Blood Cell: No significant damage to the red cell was demonstrated when in contact with the ULTI surface. This was manifested by
(1) stable red cell count and hematocrit, (2) no change in osomotic
fragility, (3) no appearance of plasma hemoglobin, and (4) absence of
fragmentation on peripheral smear. Hemolysis did occur in 25% (2/8)
of the uncoated group, manifested by a rise in plasma hemoglobin, the
appearance of fragmentation on peripheral smear and a fall in the red
cell count and hematocrit (Table 2).

TABLE 2. Changes in results of RBC assays for the 2 dogs
          showing evidence of hemolysis after 6 hours of
          perfusion in the uncoated group.

	DOG #3		DOG #7	
	Initial	Final	Initial	Final
Hematocrit	45	34%	42	33%
Plasma Hemoglobin	< 1	137 mg/dl	< 1	219 mg/dl
RBC Fragmentation	0	+	0	+
RBC Count	6.45	4.48	5.84	4.17

White Blood Cell: The ULTI group showed stable WBC counts with a progressive rise to twice the baseline levels beginning at one hour (Figure 1 a,b). This was in contrast to a rapid fall in WBC counts in the
uncoated group and a gradual return to baseline at 5 hours. Differential counts in both groups showed a relative granulocytosis. Immature
bands (the cells most susceptible to injury) were more apparent in the
ULTI group (Table 3).

TABLE 3. Final range of differential counts for white
          blood cells after 6 hours of perfusion.

	ULTI	UNCOATED
PMNs	71–85	56–74
Bands	9–15	0–5
Lymphs	12–25	17–40
Monos	0–2	0–3
Eos	0–3	0–3

<u>Platelet</u>: Whole blood platelet counts fell dramatically in the un-
coated group. The ULTI group showed minimal depression with return to
baseline in the three to six hour period (Figure 2 a,b). Although
both groups demonstrated a decreased aggregation response, the ULTI
group exhibited improved aggregation in the three to six hour period
(Figure 3 a,b).

<u>Fibrinogen</u>: Fibrinogen levels fell to 70% of baseline at 15 minutes
in both groups (Figure 4 a,b). While fibrinogen continued to decrease
to 40% of baseline with the uncoated surface, the levels appeared to
stabilize in the ULTI group.

DISCUSSION

Certain properties of the ULTI carbon have been described when applied
to the components of a membrane oxygenator. Scanning electron microscopy of the surface of an etched microchannel demonstrated a uniform
overlayer of ULTI carbon, approximately one micron thick (Borovetz et
al., 1979a). This complete coverage was verified using sequential surface analytical techniques. The ULTI surface shows a beaded appearance when applied to the microporous membrane, as a result of the
structure of the substrate material. The thickness of the ULTI carbon
varies between 0.7 and 1.7 microns. Over this range of coating thickness, there is a reduction of only 10% in oxygen permeability below
that found for the uncoated membrane. This oxygen permeability is two
orders of magnitude above that reported for silicone rubber membranes
and provides effective gas exchange through the ULTI carbon membrane
(Borovetz et al., 1979b).

Spectroscopic techniques and scanning electron microscopy confirm the
presence of a proteinaceous film on the surfaces of all membranes
after exposure to blood. After four to eight hours of perfusing the
ULTI-surfaced components, the attachment of cellular debris and fibrin
formation remains insignificant when compared to the uncoated surface
(Borovetz et al., 1978).

In this study, polytetrafluoroetheylene was chosen as the synthetic
graft material because it is a proven vascular conduit, it does not
require preclotting (which may alter blood-surface interaction), and

it can be coated successfully with the ULTI carbon. Its presence in
the circuit insured that all components in the ULTI group were composed
of animal vessel or carbon surface.

The numerical counts of the three cell types (red blood cell, white
blood cell and platelet) were more stable in experiments using the
ULTI surface. The improved platelet aggregation in the three to six
hour period for the ULTI group may have resulted from a higher count
rather than improved function of platelets. The early decrease in
fibrinogen levels in both groups can be attributed to adherence to
the foreign surface. Once these initial binding sites are covered,
further denaturation on the ULTI surface is minimal while fibrinogen
continues to decline with the uncoated surface.

ACKNOWLEDGEMENTS

The encouragement and support of Henry T. Bahnson, M.D. are deeply
appreciated. The authors wish to thank Mr. John Belhumeur and Mr.
Michael Shaver for their assistance in conducting the animal experiments and Ms. Kathleen Haupt for typing of the manuscript.

REFERENCES

Borovetz, H.S., Griffith, B.P., Phillips, L.V., Haubold, A.D., Hercules,
D.M., Hung, T-K., and Hardesty, R.L. (1978) Scanning electron microscopic and surface analytical study of an isotropic vapor deposited
carbon film on microporous membranes. Scanning Electron Microscopy, 2,
85–93.
Borovetz, H.S., Haubold, A.D., Hercules, D.M., and Hardesty, R.L.
(1979a) Development of an all carbon membrane oxygenator. 14th Bien-
nial Conference on Carbon.
Borovetz, H.S., Griffith, B.P., Mateer, D.D., Hercules, D.M., Haubold,
A.D., and Hardesty, R.L. (1979b) Carbon surfaced microporous membranes: Oxygen permeability and interactions with blood. 5th Annual
Mtg. of the Soc. for Biomaterials.
Borovetz, H.S., Mateer, D.D., Hardesty, R.L., and Haubold, A.D.
(1980) Oxygen permeability of carbon-surfaced microporous membranes.
J. of Biomed. Materials and Res., 14.2, 145–154.
Hung, T-K., Borovetz, H.S., and Weisman, M.H. (1977) Transport and
flow phenomena in a microchannel membrane oxygenator. Annals of Biomed.
Engng., 5.4, 343–361.

504 R. Debski et al

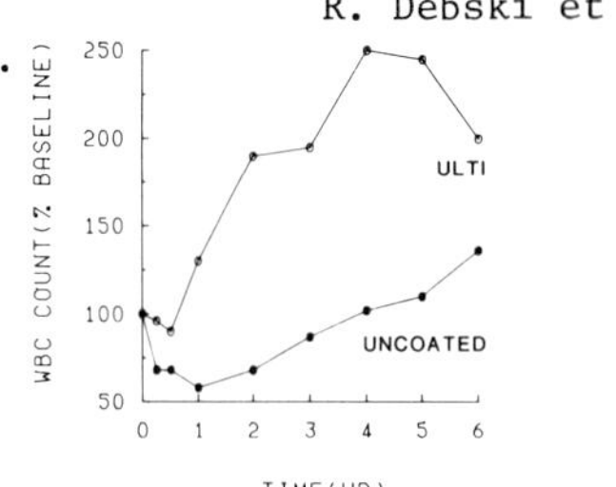
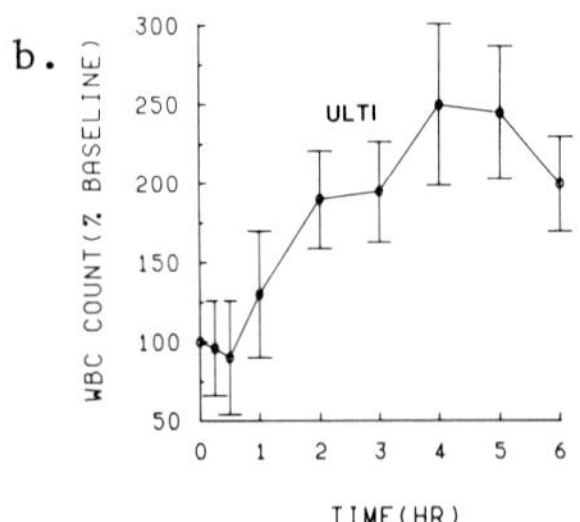

Fig. 1. White blood count expressed as percent as baseline versus time for a.) mean values for ULTI and uncoated groups, b.) mean ± 1SD for ULTI group.

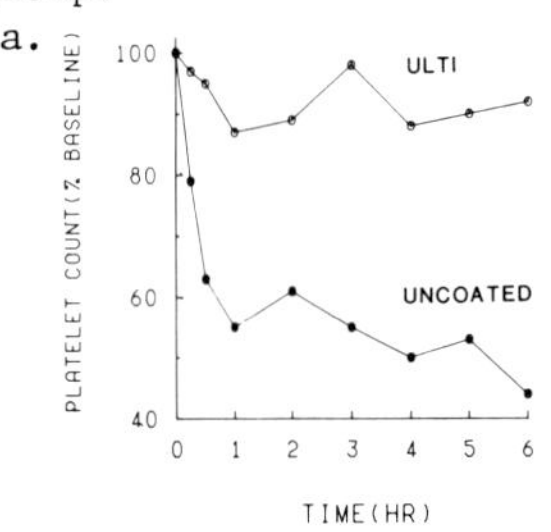
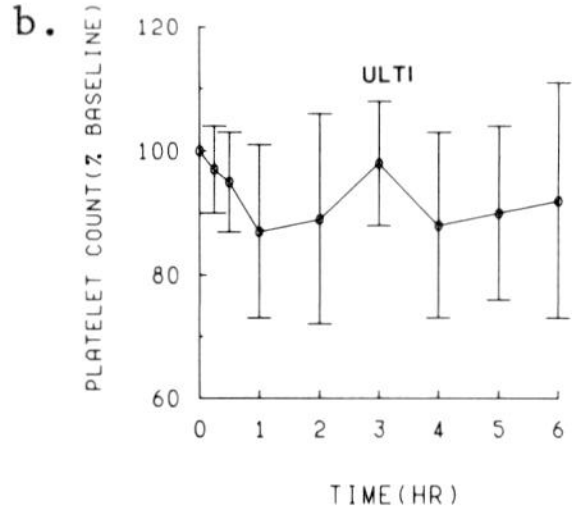

Fig. 2. Whole blood platelet count expressed as percent of baseline versus time for a.) mean values for ULTI and uncoated groups, b.) mean ± 1SD for ULTI group.

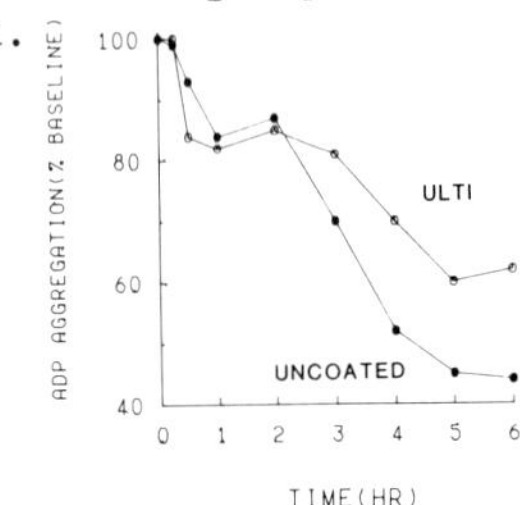
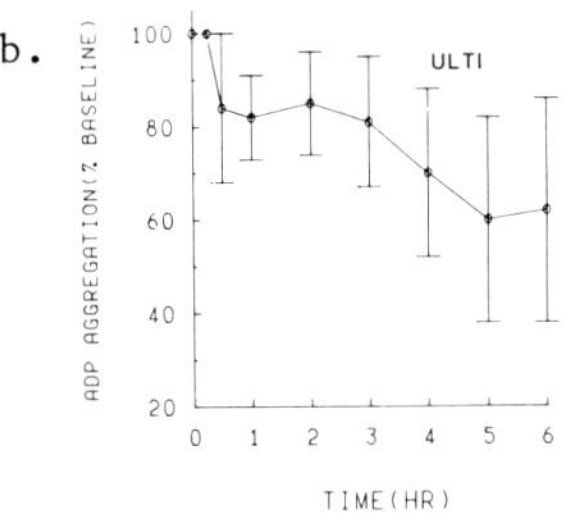

Fig. 3. Platelet aggregation induced by ADP expressed as percent of baseline versus time for a.) mean values for ULTI and uncoated groups, b.) mean + 1SD for ULTI group.

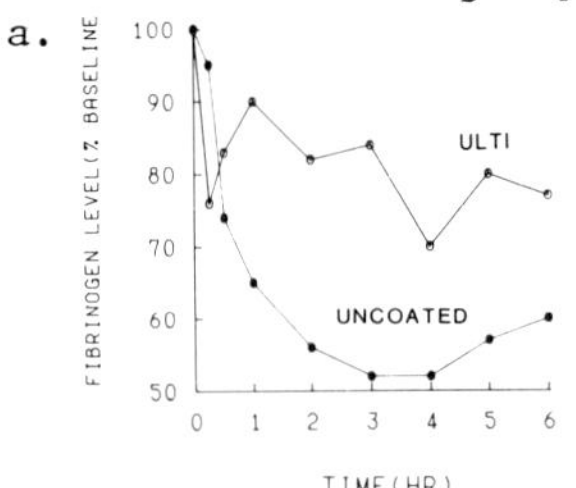
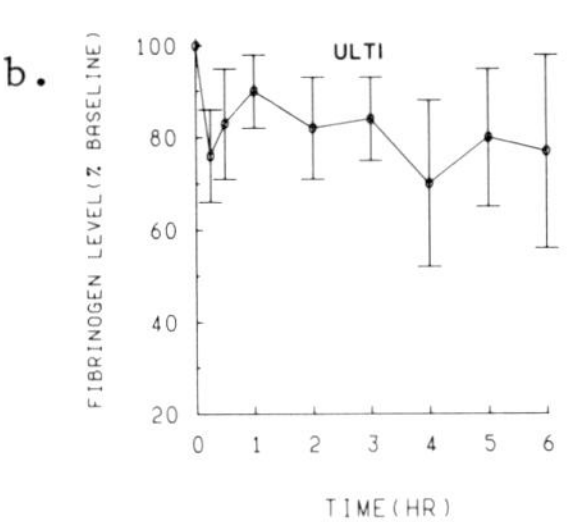

Fig. 4. Fibrinogen level expressed as percent of baseline versus time for a.) mean values for ULTI and uncoated groups, b.) mean ± 1SD for ULTI group.

Biomaterials 1980
Edited by G. D. Winter, D. F. Gibbons, and H. Plenk, Jr.

DIALYSIS–MEMBRANE – BLOOD INTERACTION

Stummvoll H.K., Graf H., Wolf A. and Leithner Ch.

2nd Medical Department, University of Vienna, Austria.

SUMMARY

A significant fall in peripheral leukocyte count, thrombocyte count, thrombocyte-aggregation index (indicating a rise in circulating thrombocyte aggregates) and arterial oxygen tension is seen during the initial phase of routine hemodialysis when cellulose dialyzer membranes are used. Mechanisms leading to these phenomena are still a matter of controversy, but cell trapping within the dialyzer contributes only little to this cytopenia since there is no significant difference in these blood cells between dialyzer-blood inlet and outlet. Sequestration of these cells in the microvasculature of the patient must be assumed.
Lung function studies and measurement of thoracic fluid content by means of transthoracic electrical impedance were performed during routine hemodialysis and gave indirect evidence that this cell sequestration mainly occurs in the pulmonary vascular bed.
Transfusion of foreign fresh plasma which was in contact with the artificial surface of the dialyzer membrane produced leukopenia and a fall in arterial oxygen tension but no thrombocytopenia and no rise in circulating thrombocyte aggregates.
It is concluded that leukopenia and hypoxemia are transferrable by a soluble plasma factor, whereas thrombocytopenia and a rise in thrombocyte aggregates depends on direct interaction between the dialyzer membrane and the thrombocytes.

INTRODUCTION

Extracorporeal hemodialysis has been in clinical use for more than 30 years but biocompatibility of dialysis membranes is still a major problem. Even after anticoagulation with heparin, numerous changes in both soluble and cellular components occur after exposure of blood to the artificial surface of the hemodialyzer membrane. Reversible leukopenia (Maher and Schreiner 1965, Kaplow and Gollinet 1968) and thrombocytopenia (Levin et al, 1978) are prominent features of this reaction of blood with the dialyzer membrane during clinical hemodialysis. Although scanning electron microscopy revealed adherence of some leukocytes and thrombocytes to the dialyzer membrane (Marshall et al, 1974), there was no significant difference in these blood cells between dialyzer blood inflow and dialyzer blood outflow. This indicates that trapping of cells within the dialyzer contributes only very little to the sharp drop

505

in peripheral cell counts which occurs during the first hour of hemodialysis. Sequestration of cells within the patient's microvasculature
seems to be the major factor leading to reversible leukopenia and thrombocytopenia. Animal studies indicate that this sequestration takes
place mainly in the pulmonary vascular bed (Toren et al, 1970).

The mechanism leading to early leukopenia and thrombopenia during hemodialysis is still a matter of controversy. Craddock et al (1977) demonstrated complement activation during hemodialysis and believe that this
is the major factor responsible for dialysis leukopenia. Others (Aljama
et al, 1978, Camussi et al, 1978) believe that direct leukocyte membrane
interaction may be involved.

The aim of this study was to find evidence that pulmonary leukocyte and
thrombocyte trapping also occurs during hemodialysis in man and to
investigate whether this cytopenia was transferable with soluble blood
factors after blood membrane contact or whether direct cellular contact
with the artificial surface was necessary.

PATIENTS AND METHODS

12 adult patients were studied during uneventful routine hemodialysis
(HD). Patients with history, clinical signs or X-ray of lung disease
were excluded. Dialysis was performed with an 1.8 m2 hollow-fiber dialyzer with a regenerated cellulose membrane (CDAK 1.8). After heparini-
sation hemodialysis was started by substituting saline for the blood
loss into the dialyzer in order to avoid acute changes in extracellular
volume. Thereafter routine HD was performed with an ultrafiltration
rate adjusted according to individual need. Leukocytes and thrombocytes
were counted in a commercial cell counter. The platelet aggregation
index (P.A.I.) was measured using the method of Wu and Hoak (1974). The
plasma complement was measured by immunohemolysis (CH 50) and arterial
blood gases were examined with an automatic blood gas analyzer. Lung
function tests were performed in an open system with a lamellar spiro-
ceptor (FD-10, Siemens FRG) for calculating respiratory volume. Concentration of oxygen in the expired air was measured paramagnetically
(Oxymat-M, Siemens FRG) and carbon dioxide concentration by the technique of ultraredabsorption (Ultramat M-CO_2, Siemens, GFR). The diffusing capacity of the lungs for carbon monoxide (D_LCO) was measured
using a steady state technique. Intrathoracic fluid changes were determined by electrical transthoracic impedance.

Prior to another HD-session, 6 of the patients received transfusion of
fresh heparinized plasma from healthy donors that had been brought into
contact with the dialyzer cellulose membrane. This was achieved by pre-
filling a hollow fiber hemodialyzer and dialyzer tubing with fresh
plasma and circulating this plasma by means of roller pumps for 20
minutes. The plasma was washed with saline and transfused into the
patient. Leukocytes, thrombocytes, P.A.I. and blood gases were measured
after plasma transfusion as well as after the subsequent HD, which was
performed on the same dialyzer.

RESULTS

Clinical hemodialysis. Figure 1 shows the effect of hemodialysis on leukocytes (WBC), platelet count and platelet aggregation index (P.A.I.). There is a significant fall in all these parameters in the early phase of HD. No arteriovenous difference could be found. The fall of P.A.I. indicates a rise in circulating thrombocyte aggregates. Total hemolytic complement (CH 50) showed a significant drop from a mean value of 24.3 U/ml before dialysis to 16.5 U/ml after 10 minutes of HD with a steady increase thereafter, reaching initial values after 60 minutes of HD.

Figure 2 shows arterial oxygen tension (p_aO_2), alveolar oxygen tension (p_AO_2), alveolar-arterial oxygen difference ($AaDO_2$) and transthoracic electrical impedance during clinical HD. p_aO_2 fell significantly whereas p_AO_2 remained unchanged giving a significant rise of $AaDO_2$. This and the significant fall of the diffusing capacity of the lung for CO (from a mean of 5.1 mmol/min/kPa before dialysis to a mean of 3.75 mmol/min/kPa after 30 minutes) indicate clearly that the cause of this hypoxemia is related to intrapulmonary changes. The same is indicated by the significant fall in transthoracic electrical impedance, which indicates an accumulation of thoracic fluid.

Plasma transfusion. Transfusion of heparinized fresh plasma that had been in contact with the dialyzer membrane produced significant leukopenia and a fall in p_aO_2. The number of platelets and the P.A.I. remained unchanged. Hemodialysis with the same dialyzer induced significant leukopenia, thrombopenia, fall in P.A.I. and fall in p_aO_2 (Figures 3).

DISCUSSION

Our results show that leukopenia may be induced by transfusion of heparinised plasma that has been in contact with a cellulose membrane. The demonstration of activated complement components in this plasma is indicative of a causative role of complement in the induction of this leukopenia, as suggested by Craddock et al (1977). The simultaneous fall in p_aO_2 indicates that complement activation, leukopenia and hypoxemia, occuring during hemodialysis with cellulose membranes, are related events. The initial fall in transthoracic impedance shows reversible pulmonary fluid accumulation which could be induced by intrapulmonary leukostasis. The rise in $AaDO_2$ as well as the fall of D_LCO are evidence of intrapulmonary disturbances leading to dialysis-related hypoxemia. The theory that hypoxemia is a consequence of CO_2 loss across the hemodialyzer during HD with subsequent hypoventilation, as proposed by Sherlock et al, (1977) and Aurigemma et al, (1977), cannot be supported because we found no drop in p_aCO_2 and no changes in minute ventilation. Dumler and Levin (1979) found leukopenia but no hypoxemia when using the hemodialyzer in ultrafiltration technique and concluded that leukopenia and hypoxemia are unrelated effects. However, with a high ultrafiltration rate interstitial (and intrapulmonary) fluid are quickly removed and this will counteract the effect of pulmonary leukostasis on oxygenation.

Thrombocytes are not affected by transfusion of plasma; neither platelet count nor platelet aggregation index show significant changes. Dialysis thrombocytopenia and a rise in circulation thrombocyte aggregation are probably induced by a direct cell membrane interaction.

REFERENCES

Aljama P., Bird P.A.E., Ward M.K., Feest T.G., Walker W., Tonboga H., Sussmann M. & Kerr D.N.S. (1978) Hemodialysis induced leucopenia and activation of complement: Effect of different membranes
Proc. Eur. Dial. Trans. Ass.,15, 144-151.
Aurigemma N.M., Feldmann N.T., Gottlieb M., Ingram R.H., Lazarus J.M. & Lowrie E.G. (1977) Arterial oxygenation during hemodialysis.
N. Engl. J. Med., 297, 871-873.
Camussi G., Segolini G., Rotunno M. & Vercellone A. (1978) Mechanism involved in acute granulocytopenia in hemodialysis: Cell membrance direct interactions.
Int. J. Art. Org., 1, 123-127.
Craddock P.R., Fehr J., Brigham K.L., Kronenberg R.S. & Jacob H.S. (1977) Complement mediated pulmonary dysfunction in hemodialysis.
N. Engl. J. Med., 196, 769-774.
Dumler F. & Levin N.W. (1979) Leucopenia and hypoxemia: Unrelated effects of hemodialysis. Arch. Int. Med., 139, 1103-1106.
Kaplow L.S. & Goffinet J.A. (1968) Profound neutropenia during the early phase of hemodialysis. JAMA, 203, 1135-1137.
Levin R.D., Kwaan H.C. & Ivanovich P. (1978) Changes in platelet function during hemodialysis. J. Lab. Clin. Med., 92, 779-786.
Maher J.F., Schreiner G.E. (1965) Hazards and complications of dialysis.
N. Engl. J. Med., 273, 370-377.
Marshall J.W., Ahearn D.J., Nothum R.J., Esterly J., Noll K.D. & Maher J.F. (1974) Adherence of blood components to dialyzer membranes.
Nephron, 12, 157-170.
Sherlock J., Ledwith J. & Letteri J. (1977) Hemodialysis induced hypoxemia: A response to loss of CO_2 across the dialyzer and increased oxygen consumption. Dialysis and Transplantation, 6, 34-35.
Toren M., Goffinet J.A. & Kaplow L.S. (1970) Pulmonary blood sequestration of neutrophils during hemodialysis. Blood, 36, 337-340.
Wu K.K. & Hoak J. (1974) A method for the quantitative detection of platelet aggregates in patients with arterial insufficiency. Lancet, 1, 924-926.

FIGURES

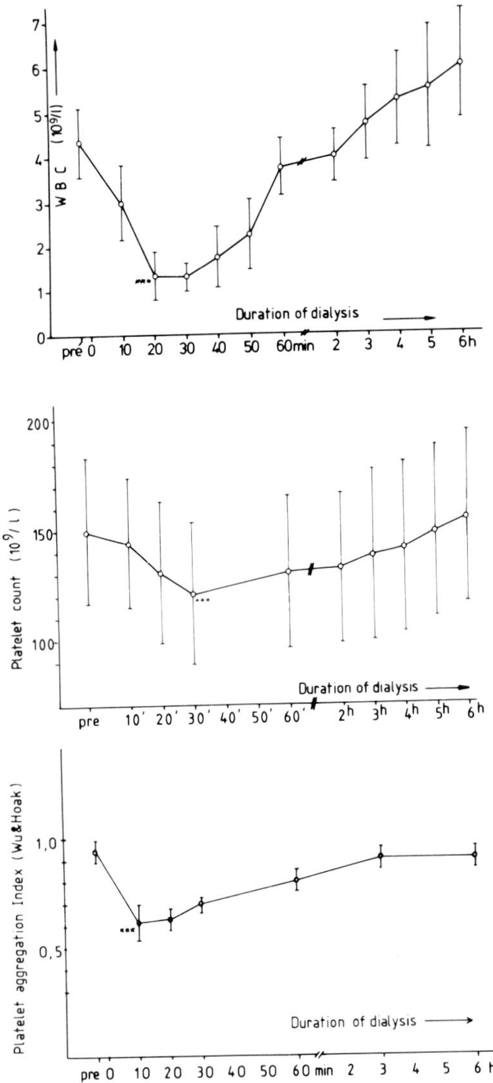

Fig. 1: Behaviour of peripheral white blood cells (WBC) platelet count and platelet aggregation index during routine hemodialysis with cellulose membrane dialyzers.

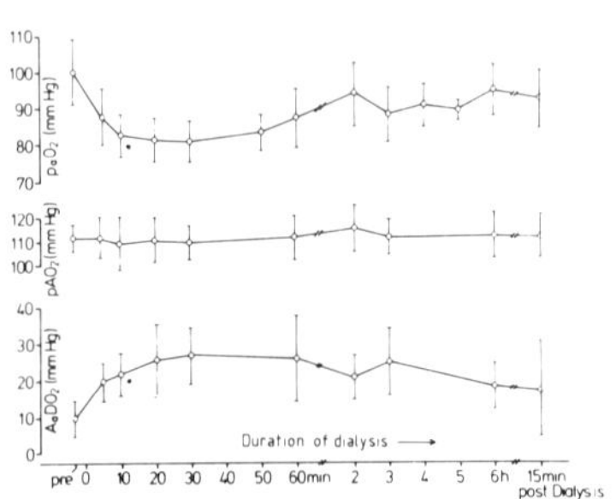
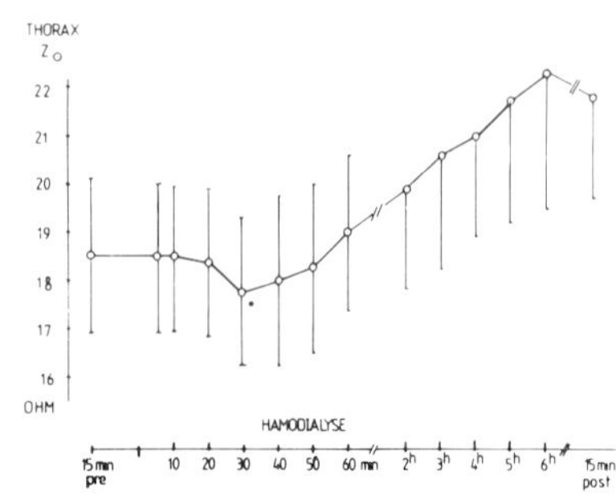

Fig. 2: Behaviour of arterial oxygen tension (p_aO_2), alveolar oxygen tension (p_AO_2) and alveolar arterial oxygen difference ($AaDO_2$) and transthoracic electrical impedance (THORAX Z o) during routine hemodialysis with cellulose membrane dialyzers.

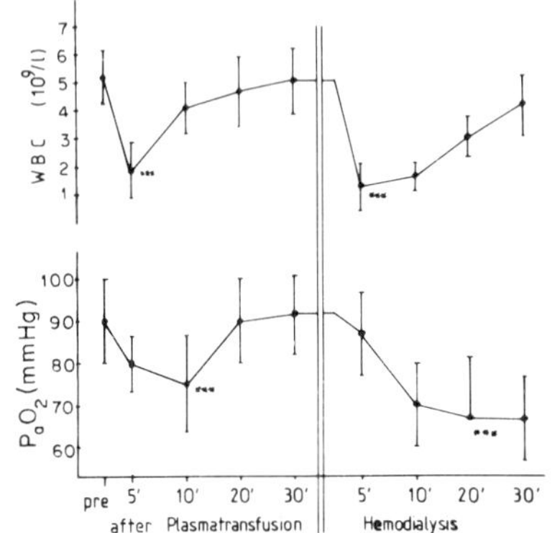
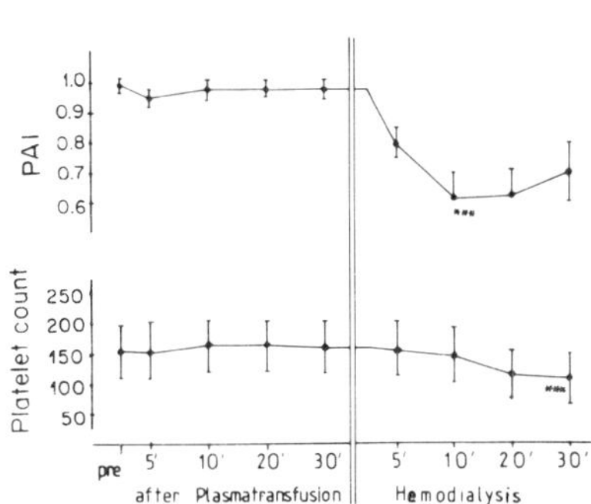

Fig. 3: Behaviour of white blood cell count (WBC), arterial oxygen tension (p_aO_2) and platelets and platelet count aggregation index (P.A.I.) after transfusion of "membrane-activated" plasma and after subsequent hemodialysis.

Vascular prostheses

Biomaterials 1980
Edited by G. D. Winter, D. F. Gibbons, and H. Plenk, Jr.
© 1982 John Wiley and Sons Ltd.

CORRELATIONS BETWEEN THE RESULTS OF IN VITRO
AND EX VIVO BLOOD COMPATIBILITY TESTS OF
BIOMATERIALS

J. P. Fischer*, U. Becker**, K. Burg*,
P. Fuhge**, and N. Heimburger**

* Hoechst AG, D-6230 Frankfurt 80

** Behringwerke AG, D-3550 Marburg

SUMMARY

Tubing of different inner diameter (ID) were prepared from
10 different polymers (Chlorinated Polyethylene,
Ethylene/Propylene/Diene/Ter-Polymer, Ethylene/Tetra-
fluoroethylene-Copolymer, Ethylene/Vinylacetate-Copolymer,
Low Density Polyethylene, Polypropylene, Polytetrafluoroethylene, Polyetherurethane, Polyvinylchloride (with
DEHP-plasticizer) and Silicone):

a) tubing of 4-5 mm ID for in vitro-blood compatibility
   tests via the determination of 9 clotting parameters
   after incubation of the polymer surface with citrated
   human blood in a rotating system,

b) tubing of 0.3-0.4 mm ID for ex vivo-evaluation of
   blood compatibility via measuring the bleeding time
   after introduction of the tubing into the ear vein
   of rabbits.

The tubing was surface modified by grafting with N-vinyl-
N-methyl acetamide (VIMA).
For both the original and the grafted tubing correlations
were established between the physical characterization
(critical surface tension, electron spectroscopy for
chemical analysis, frustrated multiple internal reflexion,
scanning electron microscopy) and the in vitro- as well
as the ex vivo-blood compatibility. VIMA-grafting led
in most cases to an enhanced blood compatibility. A good
correlation was found between the in vitro- and the
ex vivo-results.

                    J. P. Fischer et al.

INTRODUCTION

Surface grafted plastic material for biomedical applications has been attracting considerable attention in
the last decade and several concepts have been reviewed
(Bruck, 1975).

Grafting different polymeric materials with 2-hydroxy-
ethyl methacrylate (Ratner, 1975) has demonstrated the
ability to enhance the blood compatibility of conventional plastic material via hydrophilization. In a
preceeding paper (Fischer, 1979) it was shown that, of
16 different monomers, grafting with N-vinyl-N-methyl
acetamide (VIMA) resulted in the best blood compatibility
of the modified polymer surfaces.

MATERIALS AND METHODS

The following plastic materials were selected for
investigation:

CPE	=	Chlorinated Polyethylene
EPDM	=	Ethylene/Propylene/Diene/Ter-Polymer
ETFE	=	Ethylene/Tetrafluoroethylene-Copolymer
EVA	=	Ethylene/Vinylacetate-Copolymer
LDPE	=	Low Density Polyethylene
PP	=	Polypropylene
PTFE	=	Polytetrafluoroethylene
PUR	=	Polyetherurethane
PVC	=	Polyvinylchloride (with DEHP-plasticizer)
SI	=	Silicone

Tubing of 4-5 mm inner diameter (ID) and of 5-6 mm outer
diameter (OD) was prepared from each of these materials
for in vitro-blood compatibility tests and tubing of
0.3-0.4 mm ID and 0.6-0.9 mm OD for ex vivo-evaluations.
N-vinyl-N-methyl-acetamide (VIMA) with a purity of
99.8-99.9 % was used as the monomer for the grafting
reactions.

Grafting Method. Grafting was performed by filling the
tubing with monomer or a monomer/solvent mixture and
subsequent irradation under nitrogen with a high energy
^{60}Co-source. The dose rate was 400 J/kg·h and the dose
varied from 0.3 to 2.5 Mrad.

Further steps were thorough washing with different
solvents and careful drying.

Physicochemical Characterization. Whereas the total
content of the material grafted onto the base polymer
was measured by infrared spectroscopy (IR) or elemental
analysis (EA), the surface graft was characterized by

frustrated multiple internal reflexion (FMIR), by
measurements of the critical surface tension (CST), by
electron spectroscopy for chemical analysis (ESCA) and
by a specially developed microscopic evaluation of an
eosin dyeing of the grafted tubing.

CST was determined from tubing of 4-5 mm ID by contact
angle measurements and from tubing of 0.3-0.4 mm ID via
measurements of the capillary rise with pure solvents
of different surface tension (γ_L). Using the method of
Dynes and Kaelble (1974) both the polar part γ_s^p and the
dispersional part γ_s^d of CST could be determined from
tubing of 4-5 mm ID and of 0.3-0.4 mm ID.

"In vitro"-blood compatibility tests. The in vitro-blood-
compatibility test was performed with 75 cm samples of
tubing (4-5 mm ID) by equilibrating with saline solution
overnight, filling with citrated human blood, forming
a circle and incubating for 2 hours at 37 °C using a
rotating disc (Olsson, 1977). Citrated human blood from
the same donor incubated at room temperature over a
period of 2 hours in a polystyrene test-tube served as
the reference blood. A determination of 9 clotting parameters was then performed according to Becker (1976)
and the values for the reference blood were defined as
100 %. See Table 1.

TABLE 1. Determination of the in vitro-blood-
compatibility index as mean of summarized
deviations from citrated human reference blood

	In Vitro-Blood Clotting Parameters	Multi-plier	Mean deviations from Citrated Human Reference Blood = 100 % for each Parameter	
			Tubing of chlorinated Polyethylene (CPE)	Silicone-Tubing for blood transfusion
	Number of Reproductions		16	44
1	Platelet Retention (PR)	2	- 31.6 ± 3.6	- 36.6 ± 2.2
2	Platelet Factor 3 (PF 3)	1	+ 12.9 ± 1.7	+ 16.9 ± 1.8
3	Platelet Factor 4 (PF 4)	1	+115.6 ± 19.1	+113.3 ± 10.3
4	Clotting Factor XII	1	+ 7.4 ± 2.8	- 5.3 ± 1.3
5	Clotting Factor XI	1	+ 6.1 ± 3.0	- 4.2 ± 1.3
6	Clotting Factor IX	1	+ 6.8 ± 5.1	- 9.2 ± 1.6
7	Clotting Factor II	1	- 7.4 ± 2.4	- 14.3 ± 0.2
8	Recalcification Time (RCT)	1	- 8.9 ± 2.8	- 12.9 ± 2.0
9	Partial Thromboplastin Time (PTT)	2	+ 7.4 ± 0.8	+ 11.2 ± 0.8
10	In Vitro-Blood Compatibility Index = Mean of Summarized Deviations from Reference Blood =100		22.1 ± 2.35	24.7 ± 1.1

The in vitro-blood compatibility index was defined by
summarizing the deviations from 100 % of the reference
blood and calculating the mean deviation as a percentage.
PR and PTT as the most important parameters had a
multiplier of 2. PR, PF 3 and PF 4 characterize the
cellular and PTT, RCT and the clotting factors II, IX, XI
and XII characterize the plasmatic part of the in vitro-
blood compatibility index. Low values of this index
correspond to high blood compatibility and high values
to low blood compatibility.

"Ex vivo" blood compatibility tests. Tubing of 0.3-0.4
mm ID and 20 cm length were filled with airfree saline
solution and introduced into the ear vein of rabbits
(Dudley, 1976). The time till the end of bleeding was
then measured for fifteen to twenty animals.

RESULTS

"In vitro" results for VIMA-grafted tubing. VIMA-
grafting of different plastic tubing lead to an increase
of the polar contribution to the CST (γ_s^p) as well as
of the in vitro-blood compatibility. As can be seen in
Figure 1 the lower in vitro-blood compatibility index for
VIMA-grafted tubing corresponds to a higher slope $\sqrt{\gamma_s^p}$
in the Kaelble-Plot (Dynes and Kaelble, 1974).

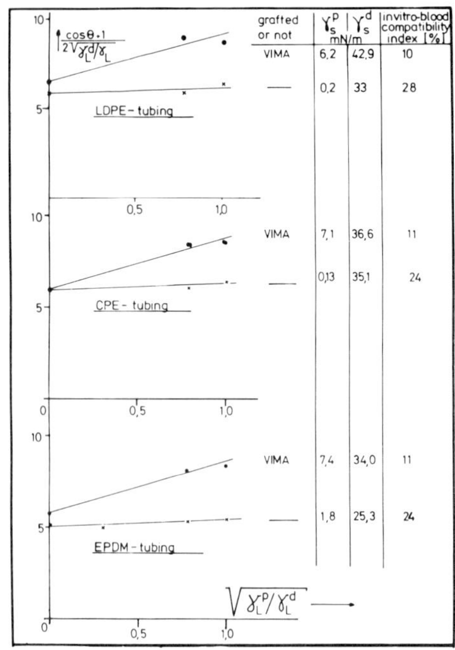

Fig. 1.   Kaelble-Plot for original and VIMA-
          grafted tubing. Correlation with the
          in vitro-blood compatibility test

In Figure 2 it is demonstrated that the degree of VIMA-grafting of 4 mm ID LDPE-tubing can be controlled by variation of the monomer conversion during the grafting step. In this case the analytical methods used were ESCA and evaluation of eosin dyeing. As can be seen further in Figure 2 the increase in the degree of grafting corresponds to an increase in CST and <u>in vitro</u>-blood compatibility.

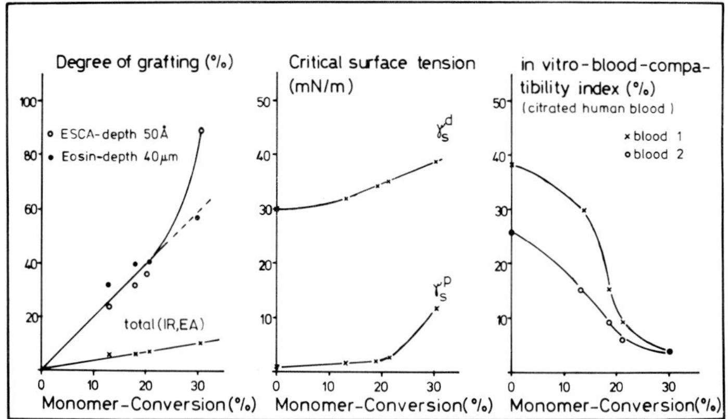

Fig. 2.   Correlation between the degree of grafting, critical surface tension and the blood compatibility of VIMA-grafted LDPE-tubing

<u>"Ex vivo" results for VIMA-grafted LDPE-tubing.</u>   As shown in Figure 3 a similiar correlation was found between the degree of grafting of VIMA-grafted 0.3 mm ID LDPE-tubing, the CST and the ex vivo-bleeding time respectively.

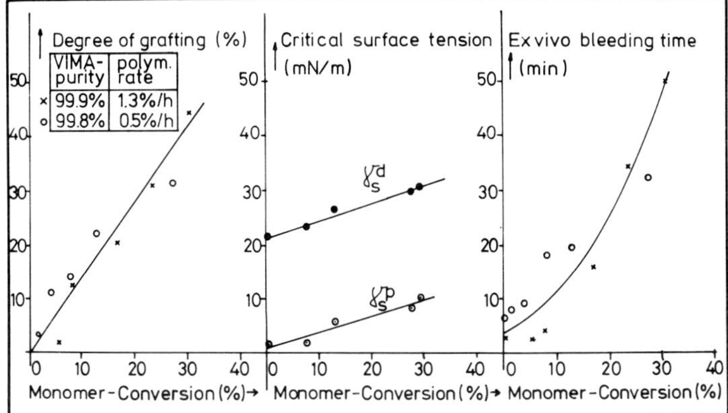

Fig. 3.   Correlations between the degree of VIMA-grafting on polyethylene-tubing (LDPE; ID : OD = 0.3 : 0.6 mm) and surface tension with the ex vivo-bleeding test on rabbits

                    J. P. Fischer et al.

Correlation of "ex vivo" and "in vitro" results. From a variety of base polymers with different degrees of grafting the in vitro-blood compatibility index and the ex vivo-bleeding time has been determined. Figure 4 shows a double logarithmic plot of these in vitro- and ex vivo-results. It can be concluded from this graph that a correlation has been established with a coefficient of 0.83. It is clear that further work has to be initiated in the direction of comparing human ex vivo-blood compatibility with the existing in vitro-methods; on the other hand we believe that these methods provide a useful tool for the initial evaluation of the blood compatibility of polymer surfaces.

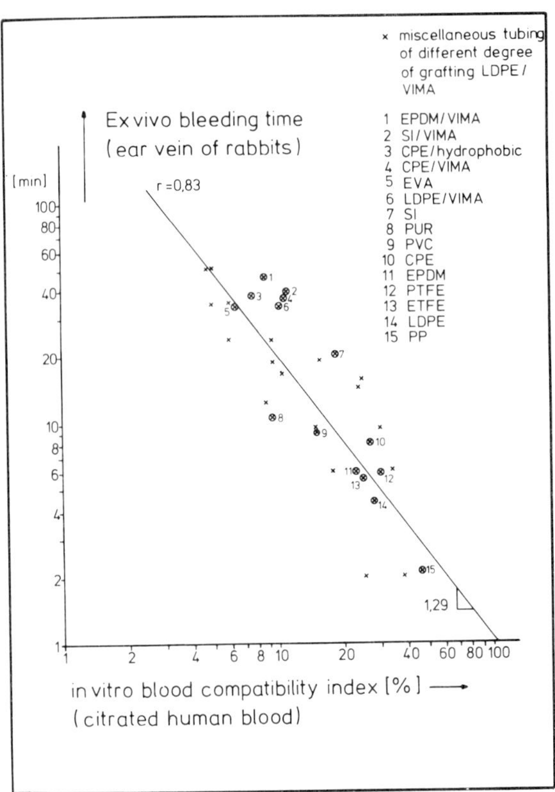

Fig. 4.   Correlation between ex vivo- and
          in vitro blood compatibility tests

<u>Comparison of "in vitro" blood compatibility of different</u>
<u>materials</u>.   Figure 5 summarizes our investigations. Since
the overall index is split into a cellular and a plasmatic response it can be stated that the cellular response
provides a better differentiation than the plasmatic
reponse.
In addition these data show that for materials presently
on the market, PUR is markedly better than PVC or SI.
With LDPE, PP, PTFE, CPE, EPDM and EVA 1 as the base
polymer it has been demonstrated that VIMA-grafting
offers an effective method to improve the poor blood
compatibility of the base polymer by a factor of between
1.5 and 14. It must be acknowledged that the grafting
technique is a rather costly and time-consuming solution
to the problem. Special formulations of CPE and additive
free EVA 2 are materials with good blood compatibility,
which could be developed as replacements for plastizer
containing PVC.

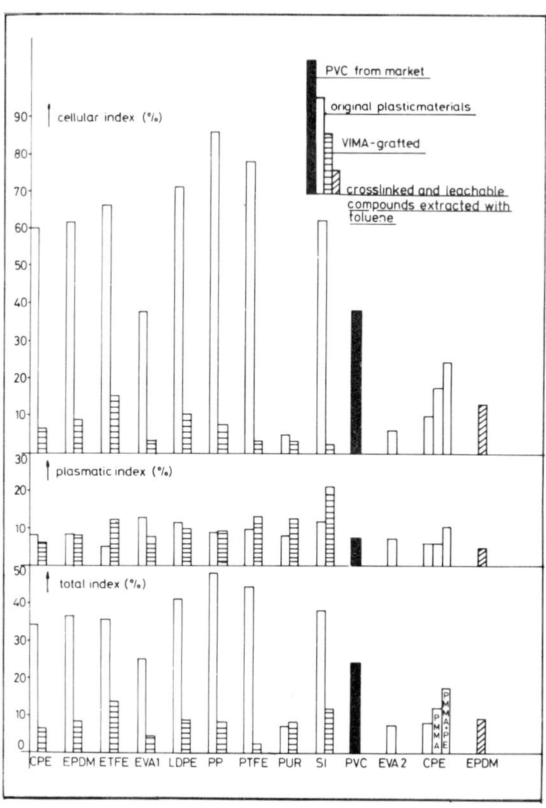

Fig. 5.   In vitro-blood compatibility index for
different plastic materials

ACKNOWLEDGEMENT

This work was sponsored by the German Government BMFT
(MSO 119).

REFERENCES

Becker, U., Karges, H. & Heimburger, N. (1976), Screening
of the blood compatibility of biomaterials with special
reference to the clotting system, Proc. Eur. Soc. Art.
Org., III, 52-56.

Bruck, S. D. (1975). Biomedical applications of polymeric materials and their interactions with blood components : A critical review of current developments, Polymer 16, 409-417.

Dudley, B., Williams, J. L., Able, K., & Muller, B.
(1976), Synthesis and characterization of blood compatible surfaces Part I : Dynamic tube test applied to
heparinized surfaces, Trans. Amer. Soc. Artif. Int. Organs,
XXII, 538-544.

Dynes, P. J., & Kaelble, D. H. (1974), Surface energy
analysis of carbon fibers and films, J. Adhesion, 6,
195-206.

Fischer, J. P., Becker, U., v. Halasz, S.-P. Mück, K.-F.,
Püschner, H., Rösinger S., Schmidt A., & Suhr, H. H.
(1979), The preparation and characterization of surface
grafted plastic materials designed for the evaluation of
their tissue and blood compatibility, J. Polymer Sci.:
Polymer Symp., 66, 443-463.

Olsson, P., Lagergreen, H., Larson, R., and Radegran, K.,
(1977), Prevention of platelet adhesion and aggregation
by a glutardialdehyde-stabilized heparin surface, Thromb.
Haemostas. (Stuttgart), 37, 274-281.

Ratner, B. D., Horbett, T., Hoffman, A. S., & Hauschka,
S. D. (1975), Cell adhesion to polymeric materials :
Implications with respect to biocompatibility, J. Biomed.
Mater. Res., 9, 407-422.

Biomaterials 1980
Edited by G. D. Winter, D. F. Gibbons, and H. Plenk, Jr.
© 1982 John Wiley and Sons Ltd.

EVALUATION OF ARTIFICIAL SURFACES USING BABOON ARTERIOVENOUS SHUNT MODEL

S.R. Hanson, L.A. Harker, B.D. Ratner and A.S. Hoffman

Departments of Medicine and Bio-Engineering
University of Washington
Seattle, Washington, USA

SUMMARY

The thrombotic response to artificial surfaces has been studied using baboons supporting femoral arteriovenous cannulae composed of various test materials. Steady-state rates of thrombus formation in vivo were assessed kinetically by measuring the survival and turnover of autologous ^{51}Cr-labeled blood platelets. Rates of platelet consumption by ten commercial polyurethane materials ranged from 2.2×10^8 - 23.3×10^8 platelets/cm^2/day and correlated inversely (r = -0.767) with measurements of the percentage of surface carbon atoms forming hydrocarbon (C-H) bonds as determined by electron spectroscopy for chemical analysis (ESCA). Comparison of these results with previous studies demonstrates that biomaterial-associated arterial thrombosis is strongly mediated by the polar character of electrostatically neutral polymeric materials.

INTRODUCTION

Platelet consumption by artificial surfaces involving the repetitive accumulation and embolization of adherent platelet masses remains a significant complication associated with the use of cardiovascular prostheses and extracorporeal devices (Allardyce et al, 1966; Berger and Salzman, 1974; Harker and Slichter, 1970, 1972; Harker et al, 1977; Lindon et al, 1980). In this context, previous studies have shown that a baboon animal model is useful for the assessment of biomaterial thrombogenesis in a manner simulating arterial thrombotic disorders in man (Harker and Hanson, 1979; Harker et al 1976, 1977; Todd et al, 1972). Specifically, rates of platelet consumption by femoral A-V

519

shunts in baboons have been shown to be reproducible and strongly dependent upon shunt surface properties, yet independent of hemodynamic and hematologic variables within the normal ranges for the test system.

In the present work this animal model has been used to assess the thrombogenicity of five additional polyurethane materials and to characterize more fully the effects of mediating variables.

METHODS

Animal and laboratory methods.   Normal male baboons (Papio cynocephalus) weighing 10-12 kg and supporting femoral A-V cannnulae composed of various test materials were maintained in restraining chairs during the period of study at the Regional Primate Research Center, University of Washington. Only male baboons were studied. With the use of methods described in detail previously (Hanson et al, 1980; Harker and Hanson 1979; Harker et al, 1976) a Silastic A-V cannula with Dacron sewing cuffs at skin exit sites was implanted between the femoral artery and vein. Cannulae were sterilized by autoclaving before surgical placement and consisted of two 35 cm lengths of Silastic tubing (0.110 inch i.d. by 0.177 inch o.d.; Dow Corning Corp., Midland Mich.) connected to Teflon vessel tips (13- to 15-guage; Seattle Artificial Kidney, Seattle, Wash.) inserted into the baboon femoral vessels. The segments of Silastic tubing were connected with a 0.5 inch length of blunt-edged Teflon tubing (0.110 inch i.d. by 0.124 inch o.d.; Zeus Industrial Products, Inc., Raritan, N.J.). Extension segments composed of various test materials were interconnected with the blunt-edged Teflon segments between the two 35 cm segments of the long-term Silastic A-V shunt. Usually four cannulations could be performed on the baboon femoral vessels, permitting multiple reuse of each animal. Each cannula remained patent an average of 4 to 6 weeks, permitting approximately 20 experiments with each animal. Studies in which cannulae occluded during the period of observation (approximately 15% of all studies) were excluded from consideration. Studies were usually initiated 5 to 7 days following the surgical procedure, although the platelet survival time in animals studied 1 day postoperatively was invariably normal. Platelet counts were measured with an electronic particle counter (Coulter Counter Model ZBI: Coulter Diagnostics, Hialeah, Fla.) on peripheral blood collected in 4 mg/ml EDTA.

Labeling procedures. Autologous baboon blood platelets were labeled with ^{51}Cr according to the ACD method described in detail elsewhere for studies with baboons (Harker et al, 1976; Harker and Hanson, 1980).

A known amount of ^{51}Cr-labeled platelet suspension was administered to the animal by intravenous injection after the preparation of a standard. Three milliter samples of whole blood, collected in EDTA were lysed with 0.5 ml of concentrated sodium dodecyl sulfate and counted for radioactivity in a gamma spectrometer (Packard Instrument Co., Inc., Downer Grove, Ill.). Blood samples were generally taken from an antecubital vein.

Analytical methods. For each study, the mean platelet survival time was determined by computer least-squares fitting of disappearance curves to gamma functions as described by Murphy and associates (Murphy and Francis, 1971). The computer program was available through the Chemical/Biological Information-Handling Program of the National Institutes of Health. This method was chosen because it is capable of modeling the variety of curves (including linear and exponential) resulting form platelet survival studies in vivo. Platelet survival time was 5.48 ± 0.11 days ($\pm$ 1.0 S.E.) in 17 normal male baboons.

The proportion of labeled platelets remaining within the systemic circulation after infusion (i.e. "recovery") was calculated from the platelet activity per milliliter extrapolated to zero time, multiplied by the estimated blood volume (ml), and divided by the platelet ^{51}Cr activity injected. Platelet turnover per microliter of blood per day was calculated from the peripheral platelet count divided by the platelet survival time in days and corrected for recovery, which averaged $85\% \pm 5$ ($\pm$ 1.0 S.D.) in 17 normal male baboons. Overall platelet turnover was calculated by multiplying platelet turnover per microliter by the estimated blood volume (70 ml/kg of body weight).

A simple mathematical model was used that allowed the separate estimation of rates of cannula-associated platelet consumption and senescent platelet removal, assuming steady-state rates of platelet production and destruction. The applicability of this approach has been described in detail elsewhere (Dornhorst 1951, Harker and Hanson 1979). Briefly, this analysis involves the assumption

                    S. R. Hanson, et al

that in the absence of cannulae or other external hazards, platelet survival curves would be linear, with all platelets having a fixed lifespan of 5.48 days. In shunt-bearing animals it is assumed that a fraction k of the total platelet population will be randomly destroyed by the cannula each day. This situation is expressed mathematically as follows:

$$\tau = \frac{1-e^{-5.48k}}{k} \qquad \tau < 5.48 \qquad (1)$$

where τ is the mean platelet survival time as determined from the computer fitting procedure. Given τ, the value of the parameter k can be determined from equation 1 by simple trial-and-error iteration. The rate of cannula platelet consumption is therefore calculated by multiplying k times the total number of platelets in the body.

TABLE I. Polyurethanes studied as A-V cannulas

Material	Length (cm)	Internal Diameter (cm)	Number of Studies
Biomer EB650	50.0	0.350	4
Superthane	37.0	0.318	4
Tygothane	50.0	0.318	4
Coextruded Renathane	50.0	0.356	4
Minor Rubber Co. Polyurethane	32.0	0.318	5
Erythrothane[1]	50.0	0.285	5

[1] Includes the results of four evaluations reported elsewhere (Hanson et al, 1980).

<u>Test Materials.</u>   The dimensions and number of studies performed with new polyurethanes are given in Table I.   Results with other materials also studied have been described elsewhere (Hanson, et al, 1980).   All materials were thoroughly washed with distilled water and prefilled with sterile isotonic saline immediately prior to insertion and testing as femoral A-V shunts. A Hewlett-Packard ESCA system (Model 5950 B; Hewlett-Packard Co., Palo Alto, Calif.) was used to take C_{1s} spectra.   Areas under the various overlapping peaks comprising the C_{1s} spectra were resolved with a computer least-squares fitting routine, assuming a Gaussian peak shape.

RESULTS

<u>Control Studies.</u>   In five normal baboons without A-V cannulae the mean platelet survival time was 5.49 $\pm$ 0.24 days ($\pm$ 1.0 S.E.).   In twelve baboons with a permanent 70 cm Silastic cannula the mean platelet survival time was not significantly reduced (5.48 $\pm$ 0.12 days, p > 0.4) demonstrating that the surgical variables were of little consequence in the model.   In those studies with permanent 70 cm Silastic shunts in which the mean platelet survival time was less than 5.48 days a value for cannula platelet consumption was calculated

TABLE II. Platelet Consumption by Erythrothane A-V Shunts

baboon number	weight (kg)	platelet count (plats/ $ul \times 10^3$)	total body platelets ($\times 10^{-9}$)	platelet survival time (days)	cannula platelet consumption (plats/cm^2-day $\times 10^{-8}$)	fraction of overall turnover
1	11.1	758	693	3.81	20.6	0.54
2	11.4	495	465	3.20	21.2	0.70
3	10.7	272	240	2.55	16.1	0.83
4	11.7	200	193	1.92	19.5	0.93
5	12.6	164	170	1.71	19.8	0.95

according to Equation I and averaged $0.6 \pm 0.2 \times 10^{10}$ platelets/day ($\pm$ 1.0 S.E.) over all studies. The mean value of 0.6×10^{10} platelets/day was considered the baseline measurement for animals with short Silastic shunts and was subsequently subtracted from measurements of cannula platelet consumption obtained when other materials were evaluated (Hanson et al, 1980).

Survival curves obtained in the five studies with erythrothane are shown in Figure I. Each study was performed in a different animal but with an identical length of tubing. The empirical and computed platelet kinetic parameters for these same studies are presented in Table II. It is apparent that baboons with lower circulating platelet concentrations also have the shorter platelet survival

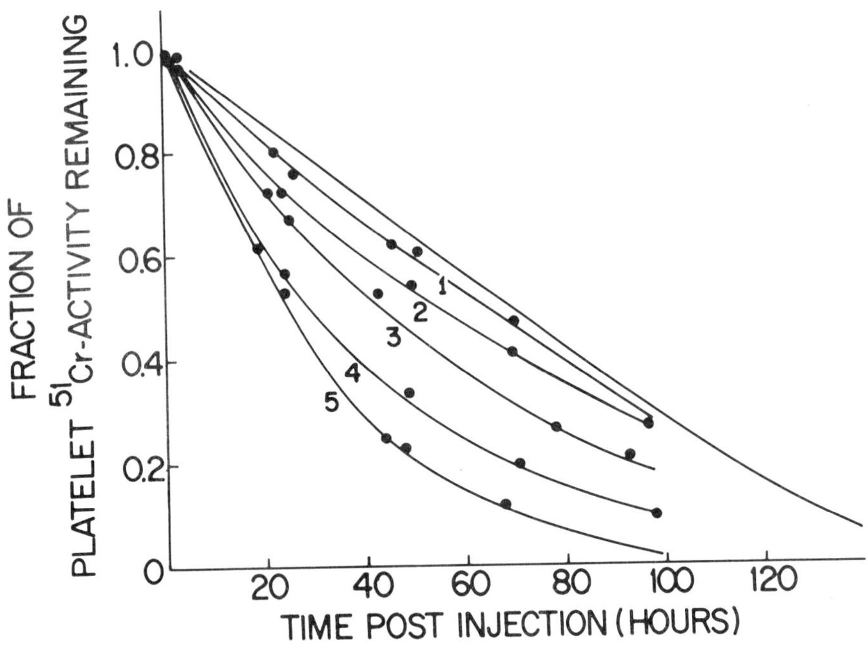

Fig. I Disappearance curves for ^{51}Cr-platelets in five baboons supporting erythrothane A-V shunts. The normal linear platelet disappearance pattern for unshunted animals is also shown (uppermost curve).

times. In those animals with the lowest platelet counts (4 and 5), greater than 90% of the overall rate of platelet turnover (which includes senescent platelet removal) could be attributed to cannula platelet consumption. Survival curves exhibited exponential behavior characteristic of random platelet utilization. Mean   platelet survival times increased with increasing platelet concentration, and platelet survival curves progressively approached the linear dissappearance pattern obtained in animals without shunts   suggesting   senescent platelet-removal. In all five studies the rate of cannula platelet consumption calculated according to equation I remained remarkably constant and independent of variations in circulating platelet concentration.   Although the variability in platelet concentration was abnormally large (Hanson et al, 1980) these studies

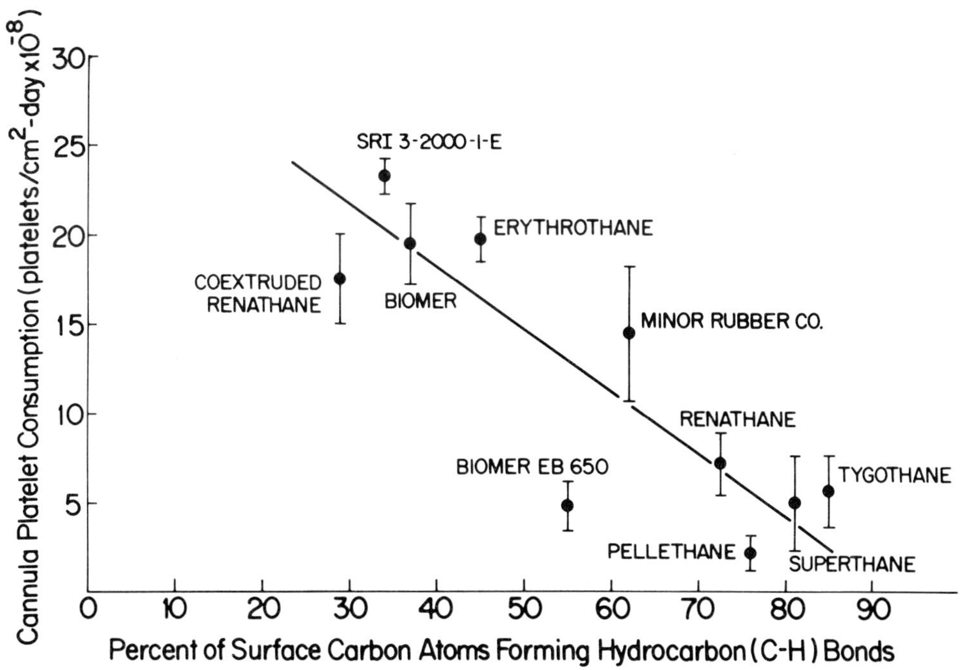

Fig. 2 Platelet consumption by polyurethanes.   Cannula platelet consumption per unit area is inversely related to the percentage surface carbon atoms forming C-H bonds, as determined from ESCA of polyurethane shunts. Mean values ± 1 S.E.

clearly demonstrate that in this system artificial surfaces consume platelets at a fixed rate which is independent of the circulating platelet concentration. Thus the impact of prosthetic surfaces, when measured as alterations in mean platelet survival time, will be determined by the prosthetic surface area and platelet-surface reactivity, relative to the size of the body platelet pool. Therefore, in the present work and previous studies (Hanson et al, 1980) measurements of cannula platelet consumption per unit area, rather than reductions in platelet lifespan, have been adopted as a more reproducible and meaningful basis for comparing the performance of artificial surfaces.

Results with ten polyurethane materials are shown in Figure 2. There was a linear inverse correlation between rates of platelet consumption per unit area and the fraction of surface carbon atoms forming hydrocarbon bonds as determined from ESCA (r = -0.767, p< 0.0001). The least reactive materials were those exhibiting the greatest proportion of nonpolar hydrocarbon-type structures.

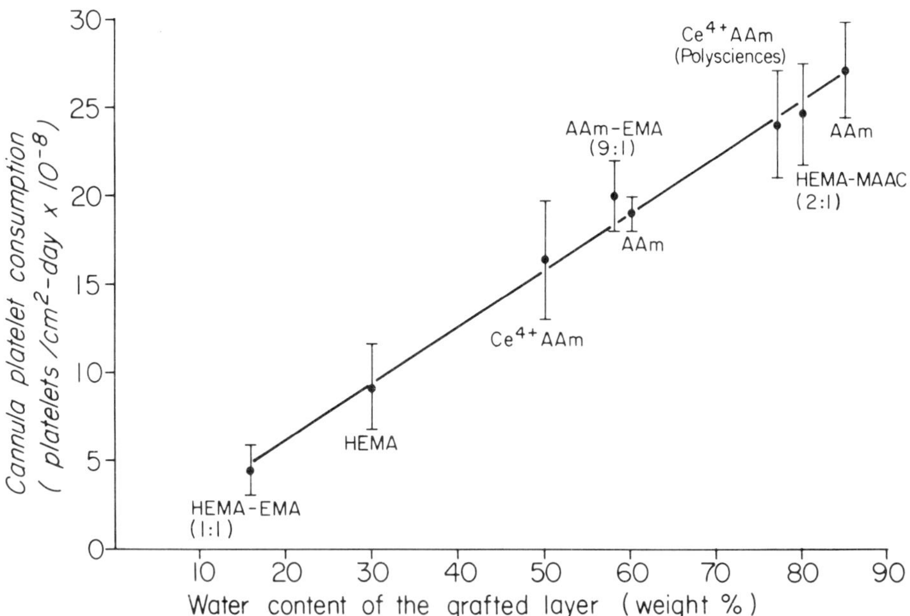

Fig. 3 Rate of cannula platelet consumption per unit area is directly related to the graft water content of shunts grafted with eight acrylic and methacrylic polymers and copolymers. HEMA, hydroxyethyl methacrylate; EMA, ethyl methacrylate; AAm, acrylamide; MAAC, methacrylic acid. Mean values are ± 1 S.E.

The results of previous studies involving acrylic and methacrylic polymers and copolymers are shown in Figure 3. Rates of cannula platelet consumption correlated directly with the water content of the luminal polymer grafts (r = 0.837). Although most of these polymers and copolymers were radiation grafted to silicone rubber (Silastic) and are electrostatically neutral, it is of interest that this correlation also includes one negatively charges copolymer poly(2-hydroxyethylmethacrylate)-poly(methacrylic acid), and two polyacrylamide grafts which were initiated chemically by Ce^{4+} ions rather than by ionizing radiation (water contents 50.8% and 77.0%). The graft substrates for these latter material were, respectively, Silastic pregrafted with poly(2-hyroxyethyl methacrylate) and pellethane. Although the effects of polymer electrical charge, substrate type, and method of initiation of polymerization were not investigated systematically, it is significant that results with the eight materials are correlated by a single variable, i.e., the water content of the grafted layer.

Results with the other four polymers studied are presented in Table III. For no material in this group did cannula platelet consumption exceed 1.6×10^8 platelets/cm^2-day. These polymers are thus relatively nonconsumptive toward platelets. Polyvinyl chloride and polyethylene values of cannula platelet consumption do not differ significantly from control values (p> 0.40). Teflon and Silastic were found to be more consumptive towards platelets, and the differences were significant (p <0.001 for Silastic and p < 0.05 for Teflon).

TABLE III. Platelet Consumption by Other Polymeric Materials

Material	Cannula platelet consumption per unit area (platelets/cm^2-day $\times 10^{-8}$)
Polyvinyl chloride (Tygon)	0.3 ± 0.2
Polyethylene (Intramedic)	0.2 ± 0.1
Polydimethylsiloxane (Silastic)	1.5 ± 0.3
Polytetrafluoroethylene (Teflon)	1.6 ± 1.0

Values are mean $\pm$ 1 S.E.

                    S. R. Hanson, et al

DISCUSSION

The present work and previous studies (Hanson et al, 1980; Harker and Hanson, 1979) have shown that thrombosis induced in the baboon by artificial surfaces is a steady-state process of selective platelet consumption that does not involve measurable utilization of circulating fibrinogen and is unaffected by heparin anticoagulation. Whereas measurements of platelet survival time and overall platelet turnover (including senescent platelet removal) may be influenced by shunt geometry (as well as type) and the circulating platelet concentration, measurements of cannula platelet consumption per unit area have been found to be reproducible and strongly dependent on material properties, yet independent of total exposed surface area, cannula blood flow rate, and circulating platelet concentration over wide ranges of these variables. Such observations thus provide a more meaningful assesment of material performance and facilitate considerably the general usefulness of this model system.

Of particular interest are results obtained with the various classes of polymeric materials which were evaluated. With the five polyurethanes studied there was approximately a 12-fold variation in the rate of platelet consumption per unit area. A good inverse correlation was obtained between the rate of platelet consumption and the percentage of surface carbon atoms forming C-H bonds, the more polar materials being the most consumptive. Further resolution of these ESCA spectra may improve the correlation significantly by incorporating parameters indicative of the relative importance of other chemical moieties present at the surface of polyurethane materials.

An excellent correlation was also found between the bulk water content of acrylic and methacrylic graft polymers and copolymers and the rate at which they consumed platelets in vivo. Approximately an eightfold variation in the rate of platelet consumption per unit area was observed, with the more fully hydrated materials being the most thrombogenic. The extent of hydration of the grafted layer appeared to be the only significant variable although materials tested included graft polymers prepared by both radiation and chemical initiation techniques, grafts on different substrates, and one graft copolymer with a net negative charge.

Four other materials, Teflon, Silastic, polyvinyl chloride, and polyethylene, were all found to consume less than 2×10^8 platelets/cm^2-day and were thus the least consumptive materials tested. Excluding polyvinyl chloride, these material exhibit relatively nonpolar surfaces to the flowing blood. However, spectroscopic analysis of polyvinyl chloride tubing indicated that the surface of this material is also nonpolar, possibly as a result of migration to the surface of plasticizers or other predominantly C-H-type additives. Thus, in general, the results of all studies suggest that polar surfaces, including surfaces which absorb water to a large extent, are consumptive towards platelets.

ACKNOWLEDGEMENT

Supported by Research Grants HL-22163,HL-1175, HL4-2970, and RR-00166 from the U.S. Public Health Service.

The technical assistance of Thomas R. Kirkman is gratefully acknowledged.

REFERENCES

Allardyce, D.B., Yoshida, S.H., & Ashmore, P.G. (1966) The importance of microembolism in the pathogenesis of organ dysfunction caused by prolonged use of the pump oxygenator, J. Thorac. Cardiovasc. Surg., 52, 706-715.

Berger, S., & Salzman, E.W. (1974) Thromboembolic complications of prosthetic devices, Prog. Hemost. Thromb., 2, 273-309.

Dornhorst, A.C. (1951) The interpretation of red cell survival curves, Blood, 6, 1284-1292.

Hanson, S.R.. Harker, L.A., Ratner, B.D., & Hoffman, A.S. (1980) Factors influencing platelet consumption by polyacrylamide hudrogels, Ann. Biomed. Eng. 7, 357-367.

Harker, L.A. & Hanson, S.R. (1979) Experimental arterial thromboembolism in baboons: mechanism, quantitation and pharmacologic prevention, J. Clin. Invest., 64, 559-569.

Harker, L.A., Ross, R., Slichter, S.J., & Scott, C.R. (1976) Homocystineinduced arteriosclerosis: the role of endothelial cell injury and platelet response in its genesis, J. Clin. Invest., 58, 731-741.

Harker, L.A. & Slichter, S.J. (1970) Studies of platelet and fibrinogen kinetics in patients with prosthetic heart valves, N. Engl. J. Med., 283, 1302-1305.

Harker, L.A. & Slichter, S.J. (1972) Platelet and fibrinogen consumption in man, N. Engl. J. Med., 287, 999-1005.

Lindon, J.N., Collins, R., Coe, N.P., Jagoda, A.,Brier-Russell, D., Merrill, E., & Salzman, E.W. (1980) In vivo assessment in sheep of thromboresistant materials by determination of platelet survival, Circ. Res., 46, 84-90.

Murphy, E.A. & Francis, M,E, (1971) The estimation of blood platelet survival. II. The multiple hit model, Thromb. Diath. Haemorrh., 25, 53-80.

Todd, M.E., McDevitt, E.L., & Goldsmith, E.I. (1972) Blood-clotting mechanisms of nonhuman primates: choice of the baboon model to simulate man, J. Med. Primatol., 1, 132-141.

Biomaterials 1980
Edited by G. D. Winter, D. F. Gibbons, and H. Plenk, Jr.
© 1982 John Wiley and Sons Ltd.

RADIATION GRAFTING OF N-VINYLPYRROLIDONE INTO SILICONE
TUBES. SYNTHESIS AND IMPLANTATION TESTS IN LAMBS

A. Chapiro, M. Foëx-Milléquant, A.-M. Jendrychowska-Bonamour
Laboratoire de Chimie Macromoléculaire sous Rayonnement,
C.N.R.S., 94320 Thiais, France

and

D. Domurado,
Laboratoire de Technologie Enzymatique, Université de
Compiègne, 60200 Compiègne, France

SUMMARY

NVP was grafted into silicone tubes using the "direct" radiation method. Homogeneous grafting in the bulk of the silicone walls (I.D. =
2 mm, O.D. = 4 mm) was achieved with 70 per cent monomer solutions in
toluene. Grafted and ungrafted tubes 7 cm long were implanted in the
carotid arteries of 6 month old lambs. It was established that after
seven days implantation a significant thrombo-resistance was reached
for samples with grafting ratios higher than 40 per cent. The bulk
grafted tubes are used for calibration of samples in which the grafting is purposely limited to a thin surface layer and for which the
grafting ratio is determined by FMIR infra-red.

INTRODUCTION

A large number of studies were devoted in the past to impart thromboresistance to various polymer substrates by grafting of hydrogels
(see for instance Bruck 1973, 1979). However, biological tests lead
to conflicting results which are at least partly caused by the fact
that any particular grafted system is governed by many parameters
which will determine a large variety of structures depending on experimental procedures. The purpose of the present work is to establish
a detailed correlation between the "fine structure" of a radiation
grafted hydrogel of poly(N-vinylpyrrolidone) P(NVP) into various polymers (silicone rubber, polypropylene and a polyurethane) and the antithrombic properties of the resulting materials. The parameters which
determine the "fine structure" are the extent of grafting (density of
grafts), the thickness of the grafted layer (depth of grafting), the
molecular weight of the grafted branches and eventually the presence
in the branches of electro-negative groups introduced by copolymerization. The present communication deals with grafted silicone rubber
tubes which are thereafter tested *in vivo* by implantation into carotid
arteries of 6 month old lambs.

EXPERIMENTAL

All samples were prepared by the direct grafting method. The experi-

532   A. Chapiro et al.

mental procedures and the kinetics of grafting are described in
detail elsewhere (Chapiro et al., 1980). The silicone tubes used were
7 cm long, 2 mm I.D. and 4 mm O.D. Their ends were cut at 45° angles
(see Fig. 2). They were subjected to gamma-rays while in contact
with a solution of NVP in a proper solvent. After irradiation the
samples were treated for 48 h with boiling methanol in order to
extract residual monomer and low molecular weight poly(NVP).The swelling ratios in water and the grafting ratios were determined gravime-
trically. The grafted tubes were sealed in double-walled polyethylene
bags containing a physiological salt solution and then sterilized
with a dose of 2.5 Mrad of gamma-rays. The grafted samples and control tubes, were implanted into lambs of average age 6 month (Préal-
pes breed). Operations were performed in the surgical unit of C.N.R.Z.
Jouy-en-Josas. Under anesthesia the carotid arteries were dissected
and one tube was inserted in each artery through two incisions and
maintained by means of two ligatures. The samples were kept in place
for 3 or 7 days. After sacrificing the animal, the tubes were withdrawn and examined. The brain was removed and dissected for evaluation of thrombi formation. The samples were fixed in a phosphate buffered 3 % glutaraldehyde solution.

RESULTS

<u>Homogeneous bulk grafting.</u> Addition of toluene to the monomer impro-
ves the swelling of silicone and allows a homogeneous grafting in the
bulk of the tubes (Chapiro et al., 1980). Best results were obtained
with a 70 per cent monomer solution in toluene which insures a fast
diffusion of the NVP into the bulk of the tube walls. The penetration of the grafted front troughout the tube wall is visualized by
staining the sample with a 0.1 per cent solution of Fuschine in
methanol (Fig. 1). It was found that the amount of water absorbed by
the grafted samples at equilibrium swelling corresponds to 11 to 12
molecules H_2O per unit of NVP in the graft. The most heavily grafted
samples (47 per cent) do not contain more than 37 weight per cent of
water a value significantly lower than the critical level assumed to
be necessary for the blood compatibility of hydrogels as described
by Bruck (Bruck 1973, see also Ratner et al. 1979).

The data summarized in Table 1 show that of the 67 tests performed 16
were unmodified silicone and only one of those control tubes remained
unclotted and clear. As the degree of grafting increases the proportion of unclotted tube increases, as does the proportion of tubes
which are free of any visible deposit. Significant improvement of
"blood-compatibility" is obtained at grafting ratios above <u>ca</u>. 40
per cent. The presence of thrombi was observed in the brains for
grafting ratios lower than 40 %. Fig. 2 represents the appearance of
the tubes after implantation : "clotted tube" (A) ; "unclotted tube
with deposit" (B), and "unclotted tube without deposit" (C). Samples
shown here were withdrawn after 7 days implantation. They were fixed
in glutaraldehyde.

The method used for preparing bulk grafted samples is limited to grafting ratios of <u>ca</u>. 50 per cent. However, for grafting ratios of 30

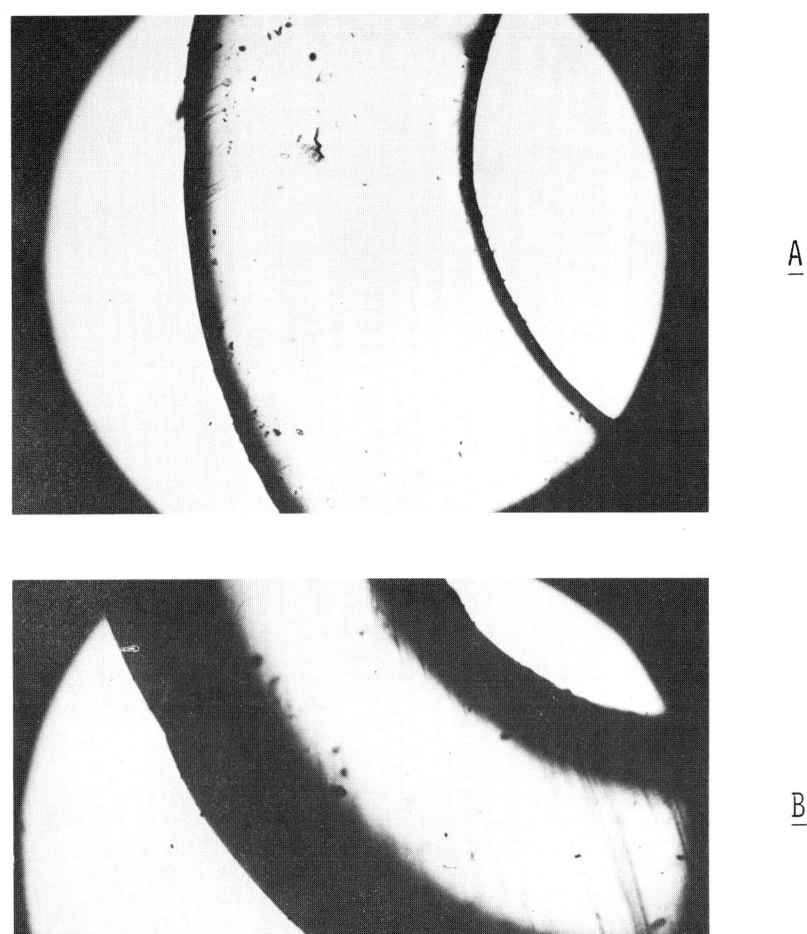

Fig. 1. Penetration of PNVP through the silicone wall
during grafting. Pictures of the cross-sections of tubes
stained in a 0,1 % Fuschine solution.
A - 45 mμ thick layer inside and outside.
B - 200 mμ thick layer inside 350 mμ outside.

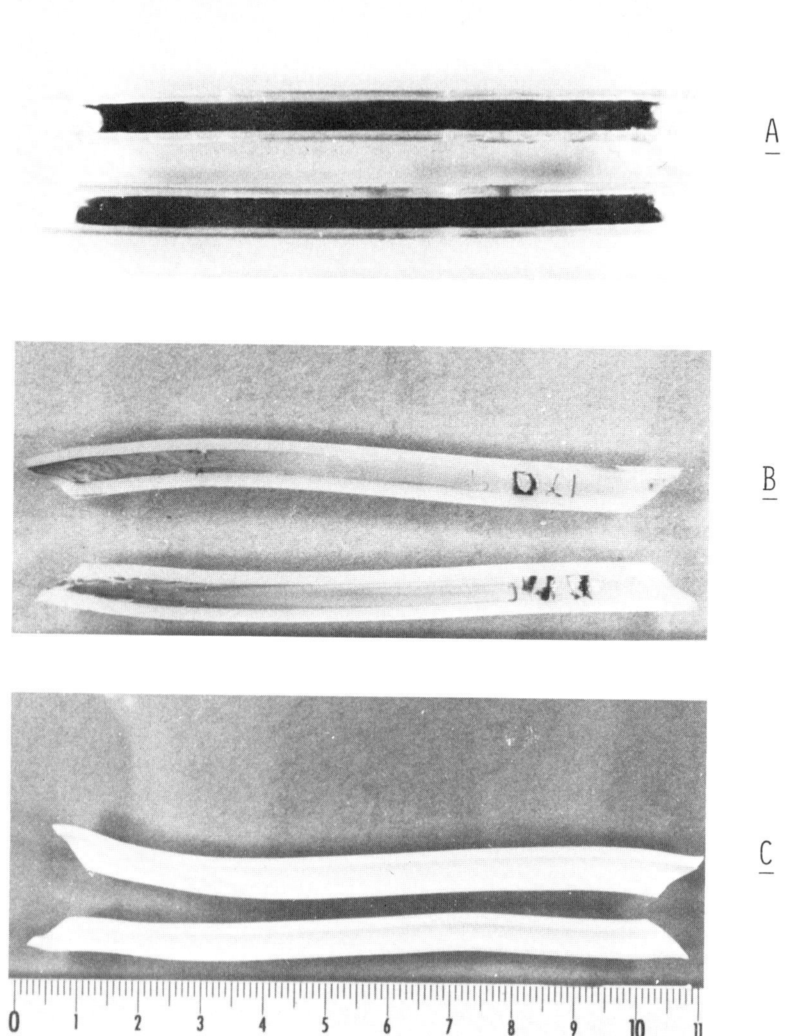

Fig. 2.   Implants withdrawn after 7 days.
A - Unmodified silicone, tube ID = 3 mm, ("clotted tube").
B - Bulk grafted silicone (22 %), tube ID = 2.4 mm,
("unclotted with deposit").
C - Bulk grafted silicone (41 %), tube ID = 2.7 mm,
("unclotted without deposit").

Table 1. Observation of tubes after seven days implantation in lamb carotid arteries

Composition of samples (per cent)			Graft ratio (per cent)	Inner diam. (mm)	Number of tests	Clotted tubes	Unclotted tubes	
Silicone	PNVP	H_2O					with deposit	without deposit
100	0	0	0	2	3	3	0	0
100	0	0	0	3	13	4	8	1
76	8	16	8–14	2.2–2.3	6	4	1	1
65	12	23	16–22	2.3–2.4	5	4	1	0
57	15	28	24–28	2.4–2.5	12	8	4	0
50	17	33	31–39	2.6–2.7	19	7	0	12
44	19	37	41–47	2.7–2.9	9	1	0	8

per cent or more the tubes become fragile in the swollen state and cannot be easily manipulated. In addition their diameter increases owing to grafting and swelling (see also Table 1), so that the flow conditions are modified.

In order to take advantage of a high hydrogel content without modifying the bulk properties and the size of the tubes, another series of samples were prepared under conditions where only the surfaces of the tubes (inside and outside) were grafted with NVP. For this purpose the tubes were irradiated in dilute aqueous solutions of NVP. A choice of experimental conditions makes it possible to control the thickness of the grafted layer. The grafting ratios on the surface of such tubes were determined using FMIR infra-red analysis after calibration with bulk grafted specimens. Samples with a surface grafting ratio of ca. 60 per cent were prepared in which the thickness of the grafted layer is 100 to 300 μm. These tubes are presently tested for their blood-compatibility.

REFERENCES

Bruck, S.D. (1973) Aspects of three types of hydrogels for biomedical applications. J. Biomed. Mater. Res., 7, 387–404.
Bruck, S.D. (1979) Physicochemical aspects of the blood compatibility of polymeric surface. J. Polym. Sci. Polymer Symposium 66, 283–312.
Chapiro, A., Foëx-Milléquant, M., Jendrychowska-Bonamour, A.-M., Lerke, Y., Sadurni, P. & Domurado, D. (1980) Polymers with improved short term hemocompatibility obtained by radiation grafting of NVP onto silicone rubber. Radiat. Phys. Chem., 15, 423–427.

Ratner, B.D., Hoffman, A.S., Hanson, S.R., Harker, L.A. &
Whiffen, J.D. (1979) Blood-compatibility-water-content relationships
for radiation grafted hydrogels. J. Polym. Sci. Polymer Symposium 66,
363-375.

Biomaterials 1980
Edited by G. D. Winter, D. F. Gibbons, and H. Plenk, Jr.
© 1982 John Wiley and Sons Ltd.

POROUS SILICONE MICROVASCULAR PROSTHESIS

C. Tizian*, K.E. Salyer** and J.L. Matthews**

*Wilheminen Hospital of Vienna, Department of Plastic and Reconstructive Surgery
** Baylor University Medical Center, Dallas, Texas

SUMMARY

The use of synthetic materials for arterial substitution and refinement of microvascular surgical techniques have made possible the treatment of certain vascular diseases which otherwise were considered inoperable. However, in small caliber vessel replacement, the autologous vein graft remained the only graft that successfully bridged microvascular defects. In this study we produced a silicone microvascular prosthesis that was evaluated in the rat abdominal aorta. The replamineform process was utilized for the production of a three dimensional fenestrated structure using silicone as the infiltrating material.

The microvascular prosthesis was inserted in the infrarenal segment of the abdominal aorta of 35 rats. The animals were sacrificed at frequency intervals of 3, 7, 9 and 14 days and 1, 3 and 6 months. Patency was studied by hemodynamic relationships from flow probe, transducer pressure tests and angiography. The tissue was subjected to histology and SEM evaluation. Antithrombogenicity was measured by fibrinolytic activator activity (FAA).

31 implants remained patent at the time of sacrifice, yielding an early patency rate of 88.6%. Thrombotic occlusion occurred in 11.4% prior to development of the neointima. The neointima developed in two stages; the intial fibrin platelet layer was reduced and after 14 days replaced with a definite neointima. Measured activity values of the FAA revealed a high antithrombotic relationship in the implant.

The patency results of this study suggest that a micrograft can remain patent over long periods of time. Silicone was compatible with other tissues and its physical characteristics contributed to the avoidance of thrombosis. This study using the rat abdominal aorta as a scientific models shows that, as long as the use of this micrograft is restricted to the replacement of arterial defects, the silicone microvascular prostheses appears to be a suitable substitute. This paper presents details of the trials that have been carried out with this micrograft and discusses future clinical applications of the prosthesis.

INTRODUCTION

The following study was prompted by the clinical need for a synthetic vascular graft as a microvessel replacement. A porous silicone microvascular prosthesis with an inside diameter of 1 mm was fabricated utilizing the replamineform principle and evaluated in the rat abdominal aorta. The replamineform principle is a technique for duplicating the porous microstructure of the carbonate skeletal components in polymeric materials. The pore structure can be replicated as a three dimensional, fenestrated structure which divides open space into two interpenetrating regions (Donnay and Pawson, 1969). When duplicated in polymers such as silicone, microstructures of this type allow the growth of periprosthetic tissue into the pores. In this study the structure of the sea urchin (Heterocentrotus trigonarius) was used for the skeletal matrix.

METHODS AND MATERIAL

After cleaning the calcite spines in water the structure was vacuum impregnated with dimethylsiloxane. The monomer was heat-polymerized and the microprosthesis machined from the spine-silicone composite. Finally, the calcite was removed by dissolution in 3% hydrochloric acid. The microvascular prosthesis had an inside diameter of 1 mm, a wall thickness of 0.3 mm and a length of 5 mm. The silicone had a pore size of 12 µ and a pore density of 50%.

Thirty-five Sprague Dawley rats, each weighing 200-250 g, were anesthetized. After exposing the infrarenal part of the abdominal aorta, which had an inside diameter of 1 mm, both iliolumbar branches were ligated. After fixing the aorta with approximator clamps, a piece 5 mm in length was resected. The defect was then bridged, inserting the tubular micrograft with two end-to-end ansatomoses by means of an everting, continuous over-and-over suture technique using 10-0 nylon for the anterior and posterior suture rows. A total of 14 stitches was required for a leak-free anastomosis. All surgical procedures were performed by the same surgeon. No anticoagulants were given prior to, during or after the operation. The animals were sacrificed after intervals of 3, 7, 9 and 14 days and 1, 3 and 6 months.

The graft patency was measured by distal aorta flow rates which were recorded with a 0.96 mm dia. electromagnetic flow probe. Flow was measured before application of the approximator clamps and at 1, 3, 7, 10 and 15 minutes after their removal. A final flow measurement was recorded on the day of sacrifice. Before retrieving the prostheses, the systolic pressures in the right carotid and femoral artery were also measured using polyethylene catheters connected to a pressure transducer and recorded on a polygraf. Finally, a thoracotomy was performed to permit insertion of a catheter into the thoracic aorta. Following this terminal event, the animal was placed under a GE 105 camera and the X-ray image of the injected contrast material was obtained.

After completion of the angiography, 1 mm areas of thoracic and mid-implant aorta walls were taken for FAA determinations. Using the fibrin-plate method, the specimens were incubated for 18 hours at 37° C. The area of fibrinolysis around each specimen was computed from direct planimetric measurements of its diameter. A 2.5% glutaraldehyde solution was perfused through the aorta and graft for fixation. The micrograft was then removed. The specimens were opened longitudinally. The anterior wall was prepared for standard histology and the posterior wall was prepared for critical point drying. Transverse and longitudinal sections were stained with H&E, Masson's trichrome, Van Giesson elastica and Wilder's reticulum stains. Critical point dried samples were also examined with a JSM-35 scanning electron microscope.

RESULTS

A total of 35 silicone microvascular prostheses were inserted in the infrarenal segment of the rat abdominal aorta. Thirty-one implants remained patent at the time of sacrifice, i.e., 3 days to 6 months, yielding an early patencey rate of 88.6% (see Table 1).

TABLE 1.

Day of sacrifice	3	7	9	14	30	90	180		
Group	1	2	3	4	5	6	7	35	(100.0%)
Occluded		x	x	x	x			4	(11.4%)
Patent	00000	000 0	00 00	000 0	0 000	00000	00000	31	(88.6%)

The average arterial flow rate in the abdominal aorta measured before implantation was 34 ml/min. Immediately after release of the clamps, the blood flow was greater than that prior to implantation and was maintained for 7 minutes. Reactive hyperemia persisted for another 15 minutes, whereupon the arterial flow rate dropped back to normal. Before sacrificing the animals, flow measurements were again performed, revealing the same values as were seen preoperatively for the patent prostheses. The four cases of occlusion showed a flow rate of 10 ml/min.

Angiography revealed that up to the ninth day a slight interruption of the contours was seen in the area of the anastomosis. Later investigations showed a plain, smooth aorta-implant junction. In the animals studied for 3 to 6 months, no stenotic alteration caused by thickening of the intima was noted in the area of the anastomosis or in the mid-portion of the prosthesis. In cases of occlusion related to thrombosis, an upgrade collateral circulation was noted.

The average value of FAA in the rat abdominal aorta was 143.1 mm^2. In the prosthesis a considerable increase in activity was seen after 3 days, reaching 420 mm^2, almost three times the value found in the aorta. Although a decrease of 340 mm^2 was observed after 7 days, this still represented a considerable increase in FAA. A linear decrease was observed after 9 and 14 days. An approximation of values in the normal aorta was seen at the end of 1 month, but after 6 months it remained consistently above the normal value in the aorta (149 mm^2).

Longitudinal and transverse sections were examined in order to assess endo-thelialization of the implant lumen, features of the interstitital spaces of the implant, adventitial reaction and the aorta-implant junction. All specimens demonstrated that the implant was functionally embedded in the structure of the aorta. The structure of the media ended abruptly at the aorta–implant junction. The adventitita was outside the prosthesis and connected to both ends of the aorta as a fibrous capsule. The development of the endothelial lining took place in two stages. Initially, fibrin, platelets and red blood cells covered the inside lining of the implant. The neointima was established and stable after one month.

DISCUSSION

Previous investigators have reported on the fate of a variety of small–caliber vessel bypass and replacement grafts (Campbell et al, 1974; Florian et al, 1976; Hastings et al, 1978). However, none of these studies utilized implants with lumen diameters of less than 2 mm.

The intial results of this study are encouraging. On the basis of patency results of 88.6%, it is evident that a micrograft (vascular prosthesis with an inside diameter less than 2 mm) can remain patent over an extended period of time. Only four implants developed a thrombotic occlusion. The ethiology of the thrombosis may have been the result of a decrease in flow rate below a critical velocity (Sauvage et al, 1974), creasting statis and thrombosis.

The patency results obtained in the present study appear to be due to different reasons. One of these involves the creation of native antithrombotic relation-ships in the implanted micrografts. Porosity (Harrison et al, 1961; Wesolowski et al, 1968) of the prothesis wall allowed the necessary tissue ingrowth though the interstices, creating a stable neointima with good attachment to the prothesis. Silicone as a synthetic material was easy to handle.

The use of microsurgical techniques was probably significant in achieving the high patency rates, since it ensured minimal surgical trauma in the area of the anastomosis.

Angiography and tissue evaluation demonstrated that an optimum hemodynamic situation had been created by the use of the end-to-end anastomosis and isodiametrics. The everting suture technique ensured that neither media nor adventitia, in which collagen is located (Acland, 1973), were exposed to the blood stream. It was possible to achieve leak-free anastomosis without tension using the continuous over and over suture technique of vascular surgery.

The future clinical application of the silicone micrograft can only be partially dealt with at this stage. When restricted to replacement of arterial defects, the silicone micrograft appears to be a suitable vascular substitute. Before implant-ing it in man, however, further experimental studies seem to be necessary. One of these is an evaluation in a peripheral artery of the dog. For this purpose, a model must be designed which assures that the blood flow does not fall below the thrombotic threshold velocity, because this immediately causes stasis and thrombosis (Sauvage et al, 1974). The rat abdominal aorta was chosen as the scientific model in this study in an effort to avoid this effect (Hebel, 1976).

However, by proving in this animal model that a synthetic micrograft can remain patent over a long period of time, the result of this experimental study provide the groundwork as well as the stimulus for additional investigations into the clinical utilisation of this implant. It is hoped that the speculation, effort and facts generated by this study can be applied in a meaningful manner towards the resolution of the questions this investigation has raised.

REFERENCES

Acland, R. (1973) Thrombus formation in microvascular surgery: An experimental study of the effects of surgical trauma. Surg 73, 766.

Campbell, C.D., Goldfarb, D. & Delton, D.D. (1974) Expanded polytetrafluoroethylene as a small artery substitute. Trans Am Soc Artif Int Organs 20, 86.

Donnay, G. & Pawson, D.L. (1969) X-ray diffraction studies of echinoderm plates. Science 166, 1147.

Florian, A., Cohn L.H., Dammin, G.J. & Collins, J.J. (1976) Small vessel replacement with Gore-Tex (polytetrafluoroethylene). Arch Surg 111, 267.

Harrison, J.H. (1961) Influence of porosity on synthetic grafts. Arch Surg 82, 8

Hastings, O., Krishna, J., Hobson, R. & Swan, K. (1978) A prospective randomized study of three expanded polytetrafluoroethylene (PTFE) grafts as small arterial substitutes. Ann Surg 188, 743.

Hebel, R. (1976) Anatomy of the Laboratory Rat, p 27. Williams & Wilkins, Baltimore.

Sauvage, L.R., Berger, K.E. & Mansfield, P.B. (1974) Future directions in the development of arterial prostheses for small and medium caliber arteries. Surg Clin North Am 54, 213.

Wesolowski, S.A., Fries, C.C. & Martinez, A. (1968) Arterial prosthetic materials. Ann NY Acad Sci, 146, 325.

Biomaterials 1980
Edited by G. D. Winter, D. F. Gibbons, and H. Plenk, Jr.
© 1982 John Wiley and Sons Ltd.

A NEW METHOD FOR DETERMINING IN VIVO COMPLIANCE OF
VASCULAR SEGMENTS

S. Klein, R. Miranda, R. Nelson, S. Elazar*, S. Austin*,
and R. White

Harbor/UCLA Medical Center, Torrance, California
* Medical Testing Systems, Fountain Valley, California

SUMMARY

Reconstruction of diseased segments of the vascular system comprises a
major area of cardiovascular surgery. A problem exists because the incidence of thrombotic occlusion of vascular substitutes remains high in
small internal diameter repairs. Low compliance has been hypothesized
as a contributing factor in graft thrombosis. This report describes a
new method for determining compliance of vascular segments, in vivo,
using electromagnetic rheoangiometry.

Ten dogs (20-30 kg.) were premedicated with morphine and anesthetized
with chloralose. A catheter was directed into the femoral artery to be
studied from an ipsilateral distal branch artery. This catheter was
utilized for blood pressure measurement and insertion of the electromagnetic rheoangiometry probe. Blood pressure measurements were confirmed in the contralateral femoral artery.

The electromagnetic rheoangiometry system consists of an intravascular
loop probe placed in an externally induced magnetic field. Changes in
the area of the loop allows measurement of intraluminal diameter.
Electrodes on the loop permit quantitation of blood velocity and flow.
Blood flow values were compared with standard electromagnetic cuff flow
probe measurements.

Simple dynamic diameter compliance (C_d) was obtained using the formula
$C_d = \frac{\Delta d}{d \cdot \Delta P}$, where ΔP is the pulse pressure, Δd is the change in internal
diameter with pulse pressure and d is the mean internal diameter of the

vessel. The compliance is expressed as a percent diameter change per
mm Hg x 10^{-2}. Using the electromagnetic rheoangiometry system, the
compliance of in situ, canine femoral artery was found to be 6.6 $\pm$ 3.5
%/mm Hg x 10^{-2}. Using this approach, long term effects of compliance
on prosthetic performance can be assessed.

INTRODUCTION

Currently used vascular prostheses are less compliant than autogenous
vessels (Kidson and Abbott, 1978). Non-compliant graft segments impede pulsatile flow and interfere with energy propagation. Kidson and
Abbott have demonstrated that autogenous vein is less than one-half as
compliant as autogenous artery and that current prostheses (Dacron,
expanded PTFE, bovine, and umbilical vein) are less compliant than
autogenous vein. Significantly decreased patency rates were demonstrated after 3 months of implantation using less compliant fabrica-
tions. Lyman et. al., (1978) confirmed these observations using co-
polyetherurethane graft materials of varying compliance.

Hokanson and Strandness (1968) determined the dynamic compliance of
woven and knitted Dacron and Teflon arterial grafts, bovine heterografts, and autogenous vein grafts after various periods of implantation. With the exception of autogenous vein grafts, implantation
reduced the compliance of each graft tested to about one-third of its
original value.

Several methods for determining the compliance of vascular segments
have been described including extraluminal cantilever transducers
(Baird et. al., 1977 and Murgo et. al., 1971), electrical calipers
(Gow, 1966), and stress-strain analysis of graft materials prior to
and following implantation (Lyman et. al., 1978 and Hokanson and
Strandness, 1968). All of these methods require isolation of the
vascular segments being studied or removal prior to analysis. Pagani
et. al., (1978) described a technique for instantaneous measurement
of the external dimensions of vascular segments using implanted
transducers and ultrasound imaging.

This report describes a new technique for quantitating, in vivo, the
compliance of vascular segments without requiring isolation of the

vessel. This is accomplished using an extension of selective angiography, electromagnetic rheoangiometry (ER) (Kolin et. al, 1978). This device consists of an intravascular loop probe placed in an externally induced magnetic field. The loop and electrodes on the loop allow simultaneous measurement of arterial internal diameter, instantaneous change in diameter, blood velocity and flow. (Figure 1)

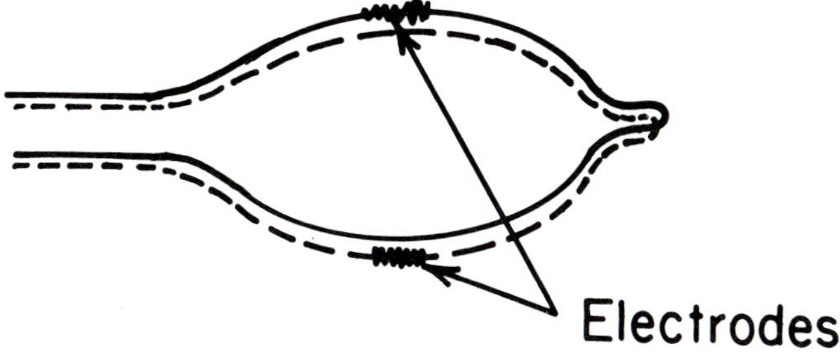

Figure 1. The loop probe consists of bifilar beryllium copper wire forming two loops side by side with each insulated from the other. One wire is exposed on one side and the other wire is exposed on the other side forming the electrodes.

Faraday's law of electromagnetic conduction describes the induced voltage that is produced when a conductive fluid (blood) passes through a magnetic field. The law states that $E = (MVd) \times 10^{-8}$ where E is the emf (volts), M is the magnetic field (gauss), V is the velocity of the liquid (cm/sec.) and d is the luminal diameter (cm.) (Figure 2)

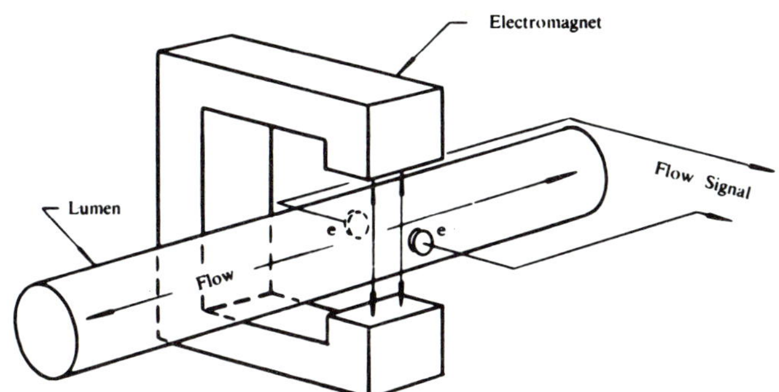

Figure 2. An induced voltage can be obtained when a conduction fluid (blood) passes through the magnetic field with direction of flow perpendicular to the field. The voltage is converted to a velocity signal by an amplifier. A linear relationship exists between the velocity of the blood and the magnitude of the voltage. Sensors (e) placed perpendicular to the field are used to record the induced voltage (E).

When a loop is introduced into a magnetic field, changes in the area
of the loop will produce a voltage (e_t) which is proportional to the
diameter within a given range (Kolin et. al., 1978). Using the electromagnetic rheoangiometry loop probe, the internal diameter of the
vessel and the velocity of the blood can be measured separately and
then multiplied to obtain flow (F). $F = \pi/4\ d^2 V$. (Figure 3)

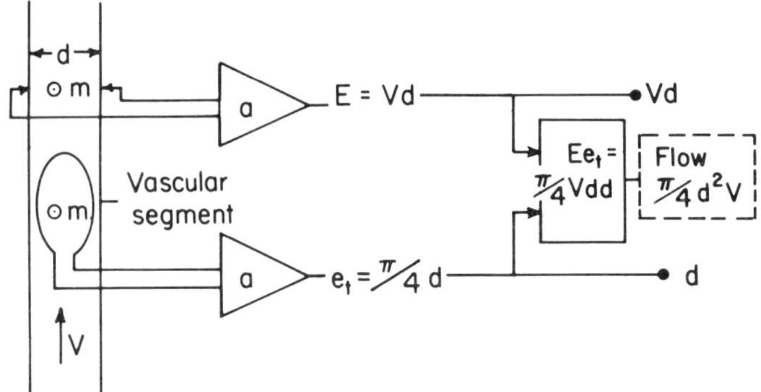

Figure 3. Electromagnetic rheoangiometry blood flow system
block diagram. Changes in the area of the loop produce a voltage (e_t) which is proportional to the diameter. Electrodes
on the loop record an induced voltage (E) produced by the
velocity of the blood. E x e_t ~ flow. ⊙M = magnetic field
perpendicular to the loop, a = amplifier.

MATERIALS AND METHODS

The electromagnetic rheoangiometry system (Medical Testing Systems,
Fountain Valley, California) utilizes a collapsible loop probe which
is introduced into the vessel being studied through a catheter.
(Figure 4) The loop probe which is contructed to match the appropriate
internal diameter of the vessel being studied exerts a distending
force which is neglegible under physiologic conditions (Kolin, 1978).
A lateral force of only 80 mg. is required to reduce the loop width
by 1 mm. Loops produce no measurable deformation on vessels until
intraluminal pressure is reduced below 6 mmHg (Kolin and MacAlpin,
1977). Histologic examination of arteries which have contained loop
probes reveal no evidence of intimal damage.

Following introduction of the probe the animal is rotated to place the
plane of the electrodes perpendicular to the electromagnetic field.

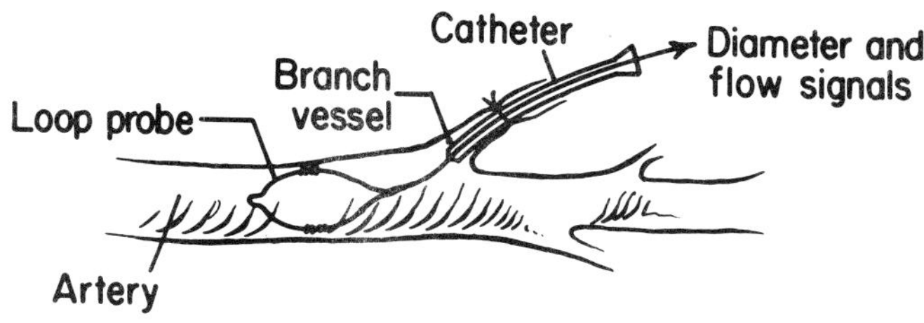

Figure 4.   Intravascular placement of loop probe.

Ten adult dogs weighin 20-30 kg. were used as the experimental animals. Prior to performing the experiments, the loop probes were calibrated for diameter in vitro by placing the loop in the lumen of precisely machined plastic cylinders. Three, four, and five mm. internal diameter measurements were calibrated by placing the probes in the
cylinders with the loop aligned perpendicular to the magnetic field.
(Figure 5)

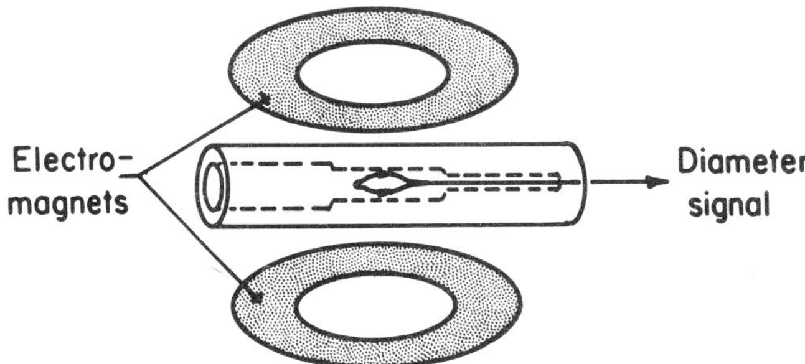

Figure 5.   Diameter calibration.

Flow calibrations were made in vivo by placing the loop probe in the
common femoral artery. An arteriovenous fistula was constructed between the femoral artery and the femoral vein distal to the probe.
Flow through the fistula was controlled using a proximally placed
Goldblatt clamp and quantitated by collecting the blood in a reser-
voir before reinfusing into the animal. (Figure 6)

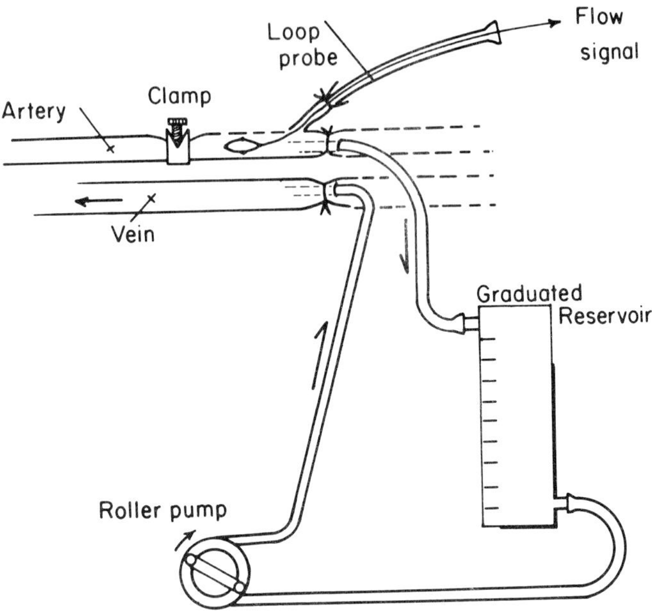

Figure 6.   Blood flow calibration.

The animals were premedicated with morphine (5 mg/kg.) and anesthetized with chloralose (75 mg/kg.) to maintain preinduction cardiovascular status (Shabethal et. al., 1963). Compliance measurements were
obtained on native artery by isolating a distal branch and introducing
the E.R. probe retrograde through a catheter (16G, 1.5 mm. internal
diameter). A specially designed adaptor was used which allowed for
introduction of the E.R. probe and for simultaneous blood pressure
monitoring. The contralateral femoral artery was also cannulated for
blood pressure measurement.

Blood pressure readings obtained from the vascular segments under
study were compared to those obtained in the contralateral femoral
artery to determine if introduction of the probe system damped the
blood pressure signal. Contralateral pressures were obtained using
two methods: 1) through a catheter placed using the same technique
as the study site, and 2) using Millar MIKRO-TIP pressure transducers

(Millar Instruments, Inc., Houston, Texas). No significant difference in blood pressure values or pulse pressure were obtained upon introduction of the probe. As a result, ipsilateral blood pressure values were used in compliance calculations.

Following introduction of the E.R. probe, the animal was rotated until the loop was perpendicular to the magnetic field as determined by maximization of the signals. Pulsatile diameter, mean diameter, blood pressure, and flow were then obtained. Experimental parameters were recorded on a six channel MFE recorder (MFE Corporation, Salem, New Hampshire). Flow values were compared with standard electromagnetic cuff flow probes (Statham Instruments, Oxnard, California). The femoral vessels were exposed to confirm the position of the probe.

Simple dynamic compliance was obtained using the formula $C_d = \dfrac{\Delta d}{d \cdot \Delta P}$ where Δd is the pulsatile diameter, d is the mean internal diameter, and ΔP is the pulse pressure. The compliance data is expressed as %/mmHg. x 10^{-2}.

RESULTS

The measured and derived compliance parameters for the ten dogs are presented in Table 1.

TABLE 1. Measured and derived compliance parameters

Parameters	Mean value $\pm$ S.D. (n=10)
Mean internal diameter	4.2 $\pm$ .8 mm
Pulsatile diameter	0.271 $\pm$ .162 mm
Mean flow	254 $\pm$ 94 cc/min
Cuff flow	192 $\pm$ 60 cc/min
Pulse pressure	100 $\pm$ 12 mmHg
Compliance	6.6 $\pm$ 3.5 %/mmHg x 10^{-2}

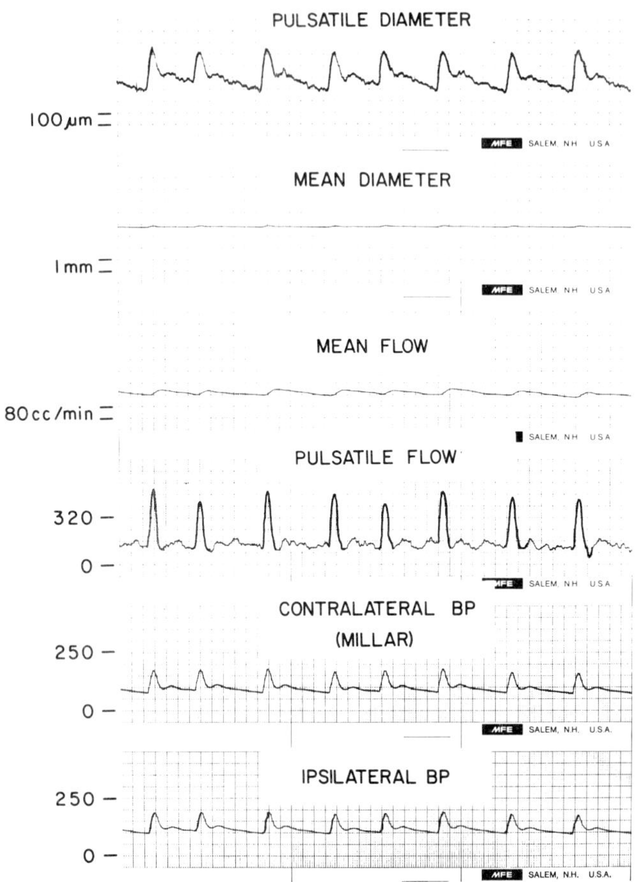

Figure 7.   A representative tracing of the variables measured
by this experimental approach.

The discrepancy between mean flow obtained with electromagnetic rheoangiometry (254 ± 94 cc/min) as compared with cuff probes (192 ± 60
cc/min) is not statistically significant.   Cuff probe flow values can
vary as much as 20-25% depending upon the amount of vascular constric-
tion produced by the cuff and by the impairment of cuff contact with
the vascular surface (Gordon et. al., 1971).

<u>DISCUSSION</u>

This study describes an intraluminal technique for quantitating the

compliance of vascular segments as an alternative to in vitro or in
vivo methods which require isolation of the segment being studied.
Using electromagnetic rheoangiometry, compliance data can be obtained
from both autogenous blood vessels and prosthetic interposition grafts
both acutely and chronically. We envision this procedure to be valuable for studying changes which likely occur with variation in the
suture technique and with progressive incorporation of microporous
graft segments.

ACKNOWLEDGEMENTS

The authors thank Dr. John Roseboro for his critique and influence in
the development of this experimental approach and Ken Johnson for his
technical assistance.

Supported by National Institutes of Health, Grant #R01 HL 24618-01
and by a grant from the American Heart Association/Greater Los Angeles
Affiliate, Grant #641.

REFERENCES

Bair, R.N., Kidson, I.G., L'Italien, G.J., and Abbott, W.M. (1977)
Dynamic compliance of arterial grafts, Am. J. Physiol, 234, 568-572.
Gordon, A.S., Elazar, S., and Austin, S. (1971) Practical Aspects of
Blood Flow Measurement, Statham Instruments, Inc., Oxnard, California.
Gow, B.S. (1966) An electrical caliper for measurement of pulsatile
arterial diameter changes in vivo, J. Appl. Physiol., 21, 1122-1126.
Hokanson, D.E. and Strandness, D.E., Jr. (1968) Stress-strain charac-
teristics of various arterial grafts, Surgery, Gynecol. and Obstet.,
127, 57-60.
Kidson, I.G. and Abbott, W.M. (1978) Low compliance and arterial graft
occlusion, Circulation, Supp. I, 58, I1-I4.
Kolin A. (1980) Absolute induction angiometry, Blood Vessels, 17, 61-
77.
Kolin, A. and MacAlpin, R.N. (1977) Induction angiometer electromagnetic magnification of vascular diameter variation in-vivo, Blood
Vessels, 14, 141-156.
Kolin, A., MacAlpin, R.N., and Steckel, R. (1978) Electromagnetic
rheoangiometry: An extension of selective angiography, Am. J. Roent-
genol., 130, 13-23.
Lyman, D.J., Fazzio, F.J., Voorhees, M., Robinson, G., and Albo, D.,
Jr. (1978) Compliance as a factor in effecting the patency rates of a
copolyurethane vascular graft, J. Biomed. Mater. Res., 12, 337-345.
Murgo, J.P., Cox, R.H., and Peterson, L.H. (1971) Cantilever trans-
ducer for continuous measurement of arterial diameter in vivo, J.
Appl. Physiol., 31, 948-953.
Pagani, M., Baig, H., Sherman, A., Manders, W.T., Quinn, P., Patrick,
T., Franklin, D., and Vatner, S.F. (1978) Measurement of multiple
simultaneous small dimensions and study of arterial pressure-dimension

relations in conscious animals, <u>Am. J. Physiol., 235</u>, 610-617.
Shabethal, R., Fowler, N.O., and Hurlburt, O. (1963) Hemodynamic
studies of dogs under phenobarbital and morphine chloralose anesthesia, <u>J. Surg. Res., 5</u>, 263-267.

Biomaterials 1980
Edited by G. D. Winter, D. F. Gibbons, and H. Plenk, Jr.
© 1982 John Wiley and Sons Ltd.

IMPAIREMENT OF GLYCOPROTEINS SYNTHESIS ON VASCULAR
PROSTHESES : A COMPARATIVE STUDY OF THREE DIFFERENT
MATERIALS.

E. Chignier[°], J. Guidollet[°°], P. Louisot[°°], J. Descotes[°°°],
and R. Eloy[°].

Unit 37 –INSERM– Cardiovascular surgery and organ transplantation laboratory.
18 av. Doyen Lépine. 69500 Bron – France. (°)

FRA INSERM– 562 and Cardiologic Hospital – Lyon – France (°°)

Cardiovascular Surgery Unity – Hospital E. Herriot – Lyon
France (°°°).

SUMMARY

The tissue which develops within vascular prostheses has been investigated in the dog by means of 1°) histological, 2°) scanning electron
microscopy and 3°) enzymic assays for cytosolic and microsomial activities involved in the biosynthesis of glycosaminoglycuronoglycans.
Dacron, Rhodergon and Goretex prostheses were compared. The enzymic
activities of the newly formed tissue were significantly lower than
those of the normal aortic wall, despite the occurrence of flattened
endothelial like cells on fibrous tissue in Dacron and Rhodergon prostheses. The complete lack of enzymes involved in glycoprotein biosynthesis was noted in Goretex prostheses and correspond to a very limited endoprosthetic tissue development.

INTRODUCTION

Vascular replacement is complicated by processes which occur at the
blood prosthesis interface and which depend upon the nature of the
tissue developed at the inner surface of the prosthesis. The intimal-
like tissue has not yet been clearly determined ; its exact nature remains a matter of controversy.
We have previously demonstrated that the normal aortic glycosyl-transferases were significantly modified in the tissue developed in contact
with vascular prostheses (Chignier et al., 1980, 1980).
Glycosyltransferases are implicated in glycoprotein and glycosaminoglycuronoglycans biosynthesis : these enzymes add successive oses and
oses derivatives to the growing carbohydrate chains ; so that, glycosyl-transferases are responsible for macromolecular constructions in
intima and involved in synthesis of new tissue. The characterization

of glycosyl-transferases, in fact, provided informations to the specificity of successive additions of carbohydrate which correspond to established models of chaining. Four enzymatic activities have been studied : N-acetyl-glucosaminyl and sialyl-transferases have a microsomal localization whereas galactosyl and xylosyl-transferases are localized in the soluble cytoplasmic phase.
The aim of the present study was to investigate the nature of tissue healing within three different types of vascular prostheses : 1) woven polyethyleneterephthalate (Dacron ®) ; 2) shaved velvet polyterephthalate diethylene glycol (Rhodergon ®) ; 3) expanded polytetrafluorethylene (Goretex ®).
Histology, scanning electron microscopy and biochemical assays for 4 enzymes implicated in the biosynthesis of the glycoprotein macromolecules were performed.

MATERIAL and METHODS

48 mongrel dogs in their second year weighing 15-20 kg were used for carotid or aortic replacements. The animals were anesthetized by intravenous injection of 0.25 g/kg Nesdonal. The abdominal aorta was replaced in 18 dogs by a Dacron ® prosthesis, and in 13 animals by Rhodergon ® prosthesis. Both types of prostheses have internal diameter of 6 to 8 mm, according to internal diameter of the aorta. Seventeen carotid replacements were carried out using a Goretex ® prosthesis with an internal diameter of 3-6 mm. All prostheses were sutured by and end to end anastomosis using monobrin 4/0 or 6/0 sutures. No drugs, anticoagulants or antibiotics were used postoperatively. The animals were sacrificed sequentially between the 30th and 80th postoperative days.
A longitudinal section of the prosthesis and of the adjacent arterial wall was fixed in Bouin's solution, embedded in parafin. Sections were stained with hematoxylin and eosin.
On the tissue which developed within the prostheses the four of the enzymatic systems implicated in the glycoprotein biosynthesis were assayed and compared with those of the normal aortic wall. The intima and tissues grown on the inside of the prosthesis are submitted to differential ultracentrifugation after congelation in liquid nitrogen and crushing. Subcellular fractionation has been controled by electron microscopy and by quantitative determination of marker enzymes characteristic of each fraction : glucose-6-phosphatase for microsomes, acid 5'-nucleotidase for lysosomes, basic 5'-nucleotidase for plasma membranes, lacticodeshydrogenase for cell sap. Glycosyl-transferases enzymatic activities are studied in acellular system in vitro accor-

ding to the general reaction : nucleoside - diphosphosugar (radio-
active) + endogenous acceptor (vascular)→(radioactive) glycosyli-
zed acceptor + nucleoside diphosphate (Richard et al., 1975).
Specimens taken from longitudinal section of the prostheses and adjacent arterial wall were fixed in a 2% buffered glutaraldehyde solution
and processed for scanning electron microscopy.

RESULTS

Microscopic examination : 60 days after implantation Dacron ® prostheses were covered inside and outside with newly formed tissue. The tissue on the luminal side of the fabrics consisted of fibrous tissue
with fibroblasts and longitudinal fibers. Flattened cells covered the
inner surface. Occasionally this layer included blood cells or thrombi.

55 days after implantation the external surface of Rhodergon ® prostheses showed minimal fibrous tissue with some inflammatory reaction
except at the suture contact points where a fibrous tissue developed
without elastin fibers. The luminal tissue consisted of fibroblasts
and fibrous tissue in close contact with the prostheses. Collagen and
elastin fibers were covered with flattened cells.

43 days after implantation of Goretex ® fabrics various types of cells
had penetrated into the pores of the prosthesis. On the luminal surface a thin fibrocellular tissue, 4-5 cell layers thick, was covered
with flattened cells.

Scanning electron microscopy : The prosthetic implants were covered
by a fibrinous deposit, fibrous tissue and fibroblastic non endothelial like cells. The cells do not have the shape and the microvillous
projections of the normal endothelial cells. Goretex R implants, particularly, were covered only by a fibrinous tissue with very few cells.
Occasionally the Goretex ® fabric was still visible even after 60
Days. (Figure 1a, 1b)

Biochemical enzymic investigations : The enzymic activities involved
in glycoprotein synthesis were evaluated in comparison with those of
normal arterial wall, which represented 100 %. (Table I). It appears
that the enzymic levels of the tissue formed on Dacron ® and Rhodergon ® are markedely decreased for the two enzymes involved in the initiation of the glucidic chain for example xylosyl-transferase and galactosyl-transferase. Galactosyl-transferase activity was markedely
increased on the Rhodergon ® prosthesis and sialyl-transferase activity was increased on both Dacron ® and Rhodergon ® prostheses. None
of the four enzymes could be detected on the Goretex ® prosthesis.

DISCUSSION

The histological and scanning electron microscopy examination leads
to the following conclusion. Rhodergon ® developed the most intense
fibrous reaction on the lumen surface. Dacron ® exhibited less fibrous reaction and Goretex ® almost no fibrous reaction. Elastin fibers were present in the tissue developed on the luminal surface of
Rhodergon ® and Dacron ® prostheses. Endothelial-like cells were
observed on Rhodergon ® and Dacron ® prostheses but were generally
absent on Goretex ® fabrics. Scanning electron microscopy demonstrated that these cellsdo not have the morphology of normal endothelial
cells, nor do they exhibit the microvillous projections of endothelial cells.(Figure 2 & Figure 3)

The biochemical investigations demonstrated : 1) the altered functional behaviour of vascular graft tissue as compared to normal intima,
with respect to the glycosylation of glycoproteins ; 2) the specific
enzyme activity was dependant upon the graft material ; 3) the complete absence of any enzymic activity in Goretex ® prosthesis.

CONCLUSION

These preliminary results demonstrate that the "neo-intimal" tissue
which had developed within the prostheses 60 days after implantation
was entirely different from normal intimal aortic tissue despite, the
presence of "endothelial-like" cells. The ability of the "neo-intima"
to synthesize structural glycoproteins has been significantly modified.
These results suggest, therefore, that a more extensive investigation
of the vascular graft tissue must to be performed in order to determine the role of the graft material and its structure.

REFERENCE

Chignier, E., Guidollet, J., Devolfe, C., Louisot, P., Descotes, J.,
(1980). Biosynthesis of glycoconjugates in polyethylene-terephthalate
aortic prostheses. Advances in Biomaterials, Vol. 1, Evaluation of
Biomaterials, Eds. Winter, Leray & DeGroot, Wiley, U.K., 529-534.
Chignier, E., Guidollet, J., Devolfe, C., Serres, M., Louisot, P.,
Descotes, J. (1980). Macromolecular and histological studies of new
tissue formation in velour vascular prostheses. Europ. Surg. Res.,
12, 130-139.
Guillaumond, M., & Louisot, P., (1975). Glycoprotein biosynthesis in
aortic wall. VI :studies of soluble xylosyl-transferase in intima.
Int. J. Biochem, 6, 491-496.
Louisot, P., (1973). Glycoprotein biosynthesis in the aortic wall :
subcellular localization and parameters of three glycosyl-transferases
of intima-media. Arterial Wall, 1, 73-74.
Richard, M., Martin, A., & Louisot, P. (1975). Evidence for glycosyl-
transferases in rat liver nuclei. Biochem. and Biophys. Res. Commun.,
64, 108-113.

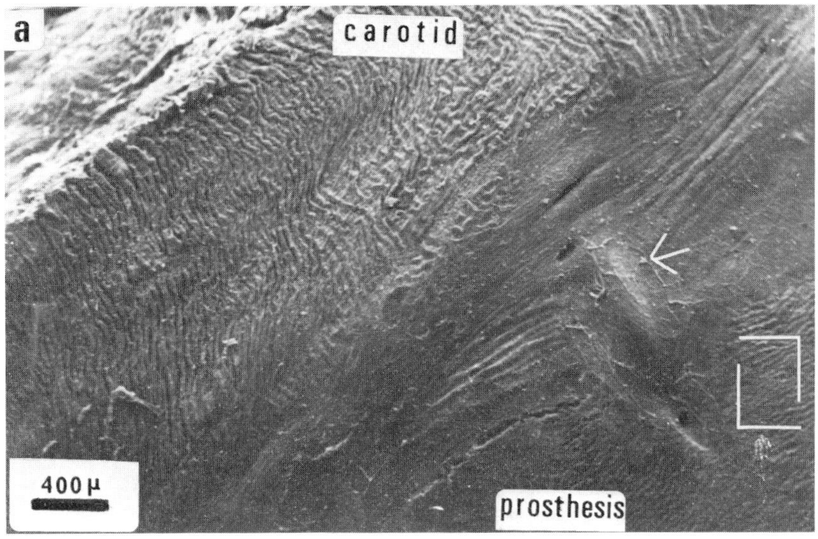

Figure 1. Goretex : 60 days.
a) Junctional zone with a stitch covered by fibrillar
tissue (↑) ; carotid endothelium is seen at the top of the
figure, and prosthesis at the bottom.

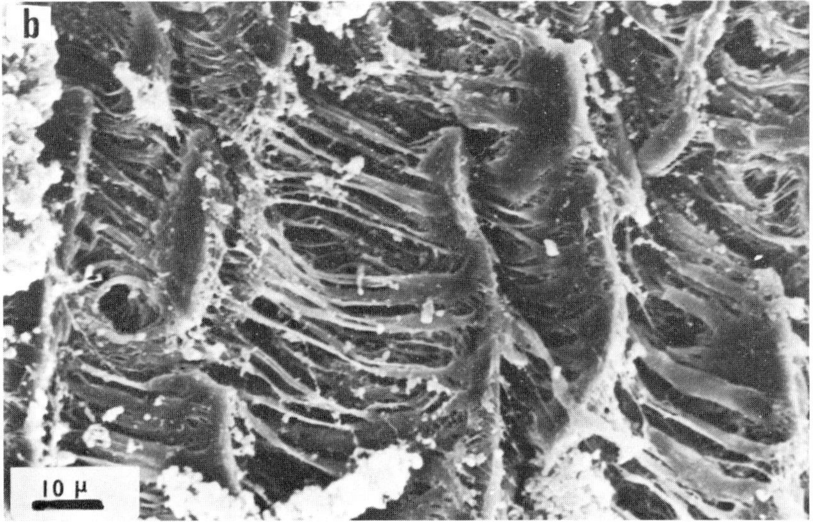

b) detail of the prosthesis not covered with fibrous tissue
or endothelial-like cells.

ENZYMIC ACTIVITIES OF GLYCOPROTEINS SYNTHESIS

	XYLOSYL TRANSFERASE	GALACTOSYL TRANSFERASE	GLUCOSAMINYL N-ACETYL TRANFERASE	SIALYL TRANFERASE
Arterial wall...	100	100	100	100
Dacron.... n:18	84	–	38	172
Rhodergon.... n:13	41	41	600	545
Gore-tex.... n:17	0	0	0	0

Table I. Graft tissue enzyme activity as per cent of normal arterial wall enzyme activities.

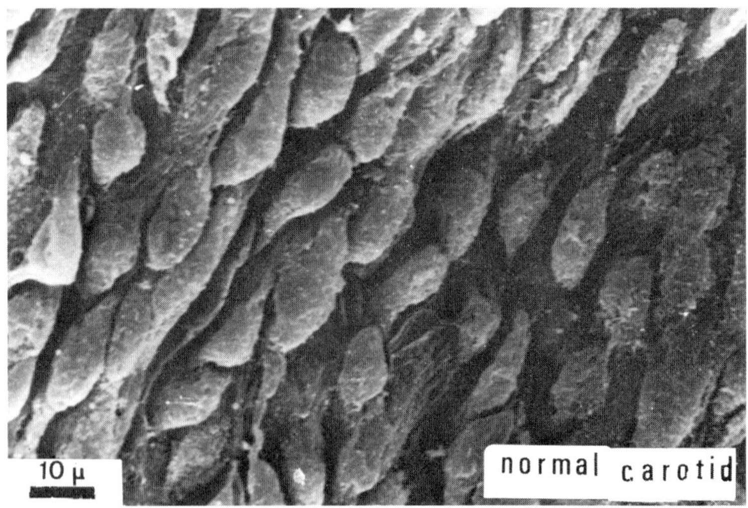

Figure 2. Morphology of normal endothelial cells observed on a dog carotid artery, with the characteristics micro-villous projections.

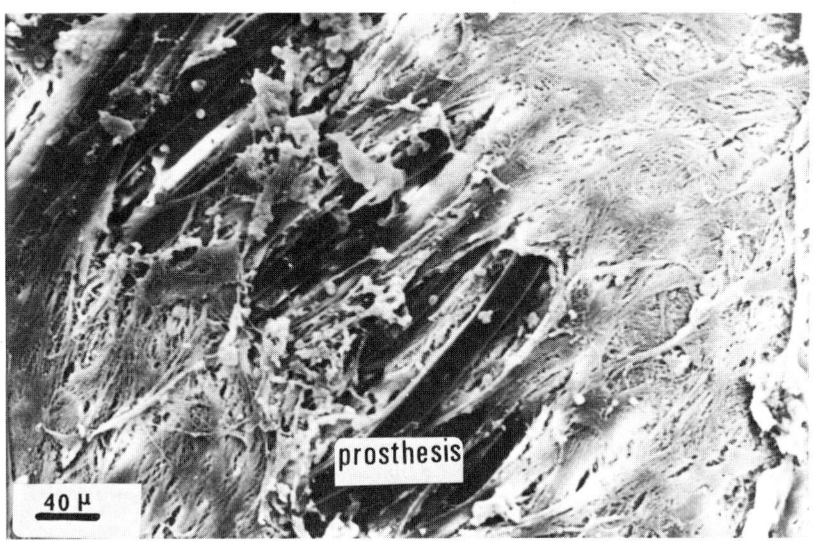

Figure 3. Woven Dacron [R] prosthesis 60 days after
implantation : no endothelial coating is observed
and fibers of the fabric are still apparent.

Biomaterials 1980
Edited by G. D. Winter, D. F. Gibbons, and H. Plenk, Jr.
© 1982 John Wiley and Sons Ltd.

MORPHOLOGICAL FINDINGS IN EXPANDED PTFE
VASCULAR GRAFTS CROSSING JOINTS

G. Geiger[*], U. Rückert[**] and B. Krempion[***]

[*]   Surgical University Clinic Mannheim, GFR
[**] Department of Surgery Landstuhl, GFR
[***] Department of Pathology, University of Heidelberg,GFR

SUMMARY

Morphological studies of long expanded polytetrafluoroethylene (PTFE)
bypasses crossing joints do not yet exist. Ten PTFE vascular grafts
were implanted in foxhounds as iliaco-femoral bypass. After 1, 3,
6 and 9 months, the grafts were studied using light microscopy,
scanning and transmission electron microscopy. There was a good
patency of all prostheses. The pre and postkinked areas showed
thrombosis leading to stenosis. After nine months endothelium was
spread over all parts of the luminal surface, including the kinked
areas. In the wall of the prosthesis there was a focal ingrowth of
fibroblastic cells with the characteristics of myocytes. Collagen
fibres could also be seen. Expanded PTFE vascular graft seems to be
a satisfactory transplant material. Prognosis of long term patency
in reconstructions crossing joints may be reduced by thrombosis of
the pre and postkinked areas.

INTRODUCTION

Expanded polytetrafluoroethylene (PTFE) is being used as a small
arterial substitute. It possesses many of the criteria required for
an ideal synthetic graft material: inertness, no biological
deterioration, primary anti-thrombogenicity and no extravasation of
blood. Because of its microporous structure, ingrowth of fibrous
tissue and capillaries is possible.

In 1972 Soyer et al successfully used expanded PTFE as a venous
substitute in piglets. Matsumoto and Hasegawa (1973) found a 100 %
patency when implanted in dogs as femoral artery substitutes. Since
that time, expanded PTFE has been in clinical use for lower extremity
arterial reconstructions. Excellent results in men were reported by
Campbell et al (1979). Veith et al (1978) found patency rates with
femoro-popliteal PTFE bypasses equal to those performed with saphenous
vein, whereas Hastings et al (1978) warned of the use of expanded
PTFE grafts in preference to saphenous veins, because he observed a
patency rate of only 56 % – 75 % in dogs after 12 weeks.

All experimental studies are based upon only short vessel interposition of synthetic grafts. Morphological investigations of long

561

bypasses, especially of joint crossing bypasses, do not yet exist.
That is why we have studied the organisation of tissue in
prostheses crossing over joints by light microscopy, scanning and
transmission electron microscopy.

MATERIALS AND METHODS

Ten expanded polytetrafluoroethylene vascular grafts (Gore-tex[R],
gas sterilised with ethyleneoxide) with an internal diameter of 6 mm
and a length of 15 cm were implanted in foxhounds (weight 25 Kg),
performed as iliaco-femoral bypass. The animals were not given pre
or post-operative anticoagulants. During the experiment angiography
was performed, showing a good patency of all straight prostheses
without stenosis, even in the acutely bent hip joint. After 1, 3, 6
and 9 months the grafts were fixed intravitally with cacodylate-
glutaraldehyde buffer solution and the animals killed under deep
anaesthesia. Then the specimens were prepared for light microscopy,
scanning and transmission electron microscopy.

RESULTS

When removed, all straight prostheses were patent. Macroscopically
at all time intervals pre and postkinked areas showed thrombosis,
leading to stenosis of the lumen. Angiography did not demonstrate
these stenoses. After one month there was a thin layer of endothelium near the anastomoses and cells were protruding into the PTFE
texture (Figure 1). In the middle of the graft, including the
kinked areas, smooth fibrin areas could be seen (Figure 2). The
pores of the expanded PTFE were filled with blood cells and a few
fibroblasts. Three and six months after implantation the kinked
areas showed islands of endothelium (Figure 3) and of fibrin.
Anastomoses were covered by a sheet of flattened endothelial cells.
There were characteristic cement lines between the cells and their
surfaces had microvilli (Figure 4). In the middle of the graft the
cells seemed to overlap and no cement lines could be observed. The
endothelium lay directly upon the expanded PTFE. In some areas
neointimal hyperplasia was found. Nine months after implantation
endothelium had spread out over the entire intimal surface of the
prostheses. Only the pre and postkinked area showed thrombi, the
kinked area itself was covered by endothelial cells (Figure 5).
Intramural pores were occupied by fibrous tissue. In transmission
electron microscopy three types of cells could be differentiated:
elongated cells, containing microfilaments and microtubules;
roundish cells with dense bodies and filapodia, enclosing PTFE
material; and cells with endoplasmatic reticulum surrounded by
collagen fibres (Figure 6).

CONCLUSIONS

Morphological studies of experimentally implanted expanded PTFE
vascular grafts had previously been carried out systematically only
on short interpositions, showing a high patency rate and total
endothelization of the luminal surface (Matsumoto & Hasegawa, 1973;
Florian et al., 1976). In our investigations with iliaco-femoral

bypasses crossing the hip joint in dogs, after nine months nearly all
the prostheses, including the kinked areas, were covered by neointima.
There was thrombosis leading to stenosis, directly before and behind
the kinked area, probably caused by turbulence. At both anastomoses
endothelium growth was orientated and seemed quiescent. In the
middle of the prostheses the direction of endothelial cells was not
orderly. These cells were often overlapped possibly because they
were migrating. In the pores of the prosthesis wall we found cells
with the characteristics of muscle cells, in part containing microtubules. A sign of cellular reaction to the PTFE, which is commonly
regarded as an inert material, was the presence of lysosomes in
some cells.

In conclusion, in our experimental studies in dogs, the expanded
PTFE vascular graft seems to be a satisfactory heterologous transplant
material for small caliber artery substitute, although there is a
luminal loss by neointimal hyperplasia, and thrombosis at the pre and
postkinked areas. These events may reduce the prognosis of long-
term patency in reconstructions crossing joints.

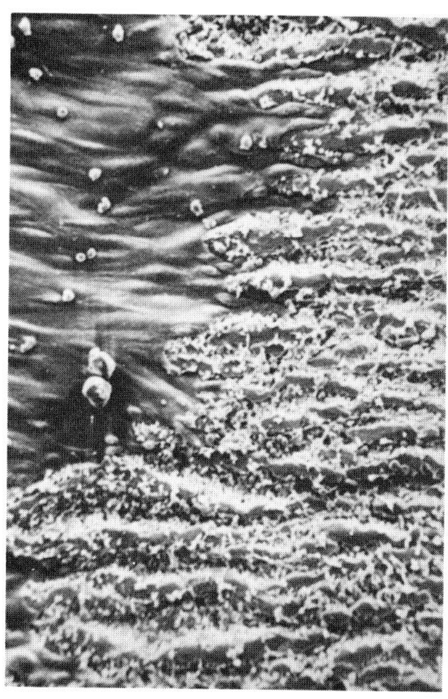

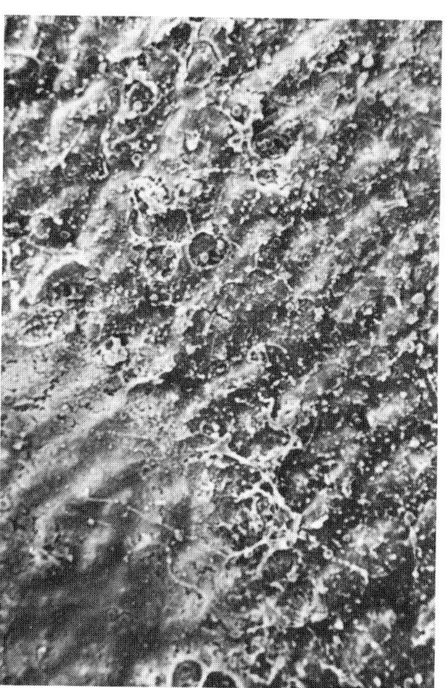

Figure 1.   Endothelial cells
protruding into the expanded
PTFE graft near the anastomosis,
one month after implantation.
Endothelium left, PTFE right.
SEM x 300

Figure 2.   Kinked area is
covered by smooth fibrin
layer one month after
implantation. SEM x 300

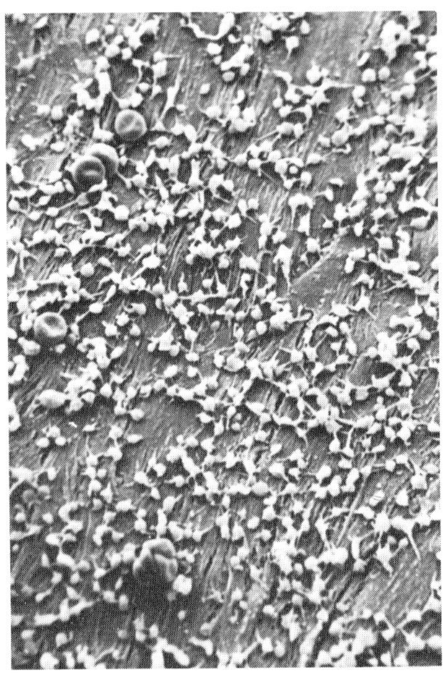

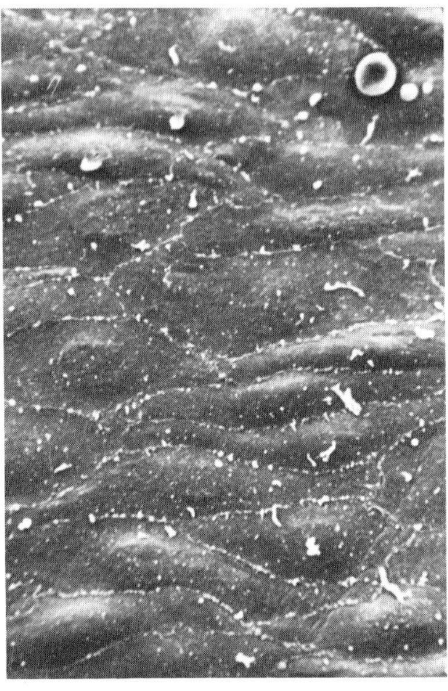

Figure 3. Surface lining cell island at the kinked area three months after implantation. Numerous thrombocytes can be seen. SEM x 1000

Figure 4. Flattened endothelial cells with microvilli and cement lines near anastomosis six months after implantation. SEM x 1000

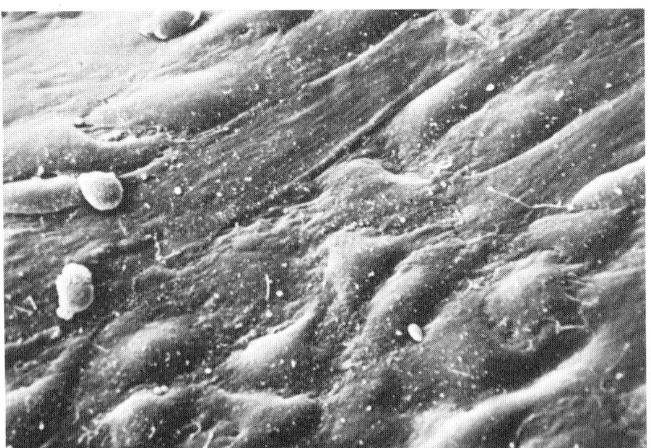

Figure 5. Unstable endothelial cells at kinked area after nine months. Cells overlap and seem to migrate. No cement lines. SEM x 1000

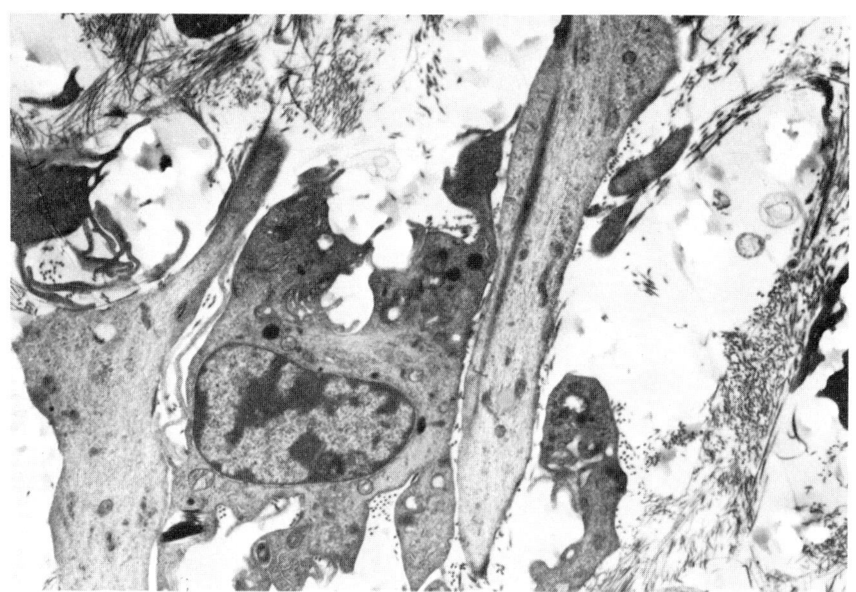

Figure 6. Cells within the wall of the prosthesis.
Note elongated cell with microfilaments and microtubules on the right; in the middle a roundish cell
with dense bodies and long filapodia; at the left
two cells with endoplasmic reticulum, surrounded by
collagen fibres. PTFE material can be seen as white
and grey amorphous areas. TEM x 10200

REFERENCES

Campbell, C.D., Brooks, D.H., Webster, M.W., Diamond, D.L., Peel,
R.L. & Bahnson, H.T. (1979) Expanded microporous polytetrafluoro-
ethylene as a vascular substitute: A two year follow up. Surgery,
85, 177-183.
Florian, A., Cohn, L.H., Dammin, G.J. & Collins, J.J. (1976) Small
vessel replacement with Gore-tex (expanded polytetrafluoroethylene).
Arch. Surg., 111, 267-270.
Hastings, O.M., Jain, K.M., Hobson, R.W. & Swan, K.G. (1978) A
prospective randomized study of three expanded polytetrafluoroethylene
(PTFE) grafts as a small arterial substitute. Ann.Surg.,188,743-747.
Matsumoto, H. & Hasegawa, T. (1973) A new vascular prosthesis for
a small caliber artery. Surgery, 74, 519-523.
Soyer, T., Lempinen, M., Cooper, P., Norton, L. & Eiseman, B. (1972)
A new venous prosthesis. Surgery, 72, 864-872.
Veith, F.J., Moss, C.M., Fell, S.C., Rhodes, B. & Haimovici, H.
(1978) Comparison of expanded PTFE and vein grafts in lower
extremity arterial reconstructions. J. Cardiovasc. Surg.,19,341-344.

Biomaterials 1980
Edited by G. D. Winter, D. F. Gibbons, and H. Plenk, Jr.
© 1982 John Wiley and Sons Ltd.

HEALING CHARACTERISTICS OF POLYETHYLENE TEREPHTHALATE VASCULAR PROSTHESES IN DOGS AS REPLACEMENT FOR THE THORACIC AORTA

R. Guidoin, P. Blais[*], L. Martin, M. Marois,
C. Gosselin, H.P. Noel, M. King and
F. Laroche

Laboratoire de Chirurgie expérimentale,
Département de Chirurgie,
Université Laval, Québec, G1K 7P4, Canada.
*Bureau of Medical Device, National
Health and Welfare, Ottawa, K1A OL2, Canada.

SUMMARY

Using canine models, a representative selection of polyethylene terephthalate (PET) vascular prostheses including woven, knitted and velour types, were evaluated for
their healing characteristics. After post-implantation
residency periods ranging from four hours to six months
at the thoracic aorta site, the grafts were excized for
pathological examination. Kidneys were also removed and
examined for trapped circulating emboli. Specimen of
prostheses and tissue were investigated using techniques
of scanning electron microscopy, light microscopy and
surface analysis. The extent of "healing", the presence
of embolizing nuclei, thrombogenicity and morphology of
the lumen wall, were assessed. Healing characteristics
of each type of devices proved similar. Velours showed
better tissue encapsulation but the internal capsule
failed to encompass all fibres. In all cases, cellular
development on the lumen was limited to areas contiguous
to the anastomosis lines. The initial water permeability
of the devices did not appear to influence healing to a
significant extent. Selection criteria and figures-of-
merit for these devices are discussed.

INTRODUCTION

Fabric cardiovascular prostheses have been in routine
clinical use for nearly two decades. Numerous types of
fabric materials, textile configurations and prostheses
designs have been developed and implanted and surgical
technics have evolved concurrently. Today, considerable
variety remains; although most devices make use of Dacron
(polyethylene terephthalate) yarn, there is no general
agreement regarding the optimum fabric characteristics

(Callow 1978). Previous works from many laboratories
have attempted to identify, evaluate and quantify the
clinical merit, the healing rate and the inherent risks
of some of these devices (Kim et al 1979, Reichle 1978,
Sawyer et al 1979). However there has been limited
activity aimed at comparing in-vivo performance in the
many currently used prostheses under standardized
conditions.

In the present work, the healing rate and the thrombogenic
character of selected prostheses were evaluated under
controlled conditions using canine models. Devices made
of woven, knitted and velour fabrics were implanted for
periods of up to six months as replacement segments for
the aorta in 86 dogs. The properties of the neoendothelium, the occurrence of embolizing nuclei, the dimensional stability of prostheses and the healing characteristics of the prosthesis-aorta interface were examined
after sacrifice of the animals.

MATERIALS AND METHODS

Prostheses. Commercial PET grafts of various fabric configurations measuring 8 to 10 mm in diameter were selected. They were autoclaved at 125°C under 33 p.s.i. for
20 minutes. These devices and their mechanical characteristics are given in Table I.

TABLE I. Prostheses Characteristics

Nomenclature	Fabric Class	Water Permeability $ml/cm^2/min.$	Bursting Strength kg/cm^2	Stitch N/cm^2
Woven de Bakey	Woven heavy wall	350	50.0	–
Knitted "	Weft knit h.wall	2530	30.9	680
Weavenit	Warp knit lt wt	2920	15.3	860
Millknit	Weft knit lt wt*	5300	19.3	910
Vasculour "D"	Internal velour	2250	17.6	520
Sauvage	External velour	3420	17.3	670
Lopor	External velour	3000	16.7	650
Microvel	Double velour	2400	11.2	550
Rhodergon	Internal velour	5790	20.2	700

*Reversed weft knit

Surgery. Healthy adult mongrel dogs (86 animals) weighing
20-30 kg each were selected. Surgical protocol included:
pre-operative fasting (24 hours), anaesthesia with sodium
pentobarbital (30 mg/kg), body temperature maintained at
37-38°C, mechanical ventilation, supplemental anaesthesia
with Fluothane, heparin anticoagulation (0.5 mg/kg). The
surgery consisted of: a left lateral thoracotomy (5th

intercostal space), a bypass blood shunt from the left
carotid artery to the right femoral artery, removal of
a one centimeter segment of thoracic aorta between two de
Bakey clamps and substitution of a preclotted 8 cm long
fabric graft using Prolene 5-0 monofilament suture for a
classical end-to-end anastomosis. Gentamycin antibiotic
was administered during the post-operative period.
Angiographies (Renograffin contrast medium) were obtained
for selected animals.

Specimen analysis. Specimen were collected after anaesthesia and anticoagulation (sodium pentobarbital,
heparin); complete grafts were removed and separated into
portions a) for light microscopy (Bouin's solution
fixation) and staining for histo-pathology (Weigart's
stain and hematoxylin, eosin and saffron). Kidneys were
also collected and fixed in 10% aqueous formalin prior
to conventional processing; b) for scanning electron
microscopy, fixation in a 2% solution of glutaraldehyde,
dehydration in graded ethanol - water and critical point
drying from CO_2, gold-palladium coated samples were examined using a Cambridge S-600 electron microscope; c)
for surface thrombogenicity segments of explanted prostheses were cut and flattened to planar surfaces of about
1 cm square using the technique of (Yates et al 1973, as
modified by Roon et al 1977). The procedure compares the
coagulation time of blood on the sample and on a reference
surface (inner wall of the animal's aorta). A coagulation
time which is close to the reference indicates a fully
hemocompatible surface; much more rapid coagulation
indicates a lack of hemocompatibility.

RESULTS

Implantations. Grafts were implanted in 86 dogs; nine
died and were excluded from this study. The 77 survivors
were separated into groups scheduled for sacrifice at
4 hours, 24 hours, 48 hours, 1 week, 2 weeks, 1 month,
2 months and 6 months.

Angiographies. Except for the heavy walled woven grafts
and the Rhodergon device all grafts were observed to
mildly expand diametrally after implantation.

Surface thrombogenicity. Variations in the thrombogenicity behavior of the graft inner wall were found. These
showed that highly thrombogenic surfaces dominate in
grafts with residence time of less than a week. Thrombogenicity diminishes rapidly during the first month and
approaches a plateau after two months. All fabric grafts
have a similar behavior.

<u>Graft healing sequence</u>. All grafts acquire a large amount
of red surface thrombi consisting of a disorganized mass
of leucocytes, platelets red cells and fibrin; this
remain for as much as 24 to 48 hours post-operative.
After one week, much of the thrombus deposit has densi-
fied to a thinner and more coherent fibrin mat in contact
with the fabric and an overlay of new thrombi can be
seen. After two weeks, cellular development becomes
evident; thin cell clusters radiate from the natural
blood vessel stumps into the prosthesis segment. After
one month, the whole lumen surface has a glistering appearance and the fibrin mat is very compact. Thrombi-
coated areas are now rare and cells resembling fibroblasts extend 2-5 mm from the anastomosis line into the
prosthesis. The appearance of the wall does not change
perceptibly after that although isolated patches of cells
are sometimes found in hydrodynamically quiescent areas
downstream from the anastomoses. On average, velour
devices take somewhat longer to produce dense fibrin
substrates. On the other hand, they are often strongly
encapsulated externally and the thickness of the neo-
formed inner capsule which embeds the fibres is much
greater than woven prostheses. Velours also show a propensity for leaving fibres and loops as "cilia" which
project above the dense surface. The anastomoses often
abound with such appendages which are probably caused by
tweezers or forceps used to aid suturing. These observations are in accord with previously described phenomena
which occur during the healing sequence of some fabric
prostheses (Stewart et al 1975, 1977). Examples of explanted prostheses with typical surfaces are shown in
Figure 1, 2 and 3.

<u>Kidney pathology</u>. Samples of kidney tissue were syste-
matically searched for evidence of infarcts which would
have arisen as a consequence of circulating microemboli.
Very few were found thus suggesting that relatively short
graft aorta segments are not significant factors in
inducing late kidney damage through infarcts when implanted according to this protocol.

DISCUSSION

The canine model appears as a satisfactory compromise
for prosthetic cardiovascular work; it permits the
evaluation of relative performance in devices if reasonable care is taken to select the animals for health and
size uniformity and to standardize the surgical conditions. However absolute performance under clinical conditions cannot be assessed reliably from such experiments; this is primarily a consequence of species-related

hematologic and healing differences (Bruck 1977). Furthermore, healthy animals do not compare well with diseased patients; in particular those with arteriosclerosis and diabetes mellitus. Such patients form the principal pool of candidates for reconstructive cardiovascular surgery.

The thoracic site may be the least critical zone for the
evaluation of grafts; the hemodynamics at 1000-2000
ml/min of blood flow are nearly ideal. The surgery,
however is more complex. The abdominal aorta is of simpler access but the blood flow rate is much less (200-400
ml/min) and only a small specimen can be accomodated.
This precludes many useful types of experiments such as
studies on mechanical properties. It is however, sufficient for healing and biocompatibility assessment.

Healing characteristics and intrinsic device thrombogenicity do not appear to vary significantly amongst the
various types of studied prostheses. Therefore, it
appears that fabric configuration and perhaps even fibre
material are not important factors in enhancing healing
and endothelialization.

It appears that cellular activity depends partly on the
existence of a dense, well organized, fibrin and/or other
protein surface. Thick "pile" fabrics such as velours do
not appear well suited for the rapid development of such
surfaces and could be at a disadvantage. The nature of
these cells, their mechanism of development and the exact
composition of their substrate are not known and are the
object of ongoing work in several laboratories. Other
than being a diagnostic of active healing processes, their
contribution to the performance of the graft is not agreed
upon; even after six months, the population of such cells
would not seem sufficient to affect the mechanical properties or the thromboresistance of the prosthesis.

Water permeability of the unused fabric, a parameter which
was given considerable attention in the early literature
(Wesolowski et al 1961, Harrison and Davalos 1961) and is
still regarded as significant, does not emerge as
a very useful criterion of performance with respect to the
development and the stability of the neoendothelium.

Pre-operative heparinization may de-emphasize the impact
of differences in surface thrombogenicity between the
different devices at implantation and may further mask
the early in-vivo behavior differences of such prostheses
or the response of the patient towards the new implant.
Heparinization has a considerable clinical merit; it
greatly reduces the occurence of early embolization
(Topping et al 1980).

The most notewortly difference in the healing characteristics of the diverse styles of fabric is the thickness
of the internal and external capsules which are very thin
for woven fabrics, moderate for knits and greatest for
velours; such a tissue encapsulation, in spite of its
thickness, also frequently fails to encapsulate all of
the fibres. It is thus suggested that thick "pile"
fabric surfaces do not contribute towards enhancing the
healing characteristics of fabric prostheses and may
contribute to the prolonged thrombogenicity of velours.

At this juncture, it is increasingly probable that the
fabric device is little more that an indifferent "exos-
kelton and/or reinforcement casing" for a tissue matrix
which eventually insulates the fundamentally hemo-incom-
patible fibres from the patient. However, the biocompatibility characteristics of the new blood contact surface
always seems inferior to native blood vessels.

ACKNOWLEDGEMENTS

We are indebted for technical assistance to J. Bastien,
S. Bourassa, G. Côté, D. Lafrenière-Gagnon and G.
Mongrain. We also wish to thank USCI, Meadox Medicals,
Golaski and Hospal for providing prostheses, Ethicon for
sutures and Schering for antibiotics. The guidance of
Drs G. Roy and L. Levasseur is also acknowledged. This
work was supported in part by grants from the Quebec
Heart Foundation and the Department of National Health
and Welfare, Canada.

REFERENCES

Bruck, S.D., (1977) Considerations of species-related
hematological differences on the evaluation of biomaterials. Biomat. Med. Dev. Art. Org 5, 97-113.

Callow, A.D., (1978) "Historical development of vascular
grafts" in Vascular Grafts ed. Sawyer P.N. and Kaplitt
M.J., Appleton Century-Crofts. New York. pp 5-22.

Harrison, J.H. and Davalos, P.A., (1961) Influence of porosity on synthetic grafts. Arch. Surg., 82, 8-13.

Kim, G.-E., Imparato, M.A., Nathan, I. et al (1979);
Dilation of synthetic grafts and junctional aneurisms.
Arch. Surg. 114, 1296-1303.

Reichle, F.A. (1978); Criteria for evaluation of new arterial prostheses by comparing vein with Dacron femoro-
popliteal bypasses; Surg. Gyn. Obst. 16, 714-720.

Roon, A.J., Moore, W.S., Goldstone, J. et al (1977);
Comparative surface thrombogenicity of implanted vascular grafts. J. Surg. Res. 22, 165-173.

Sawyer, P.N., Stanczewski, B., Hoskin, G.P. et al (1979);
In-vitro and in-vivo evaluation of Dacron velour and
knit prostheses. J. Biomed. Mat. Res. 13, 937-956.

Stewart, G.G., Essa, N., Chang, K.H.Y., Reichle, F.A.
(1975); A scanning and transmission electron microscope
study of the luminal coating on Dacron prostheses in the
canine thoracic aorta. J. Lab. Clin. Med. 85, 208-266.

Stewart, G.G., Lynch, P.R., Reichle, F.A. et al (1977);
The adhesion of leucocytes, erythrocytes and non-cellular
material to the lumen of surface of natural and artificial blood vessels in-vivo. Ann. N.Y. Acad. Sc., 283,
179-207.

Topping C., Guidoin R., Roy J. et al (1980); La précoa-
gulation des prothèses en Dacron tissé. J. Chirurgie
117, (in press).

Wesolowski S.A., Fries C.C., Karlson K.E. et al (1961);
Porosity, the primary determinant of ultimate fate of
synthetic vascular grafts. Surg. 50, 91-96.

Yates S.Q., Nakagawa Y., Berger K. et al (1973); Surface
thrombogenicity of arterial prostheses. Surg. Gyn. Obst.
136, 12-16.

DISCLAIMER

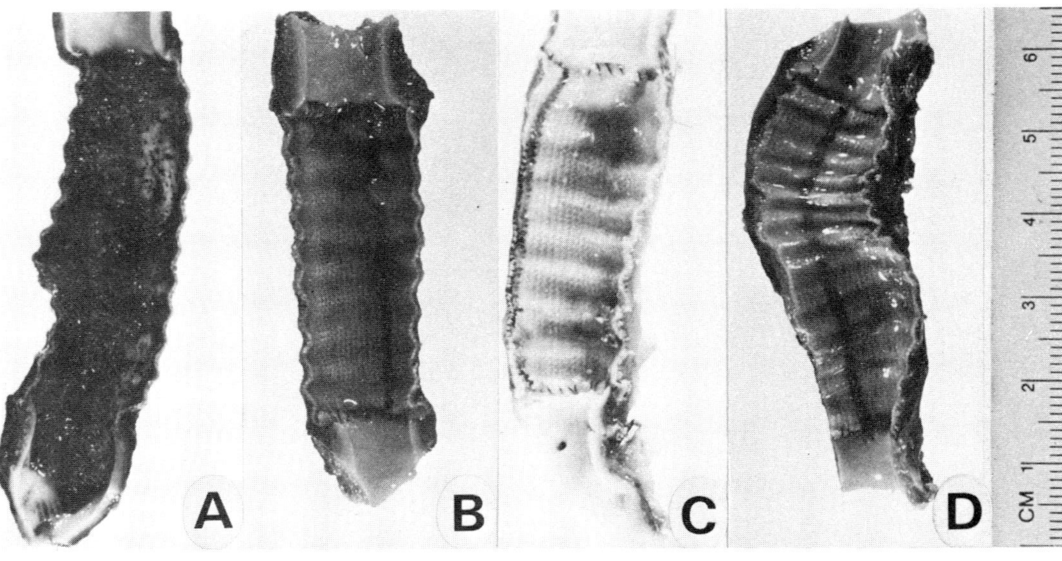

Figure 1. General view of explanted prostheses with attached aorta stumps after longitudinal slitting; postimplantation A) 4 hours B) 48 hours C) 1 month D) 6 months; note extensive blood deposits on the early explant and gradually thickening external tissue capsule during the healing process.

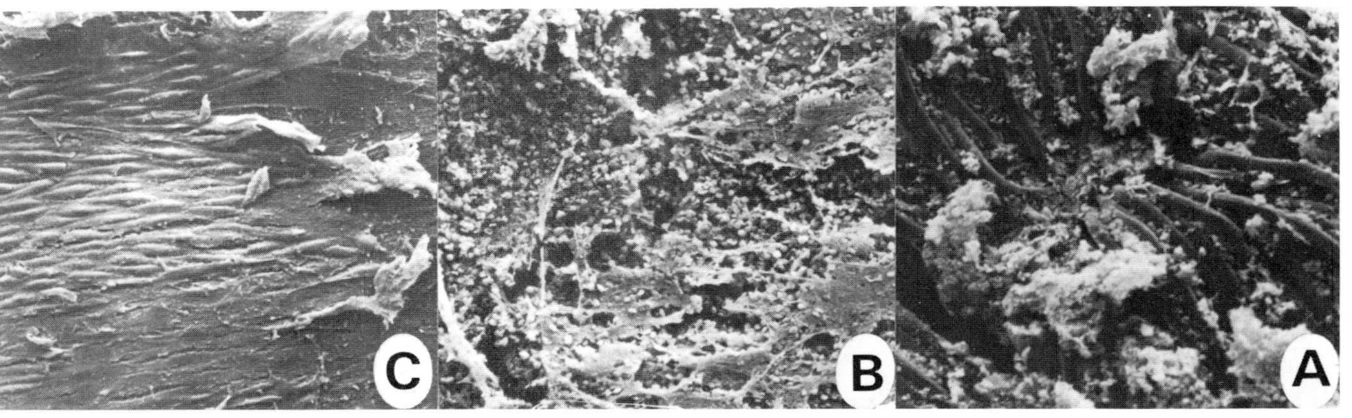

Figure 2. Typical wall surface of lumen of knitted prostheses at sites contiguous to the proximal anastomoses;postimplantation A) 48 hours; x 200, B) 1 week; x 100, C) 2 months; x 200; note gradually developing neo-endothelium which eventually covers all fibres; cells are limited to vicinity of anastomosis.

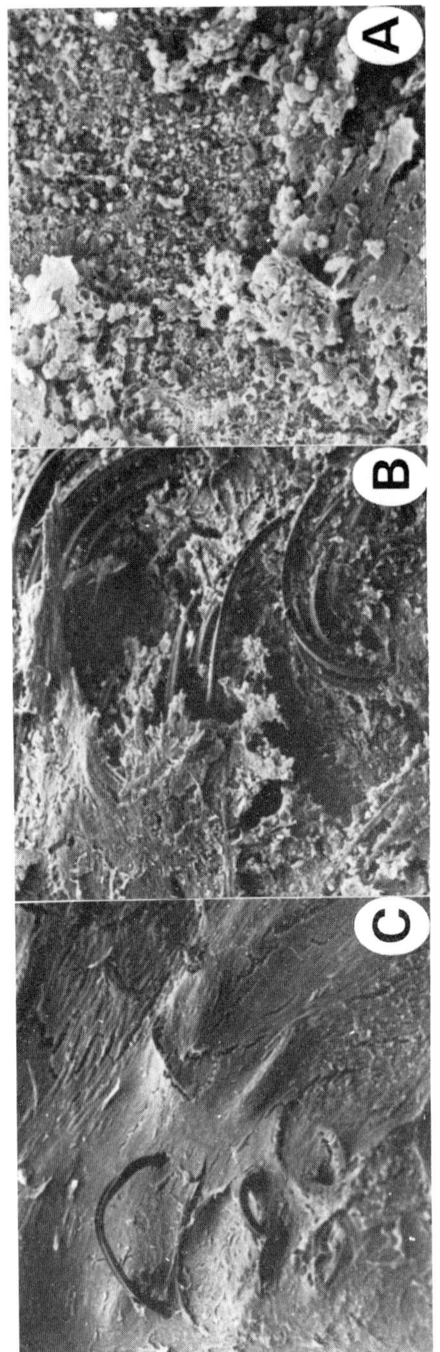

Figure 3. Typical wall surface of lumen of velour prostheses at sites contiguous to proximal anastomoses; postimplantation A) 24 hours; x 500, B) 1 week; x 100, C) 6 months; x 100; note protruding loops of Dacron in spite of the well developed tissue surface.

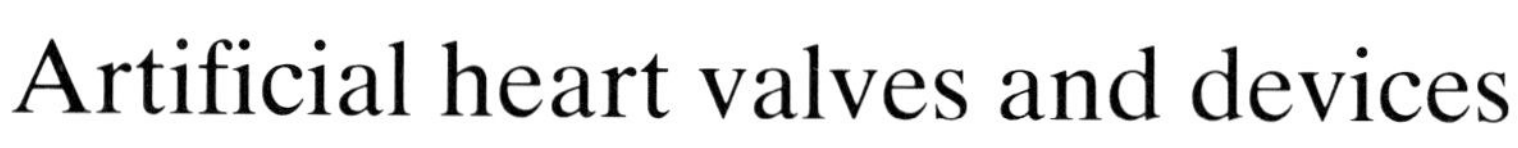

Artificial heart valves and devices

Biomaterials 1980
Edited by G. D. Winter, D. F. Gibbons, and H. Plenk, Jr.
© 1982 John Wiley and Sons Ltd.

STRUCTURE AND HISTOLOGICAL VARIABILITY OF PORCINE AORTIC VALVES

M. Galloni*, V. Ceccarelli** and V. Tavormina***

*   Istituto di Patologia Generale ed Anatomia
    Patologica Veterinaria, Università di Torino,
    Italy

** SORIN Biomedica, Reparto Chirurgia Sperimentale,
   Saluggia (VC), Italy

***Cattedra di Cardiochirurgia, Facoltà di Medicina
   e Chirurgia, Università di Torino, Italy

<u>SUMMARY</u>

Semilunar aortic valves drawn from 50 healthy pigs were
conditioned as used for valvular bioprosthesis preparation.
The samples were observed in a non-destructive way with
a stereoscopic microscope in transmitted polarizing light
and then they were prepared for optical microscopy and
for scanning electron microscopy. It was possible to
discover various alterations in the valves such as
inflammations, fibrous bundles irregularities, parasitic
protozoa and atherosclerosis in the coronary arteries.
Some of these alterations can be seen only with
destructive methods and as all of them may become weak
points in an eventual bioprosthesis, it is suggested to
prevent such lesions with a great sanitary care in
breeding the pigs whose aortic valves must be used for
bioprostheses.

<u>INTRODUCTION</u>

The porcine valvular bioprostheses are known to be very
good devices in cardiosurgery, their advantages are
recognized and their long term reliability is proved.
Failures that have occurred are of acceptable frequency
and can be attributed either to external factors, namely
the action of the host organism that can cause various
types of functional alterations, or to possible manufacture

defects or to endogenous causes connected with specific
histological defects in the animal tissue.
The aim of this research is to verify if, by normal
veterinary inspection and using common laboratory methods,
it is possible to evaluate the characteristics of the
valve tissue before its utilization. We also tried to
clarify whether, among the valves considered normal after
macroscopic examination, which necessarily must be non
destructive, there are some with alterations that can be
observed only at high magnification in the microscope.
The initial research by our group (Galloni & Ceccarelli,
1979) revealed some alterations of the valvular
endothelium consisting in small areas of erosion and
areas with abnormal surface characteristics. Later
Gobetto et al. (1979) observed some macro- and
microscopical anatomical aspects of aortic valves taken
from pigs from the moment of the birth to the age of one
year. The present work concerns the examination of 50
porcine aortic valves from one year old pigs found
healthy at clinical inspection before slaughter and at
autopsy.

METHODS

The valves were treated according the method described
for bioprosthesis preparation (Carpentier et al., 1969).
Aortic valves were taken from pigs' hearts immediately
after slaughter and kept in Hanks solution for 24hr.
Then the valves were fixed for 48 hr in a solution of
0.6% glutaraldehyde in phosphate buffer 0.1 M pH 7.3.
After the conditioning treatment the valves were
observed with a stereomicroscope in transmitted
polarizing light. Samples from each valve were prepared
for optical microscopy and for scanning electron
microscopy (SEM). For the first technique, the samples
were embedded in paraffin and sections, 5 micron thick,
were stained with hematoxilin-eosin and Weigert-
Van Gieson. For SEM the samples were fixed in 3%
glutaraldehyde in phosphate buffer 0.1 M pH 7.3, then
they were dehydrated in a graded alcohol series,
critical point dried in liquid CO_2 and sputter coated
with gold.

RESULTS

Stereomicroscopy enabled us to visualize some
characteristics of the connective tissue in the leaflets.
We observed fibrous bundles with circumferential
orientation which originate at the annulus and
progressively separate in a plexiform way towards the
center. In consequence the central area of the leaflet
has a comparatively more homogeneous structure. The
Aranzio nodule is situated in this zone, in the middle
of the free edge. The nodule consists of fibrous
connective tissue and is a strengthening element placed
in a maximal stress point. The central closure of the
lumen at the aortic root is brought about by the
juxtaposition of the three nodules.
Histological observations with the transmitted light
microscope of stained thin sections revealed that the
fibrous bundles described above are arranged in
protruding folds made by thickenings of the dense
connective tissue layer near the parietal (aortic or
outflow) surface. It was possible to see, on the
parietal side, under the endothelium, folds of smaller
dimensions containing a thin layer of loose connective
tissue. Probably these folds can be seen only when the
leaflet is not fully stressed. Ferrans et al. (1978)
and De Biasi & Pilotto (1979) suggested that these folds
had an important function in securing the elastic
extensibility of the parietal endothelium at the moment
of maximal tension.
In about 7.5% of the valves examined histologically there
were signs of inflammation in the leaflets, mostly near
the annulus. Inflammatory foci originate near the small
blood vessels in the annulus and can spread into inner
areas of the leaflet with infiltration of lymphocytes,
plasma cells and monocytes in the connective tissue.
In two cases parasitic protozoa were discovered in the
subendothelial connective tissue layer. They are round
formations of an amorphous and eosinophilic material,
surrounded by an unstainable capsule. There was no
discernable tissue reaction around the capsule. Probably
the parasites were already dead and were degenerating.
In the 10% of the pigs early atherosclerosis in the
coronary arteries was observed. The signs were

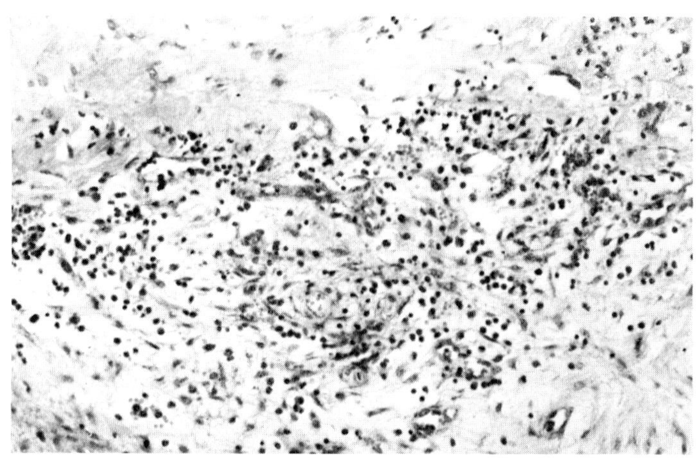

Fig. 1. Inflammatory focus in the annulus of a
porcine aortic valve. Various types of
infiltrating cells can be seen.
(H.E., medium magnification).

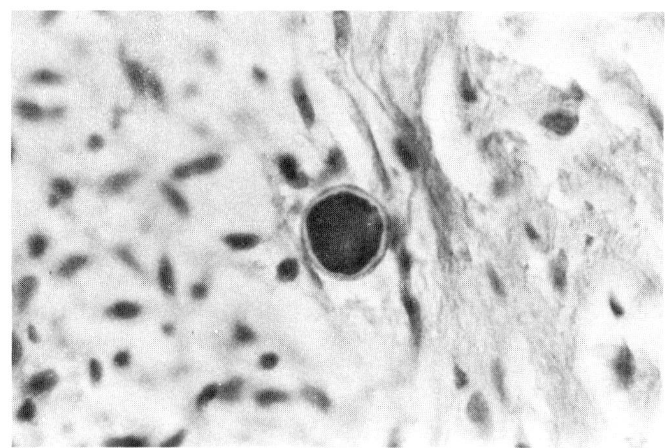

Fig. 2. Parasitic protozoan in the subendothelial
connective layer of a valvular leaflet.
(H.E., high magnification)

thickening of the arterial intima caused by lipid
deposition and an increase of connective fibres. Getty
(1965) described atherosclerosis in the aorta of hogs
less than one year of age in animals fed a normal,
controlled diet. Such phenomena are of great
significance in judging the health of the pig's whole
cardiovascular system, because of the consequences of
atherosclerosis.
The SEM allows a clear visualization of many particulars
of the surface and of inner structures of the leaflets.
On the parietal surface circumferential folds of various
sizes can be seen, covered by a continuous layer of
endothelial cells with dome-shaped bulging nuclei.
The axial surface endothelium is rather smooth and has
no folds. Observation of the internal morphology is
possible if cut leaflets are examined. The leaflet are
seen to be constructed from individual connective tissue
layers superimposed upon one another.

DISCUSSION

Selection of porcine aortic valves to be used for
bioprosthesis manufacture must be carried out with non-
destructive methods which preclude accurate histological
observations. We think that stereomicroscopy with
transmitted polarizing light may be very useful for an
easy, low magnification survey. Without causing any
damage, this method allows a good observation of the
fibrous bundles in the cusps and, increasing the image
contrast, it also permits to distinctly see some fine
characteristics of the valvular stroma and surface.
The fibrous bundles, which have strong connections to the
annulus and which divide in a close net of branches in
the center of the valvular leaflet, show, in some cases,
irregularities or small side indentations that could be
the initial causes of similar, but larger and more serious
lesions seen in long term implanted porcine valvular
bioprostheses (Guarda et al., 1980). The myocardial
septal shelf in the right coronary leaflet has variable
dimensions and should be carefully evaluated.
With the stereomicroscope it is also possible to
recognise inflammatory foci that we clearly observed in
histological sections. The most common causes of serious

endocarditis and valvulitis in one year old pigs are swine
erysipelas, septicemic streptococcosis and hog cholera.
The use of attenuated virus vaccines, for instance against
hog cholera, may bring about such undesired consequences
(Dunne & Leman, 1965). The atherosclerotic phenomena
noted in this investigation were probably caused by errors
in diet and in breeding conditions.
The number of abnormalities seen in these 50 animals is
such as to justify some doubts on the reliability of those
valves for making bioprostheses. Perhaps some of those
lesions might become weak points in an eventual
bioprosthesis and could promote malfunctionings. Our
opinion is that the pigs, the aortic valves of which must
be used for bioprostheses, should be bred in the best
environmental situations, should be fed with a carefully
balanced and hypolipic diet, should not be vaccinated
with attenuated virus vaccines and should be kept under
a close sanitary control, preferably in germ-free
conditions.

ACKNOWLEDGMENTS

The autors thank Prof. C. Benvenuti, director of the
Istituto di Anatomia e Istologia degli animali domestici,
University of Pisa, for his collaboration.

REFERENCES

Carpentier, A., Lemaigre, G., Robert, L., Carpentier, S.
& Dubost, C. (1969) Biological factors affecting long
term results of valvular heterografts. J. Thorac.
Cardiovasc. Surg., 58, 467-479
De Biasi, S. & Pilotto, F. (1979) The ultrastructure of
the leaflets of porcine aortic valves conditioned for
heterografts in man. J. Submicr. Cytol., 11, 353-364
Dunne, H.W. & Leman, A.D. (1975) Diseases of swine. fourth
ed., Iowa State Univ. Press, Ames, Iowa, USA
Ferrans, V.J., Spray, T.L., Billingham, M.E. & Roberts,
W.C. (1978) Structural changes in glutaraldehyde-treated
porcine heterografts used as substitute cardiac valves.
Am. J. Cardiol., 41, 1159-1184
Galloni, M. & Ceccarelli, V. (1979) Osservazioni in
microscopia ottica ed elettronica a scansione di valvole
semilunari aortiche porcine. Schweiz. Arch. Tierheilk.,

121, 485-491
Getty, R. (1965) The gross and microscopic occurrence
and distribution of spontaneous atherosclerosis in the
arteries of swine. in Comparative atherosclerosis
(Eds. J.C. Roberts & R. Straus), pp 11-20, Hober Medical
Division, N.Y.
Gobetto, A., Benvenuti, C., Galloni, M., Gurda, F.,
Tavormina, V. & Ceccarelli,V. (1979) Valvole semilunari
aortiche di suino e bioprotesi valvolari nell'uomo.
Modificazioni morfologiche a seconda dell'età e
variabilità della struttura istologica. Ann. Fac. Med.
Vet. Torino, 26, 50-69
Guarda, F., Morea, M., Tavormina, V., Galloni, M.,
Gobetto, A., Benvenuti, C., Ceccarelli, V., Di Summa, M.
& Casaccia, M. (1980) Valvole semilunari aortiche di suino
e bioprotesi valvolari nell'uomo. Alterazioni morfologiche
di protesi impiantate per periodi variabili nell'uomo.
Schweiz. Arch. Tierheilk., 122, 217-226

Biomaterials 1980
Edited by G. D. Winter, D. F. Gibbons, and H. Plenk, Jr.
© 1982 John Wiley and Sons Ltd.

EVALUATION OF THE MECHANICAL PROPERTIES OF STENTLESS CAR-
DIAC VALVES CONSTRUCTED FROM GLYCEROL TREATED AUTOLOGOUS
PERICARDIUM.

C. Pillot, R. Millner and G. Dureau.

Unit 37 - INSERM - Cardiovascular surgery and organ
transplantation laboratory.
18 avenue du Doyen Lépine - 69500 Bron - France.
and
I.N.S.A. Villeurbanne - France.

SUMMARY

Study of the static and dynamic properties of glycerol treated pericardium implanted in the tricuspid valve position in 7 dogs is reported
up to 28 days. Initial values for the pericardium which decreased during the first two or three days after implantation were subsequently
regained and even exceeded.

INTRODUCTION

Fresh non treated autologous pericardium when used as a cardiac valve
substitute undergoes rapid destruction due to strong inflammatory reaction (Dureau, 1978). Therefore a pretreatment of the autologous tissue is necessary : the inflammatory response of the implant is to be
suppressed. This report describes the effect of concentrated glycerol
treatment on the mechanical properties of the pericardial implants u-
sed as cardiac valves.

MATERIALS and METHODS

This work was carried out on 6 months old puppies weighing 5 to 8 kg.
After removal of the natural tricuspid valve a two leaflet valve
(bicuspid) was sutured between right atrium and ventricle. The implantation technique and surgical procedure have been described (Dureau, 1977).
At the time of operation 4 pieces of pericardium were taken from the
pericardial sac. The largest anterior aspect of the pericardium was u-
sed avoiding the apex with its fibrous attachment and the superior region near its attachment to the great vessels. Two pieces were used to
reconstruct the dog's bicuspid valve.
Seven dogs received this bicuspid valve ; in three cases one leaflet
was used directly (controls) and the other leaflet the pericardium was
treated for five minutes in 87 % glycerol at 40°C and then rehydrated
in Ringers solution prior to use. In four cases, both leaflets were
treated. The animals were sacrificed between the Ist and 28th post-
operative day. The pericardial valves were removed and the tissue

evaluated using the same tests as for the unimplanted samples, each animal being its own control.

The mechanical properties were determined from the stress-strain curve using an ADAMEL-LHOMARGY DY 14 Tensile machine and a strain rate of 5 MM/min.
The mechanical properties were characterized by their initial Young's modulus expressed as a ratio of the implanted value to that of the unimplanted material of identical pretreatment.
Dynamic properties were measured on a Rheovibron RV II B viscoelastometer (Toyo Measurements) modified to allow measurements in a 0.9 % saline solution. Measurements for each sample were made at 4 frequencies (3.5, 11, 35 and 110 Hz) and over the temperature range 10 to 40°C.
Pericardium is a viscoelastic material (Persoz, 1969) and which can be characterized by the components of a complex modulus where :
E' is the unrelaxed modulus, E'' is the relaxed modulus and $\tan \delta$ represents the viscoelastic damping of the material. E', E'', and $\tan \delta$ vary with temperature and the frequency of the applied stress (Gross, 1969). The values of E' and $\tan \delta$ at 37°C and a frequency of 110 Hz were used to compare the samples. The samples mounted on the plastic film, which gave it a certain rigidity, was placed in the saline bath and attached to the grips. The plastic film was cut before measuring.

RESULTS

The initial effect of the glycerol treatment before implantation resulted in a decrease of the biomechanical properties as expressed by the Young's modulus. The mean values of the modulus after treatment were approximately reduced by 50 %. The viscoelastic damping was also modified by the glycerol treatment from 0.053 ± 0.002 before treatment to 0.067 ± 0.003 after glycerol treatment.
After implantation : for the untreated valve pericardium there was a rapid decrease of Young's modulus as determined from stress strain curve up to day 4. Beyond day 4 no measurement was possible because of tissue deterioration (Figure 1).
For the glycerol treated valve pericardium the Young's modulus decreased during the first 24 hours but then recovered and after 6 days reached a stable value greater than that of the initial untreated pericardium (Figure 1).

Dynamic properties. The unrelaxed modulus of the untreated and glycerol treated behaved in a manner similar to that obtained from the stress strain data (Figure 2) which is to be anticipated.
The viscoelastic damping (coefficient $\tan \delta$) showed slight fluctuation around the mean value for the glycerol treated valves. However $\tan \delta$ for the untreated samples increased to 4 times their initial value

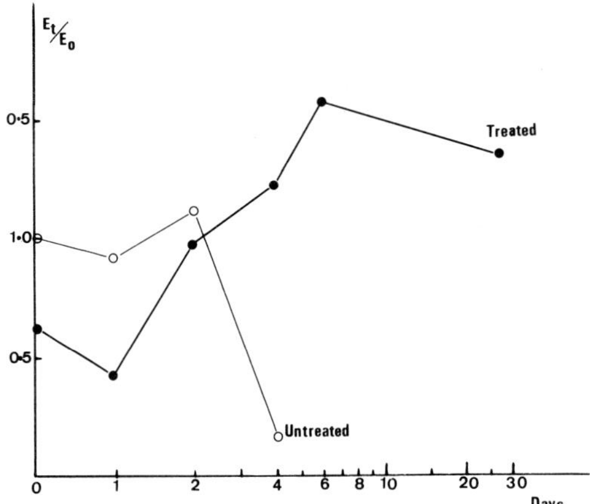

FIGURE 1. Traction tests : post-operative evolution
of the Young's modulus.

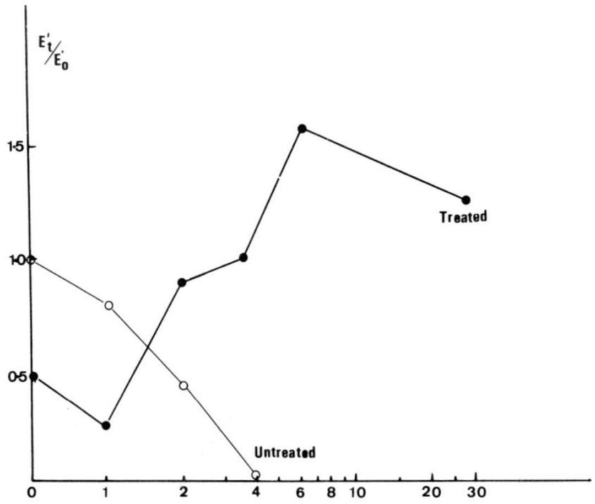

FIGURE 2. Elasticity tests : Post-operative evolution
of the unrelaxed modulus.

        C. Pillot, R. Millner and G. Dureau

by the 4th post-operative day and further measurements could not be
made because of the high damping coefficient and loss of tissue integrity (Figure 3).

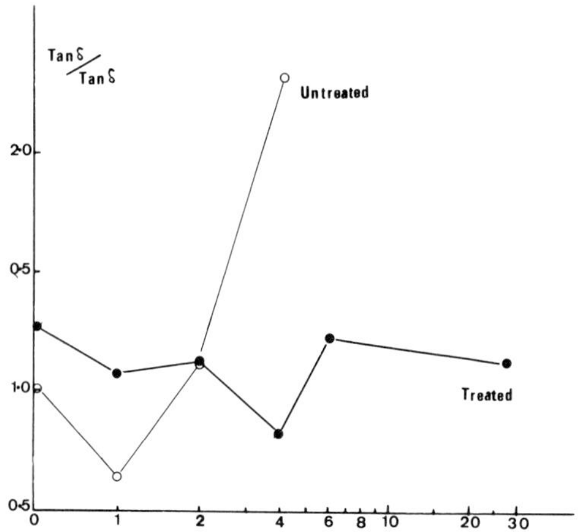

FIGURE 3. Viscoelastic damping : Post-operative evolution
of the relaxed modulus.

DISCUSSION

The biomechanical results correlate with the macroscopic and microscopic behaviour of the tissue. The rapid mechanical deterioration of the
untreated pericardium is probably due to the rapid inflammatory reaction of this tissue which confirms the pathological and clinical findings. However the relatively poor hemodynamics performance of this
valvular design in the tricuspid position must be taken into account.
Although glycerol treatment of fresh pericardium initially decreased
its mechanical properties they were regained during the next six days
and remained constant until at least 28 days. Complete degradation of
the mechanical properties occured in four days with the untreated autologous pericardium.

ACKNOWLEDGEMENT

This work was supported by Grant INSERM - CRL N° 78.5.0645 and
Institut Mérieux - Lyon - France.

REFERENCES

Dureau, G., Tabib, A. (1978) Variation de la réponse inflammatoire à
un implant autologue en fonction de sa viabilité : réponse inflamma-
toire mixte et unilatérale. C.R. Acad. Sc. Paris, 286, Série D,
1515-1518.
Dureau, G., Képénékian, G., Heynen, Y.G., Paul, J., & Belleville, J.
(1977) Development of stentless designs for biological cardiac valves.
IVth Congress of the European Society for artificial organs. London,
November.
Persoz, B. (1969) La rhéologie. Edited by Masson and Published by
Masson.
Gross, B. (1969) Mathematical structure of the theories of viscoelas-
ticity. Edited and published by E. Herman.

Biomaterials 1980
Edited by G. D. Winter, D. F. Gibbons, and H. Plenk, Jr.
© 1982 John Wiley and Sons Ltd.

DURA MATER HEART VALVES TEST:
FLOW CHARACTERISTICS AND FATIGUE LIFE DETERMINATION

P. Caminal and L. Fiz

Institut de Cibernètica,
Barcelona. Spain

SUMMARY

Several methods for _in vitro_ testing dura mater valves are described.
They include the determination of resistance to blood flow, regurgitation, mechanical properties of dura mater tissue and a fatigue life
criterium. Pressure drop and valvular incompetence level measurements
point out the good hydrodynamic characteristics of dura mater prostheses for valve replacement. In this study it is assumed that failure of a leaflet valve results from fatigue damage,and in the analysis
the Palmgren - Miner hypothesis of linear fatigue damage accumulation
is used, modified to suit a statistical analysis. The fatigue life
determination under different load conditions and with various geometric characteristics of the valves shows that a very good selection
of leaflet thickness and valve configuration is required to achieve
life times of 3.10^8 cycles (8 years at 72 bpm), assuming neither calcification nor immunological reactions are acting on the valve.

INTRODUCTION

Progress in surgical, anesthetic and postoperative care has made
possible elective cardiac valve replacement with mortality rates in
the range of five percent. However, complications (especially thromboembolism) related to the presence of mechanical prosthetic valves
or uncertainty as to the function and durability of biological valves
continue to cause surgeons and cardiologists to be cautious in re-
commending valve replacement.

The purpose of this paper is to report on _in vitro_ studies of the
prosthetic dura mater valves both made and clinically used by the
cardiac surgery service of the "Ciudad Sanitaria Francisco Franco" of
Barcelona.

The _in vitro_ test method developed considers two different parameters.
The first consists of the evaluation of the hydrodynamic performance
of dura mater valves. The second one deals with the estimation of the
mechanical durability of these valves by means of accelerated life-
tests.

METHODS

The main material of biological valves is dura mater. Preservation
and sterilization of dura mater is done in 98% glycerol and the valve is constructed by suturing 3 leaflets on a fabric-covered stent.

A ventricle and vascular system fluidic simulator has been designed
and constructed to carry out studies of longevity through variation of
the device parameters and also to make flow visualisation studies.
The pressure drop characteristics of dura mater valves is measured by
the steady flow technique (Caminal, 1980). Before developing fatigue
studies for valves the uniaxial tensile test was used to characterize
the static mechanical properties of the dura mater tissue.

The clinical history of the dura mater valve shows that fatigue has
been the prime mode of failure of prosthetic leaflet valves. In this
study it is assumed that failure of a leaflet valve results from
fatigue damage, and in the analysis the Palmgren–Miner hypothesis
(Miner, 1945) of linear fatigue damage accumulation is used, modified
to suit a statistical analysis.

From a typical set of $\underline{\text{in vivo}}$ records, it is reasonable to assume that
the net loading sustained by the valve cusp may be separated into a
periodic part with period T and a nonperiodic part. The Fourier
coefficients c_n for the periodic part can be calculated in terms of
the peak value of load (P_{max}) and period (T).

For the nonperiodic part we can assume a spectral density, with the
peaks centered about $\omega = \pm\ \Omega = 20(2\pi/T)$, a bandwith Δ and the root mean
square amplitude , a.

The loading process P(t) must be converted into the stress process
S(t).

$$S(t) = c\ P(t)$$

where c is a constant, determined   by the shell geometry, which can
be expressed as $\alpha R/h$, R and h being the valve ring radius and leaflet thickness, respectively, and α a function of the valvular meridional shape.

Following this statistical analysis of longevity for biological prosthetic valves the fatigue life (N) is obtained which is a function
of the pressure wave loading P (P_{max}, T, Ω, Δ, a), the membrane
thickness h, the valve ring radius R, the meridional shell shape fac-
tor α, and some experimentally determined constants (β, γ) which vary
with each material.

$$N = f(P_{max}, T, \Omega, a, h, R, \alpha, \beta, \gamma, \Delta)$$

The detailed analysis is published elsewhere (Caminal, 1980)

RESULTS

Experimental tests have shown that the regurgitation through the dura mater valve is of negligible hemodynamic significance. For a pressure difference of 100 mmHg, the corresponding static leak rate is 20 ml/min.

Fig. 1 shows the pressure drop characteristics for differently sized models at a steady flow of 15 l/min.

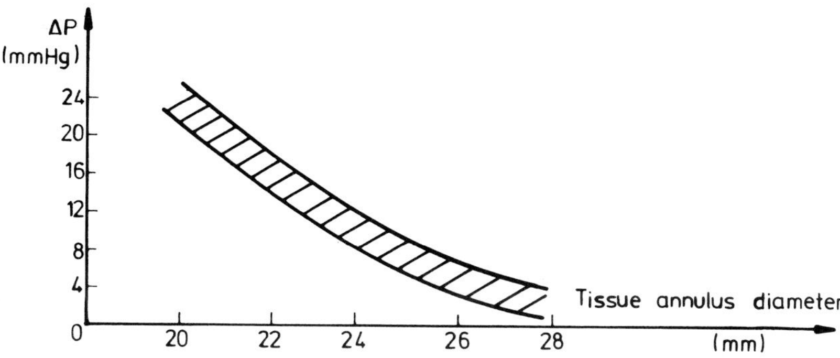

Fig.1 Steady flow pressure gradient at 15 1/min

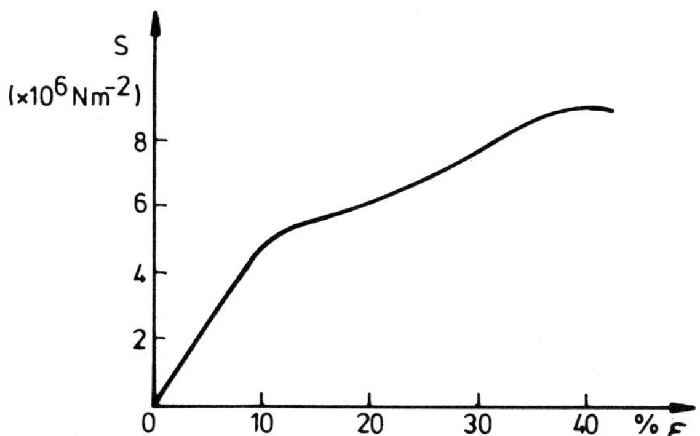

Fig.2 Stress-strain diagram

The stress–strain diagram obtained (Fig.2) by mechanical tests permits calculation of the following values: Tensile strength $8.4.10^6 \mathrm{Nm}^{-2}$; elastic limit $4.5.10^6 \mathrm{Nm}^{-2}$ and initial modulus of elasticity of the dura mater $4.5.10^7 \mathrm{Nm}^{-2}$.

The durability calculated by theoretical analysis (N_t) is

$$N_t = \beta\{\int_{So}^{\infty} S^{\gamma} \{(2\pi)^{-3/2}(\sigma_3/\sigma_1\sigma_2)(1-\alpha_\sigma^2)^{1/2}\exp\{-(S-\mu)^2(2\sigma_1^2)^{-1}(1-\alpha_\sigma^2)^{-1}\}+$$

$$+ (4\pi)^{-1}(\sigma_3/\sigma_1^2\sigma_2)\ \alpha_\sigma\ (S-\mu)\{1+g(\frac{S-\mu}{\sigma_1\sqrt{2/\alpha_\sigma^2}-2})\ \}\exp\{-(S-\mu)^2/2\sigma_1^2)\}\}dS\}^{-1}$$

where μ is the mean of $S(t) = \alpha RP(t)/h$; $\sigma_1^2, \sigma_2^2, \sigma_3^2$, are the variances of $S(t)$, $\dot{S}(t)$, $\ddot{S}(t)$, respectively; $\alpha_\sigma = \sigma_2^2/\sigma_1. \ \sigma_3$ and $g(\ )$ is the error function

The tests performed with dura mater valves at pressures from 660 to 2000 mmHg and frequencies from 60 to 120 bpm show the accuracy of the statistical analysis of longevity which is proposed to predict the lifetime of a biological valve.

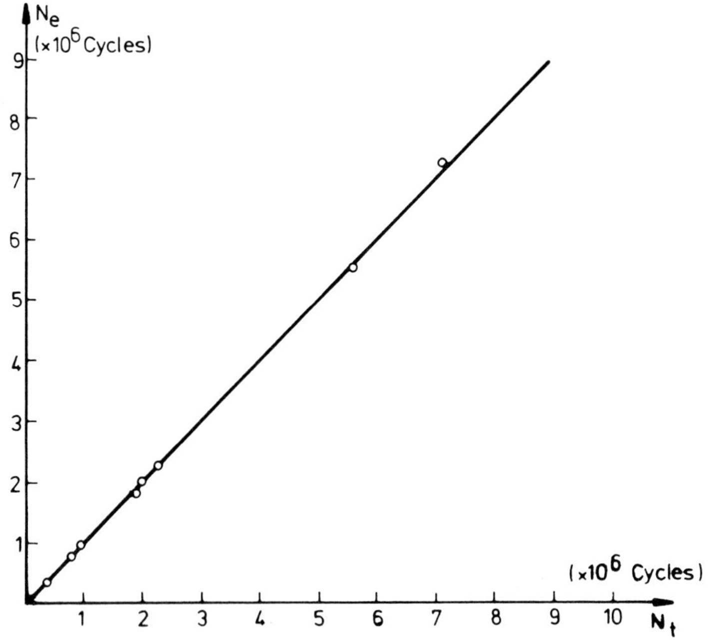

Fig. 3 Experimental versus theoretical durability

The comparison between N_t and the lifetime obtained experimentally (Ne) on the test rig is shown in Fig. 3

In studies of heart valve specimens recovered from patients,it has been found that valves failed in the _in vitro_ durability test in exactly the same manner as they did in patients.

DISCUSSION

The uniaxial tensile test shows that the static mechanical properties of dura mater tissue can be used to predict dynamic behaviour, assuming a stress process related to a pressure loading of 80-250 mmHg for physiological and pathological situations.

Measurement of dura mater valve lifetime correlates well with calculations based on statistical analysis of longevity. Given the valve size and valve leaflet thickness for a selected meridional geometry, the proposed mathematical model permits us to obtain a measure of longevity of a dura mater valve, in terms of statistical information on the pressure loading history expected across the valve after it has been implanted in a patient.

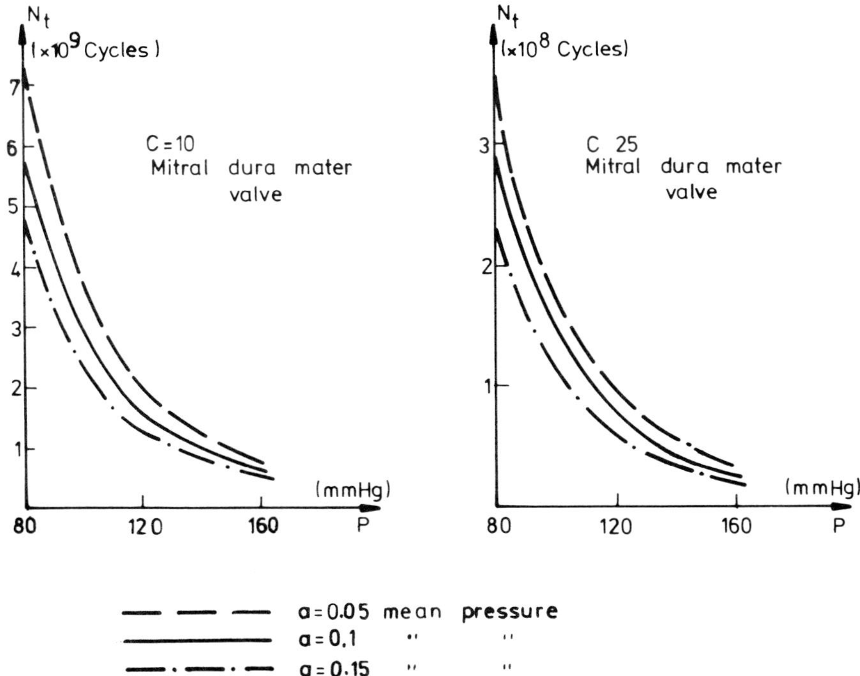

Fig. 4 Theoretical fatigue-life of dura mater valves

Fig. 4 shows the theoretical fatigue life of dura mater prostheses under different pressure loads for the mitral position with the following characteristic for the nonperiodic part of the pressure ($\Omega = 20(2\pi/T), \Delta = 0,1\Omega$, a = 0.05, 0.1, 0.15 of the mean pressure) and for different geometric characteristics of the valve (c = 10,25).

These curves show that only a very good selection of the geometric characteristic (c = $\alpha R/h$) achieves life times of 3.10^8 cycles (8 years at 72bpm). We can also conclude that these bioprostheses are contraindicated for aortic or mitral valve replacement in the presence of severe systemic hypertension.

REFERENCES

- Caminal, P. (1980) Biological Prosthetic Cardiac Valves Analysis and Characterization: Application to Dura mater Prosthesis. Ph.D. Thesis (in spanish). Universidad Politécnica de Barcelona. Instituto de Cibernética.

- Miner, M.A. (1945) Cumulative Damage in Fatigue. Journal of Applied Mechanics, 57, 159-163.

Biomaterials 1980
Edited by G. D. Winter, D. F. Gibbons, and H. Plenk, Jr.
© 1982 John Wiley and Sons Ltd.

IMMEDIATE AND LONG TERM BIOLOGICAL CONSEQUENCES OF THE
GLYCEROL PRETREATMENT OF AUTOLOGOUS PERICARDIAL CARDIAC
VALVES.

G. Dureau, Y.G. Heynen, and R. Eloy.

Unit 37 - INSERM - Cardiovascular surgery and organ
transplantation laboratory.
18 avenue du Doyen Lépine - 69500 Bron - France.

SUMMARY

Autologous pericardiac tissue has been used as valvular substitute in
dogs. Before implantation the pericardium was immersed during 10 minutes in 87 % glycerol so as to eliminate its cellular components. After
implantation the collagenous and elastin frame work was invaded by
host cells, resulting in fibroblastic cell proliferation, synthesis of
new collagen and elastin fibers, with no occurence of the classical inflammation reaction observed after implantation of non treated autologous pericardium.

INTRODUCTION

The search for the ideal valve replacement has stimulated surgical investigations for many years. Today's combined experience favours the
glutaraldehyde fixed porcine xenobioprosthesis. Nevertheless there is
no doubt from histological studies that the tissue will deteriorate
with time and valve tissue failures have been reported recently even
in young patients (Ashraf and Bloor, 1978 ; Broom, 1978 ; Ferrans et
al., 1978 ; Hetzer et al, 1978).
Fresh non-treated autologous tissue and particularly pericardium have
been evaluated with conflicting results (Ross and Olsen, 1976). In a
previous study performed in dogs we demonstrated that the intracardiac
implantation of non-vascularized living tissue is associated with the
rapid development of inflammatory lesions characterized by inflammatory cells, vegetations of the cusp, severe destruction and necrosis of
the collagen bundles.A constant clinical valve failure has been observed and death of the animals by right heart failure occured within the
first 15 post-operative days (G. Dureau and A. Tabib, 1978).
The present study investigates the biological effects of pretreatment
of autologous pericardium before implantation of cardiac valves by immersion in concentrated glycerol.

MATERIAL AND METHODS

Stentless valve replacement procedure. Mongrel puppies weighing 4-9 kg
were operated under profound hypothermia (20°C). After a careful dis-

597

section of the pericardiac tissue from the pleura covering it, autologous pericardiac fragments were immediately tailored into the desired shape and flushed in a heparinized saline solution. The pericardium was immersed in glycerol (87 % - 37°C) for 5 minutes and rehydrated in saline (18°C) for 5 minutes immediately before intracardiac implantation. Each atrioventricular valve consisted of two tennis-racket shaped fragments whose superior hemicircumference was sutured to each half of the valvular ring after resection of the natural valve. The handle of each racket was then drawn across the ventricular wall to form a tensor for each valve leaflet. These valves were implanted either in mitral (n = 54) or in tricuspid position (n = 30). The animals were killed sequentially until the 15th month.

<u>Biological investigations</u>. Histological examination of the pericardial leaflets, the atrioventricular ring insertion and the ventricular wall were performed before implantation and at time of autopsy. Hematoxylin and Weigert stain were used for the identification of elastin fibers. Pericardiac fragments before and after implantation were also cultured in Falcon disches in MEM tissue culture medium supplemented with 10 % fetal calf serum at 37°C. Cultures were maintained for at least 3 weeks and up to 8 weeks. Cell pellets were also submitted to electron microscopic investigations.
Specimens of pericardiac tissue before and after implantation as cardiac valves were also treated for scanning electron microscopy.

RESULTS

<u>Effect of the glycerol pretreatment on the pericardial tissue</u>. As compared to the non-treated pericardium, glycerol treatment resulted in immediate cell shrinkage and cell death. Mesothelial surface cells and fibrocytic cells present on and within the pericardial leaflet were lost. Collagen and elastin fibers remained the sole components of the implanted tissue as confirmed by both scanning electron microscopy and histological examinations (Figure 1) In tissue culture these pericardial glycerol-treated fragments failed to growth and no fibrocytes developed within a 3 weeks period of observation.
Immediately after implantation, these valves became very early covered with a layer of fibrin with a very moderate infiltrate of platelets and erythrocytes. Circulating histiocytes subsequently progressively invaded the fibrin layer which underwent a fibroblastic transformation and developed so as to cover the whole implanted tissue. As early as the 30th day the cellular ingrowth of the host cells extended to the cusps themselves by fibroblastic apposition. These events were not related to the site of implantation but were observed within the whole implant. Mitotic figures were seen and new collagen bundles (Figure 2) appeared by apposition on the initial fibers. New elastin fibers were also detected already at the 27th day. When placed in tissue culture

the pericardial pretreated fragments implanted 30 days before exhibited fibroblastic cell growth. No inflammatory cell reaction was detected. At the valve-blood interface, a thin flattened "endothelial-like"
cell layer developed. The exact nature of these cells was not ascertai-
ned although ultrastructural scanning electron microscopic characteristic were not incompatible with those of endothelial cells. One year
after implantation metabolically active fibrocytes were still present
within the newly formed cardiac valves (Figure 3). Collagen and elastin fibers and fibrocytes surrounded the initial fiber valve skeleton.
The newly formed collagen fibers possessed the periodic striation of
collagen at the ultrastructural level (Figure 4).
Nevertheless precocious but durable immunoblasts-like cells were regularly noted already at the 4th day and until one year after implantation (Figure 5). These plasmocytes were detected on the pericardial
tissue and even on the endocardial ventricular surface about 2-3 cm
from the valvular insertion. Using antidog immunoglobulin serum these
plasma cells were stained, acellular immunofluorescent material could
be detected in the central zone of the valvular tissue, and in some
limited areas a thin immunofluorescent deposit was present on the valvular surface itself.

DISCUSSION

Preliminary observations on the biological behaviour of glycerol pretreated autologous pericardial tissue when used as valvular leaflets
are :
The inflammatory reaction induced by the implantation of fresh autologous non treated pericardium is suppressed and is never responsible
for late valve failure.
Glycerol-treated pericardium which consisted exclusively of collagen
and elastin fibers is rapidly covered and further invaded by active
fibrocytes.
The occurrence of a humoral local reaction in response to the implantation of autologous tissue after its treatment with glycerol may be
inferred. It is possible that collagen and/or elastin of the pericardial implant have been antigenically modified by immersion in glycerol but it cannot be excluded that the latter could play the role of
an haptene or adjuvant in the induction of the observed reaction.
The newly formed tissue is able to syntesize structural proteins such
as collagen and elastin for prolonged period of time in dogs.

ACKNOWLEDGEMENT

Supported by Grant INSERM - CRL N° 78.5.0645 (Dr. Dureau).

REFERENCES

Ashraf M. & Bloor C.M., (1978) Structural alterations of the porcine heterograft after various durations of implantation. Am. J. Cardiol. 41, 1185-1190

Broom, N.D. (1978) Fatigue induced damage in glutaraldehyde preserved heart valve tissue. J. Thorac. Cardiovasc. Surg., 76, 202-211

Ferrans, V.J., Spray, T.L., Billingham M.E. & Roberts, W.C. (1978) ultrastructure of hancok porcine heterografts. Pre and post-implantation changes. Circulation, 58, suppl.I, 1-10, 1-18.

Hetzer R., Hill, D.J., Kerth, W.J., Wilson, A.J., Adappa, M.G. & Gerbode, F. (1978). Thrombosis and degeneration of Hancok valves. Clinical and pathological findings. Ann. Thor. Surg., 26, 317-322

Ross, K.J. & Olsen, E.G.J. (1976). Mitral valve reconstruction by posterior cusp advancement using a pericardial graft. Thorax, 31, 324-331.

FIGURES

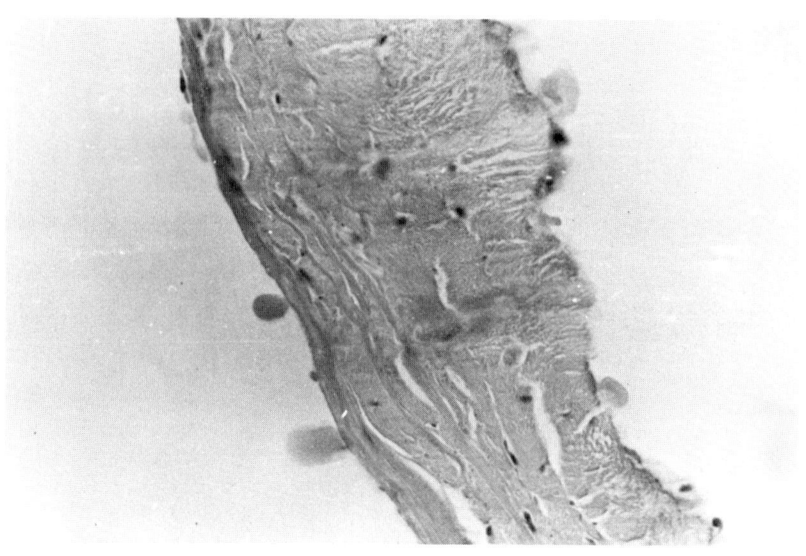

FIGURE 1. Effect of glycerol treatment on the pericardial leaflet X 218.7.

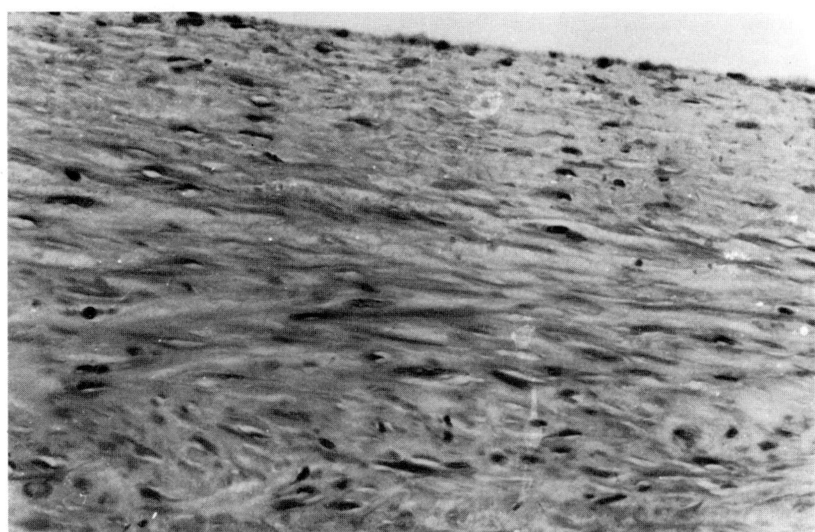

FIGURE 2. Pericardial leaflet implanted as valvular substitute 30 days before X 218.7.

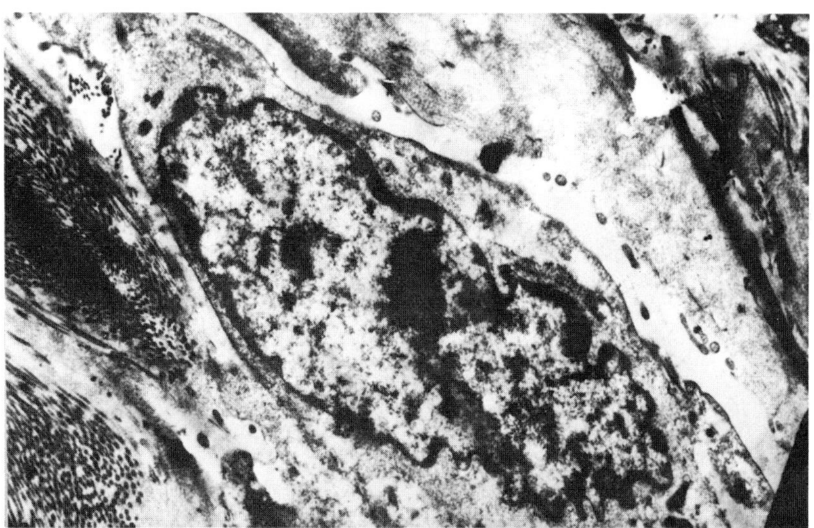

FIGURE 3. Fibroblastic cell within the implanted pericardial leaflet 140 days after implantation.

 G. Dureau, Y.G. Heynen and R. Eloy

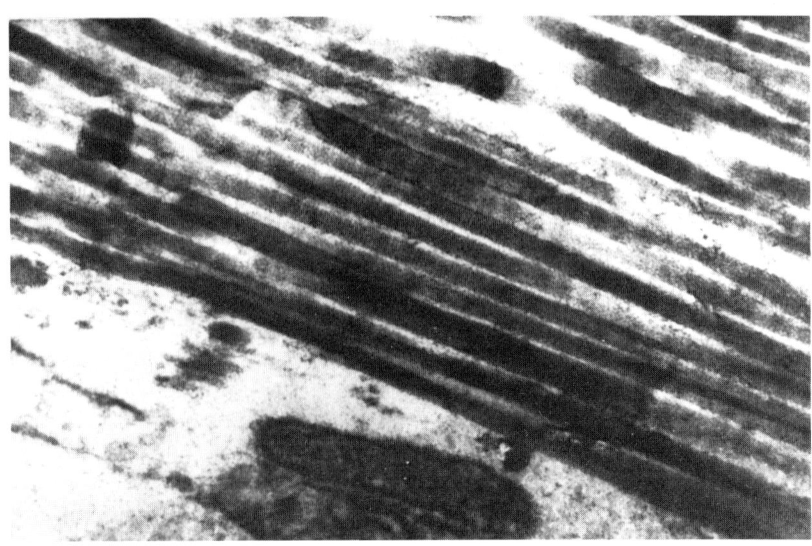

FIGURE 4. Periodic striation of newly formed collagen bundles.

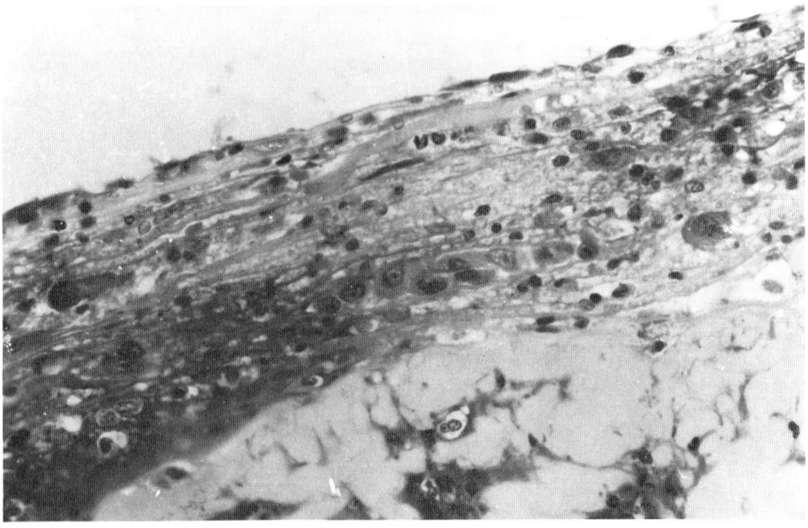

FIGURE 5. Plasma cell deposit and infiltration within pericardial tissue implanted one year X 350.

Biomaterials 1980
Edited by G. D. Winter, D. F. Gibbons, and H. Plenk, Jr.
© 1982 John Wiley and Sons Ltd.

IMMUNOGENICITY OF GLUTARALDEHYDE-TREATED TISSUE USED IN HEART VALVE REPLACEMENT

P. Bajpai, D. Russo, D. Slanczka and L. Weiskittel

University of Dayton,
Dayton, Ohio 45469

SUMMARY

Glutaraldehyde treatment is assumed to render tissues stable and
inert. Although early valve failure is rare with glutaraldehyde-
treated porcine heart valves (GTPHV), long term follow-ups indicate
that the valves undergo progressive degeneration. Since the antigenic status of GTPHV has not been resolved, studies were conducted
to determine the immunogenicity of these tissues. In the initial
study, New Zealand White rabbits were immunized with untreated
(UTPHV) or GTPHV extracts in Freund's complete adjuvant. Sera
obtained from rabbits in either group tested positive for presence
of antibodies against their corresponding antigens by capillary
tube aggregation, complement fixation, hemagglutination, and double
diffusion in gel precipitation tests. In the second study New
Zealand White rabbits were grafted subcutaneously in the abdomen
region with either UTPHV or GTPHV. Presence of circulating antibodies and cell mediated immune response was confirmed in both UTPHV
and GTPHV grafted rabbits by complement fixation, macrophage migration inhibition (MIF), and skin reaction tests. Microscopic examination of graft sections retrieved from either group of rabbits at the
end of one, two, or three months showed fragmentation and degeneration of collagen and infiltration of the grafts by inflammatory
cells. Results of this investigation show that the tanned valve is
immunogenic and may participate in autoimmune and immune-complex
diseases around and away from the implant.

INTRODUCTION

Glutaraldehyde in various concentrations and in various environments
has been used to render different kinds of microorganisms and
tissues, immobile, sterile, avirulent and biologically inert
(Carpentier et al., 1969; Stanley et al., 1973; Frost, Edwards and
Sanderson 1976; Moran and Wheeler 1976; Pricam, Fisher and Friend
1977; Relyveld 1977; Eckert and Snyder 1978; Thomas 1978 and
Brougham and Johnson 1978).

A general belief seems to exist between manufacturers of glutaraldehyde-treated heart valve heterografts and the surgeons using the
product that glutaraldehyde treatment not only renders the heart
valve more stable but also non-immunogenic. Yet glutaraldehyde
treatment of biologic material has been used effectively to produce

603

vaccines, as well as induce humoral and/or cell mediated immune
responses (Relyveld, Girard and Desormeau-Bedot 1973; Frolova et al.
1973; Frost, Edwards and Sanderson 1976; Kahan et al. 1976; Metzger,
et al. 1976; Eckert and Snyder 1978 and Bigley et al. 1980).

Frolova et al. (1973) had reported that water-soluble extracts of
glutaraldehyde-treated porcine heart valves (GTPHV) were immunogenic
but had fewer number of antigens than untreated porcine heart valve
extracts (UTPHV). Since glutaraldehyde treatment renders most of
the tissue insoluble, homogenates consisting of soluble as well as
insoluble fractions of GTPHV and UTPHV were used by Slanczka and
Bajpai (1978) and Slanczka, Russo and Bajpai (1979) to immunize rabbits. Using Capillary Tube Agglutination Test (CTAT), Complement
Fixation Test (CFT), Tanned Cell Hemagglutination Test (TCHT), Double
Diffusion in Gel Precipitation Test (DDGPT) and Immunoelectrophore-
sis, they observed that rabbits injected with either UTPHV or GTPHV
developed antibodies which reacted with both UTPHV and GTPHV antigens. Hemagglutination titers of rabbit sera fifty weeks after the
initial injections of heterograft extracts are shown in Table 1.

TABLE 1. Antibody Titers of Sera Obtained from Rabbits
          Immunized with Untreated Heart (UTPHV) or
          Glutaraldehyde-Treated Heart Valve (GTPHV)
          Antigens for Fifty Weeks.

Human '0' Erythrocytes Coated With	Hemagglutination Titers Sera From	
	UTPHV Immunized Rabbits	GTPHV Immunized Rabbits
UTPHV	> 256	> 256
GTPHV	> 256	> 256

Since the GTPHV's are grafted in patients, the validity of using
homogenate depots for releasing antigens and inducing an immune
response was questioned. On the other hand data published by Broom
(1977), Ferrans et al. (1978) and Silver (1978), suggests that
glutaraldehyde polymerized material from implanted GTPHV's leaches
out gradually into the circulation and ultimately weakens the prosthesis. Hence, the current investigation was conducted to study the
immunologic properties of UTPHV and GTPHV grafts in rabbits.

MATERIALS AND METHODS

Twenty-one New Zealand white rabbits were divided into 3 groups of 7
each. Rabbits in one group were sham-operated. Rabbits in the
other two groups were grafted subcutaneously in the abdominal region
with 1 x 2 cm sections of either untreated or glutaraldehyde-treated

porcine heart valves. Grafts were recovered after 1, 2 and 3 months
of implantation for histopathological examination. Standard histologic procedures were used for processing the tissues and staining
the sections with hematoxylin and eosin.

Glutaraldehyde-Treatment of Porcine Heart Valves. Porcine valves
were obtained fresh from the slaughterhouse and immediately placed
in cold normal saline. Valves were then trimmed to approximate
proportions of the finished product. Untreated valves were quick
frozen until use. Tanning of the trimmed porcine heart valves was
achieved by placing them in 0.5% glutaraldehyde (pH 7.4) for 2 weeks.
The glutaraldehyde-treated valves were rinsed thrice in sterile
saline and quick frozen until use. Before using the valves both
UTPHV and GTPHV were thawed slowly at 40°C.

Antigen Preparation. Valve tissue was diced and washed by repeated
centrifugations in chilled phosphate buffered saline (PBS) having a
pH of 7.35. Washed and diced tissues were subjected to successive
homogenizations and sonication in 5 mls of PBS per gram wet weight
of the tissue. The final homogenate was filtered through cheese-
cloth and Whatman #1 filter paper. Protein content of the antigen
suspension was determined by the method of Lowry et al., (1951). The
fine particulate antigen preparation was used in all serological
procedures (Slanczka and Bajpai 1978).

Complement Fixation Test. Serum obtained from the blood of each
rabbit throughout the investigation was tested for the presence
of antibodies against UTPHV and GTPHV antigens by the Complement
Fixation procedure reported by Levine (1973).

Macrophage Migration Inhibition Test (MIF). Three months after
graft implantation, MIF was performed on circulating lymphocytes
from all rabbits according to a modified procedure of Harrington
and Statsny (1973). Each rabbit's lymphocytes were tested against
GTPHV antigens.

Skin Testing. One and two months after the removal of all grafts, a
skin test for cellular immunity was performed on each rabbit according to the procedure of Hassett et al., (1977). Non-operated, un-
immunized rabbits were used as antigen controls.

       RESULTS

Four rabbits were lost during the investigation due to miscellaneous
causes including anesthesia during surgery and gall bladder obstruction.

Gross Morphology. Morphologic observations revealed that all the
implanted grafts were walled off by the host tissue. Extent of
encapsulation increased with time and after 3 months a graft-host
interface was visible. The thickness of GTPHV grafts appeared to
remain unchanged over the 3 months period, while the thickness of

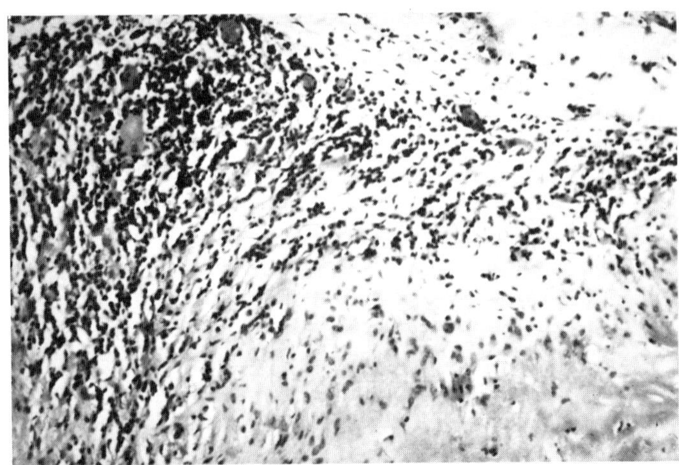

Fig. 1. Photomicrograph of a section of untreated porcine heart valve heterograft (UTPHV) implanted in rabbits for three months showing chronic inflammation with focal areas of necrosis and foreign body cells (original magnification 200 X).

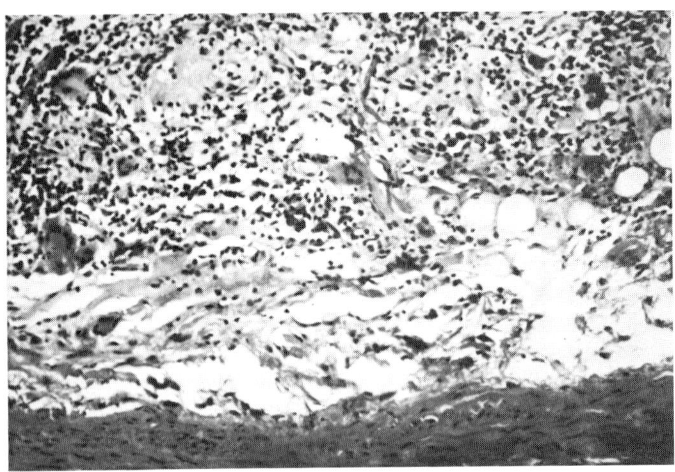

Fig. 2. Photomicrograph of a section of glutaraldehyde-treated porcine heart valve heterograft (GTPHV) implanted in rabbits for three months showing chronic inflammation with focal areas of necrosis and foreign body cells (original magnification 200 X).

UTPHV grafts decreased considerably over the same period.

<u>Histopathology</u>. Both UTPHV (Figure 1) and GTPHV (Figure 2) grafts
recovered from the rabbits at 1, 2 and 3 month intervals showed similar histopathology and processing of the grafted tissue by the host's
cellular system. Evidence of chronic inflammation with focal areas
of necrosis and phagocytosis of particulates from the implant by
foreign body cells can be observed in the photomicrographs of recovered grafts (Figure 1 and Figure 2).

<u>Antibody Response</u>. The results are shown in Table 2. All 5 rabbits
implanted with UTPHV grafts developed antibodies against UTPHV antigens. Only 2 of the 5 rabbits showed antibodies which cross reacted
with GTPHV antigens. One rabbit implanted with GTPHV grafts lost 2
of the 3 grafts three weeks after implantation and did not develop
antibodies against GTPHV or UTPHV antigens. The 4 remaining rabbits
developed antibodies which reacted with both UTPHV and GTPHV antigens. Sham operated rabbits did not develop antibodies against
UTPHV or GTPHV antigens.

TABLE 2. Range of antibody titers of rabbits grafted with
untreated heart valves (UTPHV), glutaraldehyde-
treated heart valves (GTPHV) or ungrafted control rabbits at 0, 8, and 12 weeks after graft
implantation.

		WEEK					
SERA FROM:	RABBIT NUMBER	0		8		12	
		UTPHV	GTPHV	UTPHV	GTPHV	UTPHV	GTPHV
UTPHV rabbits	5	0	0	20-160	0-10	20-80	0-10
GTPHV rabbits	4	0	0	20- 40	10-20	40-80	20-40
Control rabbits	7	0	0	0	0	0	0

Each sera sample was tested against UTPHV and GTPHV antigens by
Complement Fixation Test.

<u>Macrophage Migration Inhibition Test</u>. Lymphocytes obtained from
either UTPHV or GTPHV grafted animals on incubation with GTPHV antigens showed significant (P <.01) inhibition of macrophages from the
agar droplet (Table 3). Lymphocytes obtained from sham-operated
animals did not inhibit the migration of macrophages.

TABLE 3. Percent migration inhibition of macrophages from
an agarose droplet.

LYMPHOCYTE SOURCE:	RABBIT NUMBER	GTPHV ANTIGEN
UTPHV grafted Rabbits	5	10.5 % P <.01
GTPHV grafted Rabbits	5	14.5 % P <.01
Sham-operated Controls	4	NI

NI = No Inhibition

<u>Skin Tests</u>. Rabbits grafted with UTPHV gave a positive skin test
when challenged intradermally with UTPHV antigens (Table 4). Like-
wise rabbits grafted with GTPHV grafts gave a positive skin test when
challenged with GTPHV antigens (Table 4). One month later intradermal challenge of UTPHV grafted rabbits with GTPHV antigens and vice
versa also gave positive skin responses. All sham-operated rabbits
tested negative by the skin test with either UTPHV or GTPHV antigens.

TABLE 4. Induration in rabbits grafted with UTPHV and GTPHV
after intradermal injection of 0.1 ml saline or
0.1 ml of UTPHV or GTPHV homogenate (antigen).

Test Substance:	UTPHV Rabbits	GTPHV Rabbits
Rabbit Number	4	5
Saline	0 mm.	0 mm.
Antigen	10 ± 2 mm.	8 ± 1 mm.

Induration of 5 mm., or more indicates a positive skin reaction. UTPHV grafted rabbits were injected with UTPHV
antigen and GTPHV grafted rabbits were injected with GTPHV
antigen.

<u>DISCUSSION</u>

The results of this study suggest that glutaraldehyde treatment may
delay but does not prevent the degradation of the GTPHV grafts.
According to Broom (1978) whether a tissue has been treated with
glutaraldehyde or not, natural disintegration is inevitable. Severe
progressive disruption and/or calcification of implanted GTPHV cusps
has been reported by several investigators (Spray and Roberts 1977,
Ferrans et al. 1978; Ashraf and Bloor 1978 and Geha et al. 1979).

The presence of circulating antibodies against UTPHV and GTPHV antigens in animals grafted with these respective grafts is in accordance with the histopathological data and confirms the data published earlier by Slanczka and Bajpai (1978) and Slanczka, Russo and
Bajpai (1979). Processing of the untreated or glutaraldehyde polymerized biologic porcine heart valve by the host's defense system is
apt to induce an immune response. Moran and Wheeler (1976) and
Metzger et al. (1976) have used glutaraldehyde polymerized pollen to
induce the production of antipollen IgG. According to Bigley et al.
(1980) glutaraldehyde polymerization of antigens probably helps the
antigenic material bypass the thymocyte dependent (T) cell system.
Thus the antibodies formed against glutaraldehyde polymerized antigen by the B cells are mainly of the IgM type. Both IgM and IgG_2
fix complement in rabbits. It is important to note that sera
obtained from only 2 rabbits producing anti-UTPHV antibodies reacted
with GTPHV antigens. In contrast sera obtained from all the rabbits
producing anti-GTPHV reacted with UTPHV antigens. This observation
implies that antigens which may be masked by glutaraldehyde treatment are unmasked during the processing of the graft by the host.

According to Kahan et al. (1976) and Frost et al. (1976), glutaraldehyde-treated tissue selectively stimulates a cell-mediated immune
response due to the fixed nature of the antigen. Results of this
study show that both UTPHV and GTPHV grafts induce a cell-mediated
immune response.

Wahl and Wahl (1979) have suggested that antigenic challenge of
sensitized lymphocytes induces the production of biologic mediators
which can modulate connective tissue metabolism by releasing lympho-
kine-fibroblast activating factor (FAF) which forms collagen and lym-
phokine-macrophage activating factor (MAF) which destroys collagen.
Degradation as well as encapsulation of UTPHV and GTPHV grafts in
rabbits along with the induction of humoral as well as cell mediated
immune responses indicate that glutaraldehyde treatment does not
spare the tissue from immunologic processing.

Sheikh, Tascon and Nimmi (1980) showed that of the 35 patients implanted with Hancock heart valve porcine xenografts (HHX), 32%
showed positive leukocyte adherence inhibition on incubation with
porcine heart valve tissue extract. Variation in patient age and
the time elapsed between heart valve transplant and collection of

lymphocytes could account for some of the negative findings. They
also reported that sera of HHX and coronary bypass heart surgery
(BHS) patients developed antibodies against porcine heart valve tissue. Witebsky, Klendshoj and McNeil (1944) reported years ago that
pigs have "A" substance on their erythrocytes and tissues. Thus
sera obtained from patients having anti-A antibodies should show
reaction with porcine heart tissue. Russo (1979) observed that
glutaraldehyde treatment enhanced the inherent ability of porcine
heart valve antigens to bind with human anti-A antibodies. Russo
(1979) also observed that antisera against untreated porcine
aortic intima (UPI) and glutaraldehyde-treated porcine aortic intima
(GPI) reacted with GTPHV antigens. Russo's (1979) observations suggest the possibility that pathogenesis involving autoimmune and immune complex diseases can occur in patients implanted with glutaraldehyde-treated biologic prosthesis away from the implants.

CONCLUSIONS

Glutaraldehyde treatment stabilizes porcine heart valve tissue and
delays their eventual degradation. Glutaraldehyde treatment does not
prevent the induction of humoral or cell-mediated immune responses by
the porcine heart valve heterograft. Induction of cell mediated
immune response against glutaraldehyde-treated porcine heart valve
antigens has been confirmed in patients implanted with the tanned
tissue devices (Sheikh et al., 1980).

ACKNOWLEDGEMENTS

Acknowledgements are due to Dr. James M. Anderson for interpretation
of the photomicrographs of implanted grafts and Ann Feldmann for the
excellent typing of this manuscript.

REFERENCES

Ashraf, M. & Bloor, C. (1978) Structural alterations of the porcine
heterograft after various durations of implantations. Amer. J. Cardiol. 41, 1185-1190.
Bigley, N., Kreps, D., Smith, R. & Esa, A. (1980) Antigenic modification, rosette-forming cells, and Salmonella resistance in outbred
and inbred mice. Infec. Immun., In Press.
Broom, N. (1977) The stress/strain and fatigue behavior of glutaraldehyde preserved heart valve tissue. J. Biomechanics 10, 707-724.
Brougham, M. & Johnson, D. (1978) Studies on yeast alcohol dehydrogenase bound to solid supports. Int. J. Biochem. 9, 283-287.
Carpentier, A., Lemaigre, C., Robert L., Carpentier, S. & Dubost, C.
(1969) Biological factors affecting long-term results of valvular
heterografts. J. Thorac. Cardiovasc. Surg. 58, 467.

Eckert, B & Snyder, J. (1978) Combined immunofluorescence and high voltage microscopy of cultured mammalian cells, using an antibody that binds to glutaraldehyde-treated tubulin. Proc. Natl. Acad. Sci. 75, 334-338.

Ferrans, V., Spray, T., Billingham, M. & Roberts, W. (1978) Amer. J. Cardiol. 41, 1159-1184.

Frolova, M., Barbarash, L., Gudkova, R., & Kapinskaya, J. (1973) Effect of method of conservation on immunogenicity and antigenic composition of xenogeneic heart valve tissues. Byulletin Eksperimental noi Biologii i Meditsiny, 73, 306-309.

Frost, P., Edwards, A., & Sanderson, C. (1976) The use of glutaraldehyde fixation for the study of immune response to syngeneic tumor antigen. Ann. N.Y. Acad. Science. 276, 91-96.

Geha, A., Laks, H., Stansel, H., Cornhill, J., Kilman, J., Buckley, M. & Roberts, W. (1979) Late failure of porcine valve heterografts in children. J. Thorac. Cardiovasc. Surg., 78, 351-364.

Harrington, J. & Stastny, P. (1973) Macrophage migration from an agarose droplet: development of a micromethod for assay of delayed hypersensitivity. J. Immunol., 110, 752-759.

Hassett, A., Wood, R., Temperley, I. & Mullins, G. (1977) Cellmediated immunity to recall antigens in vivo and in vitro. Irish J. Med. Sci., 146, 167-174.

Kahan, M., Berman-Goldman, R., Saltoun, R. & Naor, D. (1976) Studies on the immune response to fixed antigens. J. Immunol., 117, 16-22.

Levine, L. (1973) Microcomplement fixation, in Immunochemistry (Ed. Weir), pp. 5B.1-5B.8. Blackwell Scientific Publications, Oxford, England.

Lowry, O., Rosenbrough, N., Farr, A. & Randall, R. (1951) Protein measurement with the folin phenol reagent. J. Biol. Chem., 193, 265-275.

Metzger, W., Patterson, R., Zeiss, C., Irons, J., Pruzansky, J., Suszko, I. & Levits, D. (1976) Comparison of polymerized and nonpolymerized antigen E for immunotherapy of ragweed allergy. N. Eng. J. Med., 295, 1160-1164.

Moran, D. & Wheeler, A. (1976) Chemical modification of crude timothy grass pollen extract: I.). Antigenicity and immunogenicity changes following amino group modification. Int. Arch. All. Appl. Immunol., 50, 693-708.

Pricam, C., Fisher, K. & Friend, D. (1977) Intramembraneous particle distribution in human erythrocytes: Effects of lysis, glutaraldehyde and poly-1-lysine. Anatomical Record, 189, 596-608.

Relyveld, E. (1977) Etude du pouvier backricide du glutaraldehyde. Ann. Microbiol., 128, 495-505.

Relyveld, E., Girard, O. & Desormeau-Bedot, J. P. (1973) Procede de Fabrication de Vaccins A L'aide du glutaraldehyde. Ann. Immunologie, Hungaricae, 17, 21-31.

Russo, D. (1979) Studies on the antigenicity of porcine intima. M.Sc. Thesis, University of Dayton, Dayton, Ohio U.S.A.

Sheikh, K., Tascon, M. & Nimmi, M. (1980) Autoimmunity in patients with Hancock Valve implant and bypass heart surgery. Fed. Proc., 39, 472.

Silver, M. (1978) Late complications of prosthetic heart valves. Arch. of Pathol. & Lab. Med., 102, 281-284.

Slanczka, D. & Bajpai, P. (1978) Immunogenicity of glutaraldehyde-treated porcine heart valves. IRCS Med. Sci., 6, 421.

Slanczka, D., Russo, D. & Bajpai, P. (1979) Immunogenicity of tanned tissue used in heart valve replacement. Proceedings of the 7th New England (Northeast) Bioengineering Conference, March 22-23, Troy, N.Y., pp. 197-200.

Spray, T. & Roberts, W. (1977) Structural changes in porcine xenografts and as substitute cardiac valves. Amer. J. Cardiol., 40, 319-330.

Stanley, W., Watters, G., Kelly, S. & Olson A. (1973) Glucoamylase immobilized on Chiton with glutaraldehyde. Biotechnol. & Bioengineering, 20, 135-140.

Thomas, S. (1978) Effects of high concentrations of glutaraldehyde on bacterial spores. Microbios. Letters 4, 199-204.

Wahl, S. & Wahl, L. (1979) Lymphokine modulation of connective tissue metabolism. Ann. N.Y. Acad. Sci., 332, 411-422.

Witebsky, E., Klendshoj, N. & McNeil, C. (1944) Potent typing sera produced by treatment of donors with isolated blood group specific substances. Proc. Soc. Exp. Biol., 55, 167-170.

Biomaterials 1980
Edited by G. D. Winter, D. F. Gibbons, and H. Plenk, Jr.
© 1982 John Wiley and Sons Ltd.

SHORT TERM RESULTS WITH XENOGRAFT BIOPROSTHESES

W.H. Wain, E. Bodnar and D.N. Ross

National Heart Hospital and
Cardiothoracic Institute, 2 Beaumont Street,
London W1N 2DX, England

SUMMARY

An estimated 400 xenograft bioprostheses used for heart valve
replacements in less than four years were associated with 30
instances of valve dysfunction within 36 months of implantation.
Infection was the most common problem (3.2%) and thromboembolism
(1.5%) and leaflet perforation (1.5%) also caused a significant
number of valve dysfunctions. Four valves were calcified (1%),
two of them in children. In spite of these problems xenograft
bioprosthetic valves continue to provide an extremely valuable
cardiac valve replacement.

INTRODUCTION

Comparative assessment of heart valve prostheses is usually based
on a long term evaluation of a large number of patients over at
least a five, and preferably ten year period. However, early observations of importance should be critically examined when they
occur rather than in the general context of a longer term evaluation.

The first commercial porcine aortic xenograft was implanted by
Cevese in 1969 and since then the three major manufacturers have
reported sales of 100,000 valves in the first ten years of their
use. There have been a number of reports of excellent long-term
results with these valves (Cevese et al 1977; Cohn et al 1976;
Angell et al 1979; Oyer et al 1979). The first xenograft valve
used at the National Heart Hospital, London, was on the 21st May
1976 and the purpose of this presentation is to illustrate 30
valves with problems seen within 36 months of implantation. There
have been 337 valve implantations during this period, and three of
the valves discussed in this presentation were implanted in other
centres. To permit the inclusion of these valves an estimate of
400 valves, rather than 337, has been made.

     W.H. Wain, E. Bodnar and D.N. Ross

OBSERVATIONS

Figure 1 shows a radiograph of a xenograft bioprosthesis with gross, diffuse intrinsic calcification.   This valve was explanted from the mitral position of a patient of 42 years old after 32 months in situ.   In the same patient the tricuspid valve had also been re-placed and this too was calcified.   There was no history of abnormal calcium metabolism or or renal dialysis.

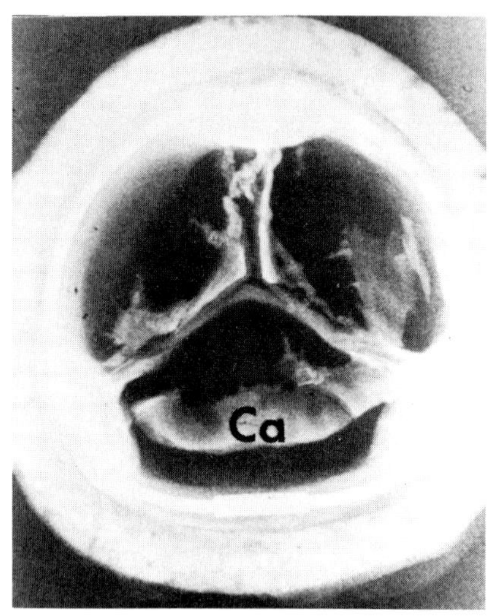

Fig. 1.   Radiograph of xenograft bioprosthesis with in-trinsic calcification.   "Ca" indicates calcification within the valve.

There were two such intrinsically calcified valves in this series, an incidence of 0.5% amongst 400 patients in less than four years.

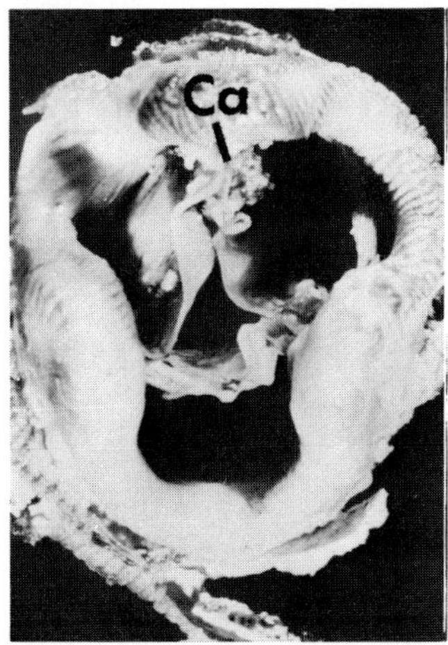

Fig. 2.   Xenograft bioprosthesis with extrinsic calcification.   "Ca" indicates extrinsic calcification at the
valve commissure.

Figure 2 shows a valve which had been implanted for 36 months in a
young man of 14 years.   There was no associated history of infection.   There have been a total of two xenograft bioprostheses with
such extrinsic calcification in young patients, an incidence of
0.5%.   Altogether there have been four valves with calcification,
an incidence of 1.0%.

Another problem usually associated with young patients is one of
valve stenosis.   In Figure 3 the xenograft bioprosthesis is
clearly seen to be compromised within the aortic root.

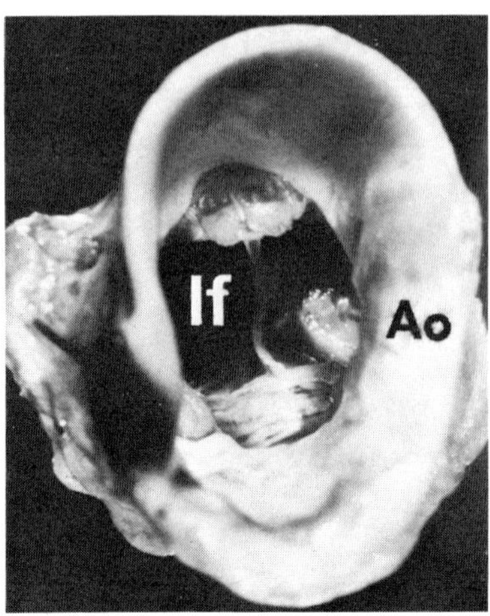

Fig. 3. Xenograft bioprosthesis in small aortic root.
"Ao" indicates the aorta: "LF" the valve leaflets.

In young patients with small aortic roots the growth potential of
the child can increase the severity of the stenosis.   In addition,
the inherent stenosis produced by the implantation within the aorta
of an effective orifice surrounded by xenograft aortic wall,
supporting frame and sewing ring will be proportionately greater for
the small sizes of xenograft valve.   Only one is reported in this
study, (Figure 3) an incidence of 0.25%

An example of perforation of a leaflet is shown in Figure 4.   It is
probable that the majority of leaflet perforations are caused by
long suture ends of stiff monofilaments.   Similar perforations have
been caused by fibrosed, stiffened braided sutures (Estes et al,
1979).

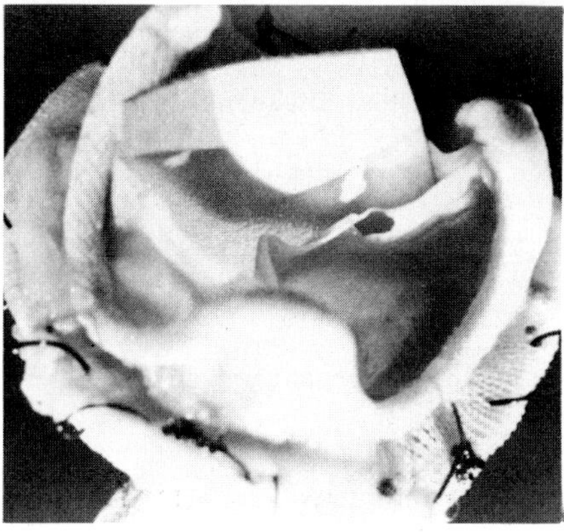

Fig. 4.   Perforations in xenograft bioprosthesis.

However, such perforations have also been found in xenograft bioprostheses explanted from the mitral position and these cannot be
explained on the basis of long suture ends.   The cause of such
perforations is a matter of speculation.   There have been six
valves with such perforations, an incidence of 1.5%.

Massive, sterile thrombotic vegetations of fibrin such as are seen
in Figure 5 cause severe haemodynamic disturbance in the absence of
any demonstrable infection.

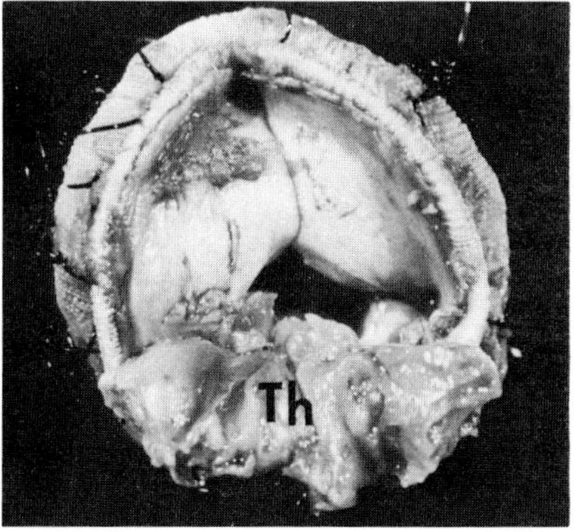

Fig. 5.   Thrombotic vegetation on xenograft bioprosthesis.
"Th" indicates the thrombus.

In addition there have been five cases of peripheral thromboemboli.
Anticoagulant therapy for patients with xenograft bioprostheses is
indicated for an initial period.   There have been six valves with
episodes of thromboembolism, an incidence of 1.5%.

There have been three cases of fungal endocarditis and ten of bacterial endocarditis.   The infections occurred within 1 to 36 months
of implantation and two were successfully treated without surgical
intervention.   There were 13 infections altogether, an incidence
of 3.25%.   The infecting organisms are listed in Table 1.

TABLE 1.   Infecting Organisms on Xenograft Bioprostheses

<u>Chaetomium</u> species	1
<u>Aspergillus</u> <u>fumigatus</u>	1
<u>Candida</u> <u>albicans</u>	1
<u>Streptococcus</u> <u>viridans</u>	1
<u>Streptococcus</u> <u>faecalis</u>	1
<u>Staphylococcus</u> <u>aureus</u>	3
<u>Staphylococcus</u> <u>epidermidis</u>	5
	13

<u>DISCUSSION</u>

Thirty xenograft bioprostheses have been reported with a variety of
valvular dysfunctions within 36 months of implantation from an estimated population of 400 valves within a four year period.   The causes of dysfunction are not unique to this study, although the proportion of the different problems does vary.

Information from Hancock Laboratories Inc. and from Edwards
Laboratories on explanted xenograft bioprostheses returned to the
laboratories for examination shows two different patterns.   The
Edwards Laboratories information (Edwards 1979) is based on a four
year period similar to this presentation and infective endocarditis
is also recognised as the most common cause of valve dysfunction.
Hancock xenograft valves have been in use for a much longer period
and an $8\frac{1}{2}$ year follow-up on 180 explanted valves has shown that calcification is the major cause of valve dysfunction although it is
recognised that calcification may be consequent upon previous infection (Hancock 1980).   Similar, late calcification has been
described by Acar et al (1976) and calcium deposits have been described in electronmicrographs (Ferrans et al 1979).

Calcification in one of our cases (Figure 1) occurred within 32
months of implantation, and so calcification should be considered in
the diagnosis of patients presenting with valve dysfunction within
three years of implantation.

There are an increasing number of reports of extrinsic calcification
at the valve commissure and consequent leaflet rupture in xenograft
bioprostheses implanted into young patients (Figure 2: Geha et al
1979; Crupi et al 1980; Smith et al 1980; & Wada et al 1980). The
causes of this are usually ascribed to a high turnover of ionised
calcium in growing children (Geha 1980).   This would almost amount
to a specific contra-indication for the use of xenograft bioprostheses in children, for whom the absence of routine long-term anticoagulation required for prosthetic mechanical valves is a great
advantage.   Calcification in young patients is a cause for concern
but the incidence of 0.5% in this report does not justify a change
in policy towards valve replacement in young patients.

Stenosis of xenograft bioprostheses in growing children (Figure 3)
is exacerbated by the requirement for small sizes of valve in small
aortic roots of children.   In these cases it is not possible to use
a larger valve implant and another type of valve replacement may be
required.   In order to overcome the stenosis seen in Figure 3 it
was necessary to carry out a total root replacement with a homograft
aortic valve and reimplantation of the coronary arteries.   Selection of the correct size of valve for replacement, or an alternative
type of valve is obviously important in young patients.

Size selection, the length of suture ends and the placing of knots
are under the control of the surgeon.   A change in suture technique has reduced the incidence of leaflet perforations seen in
Figure 4.   It should be emphasised that these small perforations
are not often seen at surgery for the removal of the valve but
usually during a subsequent detailed laboratory investigation.

Anticoagulation therapy for xenograft bioprostheses has been introduced by some centres (Oyer et al 1979).   There have been reports
of long-term follow-ups without anticoagulation therapy (Pipkin et
al 1976).   Thromboemboli are reported from both of these series,
and thrombotic apposition of fibrin on the xenograft bioprosthesis,
as seen in Figure 5, is an occasional cause of valve dysfunction.
The recommendation for anticoagulant therapy varies between centres
and even between surgeons at any one centre.   The introduction of
xenograft valves followed a decade of homograft valve implantation
in which thromboembolism did not occur (Ross et al 1979).   It was
hoped that xenograft valves would have a similar embolus-free experience but this has not been the case (Figure 5 and Klovekorn et

al 1980).   Possibly the requirements for a supporting frame and a
sewing ring in xenograft valves provide thrombogenic circumstances
within the first few weeks after implantation.   Nevertheless, em-
bolic rates for xenograft valves are generally lower than those
reported for prosthetic mechanical valves (Starr et al 1977).

Infective endocarditis was the major cause of xenograft valve dysfunction.   The pattern of organisms was similar to that reported
by Rossiter et al (1978) and the prevalence of <u>Staphylococcus
epidermidis</u> as the causative organism(Table 1) is a trend associated with mechanical and xenograft valves.   This may be related to
the handling required during the washing procedure for the xenograft
valves.

Other problems have been reported following xenograft bioprosthesis
implantation which were not seen in this series.   These include
anticoagulant-associated bleeding (Struck et al 1979; Klovekorn et
al 1980)and ventricular perforations (Edwards 1979).

<u>REFERENCES</u>

Acar, J., Carpentier, A., Chomette, G., Lelugen, C., Geschwind, H.
& Starkman, S. (1976) Evolution stenosante des heterograffes en
position aortique ou mitrale. A propos de deux cas. <u>Arch Mal
Coeur, 69</u>, 929-
Angell, W.W., Angell, J.D. & Sywak, A. (1979) The Angell-Shiley
porcine xenograft. <u>Ann Thorac Surg, 28</u>, 537-552.
Cevese, P.G., Gallucci, V., Morea, M., Volta, S.D., Fasoli, G. &
Casarotto, D. (1977) Heart valve replacement with the Hancock bioprosthesis. Analysis of long-term results. <u>Circulation, 56</u>, Suppl
2, 111-116.
Cohn, L.H., Sanders, J.H. & Collins, J.J. (1976) Aortic valve replacement with the Hancock porcine xenograft. <u>Ann Thorac Surg, 22</u>,
221-227.
Crupi, G., Gibson, D., Heard, B. & Lincoln, C. (1980) Severe late
failure of a porcine xenograft mitral valve: clinical, echocardio-
graphic and pathological findings. <u>Thorax, 35</u>, 210-212.
Edwards Laboratories (1979) <u>Clinical report</u>: Carpentier-Edwards Bio-
prostheses.
Estes, M.S., Komatsu, S.K., Nashef, A. & Lane, E. (1979) In-vitro
testing of bioprostheses, in <u>Bioprosthetic Cardiac Valves</u> (Eds.,
Sebening, Klovekorn, Meisner & Struck), pp 271-277. Deutsches
Herzzentrum, Munchen.
Ferrans , V.J., Boyce, S.W., Billingham, M.E., Spray, T.L. & Roberts
W.C. (1979) Ultrasound alteration in porcine valvular heterografts,
in <u>Bioprosthetic Cardiac Valves</u>, (Eds., Klovekorn, Meisner, Struck,
Sebening), pp 295-315. Deutsches Herzzentrum , Munchen.

Geha, A.S. (1980) Valve replacement in children. <u>Ann Thorac Surg</u>, <u>29</u>, 500-501.

Geha, A.S., Laks, H., Stansel, H.C., Cornhill, J.F., Kilman, J.W., Buckely, M.J. & Roberts, W.C. (1979) Late failure of porcine valve heterografts in children. <u>J Thorac Cardiovasc Surg, 78</u>, 351-364.

Hancock Laboratories Inc. (April 1980) <u>Durability Assessment of the Hancock Porcine Bioprosthesis: Dysfunction and Durability</u>.

Klovekorn, W.P., Struck, E. & Sebening, F. (1980) Early and late results after bioprosthetic cardiac valve replacement. <u>Europ Heart J, 1</u>, 129-135.

Oyer, P.E., Stinson, E.B., Reitz, B.A., Miller, D.C., Rossiter, S.J. & Shumway, N.E. (1979) Long-term evaluation of the porcine xeno-graft bioprosthesis. <u>J Thorac Cardiovasc Surg, 78</u>, 343-350.

Pipkin, R.D., Bach, W.C. & Fogarty, T.J. (1976) Evaluation of aortic valve replacement with a porcine xenograft without long term anticoagulation. <u>J Thorac Cardiovasc Surg, 71</u>, 179-186.

Ross, D.N., Martelli, V. & Wain, W.H. (1979) Allograft and auto-graft valves used for aortic valve replacement, in <u>Biological Tissue Valves</u>, (Eds., Ionescu), pp. 127-172, London, Butterworth.

Rossiter, S.J., Stinson, E.B., Oyer, P.E., Miller, D.C., Schapira, J.N., Martin, R.P. & Shumway, N.E. (1978) Prosthetic valve endo-carditis: A comparison of heterograft tissue valves and mechanical valves. <u>J Thorac Cardiovasc Surg, 76</u>, 795-803.

Smith, J.M., Cooley, D.A., Ferreira, W. & Reul, G.J. (1980) Aortic valve replacement in preteenage children. <u>Ann Thorac Surg, 29</u>, 512-518.

Starr, A., Grunkemeier, G.L., Lambert, L.E., Thomas, D., Sugimura, S. & Lefrak, A. (1977) Aortic valve replacement: A ten-year follow-up of non-cloth covered vs cloth covered caged ball prostheses. <u>Circulation, 56</u>, Suppl 2, 133-

Wada, J., Yokoyama, M., Hashimoto, A., Imai, Y., Kitamura, N., Takao, A. & Momma, K. (1980) Long term follow-up of artificial valves in patients under 15 years old. <u>Ann Thorac Surg, 29</u>, 519-521.

Struck, E., Meisner, H., Schmidt-Habelmann, P. & Sebening, F. (1979) Cardiac valve replacement with Hancock and Carpentier-Edwards bioprosthesis in, <u>Bioprosthetic Cardiac Valves</u> (Eds., Sebening, Klovekorn, Meisner & Struck), pp 61-67. Deutches Her-zzentrum, Munchen.

Biomaterials 1980
Edited by G. D. Winter, D. F. Gibbons, and H. Plenk, Jr.
© 1982 John Wiley and Sons Ltd.

CHARACTERIZATION OF HIGH FLEX-LIFE POLYOLEFIN
IMPLANT ELASTOMER

J.B. Koeneman, R.A. Auerbach, D.B. Berry

Lord Corporation
Erie, Pennsylvania U.S.A.

SUMMARY

Dynamic mechanical property measurements were made on BION™ elastomer,
a high flex-life polyolefin implant material. The material was shown
to be highly damped and the elastic moduli increase with frequency.
The elastic moduli show a significant increase at mean strains over
40 percent. A phase transition at -30°F is indicated. To have a
meaningful comparative accelerated life test of elastomers, the effect
of the means of accelerating the test (mean strain, dynamic strain,
temperature) on the elastic properties must be considered. For viscoelastic materials, prototype testing which accurately simulates
service conditions is necessary.

INTRODUCTION

A relatively new elastomer has been used as the diaphragm for an
artificial heart and the flexible part of an artificial finger prosthesis. The material has been called Hexsyn™ or BION™ elastomer in
the literature. It is a stereoregular synthetic polyolefin and is
sulfur vulcanizable by virtue of a low level of residual unsaturation.
The exceptional flex-fatigue results of the previously-reported constant displacement (DeMattia) tests are probably due to the fully
saturated backbone and self-plasticizing nature of the pendant alkyl
chains.

To more fully characterize the material, dynamic mechanical measurements were made. Efforts are also being made to develop accelerated
fatigue life test methods for elastomers to be used in medical
devices. (McMillin et al, 1979, Kardos et al, 1979, Penn et al,
1979)

The viscoelastic property data contained in this report are necessary
to judge the validity of extrapolating the results of any accelerated
test to service performance.

623

EXPERIMENTAL PROCEDURE

The room temperature tests were performed on a motion-controlled servo-hydraulic test stand and a Gilmore Model 645 command/analysis digital computer. The test specimen shown in Figure 1 had two rectangles of the elastomer bonded between three pieces of metal in a double lap shear configuration. To profile the viscoelastic properties of the elastomer, 30 individual tests were run. Each test was conducted with a unique combination of frequency, mean amplitude, and dynamic amplitude parameters.

Analysis was performed within the Gilmore Model 645 analyzer by subjecting the motion and force signals first to conversion to digital form, then to Fourier analysis where the fundamentals of each were extracted. This method makes possible very accurate determination of the angle "delta", the phase angle between complex force and the motion which caused it. The tangent of this angle is the "loss factor". The moduli reported are based on the complex spring rate K^* and the angle delta, from which are derived K' and K''. These are in turn scaled for the geometry of the sample to arrive at the shear moduli G' and G''. All calculations were based on the fundamental frequency component of the complex force and motion; all higher harmonics were ignored. The effect of temperature on the dynamic properties was measured with a "Rheovibron" dynamic testing machine.

RESULTS

The effect of frequency on elastic modulus, G', damping modulus, G'', and loss factor, $\eta=G''/G'$, is shown in Figure 2. This test sequence had 0% mean strain and ±10% dynamic strain. The effect of mean strain on viscoelastic properties is shown in Figure 3 and the effect of dynamic strain range is shown in Figure 4. The Rheovibron temperature effect data is shown in Figure 5.

DISCUSSION

BION™ elastomer is a highly damped material. The increase in moduli with frequency as shown in Figure 2 is much more than for most elastomers. For example, the increase in G' between 1 Hz and 100 Hz is six times that of a standard natural rubber compound. This means that accelerating the fatigue life testing by increasing the rate of flexing applies a much higher stress on this material than on most other elastomers. Similarly, extrapolating high strain fatigue life data to actual service conditions can misrepresent this material because of the significant increase in elastic modulus with mean strain as shown in Figure 3. Unnotched, accelerated fatigue tests often go over 100% mean strain. The effect of dynamic strain amplitude on elastic properties must also be considered when comparing materials in a fatigue test. The decrease in elastic moduli values is shown in Figure 4. The variation of viscoelastic properties with temperature as shown in Figure 5 must be taken into consideration when comparing materials. Certainly, test temperatures below the peak in the E'' curve would not be appropriate.

Methods of accelerating life testing of elastomers are to, a) increase the static strain above service levels, b) increase the dynamic strain above service levels or c) increase or decrease the temperature from the service temperature. Before a meaningful comparison of materials can be made in any of these accelerated tests, a complete dynamic material property profile of each material must be made. The amount of acceleration (e.g. the increase in stress caused by an increase in stiffness of modulus) of each material can then be estimated.

High strain and accelerated frequency testing are often necessary to obtain results in a reasonable period of time. However, predictions of service life or ranking of materials in such tests may not be valid unless the effects of these variables on the dynamic moduli are measured and accounted for. A possible method of accelerating a life test without increasing strain or frequency is by introducing cuts in the material before testing. This assumes that service life is determined by flaw growth rather than flaw initiation.

For viscoelastic materials, prototype testing which accurately simulates service conditions is necessary.

<u>REFERENCES</u>

Kardos, J.L., Sanson, W.M. & Clark, R.E. (1979) Physical testing of polymers for use in circulatory assist devices. NIH, National Heart, Lung and Blood Institute, Devices and Technology Branch Contractor's Meeting program, pp 79-80.
McMillin, C.R., Orofino, T.A. & Shepperd, D.L. (1979) Physical testing of polymers. NIH, National Heart, Lung and Blood Institute, Devices and Technology Branch Contractor's Meeting program, p 81.
Penn, R.W. & McKenna, G.B. (1979) Physical testing of polymers for use in circulatory assist devices. NIH, National Heart, Lung and Blood Institute, Devices and Technology Branch Contractor's Meeting program, p 82.

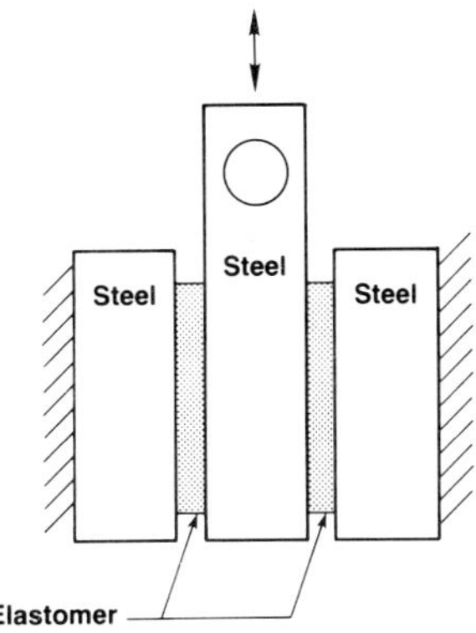

Figure 1. Test Specimen

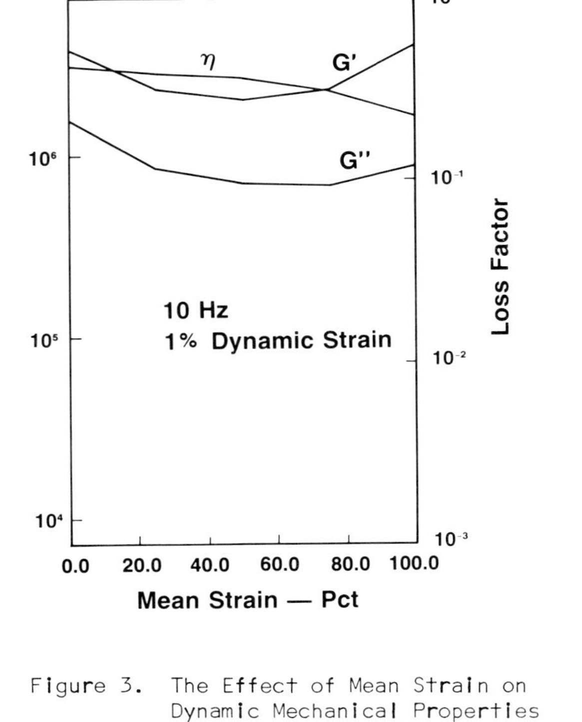

Figure 3.   The Effect of Mean Strain on Dynamic Mechanical Properties

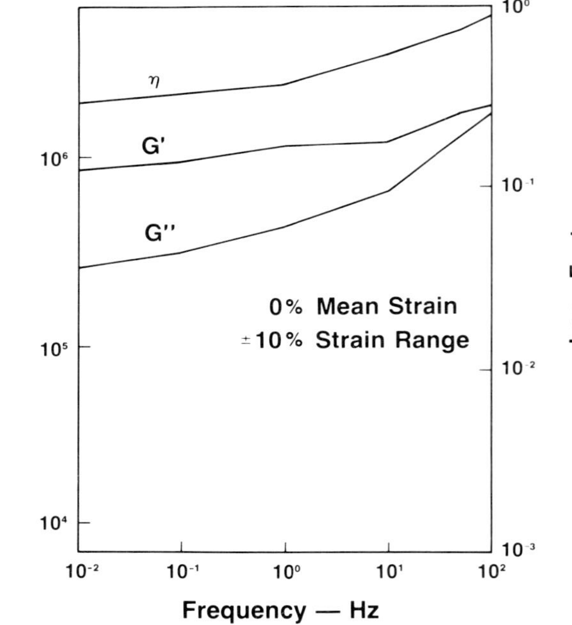

Figure 2.   The Effect of Frequency on Dynamic Mechanical Properties

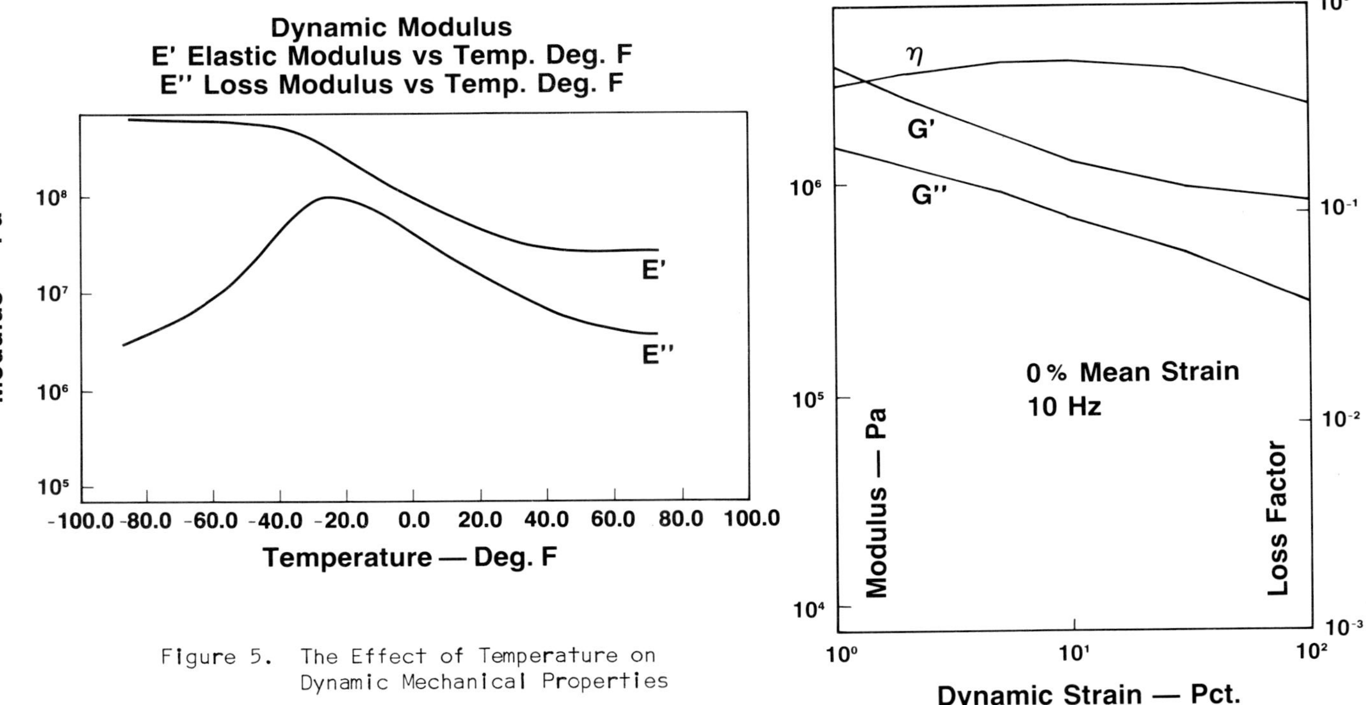

Figure 5.   The Effect of Temperature on Dynamic Mechanical Properties

Figure 4.   The Effect of Dynamic Strain on Dynamic Mechanical Properties

Biomaterials 1980
Edited by G. D. Winter, D. F. Gibbons, and H. Plenk, Jr.
© 1982 John Wiley and Sons Ltd.

MECHANICAL DURABILITY OF CANDIDATE ELASTOMERS
FOR BLOOD PUMP APPLICATIONS

G. B. McKenna and R. W. Penn
Polymer Science and Standards Division
National Bureau of Standards
Washington, D. C. 20234

SUMMARY

This paper describes a test methodology which we have developed for
the characterization of the durability of elastomers which are
candidate materials for blood pump applications. The testing approach
is based upon a cumulative damage rule which we have used to describe
the time dependent failure of glassy and semicrystalline polymers.
We are characterizing the lifetime behaviors of polyolefin, segmented
polyurethane and urethane-silicone copolymer elastomers which are
candidate materials for blood pump applications. In addition, work
is being done to characterize the durability of a standard butyl
rubber for use in interlaboratory comparisons with other labs working
on this contract. Uniaxial and equi-biaxial test results are reported.

INTRODUCTION

The mechanical durability of an elastomer is a critical factor in its
suitability for blood pump applications. In such applications an
elastomeric bladder is expected to undergo cyclic stress or strain
histories at a frequency of approximately 2 Hz for periods of several
years. Test methodologies for characterizing the mechanical durability of such materials do not exist. Based on previous work using
an additivity of (or cumulative) damage rule as a model to describe
time dependent failure of both glassy and semi-crystalline polymers
(Penn and McKenna, 1979; McKenna and Penn, 1980), we have developed
a useful methodology for describing the mechanical durability of
elastomers which are candidate materials for blood pump applications.

The concept of cumulative damage depends on the assumption that
material failure is the result of damage accumulation due to stress.
When the damage reaches a critical value failure occurs. The Bailey
(1939) criterion and the form of the rule which we will use assumes
that the rate at which damage accumulates is a function only of the
current stress, σ. Then the time to fail, t_B, is related to the
stress history, $\sigma(\xi)$, by the following equation:

$$\int_{o}^{t_B} \frac{d\xi}{\tau_B(\sigma(\xi))} = 1 \qquad (1)$$

where $\tau_B(\sigma)$ is the time to fail in constant stress experiments. Thus, each increment of time, $d\xi$ during which the load is $\sigma(\xi)$, is weighted inversely as the lifetime, $\tau_B(\sigma)$, which the specimen would have had under a constant stress, σ, and the sample should fail when the value of the integral reaches one.

Although our previous work has shown that this simple form of the additivity of damage rule has limited applicability as a tool for predicting material lifetime, the model does suggest that in assessing material durability one should examine three aspects of failure: a.) Failure times in static loading; b.) failure times in dynamic loading; and c.) Frequency dependence of failure times in fatigue.

MATERIALS AND METHODS

The elastomers which we are evaluating include a carbon black filled polyolefin rubber used by the Cleveland Clinic[*] in their artificial heart program, a urethane-silicone copolymer which is manufactured by Avco Everett Laboratories[*] under the trade name Avcothane 51[*], and a segmented polyurethane elastomer which is known by the trade name Biomer[*]. In addition, we have been testing a carbon black filled butyl rubber which was manufactured in our laboratories as an inter-laboratory control material. All materials were obtained in the form of sheets. Nominal sheet thickness ranged from 0.5 to 1 mm depending upon material. The reader is referred to Penn, et.al (1979) for further description of the materials.

Both uniaxial and equibiaxial testing have been used to evaluate the candidate elastomers. The testing apparatus and methods are described in detail in earlier work (Penn, et.al., 1979). Uniaxial creep experiments were conducted by hanging weights from samples directly or through a system of pulleys. Uniaxial fatigue experiments were conducted using a servo-hydraulic testing machine. Sinusoidally varying loads were applied to dumbbell specimens at frequencies of 0.002, 0.01 and 0.09 Hz.

Equibiaxial static data were obtained by using constant regulated air pressure to inflate a circular membrane which was clamped at the edge. Biaxial fatigue testing was conducted by applying a pulsatile air pressure to such a clamped membrane by means of a motor driven spool valve. The pressure varied between zero and a peak value at a frequency of 3 Hz. The reduced pressure, which is the applied pressure divided by membrane thickness, was used as the stress variable.

---

[*]Certain commercial materials and equipment are identified in this paper in order to specify adequately the experimental procedure. In no case does such identification imply recommendation or endorsement by the National Bureau of Standards, nor does it imply necessarily the best available for the purpose.

RESULTS AND DISCUSSION

Uniaxial failure data has been obtained for all four elastomers.
Static failure results for the butyl and the polyolefin rubbers in
air at 23°C are presented in Figure 1. The lines represent least
squares fits to the data of the form

$$\ln t_B = A + B\sigma \tag{2}$$

where t_B is the time to fail, σ is the stress and A and B are the
intercept and slope respectively. As can be seen from Figure 1, the
lifetime of the butyl rubber at high stresses is longer than that of
the polyolefin rubber, while at low stresses the opposite is true.
We also note that the scatter in the polyolefin failure time data is
much greater than it is for the butyl rubber.

Figure 2 shows uniaxial static test results for the urethane-silicone
copolymer and the segmented polyurethane elastomer. The results for
the urethane-silicone material were obtained at both 23°C and 37°C in
a .15N saline solution. Limited results at 23°C in saline indicate
that there is little difference between behavior in air and saline
for the segmented polyurethane. Unlike the butyl and polyolefin
rubbers, the data for the urethane-silicone and segmented polyurethane
materials do not fit a curve of the form of equation (2). The lines
in Figure 2 are "eyeball" fits to the data. The urethane-silicone
copolymer shows shorter lifetimes at the same stresses than does the
segmented urethane. Both materials show longer lifetimes than do the
polyolefin or butyl rubbers.

The polyolefin and butyl rubbers were tested in zero-tension sinsoidal
fatigue in air at 23°C. The lifetimes under cyclic loading conditions
were lower than both the predictions obtained by integrating equation
(1) and the static lifetimes. Lifetime also varied with test
frequency, contrary to what is predicted by the cumulative damage
model.

To illustrate the frequency dependence of the fatigue lifetimes, we
fit the fatigue data to a multiple regression model of the form

$$\ln t_B = A + B\ln \omega + C\sigma \tag{3}$$

Statistical methods were used to test two hypotheses: that for a given
peak stress and independent of test frequency either 1) fatigue
failure occurs at a constant time (from equation 1) or 2) fatigue
failure occurs at a constant number of cycles (cycle dependent
fatigue). The coefficients from the model of equation (3) are shown
with their standard errors in Table 1. If fatigue lifetime were
constant, as predicted from the additivity of damage model, then the
coefficient B would be zero. If, on the other hand, fatigue were a
"cycle dependent process" B would be -1. Based on a student's "t"
test both hypotheses can be rejected at the 97.5% confidence level.
Thus, the frequency dependence of the behavior of the butyl and

polyolefin rubbers is intermediate between that predicted by the
"cumulative damage" and "cycle dependent" fatigue models. An
important aspect of the fact that the frequency dependence of lifetime is intermediate between the cumulative damage model represented
by equation (1) and that described by cycle dependent fatigue is that
if an accelerated test method depends upon high test frequency to
accelerate failure, it will over estimate the lifetime at lower
frequencies.

TABLE 1   Time to Fail Parameters for Uniaxial Dynamic Tests

Parameter[*]	Polyolefin Rubber, N = 35		NBS Butyl Rubber, N = 11	
	Value	E_s	Value	E_s
A	13.244	$\pm.928$	7.41	$\pm.187$
B	-.748	$\pm.107$	-.644	$\pm.519$
C	-.755	$\pm.101$	--	--

[*]Fit to $\ln t_B = A + B\ln \omega + C\sigma$, where t_B is the time to fail in
seconds, ω is the frequency in Hz, σ is the peak stress in MPa, E_s
is the standard error of the coefficient and N is the number of
data points.

Biaxial static test data have been obtained for the NBS butyl and
polyolefin rubbers at room temperature in air. Biaxial dynamic data
have been obtained for the NBS butyl rubber and for the urethane-
silicone copolymer at 23°C and 37°C in .15N saline solution. Dynamic
data have also been obtained for the polyolefin rubber at 23°C in
.15N saline solution.

The static test results are depicted in a plot of the logarithm of
time to fail vs. reduced pressure in Figure 3. The lines represent
least squares fits to the regression model:

$$\ln t_B = A + B(P/h) \tag{4}$$

where t_B is the time to fail in seconds and P/h is the reduced
pressure in MPa/m. These results indicate that under static loading
and at 23°C in air the polyolefin rubber has a longer lifetime than
does the butyl rubber over the range of reduced pressures applied.
Again the scatter of the polyolefin rubber test data is greater than
that of the butyl rubber data.

The dynamic (fatigue) test results are depicted in Figure 4. The
data were fitted to equation (4) using linear regression analysis
and the resulting parameters are shown in Table 2. Several significant features can be observed from the results:

1. The slopes are not significantly different at 23 and 37°C for the
two materials for which data are available. This fact allows us to
calculate activation energies for the fatigue failure process. We
obtained activation energies of 22 and 25 kcal/mole for the butyl and
urethane-silicone copolymer elastomers, respectively.

2. The lifetimes are very much shorter in dynamic testing than in static testing when they are compared at the same reduced pressure. This conflicts with the simple additive damage rule.

3. The deviations of the logarithm of the failure times from the regression line of equation (4) give an estimate of the probability distribution function for failure times. At the 95% confidence level the distribution of failure times in fatigue testing is narrower than in static testing. This is consistent with the behavior observed by Halpin and Polley (1967) in a filled SBR rubber.

TABLE 2   Regression Parameters for Biaxial Tests[*]

	$\underline{A}$	$\underline{B}$	$\underline{E_s}$	$\underline{N}$
Static, 23°C				
NBS Butyl	24.62	−.154	+.863	25
Polyolefin	27.20	−.118	+1.55	17
Fatigue, 23°C				
NBS Butyl	19.68	−.153	+.619	33
Polyolefin	20.94	−.110	+1.01	19
US Copolymer	27.79	−.136	+.980	4
Fatigue, 37°C				
NBS Butyl	18.33	−.156	+.491	10
US Copolymer	22.52	−.104	+1.34	7

[*] Fit to $\ln t_B = A + B\, P/h$, where t_B is the time to fail in seconds and P/h is the reduced pressure in MPa/m. E_s is the standard error from the regression line and N is the number of data points.

<u>ACKNOWLEDGEMENTS</u>

This work was supported by the National Heart, Lung and Blood Institute, National Institutes of Health, under contract No. Y01-HV-8-0003.

<u>REFERENCES</u>

Bailey, J. (1939) "An Attempt to Correlate Some Tensile Strength Measurements on Glass: III". <u>Glassy Industry, 20</u>, 94-99.

Halpin, J. C. and Polley, H.W. (1967), Observations on the Fracture of Viscoelastic Bodies. <u>Journal of Composite Materials, 1</u>, 65-81.

McKenna, G.B. and Penn, R.W. (1980), "Time Dependent Failure Behavior of Poly(methyl methacrylate) and Polyethylene", <u>Polymer 21</u>, 213-220.

Penn, R.W. and McKenna, G.B. (1979) "Fatigue Effects in Poly(methyl methacrylate)", in <u>Durability of Macromolecular Materials</u>, ed. by R. K. Eby, ACS Symposium Series, 95, ACS, Washington, D.C. pp. 331-339.

Penn,R.W., McKenna, G. B., and Khoury, F.A. (1979), "Physical Testing of Polymers for Use in Circulatory Assist Devices", Second Annual Report to NHLBI, Contract No. Y01-HV-8-0003, Octo., 1979.

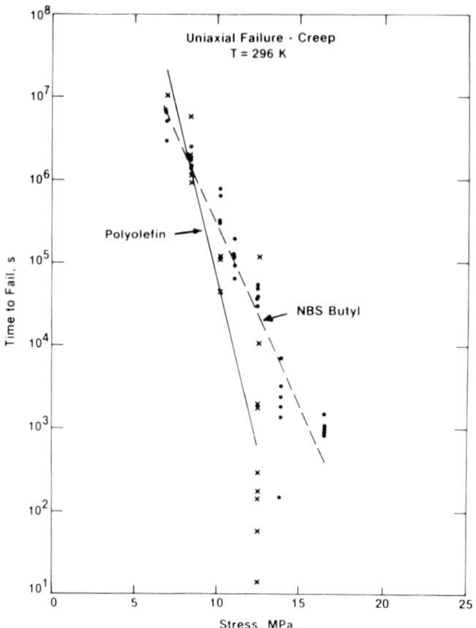

Figure 1. Time-to Fail vs. Stress
in Uniaxial Creep for Butyl and
Polyolefin Rubbers. Tests were
conducted in air at 23°C.

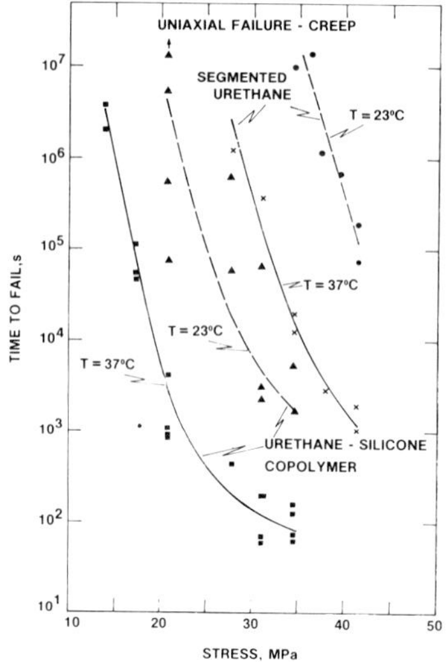

Figure 2. Time-to-Fail vs. Stress
in Uniaxial Creep for Segmented
Polyurethane and Urethane-Silicone
Elastomers. Urethane-Silicone Copolymer: (▲)23°C in .15N Saline;
(■)37°C in .15N Saline. Segmented
Polyurethane: (●)23°C in air;
(✕)37°C in .15N Saline.

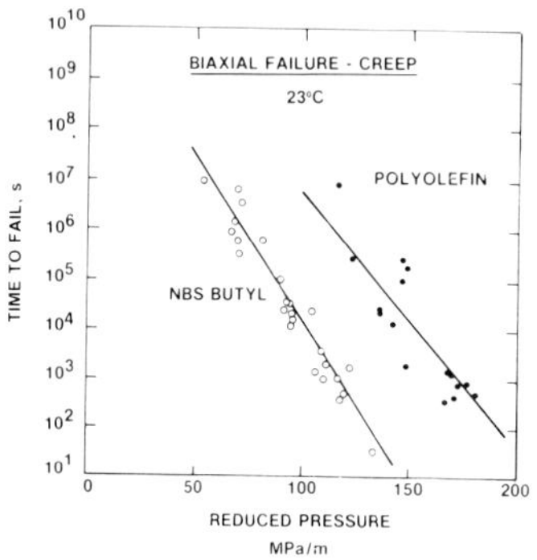

Figure 3. Time-to-Fail vs.
Reduced Pressure in Equi-biaxial
Creep for Butyl and Polyolefin
Rubbers. Tests were conducted
in air at 23°C.

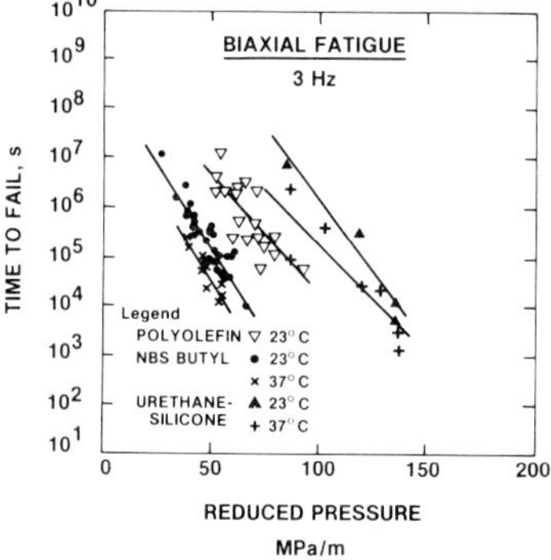

Figure 4. Time-to-Fail vs. Peak
Reduced Pressure in Equi-biaxial
Fatigue Experiments for Three
Candidate Elastomers. Tests were
conducted in .15N saline solution.

PART 3

SPECIAL APPLICATIONS OF BIOMATERIALS

Dressings and structures

Biomaterials 1980
Edited by G. D. Winter, D. F. Gibbons, and H. Plenk, Jr.
© 1982 John Wiley and Sons Ltd.

ARTIFICIAL SKIN DESIGN: PERMANENT CLOSURE
OF FULL THICKNESS SKIN WOUNDS

I.V. Yannas and J.F. Burke

Fibers and Polymers Laboratories
Department of Mechanical Engineering,
Massachusetts Institute of Technology,
Cambridge, MA 02139
Shriners Burns Institute and
Harvard Medical School, Boston, MA 02114

SUMMARY

We have achieved permanent closure of full-thickness skin wounds in
guinea pigs without use of an autograft. The results of our extensive experiments show that single application of a cell-free bilayer
polymeric membrane closes up the full-thickness wound, reliably controlling both fluid loss and infection. The membrane consists of a
top layer of conventional crosslinked silicone elastomer bonded onto
a highly porous layer fabricated from a novel collagen/glycosamino-
glycan graft copolymer. Results of extensive animal studies show
that the graft is not rejected, nor does it require removal or other
traumatic manipulation. Instead, the silicone layer is spontaneously
ejected by the advancing epidermis while the collagen-glycosamino-
glycan layer is metabolically replaced in 40-50 days by epithelialized
scar tissue. Preliminary studies with several human subjects, all
victims of deep burns, have shown very encouraging results.

INTRODUCTION

Over the past 10 years we have undertaken the design of a membrane
for treatment of patients with extensive full-thickness skin loss.
The design has been divided in two stages, respectively corresponding
to the short-term and long-term needs of the patient. Stage 1 is a
wound closure which prevents bacterial infection and controls moisture
loss to physiological levels without requiring surgical removal or
other traumatic manipulation. Stage 2 membranes are advanced versions
of the above, capable of controlling scar formation. Stage 1 membranes have been extensively studied with an animal model and to a
limited extent recently with humans. This paper outlines the preliminary performance characteristics of Stage 1 membranes. Work is
in progress to complete the design of Stage 2.

The physics of wound closure must be carefully taken into account in
the design of Stage 1. Efficient wetting of the woundbed by the graft
has been cited (Yannas and Burke, 1980) as a prerequisite of an interface which remains free of infection. An early bond of finite

635

strength between graft and woundbed assures continuing intimacy of
contact over the entire wound area, while the graft perimeter may
be sutured onto the woundbed. To achieve intimate contact it is necessary to control the surface energy, modulus of elasticity, thickness
and moisture permeability of the suturable membrane within certain
bounds (Yannas et al., 1977). It is also necessary to remove weak
boundary layers potentially arising from necrotic tissue which has
not been excised.

Once intimate contact between graft and woundbed has been achieved,
attention focuses on the biochemical interactions between the apposed
surfaces. These interactions predominantly result from migrations of
mesenchymal cells (primarily fibroblasts and endothelial cells) in a
direction normal to the plane of the graft and of epithelial cells
parallel to the plane of the graft (Figure 1).

MATERIALS AND METHODS

Bilayer membranes (Figure 1) were fabricated by the following procedure (Yannas et al., 1975. Yannas et al., 1980). Insoluble particles
of bovine hide collagen were dispersed in 0.05M acetic acid, pH 3.
An acidic solution of chondroitin 6-sulfate, a glycosaminoglycan
(GAG), was added dropwise to the stirred collagen dispersion until the
desired level of collagen/GAG ratio was reached. GAG addition caused
precipitation of collagen out of the acid medium into a fibrous mass,
which was homogenized. The homogenized dispersion of coprecipitated
collagen/GAG particles (ave. diam. 120 μm) was directly freezed-dried
to a highly porous solid (Dagalakis et al., 1980) and it was then
lightly crosslinked by exposure to a vacuum oven at 105°C. This
treatment also amounted to a first antibacterial treatment. A room-
temperature-curing silicone polymer (Dow Corning Silastic Medical
Adhesive Silicone Type A) was then spread over the membrane, the
thickness of the silicone layer, usually 0.3 mm or less, adjusted
to provide a bilayer membrane with the desired flexural rigidity.
The bilayer was then immersed in a glutaraldehyde bath where it was
crosslinked additionally while also being subjected to a second antibacterial treatment. Following exhaustive rinsing in sterile physiological saline to remove traces of free glutaraldehyde, the sterile
bilayer membrane was stored in 70/30 isopropanol/water or in the
freeze-dried state until ready to be grafted.

Using methods which have been described elsewhere (Yannas et al.,
1980) in detail, it is possible to determine several structural
parameters of the lower layer. This membrane is a collagen-GAG graft
copolymer, bound GAG content 8.2 ± 0.8%-wt., average molecular weight
between crosslinks 12750 ± 3300, lattice order of collagen fibers
currently under study, pore volume fraction about 95% and mean pore
size 50 ± 20 μm. Bilayer membranes currently in use have Young's
moduli in the range 7-40 x 10^4 N/m^2 with moisture permeabilities
ranging between 1-10 mg/cm^2/hr (values obtained in hydrated state).

Animal skin grafting studies were performed with female white Hartley

guinea pigs weighing 300-400 g each. The grafting operation was
carried out under aseptic conditions. Full-thickness skin down to,
but not including, the panniculus carnosus was excised from the back
of the anesthetized animal over an area 3 x 1.5 cm and a segment of
bilayer membrane was placed on the woundbed and sutured in place with
ten nylon stitches. The graft was covered with a 10-cm Elastoplast
bandage onto which a sterile gauze pad had been attached.

Two types of graft controls were commonly used in these studies.
The first was an allograft. The second was an ungrafted wound, prepared identically as above, but covered with a piece of sterile vas-
eline impregnated gauze (Xeroform, Chesebrough Ponds, Greenwich,
Conn.) prior to application of the remainder of the dressing. The
gauze was changed approximately every four days. Animal wounds were
carefully unbandaged and inspected ever 3-7 days for infection and
for exudation. The geometry of the wound was recorded photographic-
ally and a new dressing was applied. Specimens for histopathological
examination were prepared using standard procedures and were stained
with Mayer's hematoxylin, counterstained with eosin, and mounted for
viewing.

Human subjects were grafted with segments of the bilayer membrane
following primary excision of burned eschar. Techniques previously
described with autografting (Burke et al., 1974) were generally used.
Grafts were applied on the excised surface, free from devitalized
tissue, on which meticulous hemostasis had been obtained. Following
placement on the woundbed, grafts were carefully sutured under slight
tension, avoiding wrinkling of the thin membrane.

RESULTS AND DISCUSSION

<u>Grafting of full-thickness wounds with guinea pigs.</u> Results obtained
by grafting over 80 animals showed clear differences between the performance of the bilayer membrane described here and that of the allograft. By Day 14 the allograft was generally well on its way to being
rejected as the wound was undergoing strong contraction. By contrast,
wounds covered with the bilayer membrane showed little contraction and
no evidence of rejection. Histopathological slides of the
region grafted with the bilayer membrane also showed no evidence of
rejection over the entire course of the grafting experiments (up to
400 days).

An interesting and reproducible finding which is currently under scru-
tiny is the 10-day delay in onset of wound contraction which was
observed with wounds grafted with the bilayer membrane compared to the
ungrafted controls. The result amounts to a delay in "half-life" of
the wound (the time necessary for the wound area to contract to 50% of
the original area) from about 12 days with the ungrafted controls to
about 30 days with grafted wounds.

The histopathological evidence is that epidermal migration consistently occurs over, rather than under, the bottom layer of the

bilayer graft. Coverage of the bottom layer of the graft by the
advancing epidermis is complete by Day 30 to 40. The top (silicone)
layer of the graft is spontaneously ejected at about the same time,
revealing a scar, while the histopathological evidence clearly indicates completion of epithelialization over the entire area.

Experiments with over 80 animals have shown that closure of 3 x 1.5 cm
full-thickness wounds with a single piece of the bilayer membrane
described above provides reliable protection against infection and
fluid loss. Preliminary experiments with animals have shown that
much larger wounds can be effectively epithelialized by innoculation
of autologous epidermal cells, previously cultured _in vitro_ for about
ten days or less, just below the silicone layer of the sutured graft.
This finding suggests that this additional manipulation of innoculat-
ing our membranes with cultured autologous epidermal cells extends
indefinitely the area of skin loss which can be permanently closed
with the bilayer membrane in its present state of development.

Grafting of human subjects. Seven extensively burned (50 to 95% body
area) human subjects, five to twelve-year-old males and females, were
grafted with rectangular pieces of membrane ranging from 5 x 10 to 15
x 25 cm (Figure 2). The grafts remained in place from 15 to 40 days.
During this period no infection or inflammation were noted. Occasional lifting of the edge of the graft was treated as with an autograft,
by cutting off. Whenever the graft was next to intact epidermis the
epidermal edge migrated between the two layers of the membranes over
a distance of a few mm. At about the 40-day level, the lower layer
of the membrane described above had been apparently biodegraded
entirely without sign of inflammation while the top (silicone) layer
became loose and separated off. Due to the limited availability of
the bilayer membrane at this stage of our work, we have grafted so
far up to 4% only of total individual body surface with it.

On the basis of these preliminary studies it appears that the bilayer
membrane described above performs clinically at a level clearly
superior to that attained with pigskin, which is normally removed
after 4-9 days of use, or cadaver skin (allograft), which is often
removed after a period of 15-25 days. Work is currently under way
to increase the availability of the bilayer membrane and to extned
its use clinically to the permanent closure of the largest full-
thickness wounds.

ACKNOWLEDGEMENTS

We thank Dr. R.L. Trelstad for useful discussions of the histopathological evidence as well as Dr. M. Warpehoski, Mr. E. Skrabut and
Mr. P. Stasikelis for preparing most of the membranes used in the
work reported here and collecting the data on most of the animal
experiments. This work has been partly supported by the Department
of Mechanical Engineering, MIT (H.H. Richardson, Head) and partly by
the National Institutes of Health (Grant GM 23946).

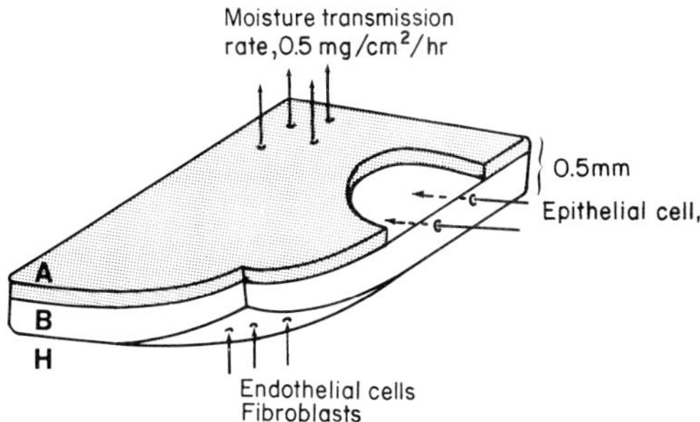

Fig. 1. Schematic representation of bilayer membrane
indicating the flux of moisture and cells, originating
with the host (H), through layers A (silicone) and B
(collagen-GAG).

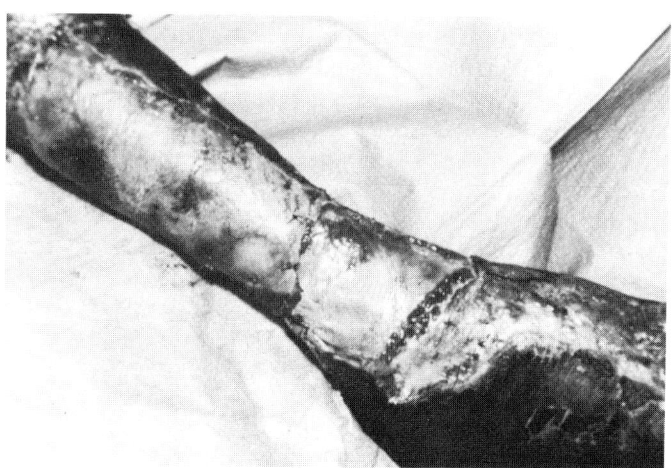

Fig. 2. Closure of full-thickness skin wound, resulting
from burn, in a 9-year-old human male. Age of graft: 18 days.

REFERENCES

Burke, J.F., Bondoc, C.C. & Quinby, W.C., (1974) Primary Burn Excision
and Immediate Grafting. A Method of Shortening Illness, J. Trauma
14, 389-394.
Dagalakis, N., Flink, J., Stasikelis, P., Burke, J.F. & Yannas, I.V.,
(1980) Design of an Artificial Skin. Part III. Control of Pore
Structure. J. Biomed. Mat. Res., 14, 511-528.
Yannas, I.V., Burke, J.F., Gordon, P.L. & Huang, C., (1977) Multilayer
Membrane Useful as Synthetic Skin, US Patent 4,060,081.
Yannas, I.V., Burke, J.F., Huang, C. & Gordon, P.L., (1975)
Suppression of In Vivo Degradability and of Immunogenicity of Collagen
by Reaction with Glycosaminoglycans, Polymer Preprints, Pol. Chem.
Div. Amer. Chem. Soc. 16(2), 209-214.
Yannas, I.V. & J.F. Burke, (1980) Design of an Artificial Skin.
Part I. Design Principles. J. Biomed. Mater. Res. 14, 65-81.
Yannas, I.V., Burke, J.F., Gordon, P.L., Huang, C. & Rubenstein, R.H.,
(1980) Design of an Artificial Skin. Part II. Control of Chemical
Composition. J. Biomed. Mat. Res. 14, 107-131.

Biomaterials 1980
Edited by G. D. Winter, D. F. Gibbons, and H. Plenk, Jr.
© 1982 John Wiley and Sons Ltd.

A COMPARATIVE STUDY OF TEMPORARY
SKIN COVERS ON CONTAMINATED WOUNDS
AND BURNS: CONTROL OF INFECTION,
ADHERENCE AND EFFECT OF ADDITIONAL
TOPICAL ANTISEPTICS

W. Mutschler, C. Burri, L. Claes,
R. Frankenhauser and E. Plank

Dep. of Emergency and Plastic and
Reconstructive Surgery,
University of Ulm, D-7900 Ulm, G.F.R.

SUMMARY

The result of different skin dressings on the wound
healing was tested on infected wounds and burns. Infected wounds were made by circular excision on the back of
pigs and infection with 10^8 Pseudomonas aeruginosa. Full
thickness burns were set using a heated steel stamp. The
wounds were covered with polyurethane foam laminated to
a PTFE film, microporous polyvinylalcohol foam, lyophilised pig skin or cotton compresses. The main differences between the dressings concerned (i) the epithelisation, which was more complete under polyurethane foam
and polyvinylalcohol foam as compared to lyophilised
pig skin and cotton compresses (ii) the bacterial contamination which was significantly lower in wounds covered
with polyvinylalcohol foam (iii) the adherence of the
dressings to the wound surfaces which was 2 to 3 times
higher for polyvinylalcohol foam than for polyurethane
foam and cotton compresses. The adherence was measured
by determination of the tensile forces necessary to tear
the dressings free of infected wounds of rats. The bacterial contamination of Pseudomonas aeruginosa infected
skin defects of rats could be further reduced when
polyvinylalcohol foam was moistened with different local
antiseptics, namely Isopropanol-quaternary-Ammonium-
compound, PVP-Iodine or Taurolin.

INTRODUCTION

Temporary skin dressings are designed to cleanse wounds
and stimulate good granulation tissue, to prevent or
control bacterial colonization of the wound and to avoid
excessive loss of fluid (Tavis et al., 1978). Today they

641

are not only used in the treatment of full thickness
burns but also as short term coverage on granulating
surfaces, infected wounds or infected open fractures.

In the present study the wound healing of infected
wounds and burns was compared in an animal test using
different skin dressings. The cleansing effect of these
different skin dressings was correlated with their
adherence to the surface of the wounds. Additionally we
tested, whether the bacterial numbers in infected wounds
could be reduced using a combination of topical antiseptics and synthetic skin dressings.

<u>MATERIALS AND METHODS</u>

Polyurethane foam laminated to Polytetrafluorethylene
film (Epigard[R], Parke-Davis, Detroit, USA), microporous
polyvinylalcohol foam (PVA; Coldex[R], Temca, Nürnberg,
F.R.G.) and lyophilised pig skin (Corethium[R], Ethicon,
Hamburg, F.R.G.) were compared with regard to wound
healing and prevention or lowering of bacterial contamination. Cotton compresses (DIN 61630, Hartmann,
Heidenheim, F.R.G.) served as control. Each of 10 pigs
received 10 full thickness burns with a diameter of
5 cm on the back by impressing a steel stamp with a
temperature of 800°C for 10 seconds. After 4 days the
necrotic tissue was excised to the muscle fascia. The
4 different skin dressings were then sutured in pairs.
To generate infected wounds 10 skin defects were set
by 5 cm circular excisions to the fascia on the backs
of 10 pigs. Each wound was infected with 10^{8} colony
forming units of Pseudomonas aeruginosa in 0,1 ml
physiological saline. In both series of experiments
the skin dressings were changed every 2 days. The wound
areas were measured every 2 days over a period of 18
days. For histological examinations 5 biopsies per pig
were taken after 2, 4, 12 and 18 days, fixed in 3,5 %
formaline and imbedded in paraffin. 5 µm slices were
stained with hematoxylin eosin. Bacteriological evaluations were performed after 4, 8, 12 and 18 days using
wet swabs which were rolled once over the total wound
area. Bacteria were eluted from the swabs and the number of colony forming units was determined on blood
agar plates.

To establish baseline adherence values for synthetic
dressings on infected wounds, a method was devised to
quantitate the adherence using a rat model. In 48 rats,
skin defects of 3 x 5 cm were inoculated with 10^7 Pseudomonas aeruginosa and covered 24 hours later, when the
infection was established, with cotton compresses,
Epigard[R] or PVA. The dressings were kept in place with
wound clips. The force necessary to tear the dressings
free was investigated after 2 or 4 days. To do this,
the necks of rats were fixed in a special clamp, which
presented the covers at a 180° angle to the tearing
force. The posterior ends of the dressings were freed
from tissue and attached to a material testing machine
by means of a second clamp. The covers were drawn in an
anterior-posterior direction with a constant velocity
of 60 mm/min. The tensile force was directly measured
and plotted on a x-y-writer. Thus maximal tensile forces as well as the energy needed to tear the dressing
free could be calculated.

To prepare infected wounds more quickly for grafting we
tried to combine the cleansing effect of synthetic skin
covers with the bactericidal effect of different local
antiseptics. Because of its open porous structure PVA
was highly suitable for continuous moistening of wounds.
A dorsal 3 x 3 cm infected surface wound on 120 rats
was established by inoculation of the panniculus carnosus with 10^7 P. aeruginosa. Twenty-four hours later
the greenish purulent tissue was covered with PVA and
soaked with either an Isopropanol -quaternary-Ammonium-
compound, (Avitracid[R], Adroka AG, Basel, Swiss), PVP-
Iodine (Braunol[R], Braun, Melsungen, F.R.G.), Taurolin
1 % (Drainasept[R], Geistlich, Wolhusen, Swiss) or physiological saline as a control. Wounds were moistened
every 6 or 12 hours and the PVA was changed every 2
days. Rats were sacrificed after 2, 6 or 10 days. Then
part of the panniculus carnosus and the underlying
muscle tissue was homogenized separately and bacterial
colonies were counted after 24 hours of growth on agar
plates. Another part of each tissue was examined histologically.

<u>RESULTS</u>

In pig experiments, the results are very similar for
both infected wounds and burns: Using PVA and Epigard[R]
about 70 - 90 % of wound areas were reduced and epithelialized after 18 days as compared to lyophilised pig
skin and cotton compresses where wound areas showed an
epithelisation of only 50 - 60 %. Histologically a cell
rich granulation tissue could be observed beginning
from the 4th day. On its surface detritus from necrotic
cells and clusters of bacteria could be seen. These
contaminations which disturb the wound healing were
removed by the two synthetic dressings thus favoring a
good epithelisation but not by lyophilised pig skin and
cotton compresses. With the synthetic skin covers
epithelisation started at the 8th day and was nearly
complete at the 18th day, accompagnied by an increase
of fibrillogenesis and growth of small vessels in the
granulation tissue. Bacteriological investigations
showed that Staphylococcus epidermitis was predominant
in burns while infected wounds predominantly contained
Pseudomonas aeruginosa up to the 4th day. After 4 days
Pseudomonas aeruginosa disappeared and Staphylococcus
epidermitis predominated. The development of bacterial
numbers in burns is demonstrated in figure 1. The statistical significance of the different bacterial numbers in dependence of the skin dressing used was proved
by orthogonal linear contrast variance analysis. Only
wounds covered with PVA showed significant lower bacterial numbers when compared with the other skin dressings ($p < 0.001$). Between Epigard[R] lyophilized pig skin
and cotton compresses no significant differences could
be observed. Similar results were obtained with infected wounds. Only wounds covered with PVA showed significant lower amounts of bacterial numbers when compared
with the other skin dressings ($p < 0.05$) (data not shown).

The wound cleansing effect of skin dressings has been
suggested to depend on the adherence of the dressings
to the surface of the wound, thus providing a framework penetrated by bacteria and fibroblasts (Tavis et
al., 1978). Therefore we examined whether the tensile
forces necessary to tear the dressings free were
different.
Median values of the maximal tensile forces after 2 or
4 days were 10.48 Newton (N) or 7.22 N for compresses,
9.22 N or 4.3 N for Epigard[R] and 23.58 or 24.6 N for

PVA (Fig. 2). The significant ($p < 0.001$) difference between the tensile forces of PVA as compared to Epigard[R] and compresses corresponded well to the macroscopic aspect: Tissue was adherent to PVA and not adherent to compresses or Epigard[R], where an uncleansed wound remained.

How bacterial numbers are reduced in infected wounds by a combination of PVA and 3 different topical antiseptics was the aim of the third series of experiments. Figure 3 shows, that within 6 or 10 days all antiseptics significantly reduced the bacterial number. Taurolin gave the best result within 10 days. However, the high numbers of P. aeruginosa demonstrate that the tissue was still infected and not suitable for grafting. On the other hand, on the second day, wounds treated only with physiological saline, had a lower bacterial content as compared to PVP-Iodine or Taurolin treated wounds.
Our impression was, that a rapid evaporation of the antiseptics was responsible for both observations. Therefore we moistened PVA every 6 hours over 2 days and got a remarkable reduction of bacteria (Fig. 4). In contrast, saline treated wounds showed an increase of bacteria, a consequence of increased humidity favouring bacterial growth.
The underlying muscles contained about 10^7 P.aeruginosa per g tissue if treated with physiological saline over 2 days, and only 10^3 to 10^4 bacteria per g tissue if treated with Isopropanol-quaternary-Ammonium, PVP-Iodine or Taurolin. This is below the "critical point" of 10^5 organisms per g tissue for grafting (Saymen et al., 1973).

DISCUSSION

The wound cleansing effect of skin dressings most likely depends on a regular removal of wound exudate and the adherence of the materials to the wound surface, providing a framework in which fibroblasts and bacteria can penetrate (Tavis et al., 1978). In the present study we compared the efficacy of different skin dressings (Corethium[R], Epigard[R], Coldex[R], cotton compresses) on infected wounds and burns in an animal test. The main differences between the skin dressings concerned (i) the epithelisation of wounds, which was more complete under Coldex[R] and Epigard[R] as compared to

Corethium[R] or cotton compresses (ii) the bacterial
contamination, which was significantly lower in wounds
covered with Coldex[R] than in wounds covered with the
other skin dressings (iii) the adherence of the skin
dressings to the wound surfaces, which was 2 to 3 times
higher for Coldex[R] than for Epigard[R] or cotton compresses.
These results are consistent with the hypothesis that
the adherence of skin dressings might be important for
their wound cleansing effect.
The bacterial contamination of skin defects of rats
could be reduced further when Coldex[R] was humidified
with different topic antiseptics. So an additional
frequent moistening with antiseptics may accelerate
the preparation for grafting in severely infected
wounds (Burleson and Eiseman, 1973). Since the adherence of Coldex[R] to the wound surfaces was greatly
reduced by moistening with antiseptics the removal of
wound exsudates was decreased. To overcome this disadvantage we recommend an alternated therapy of infected wounds using skin dressings moistened with antiseptics followed by skin dressings without antiseptics.
Preliminary clinical observations using a combination
of Coldex[R] and Coldex[R] humidified with Taurolin gave
positive results.

REFERENCES

Burleson, R., & Eiseman, B. (1973): Effect of skin
dressings and topical antibiotics on healing of partial
thickness skin wounds in rats. Surg.Gyn.Obstet. 136,
958-960.
Saymen, D.G., Nathan, P., Holder, J.A., Hill, E.O. &
Macmillan, B.G. (1973): Control of surface wound infection: Skin versus synthetic grafts. Appl.Microbiol.,
25, 921-934.
Tavis, M.J., Thornton, J., Danet, R. & Bartlett, R.H.,
(1978): Current status of skin substitutes. Surg.Clin.
North Am. 58, 1233-1248.

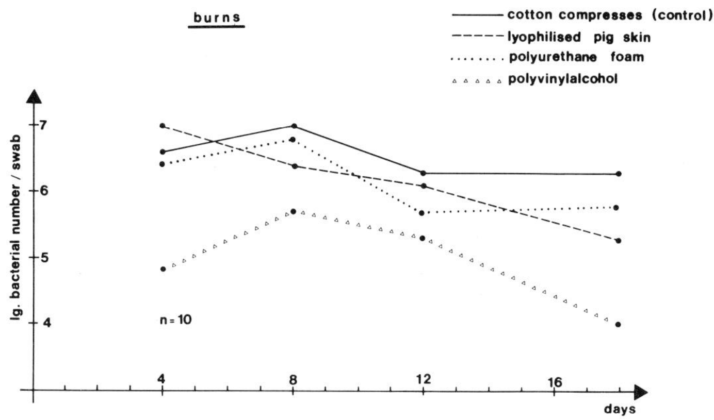

Fig. 1. Mean $\langle \log_{10} \rangle$ bacterial count per swab 4,8, 12 and 18 days after excision of burns.

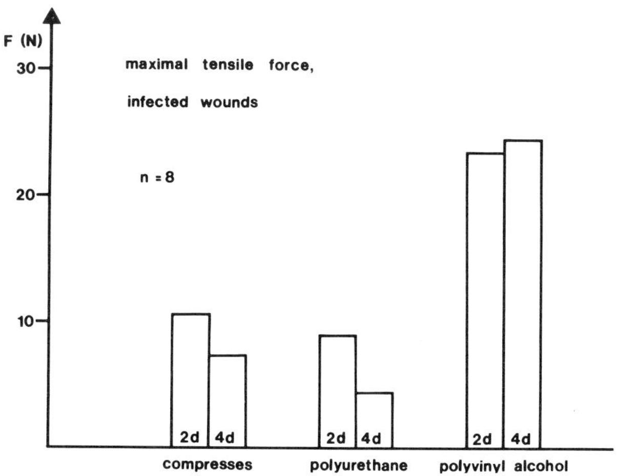

Fig. 2. Median values of maximal tensile forces after 2 or 4 days, infected wounds.

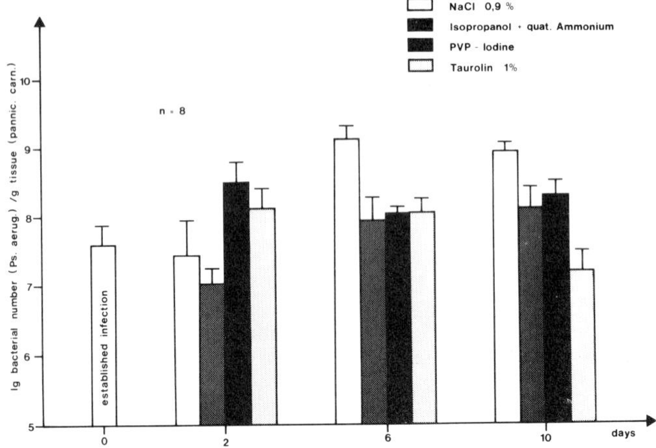

Fig. 3. Mean Pseudomonas aeruginosa content per g panniculus carnosus (mean $\langle \log_{10} \rangle$ $\pm$ s.d.), 2, 6 or 10 days after soaking PVA every 12 h with three different topical antiseptics.

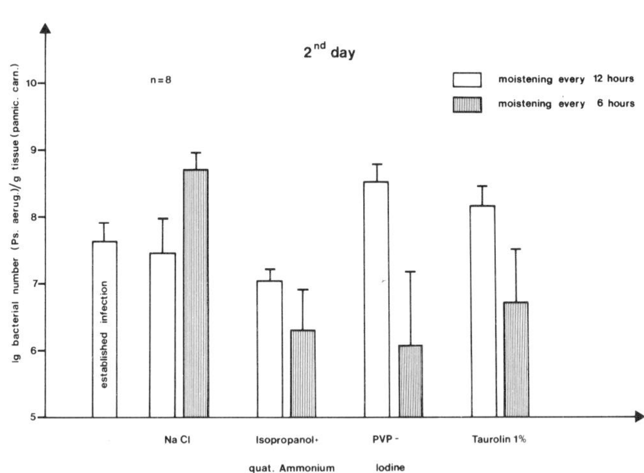

Fig. 4. Comparison of the mean Pseudomonas aeruginosa content per g panniculus carnosus (mean $\langle \log_{10} \rangle$ $\pm$ s.d.), 2 days after soaking PVA every 12 rsp 6 h with three different topical antiseptics.

Biomaterials 1980
Edited by G. D. Winter, D. F. Gibbons, and H. Plenk, Jr.
© 1982 John Wiley and Sons Ltd.

MODIFIED CELLULOSE SUTURE MATERIAL WITH A
MECHANOCHEMICAL EFFECT ON THE HEALING WOUND

V.K. Kalnberzs, L.I. Slutskii, L.E. Dombrovska,
Y.K. Vilks, A.Z. Amelin, L.M. Vantsevitch,
S.V. Tkatchev, F.N. Kaputskii.

Research Institute of Traumatology and
Orthopaedics, Riga, USSR.

SUMMARY

This paper reports the results of the study of "Rimine", a new suture
material obtained by chemical modification of cellulose (cotton).
The experiments in which linear skin incisions in rats were closed
with modified cellulose sutures showed that these sutures rapidly
absorbed, resulted in an excellent early wound scar, and significantly
improved its biomechanical parameters. During the wound healing
process a pronounced accumulation of glycosaminoglycans in wound
tissue was observed.

INTRODUCTION

The choice of suture materials for surgery is made mainly on the
basis of the mechanical properties of the suture. The biological
interaction with tissues is considered only from the point of view
of the intensity of the inflammatory reaction caused by the suture
(Nockemann, 1968; Van Winkle & Hastings, 1972; Furmanov, 1978). Such
an approach found its expression in Furmanov's definition of an ideal
suture material: "A non-allergenic thread of sufficient strength and
small diameter, absorbable and not causing inflammatory reaction is
the ideal variant of surgical suture material." This definition
disregards the fact that all known suture materials slow down the
process of wound healing mainly because of the stress protection which
they impart to the wound (Brunius, 1968; Lamborn et al., 1970). An
ideal suture is one that does not merely avoid negative reactions,
but should stimulate the process of healing.
This paper presents studies of the new suture material "Rimine"
which was obtained by a special chemical processing of cellulose
(cotton) and which possesses the ability to be rapidly absorbed
(Comper & Laurent, 1978).

METHODS AND RESULTS

Modified cellulose suture, sterilized by gamma irradiation (1.5 Mrad)
was studied in our experiment utilizing a total of 114 laboratory
rats. A linear incision 3 cm in length was made through the entire
thickness of skin along the midline of back and closed using 5

interrupted sutures. Modified cellulose suture was used in 57
animals. As a basis of comparison, catgut sutures were used in an
additional 26 rats and silk sutures in 31 rats.

Suture absorbability. The absorbability of the modified cellulose
suture was demonstrated macroscopically by knot disintegration that
began on the second and ended on the fifth day. Silk knots were
completely preserved until the 44th day and those of catgut
persisted until the 28th day (in cases where the sutures were not
removed earlier). The absorbability of the modified cellulose was
confirmed by histological studies on the basis of its birefringence
in polarized light. Few birefringent fragments of the modified
cellulose threads were found in histological sections after seven
days.
Gross wound appearance. The use of the modified cellulose suture
did not cause wound purulence or separation of the wound margins in
spite of its rapid disappearance. The excellent cosmetic features
of the wound scar were apparent by the seventh day. The scar was
very thin, threadlike and soft, and there were no marks where the
sutures had been. Fourteen days after the operation the scar was
hardly distinguishable from the surrounding skin. The wound closed
by silk, after removal of the sutures on the seventh day, was covered
with a scab that subsequently became considerably rougher and there
were persistent scars where the sutures were placed.
Histological evaluation. Histologic examination of those incisions
which were closed with modified cellulose sutures showed that at
seven days an extremely thin zone of granulo-fibrous tissue with a
sharply positive reaction for glycosaminoglycans (alcian blue) was
observed under the epithelized scar. After two weeks the completely
epithelized skin scar was imperceptible and the granulation tissue
had disappeared. By contrast, on the seventh day after application
of silk sutures, the wound scar was uneven and wide and only
partially epithelialized. The skin defect was filled with granulation
tissue covered with scab and the proliferating granulation tissue
penetrated into the adjacent muscle. At 14 days, invasion of the
granulation tissue with foreign body cells and fibrosis in the
areas of thread introduction were observed.
Biomechanical results. A comparison of the mechanical properties of
the linear incisions closed with modified cellulose and silk sutures
was made. The tests were performed on a specially designed stand,
enabling the tensile load to be measured to a precision of 1.0 g with
strains up to 300 percent. Breaking stress (σ^*), strain at break
(ϵ^*), secant modulus (E^*), and tangent modulus at 50 percent breaking
stress (E^T) were calculated from the recorded data. In the first
series of tests the modified cellulose suture had completely absorbed
by the seventh day. The breaking stress of wounds closed with the
modified cellulose sutures exceeded the breaking stress of wounds
closed with silk (Table 1). This was the case even though the
modified cellulose sutures were absorbed at this time and no longer
acting to appose the wound margins.

TABLE 1. Results of biomechanical tests of skin wound scar

	Days	Modified cellulose		Silk		
		X	S_x	X	Sx	P
σ* C		657.0	76.0			
g/mm^2	7	15.6	2.1	10.3	2.3	0.05
	14	31.7	1.2	29.6	4.7	0.05
stress	21	75.4	16.7	38.5	13.2	0.05
	30	184.3	34.2	79.2	6.6	0.02
	44	610.0	70.0	370.0	50.0	0.05
ε* C		0.74	0.18			
strain	7	0.52	0.11	0.57	0.03	0.05
	14	0.61	0.06	0.85	0.06	0.05
	21	0.49	0.08	0.44	0.09	0.05
	30	0.51	0.04	0.46	0.02	0.05
	44	0.46	0.04	0.69	0.12	0.05
E* C		901.0	138.0			
g/mm^2	7	35.4	8.3	18.5	3.7	0.05
secant	14	59.1	9.5	36.3	16.4	0.05
modulus	21	163.0	32.1	87.0	18.3	0.05
	30	338.0	75.0	196.0	24.2	0.05
	44	1360.0	240.0	610.0	110.0	0.05
E^T C		3922.0	721.0			
g/mm^2	7	53.2	5.3	29.5	5.2	0.05
tangent	14	113.2	7.6	66.9	17.0	0.01
modulus	21	237.0	25.9	138.0	37.2	0.02
	30	508.0	51.0	301.0	44.0	0.05
	44	3300.0	600.0	1180.0	380.0	0.02

C - control (intact skin)
X - mean
S_x - standard deviation
P - probability

Subsequently the difference in breaking stress increased and on the
44th day after operation the breaking stress of the modified
cellulose closed wound scar was double the breaking stress of the
silk closed wound scar, and practically that of intact skin. Tauber
et al (1974) claim that for all previously known suture materials,
the breaking stress of the wound scar at this time attains only
70 percent of the strength of the intact skin. The secant modulus
also normalises on the 44th day after the operation when the wound
is closed with the modified cellulose. At this time the tangential
modulus of elasticity is three times higher in those wound closed
with the modified cellulose than in silk closed wounds.

DISCUSSION

What is the mechanism of such a benefitial influence of modified
cellulose sutures on the process of wound healing? The very rapid
absorbability of modified cellulose sutures may be one of the factors
for rapid strengthening of the wound scar and the excellent cosmetic
results. Such a conclusion follows from findings that early suture
removal (or dispensing with their use altogether) promotes wound
healing (Myers et al., 1970).
This, however, should not be regarded as the only factor, because
both early suture removal (rarely possible in clinical practice) and
substitution of sutures by plaster or glue are not as effective as
the modified cellulose suture. It may be assumed that the effectiveness of modified cellulose is connected with peculiarities of the
connective tissue reaction caused by this material. In our experiments
using rats subcutaneously implanted with lumps of the modified
cellulose sutures we saw the development of new tissue which underwent
rapid involution. This tissue differed from all known varieties of
granulo-fibrous tissues by having a very high content of glycosaminoglycans. We found the same high content of alcian blue staining
material in the modified cellulose closed wound, as reported above.
Quantitative biochemical analyses showed that the content of hexur-
onic acids, a component of glycosaminoglycans, in the dried, defatted
modified cellulose granulation tissue reached 1.2 - 1.3 g/100.
Glycosaminoglycans are physiological activators of collagen fibrillogenesis (Comper & Laurent, 1978) resulting in rapid formation of the
wound scar and optimizing its biomechanical properties.
We conclude that the modified cellulose suture influenced metabolic
processes in the developing scar and brought about a desirable
improvement in the biomechanical properties of the sutured wounds.

REFERENCES

Brunius, U. (1968) Wound healing impairment from sutures. A tensio-
metric and histologic study in the rat. Goteborg.
Comper, W.D. & Laurent, T.C. (1978) Physiological function of
polysaccharides. Physiol. Rev., 88, 255-315.
Furmanov, I.A. (1978) Sozdanije i primenenije rassasivajuschkhsya
njitej dlja nalozenija khirurgicheskikh shvov. Klinicheskaja
khirurgija, 8, 71-75 (in Russian).
Lamborn, P.B., Soloway, H.B., Matsumoto, T. & Aaby, G.V. (1970)
Comparison of tensile strength of wounds closed by sutures and
cyanoacrylates. Am. J. Vet. Res., 31, 125-130.
Myers, M.B., Cherry, G. & Heimburger, S. (1969) Augmentation of
wound tensile strength by early removal of sutures. Am. J. Surg.,
117, 338-341.
Nockemann, P.F. (1968) Die chirurgische Nacht. G.Thieme Verlag,
Stuttgart.
Tauber, R., Seidel, W., Heller, E.J. & Stadler, C. (1974) Die
Bedeutung des Nahtmaterials furdie ressfetigkeit heilender fascien
und hautwunden. Langenbecks Arch. Chir., 333, 273-282.
Van Winkle, W.J. & Hastings, J.C. (1972) Considerations in the
choice of suture material for various tissues. Surg. Gynec. Obstet.
135, 113-126.

STRESS RELAXATION OF SYNTHETIC SUTURES

C. C. Chu

Department of Design & Environmental Analysis
Martha Van Rensselaer Hall
Cornell University
Ithaca, NY 14853 USA

SUMMARY

The stress relaxation of 6 commonly used sutures Ethilon, Nurolon,
Dexon, Vicryl, Silk and Prolene was examined for the purpose of identifying the suitability of suture materials in closing surgical
wounds having severe edema. The tests were conducted in a chamber of
constant temperature ($70°F + 2°F$) and humidity ($65\% + 2\%$) and stress
relaxation was measured at 1, 2, 4, 6, and 10% extensions. It was
found that 1) except for sutures made of Nylon 66 the relationship of
stress relaxation with time was nonlinear even at low strain levels;
2) the construction of the sutures seemed to have some effects on
stress relaxation; and 3) a faster stress relaxation was observed at
a higher strain level. On the basis of reduced stress relaxation,
Prolene showed the largest percentage decrease in forces at both
small and large strain levels. Silk showed the least changes in reduced stress relaxation at the small strain levels while behaved second to worst at the large strain levels. Dexon and Vicryl exhibited
very similar reduced stress relaxation at the small strain levels.
Data from experiments in saline solution should be obtained prior to
a better distinguishing the suitability of these sutures in closing
wounds having severe edema.

INTRODUCTION

Viscoelasticity is a fundamental property of suture materials made
from fibrous polymers. Published information on the viscoelastic behavior of braided fibers hardly exist. Knowledge of the vicoelastic
properties of synthetic suture materials should promote a better understanding of the time dependence of suture stress and strain.
These time-dependent mechanical properties of sutures may have clinical consequences. When a suture is used to close a wound, the suture
material experiences the same forces that the body normally does, especially during the lag phase of wound healing. In some clinical
cases, such as edema, the swelling of the tissue of the wound elon-
gates the suture (Price 1948). The resulting stress on the elongated
suture material decreases continuously with time, disrupting the
wound as stress on the suture material reduces to the level that cannot approximate the wounded tissues. An understanding of the time-
dependent behavior of stress and strain on the suture material is im-

portant also because the soft tissues that suture material unites are
viscoelastic (Fung 1972). Information on the viscoelastic behavior
of suture materials can be combined with information on the viscoelastic behavior of soft tissues to help in the selection of sutures
for closing surgical wounds, especially for wounds with severe edema.
The viscoelasticity of polymeric fibers can best be studied in terms
of stress relaxation and the creep phenomenon (Hall 1967). This is a
report on the in vitro experimental work on the stress relaxation of
six suture materials.

MATERIALS AND METHODS

The suture materials studied were Ethilon, Nurolon, Prolene, surgical
Silk, Dexon, and Vicryl. Except for the monofilments Ethilon and
Prolene, the rest were in braided form. All have size 2-0 and are
manufactured by Ethicon, except Dexon, which is manufactured by Davis
and Geck.

Suture materials were conditioned before testing by storage in a
chamber at a constant temperature (70°F $\pm$ 2°F) and humidity (65% $\pm$ 2%)
for 24 hours; they were tested under the same conditions. The stress
relaxation of all suture materials was determined on an Instron Tens-
ometer Table Model TM. The testing conditions were: gauge length, 3
in.; crosshead speed, 1 inch/min.; and chart speed, 10 inches/min.
The strain levels used to obtain stress relaxation were 1, 2, 4, 6,
and 10%. These five levels of elongation were chosen because, although the actual elongation of a suture in a clinical situtation is
not known, it is believed that an increase in length of less than 10%
would be the most probable clinical condition in severe edema.

RESULTS

The effect of strain level on stress relaxation of selected suture
materials is shown in Fig. 1-4. These show the amount of stress remaining at time plotted against the logarithm of time (in seconds) at
the 1 - 10% strain levels. Two general characteristics were found.
First, except for Ethilon and Nurolon, the relationship of stress relaxation with time was nonlinear even at 1% strain level. The non-
linearity became more pronounced at higher strain levels and was most
obvious with Prolene, surgical silk, and Dexon. Sutures made of Nylon 6,6 showed a linear viscoelastic behavior at a strain level of 1%,
but at higher strain levels the viscoelasticity became nonlinear.

Second, a faster stress relaxation was observed at a higher strain
level and various degrees of dependence of stress relaxation on
strain levels were observed for suture materials of different chemical nature. Silk showed the most pronounced dependence of stress relaxation on strain levels, while Ethilon and Nurolon showed the least
dependence. Prolene, Vicryl and Dexon fell between silk and nylon.

In order to compare the stress relaxation of different suture material at different strain levels, the reduced stress relaxation, represented by $R(t) = T(t)/T(t_o)$ in which $T(t_o)$ was the tension in the su-

ture at the instant t_o, the time at which the crosshead of the Instron stops at a specified extension level, and T(t) was the tension at time t - t_o and at the corresponding extension level, was calculated and are shown in Fig. 5 & 6. At the 2% strain level (Fig. 5), the differences in stress relaxation among different suture materials were large. The construction of the suture seemed to influence stress relaxation. The stress relaxation curves of a braided nylon suture (Nurolon) were different from the monofilament nylon (Ethilon) at the corresponding strain levels. At all strain levels, Nurolon exhibited less stress relaxation than Ethilon. Whether this observation will be confirmed for other suture materials cannot be determined. Prolene showed the greatest percentage decrease in force with time. Dexon and Vicryl, showed the least R(t) among the six sutures.

When the strain level increased to 10% (Fig. 6), the differences in R(t) became more apparent, and the order of the magnitude of R(t) was different from 2% strain level. Prolene still showed the largest drop in percentage of force with time. But silk became the second to the largest. The differences between Dexon and Vicryl became gradually large, and Vicryl exhibited the least change of R(t). Ethilon and Nurolon still showed different reduced stress relaxation at this strain level, and Nurolon was better than Ethilon.

DISCUSSION

The results indicate that although linear viscoelasticity appears at very small elongation in some polymers, no linear relationship was found in the fibrous polymers tested under the specified conditions. On the basis of reduced stress relaxation, the suture materials at a low level of strain could be divided into three groups: those with a large stress relaxation, such as Prolene; those with a small stress relaxation, such as silk; and those with a moderate amount, such as Nurolon, Ethilon, Vicryl and Dexon. This order, however, depends on the strain level. Obviously, the different behavior of the suture materials was the result of chemical differences in the materials. The behavior of faster stress relaxation at the higher extensions is believed to be due to a temperature effect. An extension of 10% is normally beyond the yield point of most suture materials. Consequently, it results in a rise in temperature due to a large energy loss. It would take several seconds for the excess heat to be dissipated from the suture materials. This behavior was also observed in viscose rayon yarn (Meredith 1954).

Since stress relaxation is a result of segmental mobility of the constituent polymeric chains, which enables them to achieve a new equilibrium position, polymers that are highly cross linked or possess high crystallinity or molecular weight associated with physical entanglement of the segments will show restricted mobility of chain segments and smaller stress relaxation. For Nylon 6,6, the chains are in planar zigzag conformation and are fully extended (Holmes 1955). This conformation, facilitates strong intermolecular interactions between two adjacent chains. This might be why Ethilon and Nurolon showed the small amount of stress relaxation. The reason that Nurolon

                                C. C. Chu

exhibited less stress relaxation than Ethilon might be due to the
braided structure of Nurolon. The frictional forces at the crossover
points in braid might retard the relaxation of stress and hence renders less degree of stress relaxation.

The differences in stress relaxation behavior among the different suture materials has clinical implication. Based on stress relaxation
data alone, sutures having large stress relaxation may not be a good
choice for closing surgical wounds that have or will develop severe
edema, because edema causes swelling of the wound tissue and stretches
the suture materials which support the wound. Should the tissue be
strong enough to resist cutting by the suture materials, the materials will experience stress relaxation, and the actual strength of the
suture should decrease with time. If the force of the suture material decreases so much that the material cannot precisely approximate
the suture line, the wound could be disrupted. Of the sutures studied, Prolene had the greatest and fastest stress relaxation; it may
therefore disrupt the wound more easily in case of marked edema.
However, no clinical data are available at the present time on the
effect of stress relaxation on disruption of wounds. At a small level
of edema (corresponding to small strain level) silk sutures may be a
better choice than others, because they showed the least percent
change of force with time. However, Vicryl, Dexon and Nurolon are
better than other sutures at a severe edema condition. But it is premature to draw a preference order without additional data from stress
relaxation experiments in saline or a simulated extracellular fluid
condition.

ACKNOWLEDGMENT

We are grateful to the financial support of the College of Human
Ecology, Cornell University.

REFERENCES

Fung, Y.C. (1972). 'Biomechanics - Its foundation and objectives',
Prentice Hall, NJ.
Hall, I.H. (1967). 'Viscoelasticity of textile fibers at finite
strains', J. Polym. Sci., A-2, 5, 119.
Holmes, D.R., Bunn, C.W., Smith, D.J. (1955). 'The crystal structure
of Polycaproamide: Nylon 6', J. Polym. Sci., 17, 159.
Meredith, R. (1954). 'Relaxation of stress in stretched cellulose
fibres', J. Text. Inst., 45, T438.
Price, P.G. (1948). 'Stress, strain and sutures', Ann. Sug., 128(3),
408.

Biomaterials 1980
Edited by G. D. Winter, D. F. Gibbons, and H. Plenk, Jr.
© 1982 John Wiley and Sons Ltd.

C. C. Chu

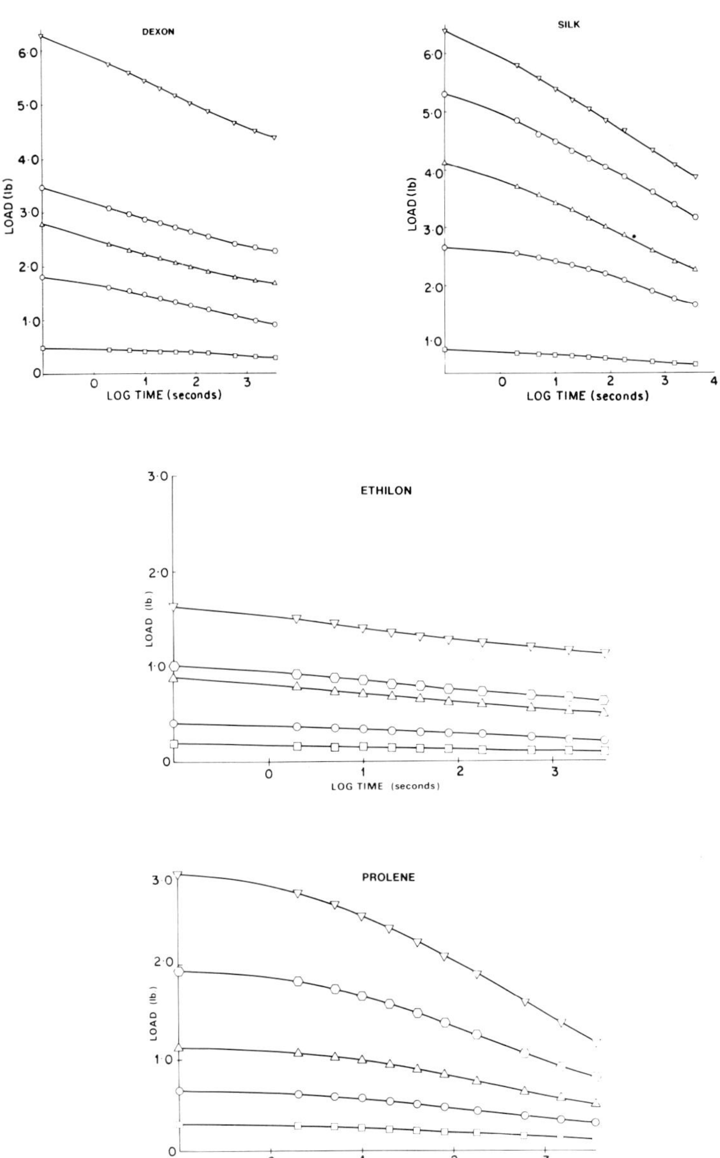

Fig. 1-4. Stress Relaxation of 2-0 Dexon, Silk, Ethilon and Prolene Sutures at various strain levels. □ - 1%; ○ - 2%; △ - 4%; ◇ - 6%; ▽ - 10%.

C. C. Chu

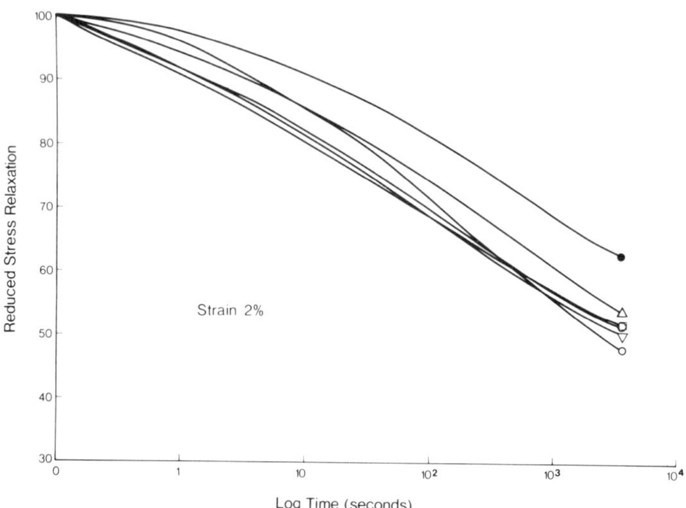

Fig. 5. Reduced Stress Relaxation of 2-0 Sutures at 2% Strain Level. ● - Silk; △ - Nurolon; □ - Ethilon; ⬡ - Vicryl; ▽ - Dexon; ◯ - Prolene.

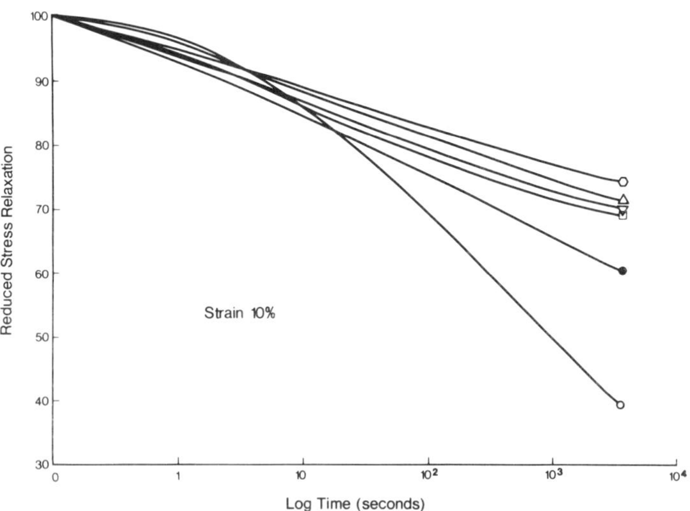

Fig. 6. Reduced Stress Relaxation of 2-0 Sutures at 10% Strain Level. ● - Silk; △ - Nurolon; □ - Ethilon; ⬡ - Vicryl; ▽ - Dexon; ◯ - Prolene.

Biomaterials 1980
Edited by G. D. Winter, D. F. Gibbons, and H. Plenk, Jr.
© 1982 John Wiley and Sons Ltd.

AN ANALYSIS OF SURGICAL KNOT SECURITY IN SUTURES

B. S. Gupta
School of Textiles, North Carolina State University
Raleigh, North Carolina

and

R. W. Postlethwait
V. A. Hospital, Durham, North Carolina

SUMMARY

Security of square surgical knots was examined in sutures of four
different types; namely, Mersilene®, Polydek®, Ti-cron®, and silk.
The first three of these were of polyester fiber material but varied
in terms of the surface finish. Knots were constructed under
controlled conditions on a special device. The variables employed
were the suture type, suture size, number of throws, tying tension,
and the suture environment. The latter varied between dry, saline
and animal. Knot performance was assessed from the force-deformation
curves obtained in Instron® tensile tests. The parameter emphasized
was the knot holding force - the force generated at slippage or, in
the absence of slippage, breakage. The major conclusion arrived was
that inter-fiber friction plays an important role in governing
security of surgical knots. Sutures with lower frictional
coefficients slipped at lower forces and required additional throws
to develop a secure knot construction. Based upon this hypothesis,
it was possible to propose a workable model of a secure knot.

INTRODUCTION

Although surgery has made great advances over the years, the ancient
method of using a suture material and holding it in place by
mechanical interlacing are still the most widely used current
practices in holding repaired or torn tissues together or implanting
a prosthetic device. The surgical knot, holding the suture loop in
place, is indeed the weakest and the most unreliable element in the
assembly, always threatening to break or slip prematurely.
Described here are selected results from an on-going study the
objectives of which are to identify conditions and variables, both
material related and clinical, which influence knot strength and
security. The main emphasis of this paper will be to show that one
of the most important variables which influence performance of knots
in surgery is the coefficient of friction. Based on this result, a
general model of a secure surgical knot will be proposed and
discussed.

MATERIALS AND METHODS

<u>Suture Materials</u>. The sutures selected for this investigation were all multifilament braided structures of four different types. Two of these were uncoated and two coated. One of these was a natural suture material and the other three synthetic. These were: silk (Ethicon); Mersilene®, uncoated polyester (Ethicon); Polydek®, Teflon® impregnated polyester (Deknatel); and Ti-cron®, silicone treated polyester (Davis and Geck).

<u>Suture Sizes</u>. The sizes used were: 1-0, 2-0, 3-0 and 4-0.

<u>Knot Construction</u>. The knot configuration was square, with the number of throws varying from 2 to 5. The tension used in constructing knots was varied under controlled conditions from half a pound to near the suture breaking load in half pound increments.

<u>Testing Environment</u>. This was varied between dry, saline and animal.

<u>Device for Construction Knots and Dry Procedure</u>. The schematic of the device used is shown in Figure 1. A loop is tied around two

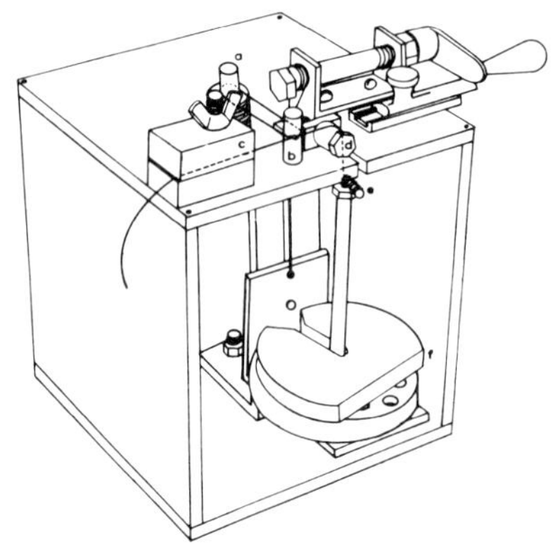

Fig. 1. Device for constructing controlled knots.

metal posts set at 2 inches apart. One end is clamped securely in place while the other subjected to the desired tensioning force. The latter was applied to each successive throw beginning with the second. The free ends were cut to approximately 3 mm from the knot.

<u>Procedure Utilizing Saline and Animal Environments</u>. For saline tests, the suture was immersed in 5% saline solution for 5 seconds before constructing the knot, and the knot was immersed in saline solution for 3 minutes before testing on Instron®. For animal tests, sutures containing controlled knots were implanted inside the stomach

wall of dogs. The knots were placed such that they were easily
impregnated by body fluids but no tension was applied to the knots
while inside the animal. The test periods were 5 and 21 days. In
order to prevent tissues surrounding sutures and making retrieval
difficult, the sutures for the 21 day tests were encased in metallic
blood filters, allowing easy body fluid penetration, and tacked in
the stomach wall.

Knot Performance Tests. All tests of knot performance were carried
out on an Instron® tensiometer using 2" gage length and 2"/min rate
of jaw separation. Two types of tests were carried out, loop and
straight. In the former, which simulates more nearly the actual
conditions, the loop formed by tying a knot was placed over two pegs
held in the Instron® jaws and stretched. In the straight tests,
specially convenient when using animal environment, the loop obtained
was cut in the center and tested as a straight strand with the knot
in the middle. The force values obtained in loop tests are
approximately twice the values obtained in straight tests.

Knot Parameters. From the force-deformation curves, four parameter
of interest could be assessed. They are: (1) knot breaking
strength, the force at which knot ruptures; (2) knot holding force,
the average force at which knot slips; (3) slippage, the amount by
which a knot slips before retightening and finally breaking; and (4)
knot efficiency, the fraction of suture strength retained by a
knotted suture. If in a knot tensile test, there was no measurable
slippage then the knot holding force was considered as being equal to
the knot breaking strength. In some tests, a knot first slipped to
some extent, then retightened and finally ruptured. In such tests,
values of the above mentioned first three parameters could be
assessed. If a knot slipped all the way, then the value of only the
knot holding force could be regiestered. Although a more thorough
understanding of the behavior of a surgical knot would be given by
the results based upon all the above four parameters, only one aspect
could be adequately covered here. The parameter of greatest interest
and the one most directly related to knot security, is the knot
holding force and is the one emphasized in this paper.

RESULTS AND DISCUSSION

The data obtained from tensile tests was subjected to the statistical
analysis of variance. It was found that the value of knot holding
force (KHF) was most highly influenced by the size of the suture,
the number of throws and the type of the suture, but, somewhat
unexpectedly, was little affected by the amount of tension used in
tying of knots (Good, E. D., 1978). Whatever effect observed was
mostly in Mersilene® and the general trend found was a slight
increase in KHF with tying tension.

From the rest of the analysis, tension was omitted as a variable.
Figure 2 shows the effect of throws on the knot holding force values

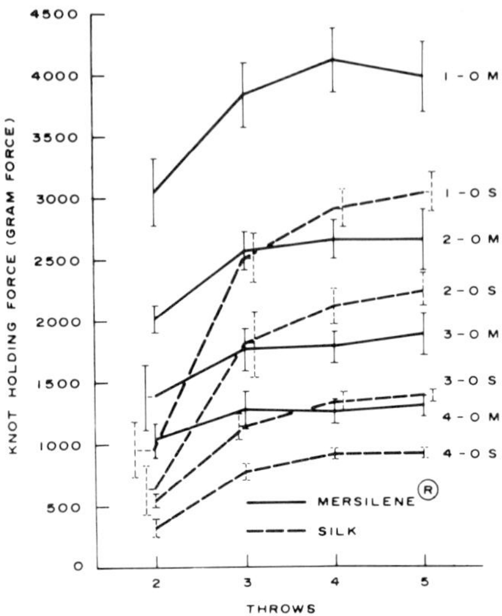

Fig. 2. Effect of number of throws on knot security of
Mersilene® (M) and silk (S) in dry straight tests.
Sizes, 1-0 to 4-0.

of Mersilene® and silk in dry straight tests. For any given size of
suture, the optimum KHF value of silk is much lower than that of
Mersilene®. This difference obviously comes from the differences in
the structures of the two polymers. The 2-throw knot in silk slips
at a very low load and there is a substantial increase in the KHF
value as the number of throws increase from 2 to 3. Further addition
of throws continue to improve knot security in silk. In contrast,
the 2-throw knot in Mersilene® is relatively secure and reaches
optimum KHF value in all cases at 3 throws, except size 1-0.

The KHF values of the three polyester sutures, differently finished,
are compared in Table 1.

TABLE 1. Knot holding force (gram-force) of three polyester sutures, size 2-0

	Number of throws		
	2	3	4
Polydek®	1015	2329	2657
Mersilene®	2003	2534	2621
Ti-cron®	224	1135	2443

It is obvious that special coatings on the Polydek® and the Ti-cron® sutures are greatly responsible for the relatively much lower KHF values at 2 throws and, for Ti-cron, also at 3 throws, as compared to the corresponding values in Mersilene®. In Ti-cron®, specially, the change from 2 to 3 and then to 4 throws is dramatic and the optimum value is perhaps not reached until after an additional throw or two are added. It is interesting to note that these three sutures, being the same chemically, reach nearly the same optimum value of KHF.

Table 2 summarizes the number and percentages of knots that slipped

TABLE 2. Comparison of knots slipping partially and completely in silk and Mersilene® sutures

Suture	Conditions	Number of total tests	No. slipped partially (%)		No. slipped completely (%)	
Mersilene®	Dry	464	70	(15)	2	(1)
	Saline	216	25	(12)	11	(5)
Silk	Dry	384	7	(2)	97	(25)
	Saline	192	5	(3)	79	(41)

partially or completely in Mersilene® and silk, under dry and saline test conditions. In silk, in dry tests, 25% of the knots slipped completely, and, in saline, 41% slipped completely. In contrast, in Mersilene®, only 1% slipped completely in dry and 5% slipped completely in saline. One interesting effect of partial slippage, i.e., slipping to some extent, retightening, and then finally breaking, found in this investigation, was that the knots that slipped partially gave a lower breaking strength than the knots which did not slip at all. The difference in some cases was nearly 20%. This reduction was evidently due to physical damage from abrasion of the surface structure.

The next set of experiments involved animal tests in which silk and Mersilene® sutures containing control knots were implanted in dogs

for 5 and 21 days, removed and then tested for KHF values (Good,
E. D., 1978). The results are compared with dry test values in
Figure 3. It is seen that the animal test values are lower than

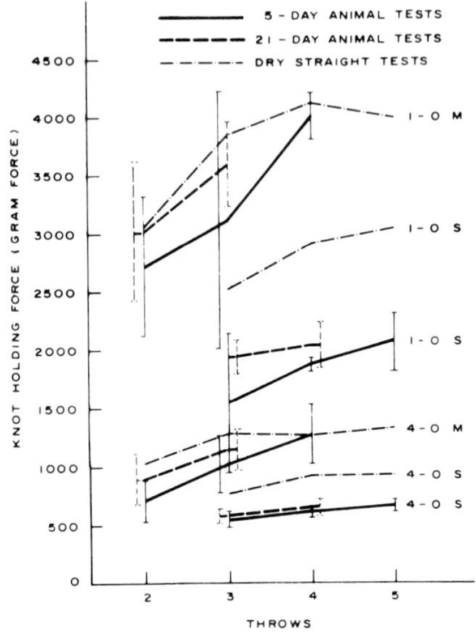

Fig. 3. Comparison of animal and dry test knot security
in Mersilene® (M) and silk (S). Sizes, 1-0 and 4-0.

the dry test values. The 21-day animal test value is higher than the
5-day animal test value but still lower than the dry test value. In
Mersilene®, at about 4 throws, the animal and the dry test values
become equal. This is not the case with silk wherein a large gap
exists between the dry and the animal test values. This difference
in silk comes from the structural degradation commonly observed. The
relatively lower KHF values in animal tests is undoubtedly due to
lubricity of the surface making it more slippery, an effect which can
be overcome by putting more throws, as noted in Mersilene® at 4
throws. The higher KHF value in the 21-day tests, as compared with
the 5-day tests, was most likely due to increased frictional
restraints coming from the coagulation of body fluids, or fine
tissues growing in and around the structure of the knot making it
more secure.

In summarizing the results thus far, it was quite clear that friction
had played an important role in governing the differences found in
the KHF values between (1) the coated and the uncoated polyester
sutures, (2) the saline and the dry test values, and (3) the animal
and the dry test values. That, friction could also account for the
differences in the KHF values noted between the silk and the
Mersilene® sutures was confirmed from frictional tests (Wolf, K. W.,

1979) carried out by the classical twist method (Lindberg and Gralen, 1948), the results of which are shown in Table 3. These results show

TABLE 3. Friction tests of Mersilene® and silk sutures

Suture Type	Applied tension To (lbs.)	Coefficient of friction			
		Size 1 - 0		Size 4 - 0	
		n=1	n=4	n=1	n=4
Silk	0.125	0.30	0.32	0.24	0.18
	0.500	0.21	0.25	0.15	0.15
	1.000	0.17	0.21	0.14	0.13
	1.500	0.12	0.20	0.09	0.12
	2.000	0.14	0.18	0.12	0.12
Mersilene®	0.125	0.32	0.36	0.26	0.20
	0.500	0.21	0.30	0.16	0.17
	1.000	0.17	0.27	0.13	0.15
	1.500	0.15	0.25	0.12	0.13
	2.000	0.15	0.24	0.11	0.12

n = turns of twist

that the coefficient of friction of silk sutures, used in present investigation was, in general, lower than that of Mersilene®.

Based on these findings, it is possible to put together a friction based hypothesis of a secure knot. A suture is looped around cut vessels or tissues, the ends pulled tightly together and tied with a knot. The tissues exert outward pressure on the loop tending to expand its size (Figure 4) and as a result exert a tension Ta on

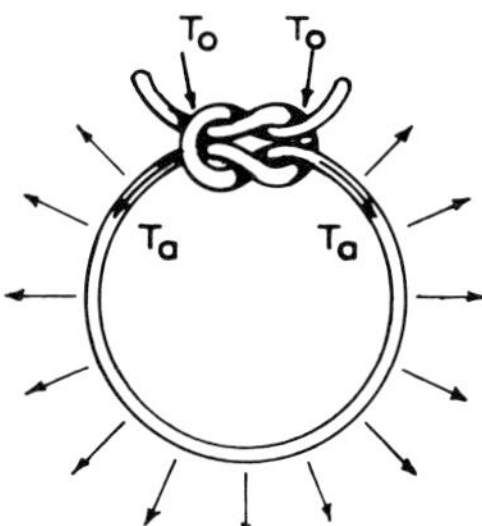

Fig. 4. Model of a secure knot.

each of the two inner loop ends. The interlacing of the knot more or less coincides with the geometry of the twist method and, thus, the tension T necessary to cause slippage could be approximately given by the Lindberg and Gralen's (1948) equation:

$$T = To \exp(\pi n\beta\mu)$$

In this equation, To will be the tension at the entrance to or the exit from the knot where the suture ends are positively gripped by the compressive forces within the knot, n will be equivalent to the number of throws, β is the twist angle, and μ is the coefficient of friction.

The tension T can be obtained theoretically by relating each of the other components of equation to the parameters of suture and knot construction. Alternatively, the value of T can be obtained directly from measurements of knot holding force by the loop method and could be equated by impirical means to suture size and tensile and frictional properties, and parameters of knot construction. The major problem in quantifying knot security in a given clinical situation is to determine or predict the value of tension Ta existing in the loop. Its value will depend upon, among other factors, the size of the suture loop, the tension applied in tying of knot and the mechanical and visco-elastic properties of tissues being joined. The data on this last aspect is lacking in the literature but its availability will play an important role towards further progress in knot security studies.

The criteria for a secure knot will be simply that the knot holding force T and the knot breaking strength F are greater than Ta, or the ratios, T/Ta and F/Ta, are greater than 1, at the time the wound is closed and during the period of healing. One could also assign, in an effort at standardization, appropriate ranges of values for these ratios and define a fully reliable, a partially reliable and an unreliable surgical knot.

ACKNOWLEGEMENTS

This work was supported by funds from the North Carolina State University's Biomedical Research Support Grant, BRSG #RR07071, the organized research funds of the School of Textiles, North Carolina State University, and the material supplies from and the clinical facilities of the Veterans Administration Hospital. The authors gratefully acknowledge these assistances.

REFERENCES

Good, E. Dale (1978) Mechanical analysis of knot strength and security in polyester and silk surgical sutures, unpublished Master of Science thesis, School of Textiles, North Carolina State University, Raleigh, North Carolina.
Lindberg, J. & Gralen, N. (1948) Measurement of friction between single fibers, Textile Res. J., 18, 287-301.
Wolf, K. W. (1979) An experimental study of interfiber friction in surgical sutures by the twist method, unpublished Master of Science Thesis, School of Textiles,North Carolina State University, Raleigh.

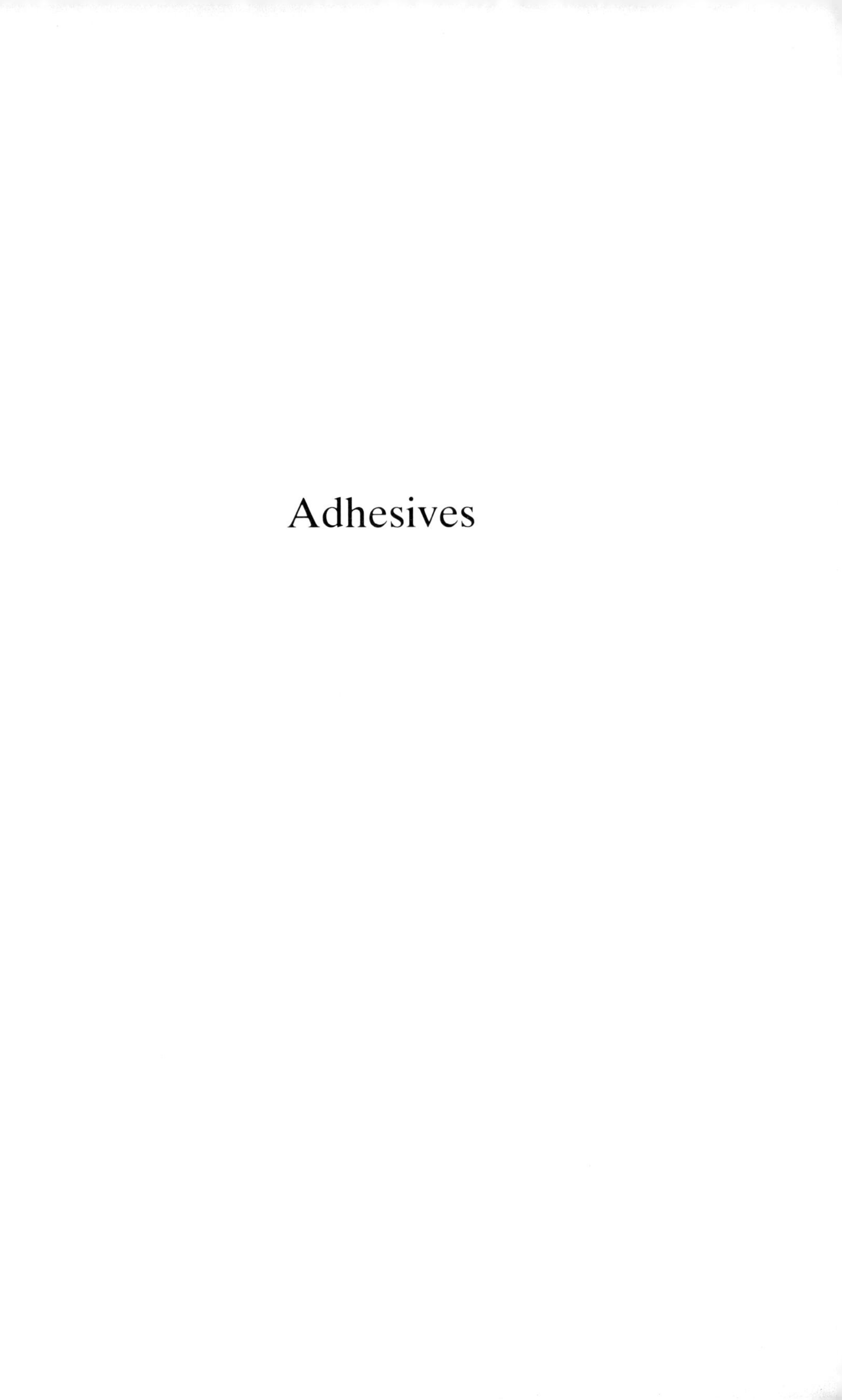

Adhesives

Biomaterials 1980
Edited by G. D. Winter, D. F. Gibbons, and H. Plenk, Jr.
© 1982 John Wiley and Sons Ltd.

BACKGROUND AND METHODS OF "FIBRIN SEALING"

H. Redl[1], G. Schlag[1], H. Dinges[2], H. Kuderna[3] and T. Seelich[4]

1) Ludwig Boltzmann-Institut für experimentelle Traumatologie, Vienna, Austria
2) Pathologisch-bakteriologisches Institut des Kaiser Franz Josef-Spitals, Vienna, Austria
3) Unfallkrankenhaus-Lorenz Böhler, Vienna, Austria
4) IMMUNO AG, Vienna, Austria

SUMMARY

A biological two-component sealant has proved effective in face to face sealing of tissue, wound sealing, or in establishing haemostasis. The two components of the system comprise a) highly concentrated human fibrinogen, factor XIII and other human plasma proteins, and b) thrombin and $CaCl_2$. A fibrinolysis inhibitor is generally added to one of the two components. The essential reactions after mixing of the two components are coagulation, fibrin cross-linking and, finally, lysis and absorption of the clot material during the wound healing process. In an attempt to control and optimize the method, these reactions, and the dependence of the tensile strength of standardized clots on fibrin cross-linking were examined in vitro. A new application device was developed which makes it possible to mix and apply the two components of the system simultaneously either through a needle or by spraying.

INTRODUCTION

A fibrin sealant produced from human plasma (Tisseel®, Fibrin Seal (Human), Immuno AG, Vienna, Austria) has proved effective in face to face sealing of tissue, wound sealing, and in establishing haemostasis. It is a two-component system comprising the sealant proper which contains highly concentrated fibrinogen and factor XIII (F XIII) in addition to other plasma proteins such as albumin and cold-insoluble globulin (CIG), and a second component, the hardener, which is a solution of thrombin and calcium chloride. A fibrinolysis inhibitor is generally added to one of the two components. When the two components are mixed, coagulation occurs, and in the further course of the process, the activated factor XIII (F XIIIa) causes cross-linking of the fibrin (Laki, 1972, Schwartz et al, 1973). A clot of increasing rigidity is formed, which is gradually lysed and absorbed during the wound healing process (Fig. 1). In an attempt to control and optimize the method, we examined the mode of action and properties of the sealant in greater depth.

METHODS, RESULTS AND DISCUSSION

The coagulation time (at 37° C) depends on the chosen thrombin concentration; with a final concentration of 2 NIH units/ml, coagulation will occur within 30 to 120 seconds; if the final concentration is 50 NIH units/ml or higher, the sealant will harden in less than 10 seconds. Some antibiotics, like gentamycin, polymycin B, and neomycin, double or triple the coagulation time if a low thrombin concentration (2 NIH units/ml reaction mixture) is used (Table 1).

Table 1:   **Influence of various antibiotics on the coagulation time of the fibrin sealant**

2 NIH units thrombin/ml clot

Control	~ 30 sec.
GENTAMYCIN (10 mg/ml clot)	~ 80 sec.
POLYMYCIN B (10 mg/ml clot)	~ 56 sec.
NEOMYCIN (50 mg/ml clot)	~ 56 sec.

A similar coagulation inhibiting effect of penicillin, streptomycin, and aureomycin has already been described (Mlczoch and Vinazzer, 1952).

The cross-linking reaction of fibrin can be demonstrated by Na–dodecylsulfate-polyacrylamide gel electrophoresis (SDS–PAGE) (Schwartz et al, 1973, Weber and Osborn, 1969). Figure 2 shows the mode of reaction of a typical batch under conditions of practical application, i.e. at 37° C upon mixing (1:1) with a thrombin-$CaCl_2$ solution (15 NIH units of thrombin/ml, 40 mmol of $CaCl_2$/l), without addition of F XIII. Aprotinin was added to series A (50 KIU/ml of fibrin sealant), while no fibrinolysis inhibitor was added to series B. After given periods of time, the reaction was stopped by the addition of a solution consisting of 9 M urea, 4.5% SDS and 5.0% β-mercaptoethanol under heating to 70° C (Seelich and Redl, 1979). As can be seen, the fibrin seal itself contains sufficient F XIII to produce a high degree of cross-linking. After a few minutes, the fibrin-γ-chains are completely cross-linked. The process of fibrin α-chain cross-linking is shown graphically in Figure 3. In conformity with the results of Mosher (1975), the cross-linking reaction of the CIG can also be seen (Figure 2). To achieve an optimum rate of cross-linking, however, the $CaCl_2$ concentration must at least be 5 mmol/l (Seelich and Redl, 1980).

Gentamycin substantially inhibits this cross-linking reaction. The addition of gentamycin (17.5 mg/ml clot) to otherwise identical samples reduced the degree of α-chain cross-linking from 36.0% to 6.0%. However, the rate of fibrin cross-linking in the presence of antibiotics can be normalized by incorporating additional factor XIII (20 units/ml) into the reaction mixture.

The importance of fibrin cross-linking lies in the resulting increase in clot rigidity (Shen et al, 1974). Dependence of the tensile strength of standardized fibrin seal clots on fibrin α-chain cross-linking is illustrated in Figure 4 (Guttmann, 1978). The tensile strength increases up to an α-chain cross-linking degree of about 70% and reaches a plateau around 35 kPa: however, at a degree of 35%, i.e. after a reaction time of about 10 minutes, about 70% of the maximum tensile strength has already been reached. Stemberger (1979) found similar maximum values of tensile strength.

However, the importance of F XIII in the fibrin seal system is not limited to fibrin cross-linking. The investigations of Duckert and Nyman (1978) show that the presence of F XIIIa also causes collagen to cross-link with fibrin. Collagen is a major component of connective tissue and it may be assumed that the adhesion of the seal to the tissue, which has proved very good, results from covalent links between collagen and fibrin.

In the first phase of the wound healing process, fibroblasts proliferate into the fibrin clot. In vitro experiments by Beck et al (1962), Bruhn et al (1979) and Turowski et al (1979) have shown that both F XIII and fibrin (but not fibrinogen), stimulate fibroblast growth and that the presence of a stabilized fibrin structure is essential for the formation of a fibroblast network. Animal experiments carried out by Knoche and Schmitt (1976) corroborate the stimulating effect of F XIII on wound healing: they attribute this effect to the growth of fibroblasts.

We also investigated the resistance of the fibrin sealant to fibrinolysis. As shown in Figure 2 (series B), after 24 hours of incubation at 37° C, slight fibrinolysis may occur in fibrin seal clots to which no protease inhibitor has been added. The presence of fibrin split products is proof that some of the fibrin lysed. This process can be suppressed by the addition of as little as 30 to 50 KIU of aprotinin per ml of fibrin seal. In practice, therefore, it is the fibrinolytic activity of the sealing area which is the determining factor, and this activity may vary widely.

In an attempt to simulate this situation, fibrin seal clots containing various fibrinolysis inhibitors in different concentrations were topped with isotonic saline or urokinase solution and incubated at 37° C. The protein content of the supernatant was determined at intervals of 24 hours, the supernatant replaced with fresh saline or urokinase solution, and the procedure repeated to determine the resistance of the clot until fully lysed (Guttmann, 1978).

The fibrinolysis inhibitors used in this test were ε-aminocaproic acid (EACA), trans-4-(aminomethyl)-cyclohexanoic acid (trans-AMCHA) and the natural polyvalent protease inhibitor aprotinin.

A typical test is diagrammatically represented in Figure 5. 0.1 ml of fibrin seal was mixed with 0.05 ml of inhibitor solution and 0.1 ml of a thrombin calcium chloride solution (40 mmol of $CaCl_2$/l,5 mmol of NaN_3/l, 4 NIH units of thrombin/l), then incubated for 30 min. at 37° C and topped with 2.0 ml of urokinase solution (7.5 CTA units/ml). The further procedure was as described above.

With an aprotinin content of 250 KIU/ml of fibrin seal and daily topping with fresh urokinase solution, pronounced fibrinolysis (E_{280} in supernatant > 0.1) developed on the 5th day only. By increasing the aprotinin dose, resistance of the clot could be prolonged almost arbitrarily. This long-term effect could not be achieved with EACA or trans-AMCHA, not even if higher concentrations were used. With 20 KIU aprotinin per ml of fibrin seal and topping with isotonic saline, pronounced fibrinolysis occurred from the 5th day; with a concentration of 100 KIU per ml, from the 7th day. Of all the fibrinolysis inhibitors tested, aprotinin proved the most effective. Animal experiments in which the fibrin seal was detected histochemically (Dinges, 1979) corroborate this result (Dinges et al, 1980).

However, excessively long survival of the sealant is not desirable. It should eventually yield to wound healing and one of the remarkable advantages of the sealant is its complete absorbability. Provided that it is possible to evaluate the fibrinolytic activity in the sealing area, the life of sealings can be roughly controlled by appropriate dosages of aprotinin.

Finally, we would like to discuss various modes of application of the seal and introduce a new device which facilitates and improves application.

It goes without saying that in order to obtain maximum rigidity the two components need to be thoroughly mixed. The classical method involves the use of high thrombin concentrations (several 100 NIH units/ml) and consecutive application of the two components. This results in fast rate coagulation on the interface of the two components, but consequently poor intermingling and poor rigidity of the resulting clot.

The method of premixing was introduced by Kuderna (1979) for nerve sealing. It can also be used for skin transplantation and bone sealing. A drawback of the method may be that it requires the surgeon to work rather fast. Coagulation occurs slowly and the technique cannot be recommended when it is desirable to achieve haemostasis.

For these reasons we developed a new application device consisting of a double syringe and two detachable heads, which makes it possible to mix and apply the two components simultaneously either through a needle or by spraying (Figure 6). Both techniques are simple to use, high and low thrombin concentrations can be employed and the two components are well enough mixed to ensure high rigidity of sealing. Spraying in combination with a high thrombin concentration (500 NIH units/ml, second component) has proved particularly effective in establishing haemostasis.

REFERENCES

Beck, E., Duckert, F. & Ernst, M. (1962) Der Einfluß des fibrinstabilisierenden Faktors (FSF) auf Funktion und Morphologie von Fibroblasten in vitro. Z. Zellforsch 57, 327-346.
Bruhn, H.D., Christopers, E., Pohl, J. & Scholl, G. (1980) Regulation der Fibroblastenproliferation durch Fibrinogen/Fibrin, Fibronectin und Factor XIII.

Fibrinogen, Fibrin und Fibrinkleber, (Ed. Schimpf), 217-226. F.K. Schattauer Verlag, Stuttgart, New York.

Dinges, H.P., Redl, H., Kuderna, H. & Matras, H. (1979) Histologie nach Fibrinklebung. Dtsch. Z. Mund-Kiefer-Gesichts-Chir. 3, 29-31.

Dinges, H.P., Redl, H., Matras, H. & Kuderna, H. Water-tight closure of the spinal dura (with special reference to inhibition of fibrin clot lysis). Presented at the Joseph Society International Meeting, Salzburg, June 1980, paper in press.

Duckert, F. & Nyman, D. (1978) Factor XIII, fibrin and collagen. Collagen-Platelet Interaction, Proceedings of the First Munich Symposium on Biology of Connective Tissue, July 1976 (Ed. Gastpar) 391-396. F.K. Schattauer Verlag, Stuttgart, New York.

Guttmann, T. (1978) Untersuchungen eines Fibrinklebers für die Anwendung in der Chirurgie peripherer Nerven. Diplomarbeit, Inst. f. Botanik, Techn. Mikroskopie u. Organ. Rohstofflehre, Techn. Univ. Wien.

Knoche, H. & Schmitt, G. (1976) Autoradiographische Untersuchungen über den Einfluß des Faktors XIII auf die Wundheilung im Tierexperiment. Arzneim. Forsch. (Drug Res.) 26, 547-551.

Kudnera, H. (1979) Das Fibrinklebesystem. Nervenklebung. Dtsch. Z. Mund-Kiefer-Gesichts-Chir. 3, 32-35.

Laki, K. (1972) Fibrinoligase: The fibrin-stabilizing factor system of blood plasma. Ann. N.Y. Acad. Sci., 202, 6-30.

Mlczoch, F. & Vinazzer, H. (1952) Die Beeinflussung der Thrombin-Fibrinogen-Reaktion durch Penicillin, Streptomycin und Aureomycin. Experientia 8, 150-157.

Mosher, D.F. (1975) Cross-linking of cold-insoluble globulin by fibrin-stabilizing factor. J. Biol. Chem. 250, 6614-6621.

Schwartz, M.L., Pizzo, S.V., Hill, R.L. & McKee, P.A. (1973) Human factor XIII from plasma and platelets. Molecular weights, subunit structures, proteolytic activation and cross-linking of fibrinogen and fibrin. J. Biol. Chem. 248, 1395-1407.

Seelich, T. & Redl, H. (1979) Das Fibrinklebesystem. Biochemische Grundlagen der Klebemethode. Dtsch. Z. Mund-Kiefer-Gesichts-Chir. 3, 22-26.

Seelich, T. & Redl, H. (1980) Theoretische Grundlagen des Fibrinklebers. Fibrinogen, Fibrin und Fibrinkleber, (Ed. Schimpf), 199-208. F.K. Schattauer Verlag, Stuttgart, New York.

Shen, L.L., McDonagh, R.P., McDonagh, J. & Hermans, J.Jr. (1974) Fibrin gel structure: influence of calcium and covalent cross-linking on the elasticity. Biochem. Biophys. Res. Comm. 56, 793-798.

Stemberger, A. (1979). Personal communication.

Turowski, G., Schaadt, M., Barthels, M., Diehl, V. & Poliwoda, H. (1980) Unterschiedlicher Einfluß von Fibrinogen und Faktor XIII auf das Wachstum von Primär- und Kulturfibroblasten. Fibrinogen, Fibrin und Fibrinkleber, (Ed. Schimpf), 227-237. F.K. Schattauer Verlag, Stuttgart, New York.

Weber, K. & Osborn, M. (1969) The reliability of molecular weight determinations by dodecylsulfate-polyacrylamide gel electrophoresis. J. Biol. Chem, 244, 4406-4412.

FIGURES

Figure 1: Reaction scheme of fibrin seal

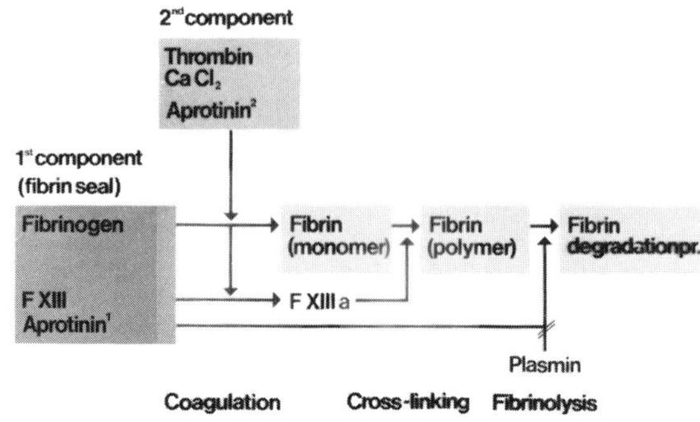

Figure 2: Cross-linking reaction of fibrin seal, a) with, and b) without aprotinin, as shown by SDS-polyacrylamide gel electrophoresis (in 5% gels) of the reduced samples. Coomassie-blue staining. Reaction times in each series: 0 min, 3 min, 10 min, 30 min, 5.00 hr, and 24.00 hr.

α, β, γ: fibrin(ogen) chains

CIG: cold-insoluble globulin

FDP: fibrin degradation products

For further details, see text.

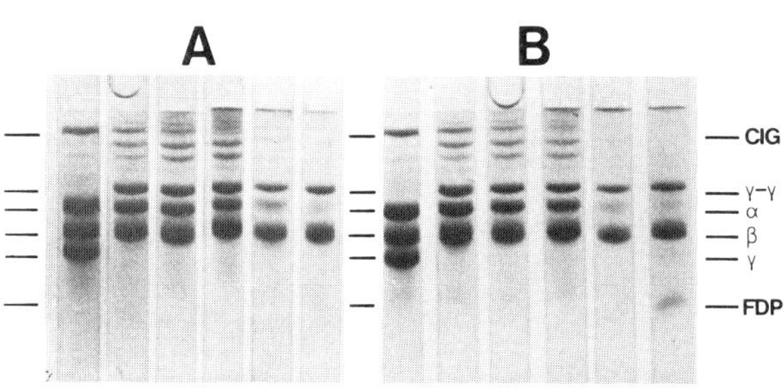

A with 50 KIE aprotinin/ml fibrin-seal
B without aprotinin

reaction time 0 min. 3 min. 10 min. 30 min. 5,00 h 24,00 h

Figure 3: Cross-linking reaction of fibrin α-chains as obtained by densitometric evaluation of gels shown in Figure 2. For each gel, the fibrin β-chain band was taken as an internal standard, and the relative decrease of α-monomer used for the calculation of α-chain polymerization.

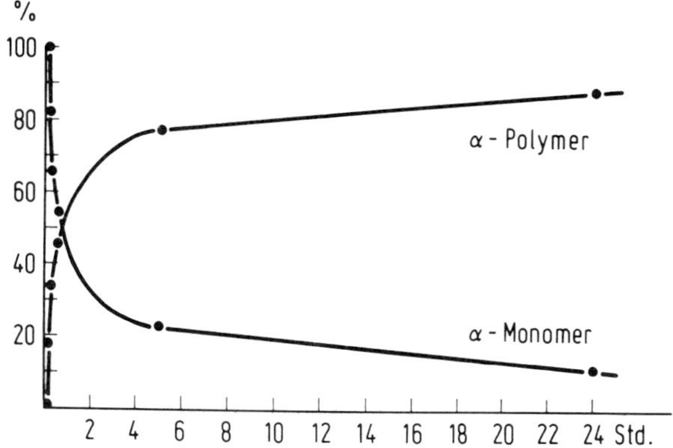

Figure 4: Dependence of tensile strength of standardized fibrin seal clots on the degree of fibrin α-chain polymerization. Clots were prepared by mixing equal volumes of fibrin seal and a solution containing 4 NIH units of thrombin/ml and 40 mmol of $CaCl_2$/1. For experimental details, see J. Guttmann (1978).

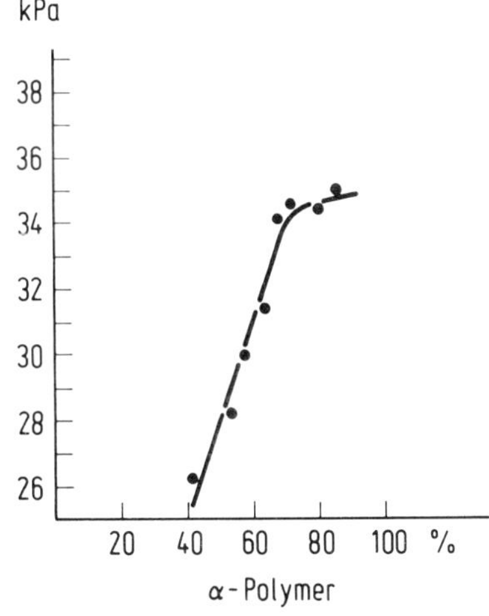

Figure 5: In vitro lysis of standardized fibrin seal clots in the presence
of different fibrinolysis inhibitors in
the clot and urokinase in the supernatant: inhibitor content per ml of
fibrin seal:
a) 20 mg EACA
b) 200 mg EACA
c) 5 mg trans-AMCHA
d) 50 mg trans-AMCHA
e) 250 KIU aprotinin
f) 1000 KIU aprotinin
For further details, see text.

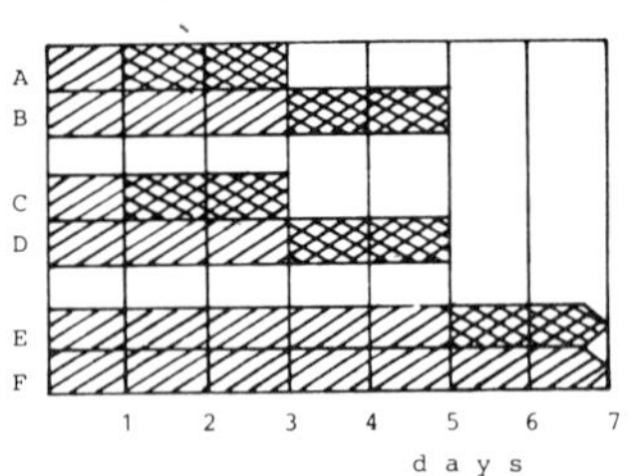

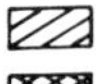

Figure 6: Double syringe for simultaneous mixing and application of the
two components of the sealing system with two detachable heads:
needle, attached (right) and spraying
head (left).

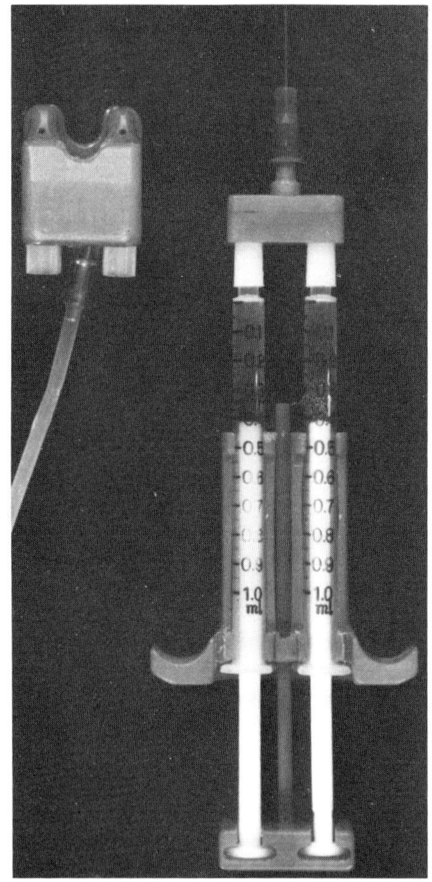

Biomaterials 1980
Edited by G. D. Winter, D. F. Gibbons, and H. Plenk, Jr.
© 1982 John Wiley and Sons Ltd.

MECHANICAL PROPERTIES
OF FIBRINOGEN-ADHESIVE MATERIAL

R. Nowotny*, A. Chalupka**, Ch. Nowotny*** and
P. Bösch****

*Institut für Radiumforschung, **Institut für
Festkörperphysik, ***2. Univ.-Frauenklinik and
****Orthopädische Univ.Klinik, University of
Vienna, A-1090 Vienna, Austria

SUMMARY

The objective of this study was to establish a method for the
determination of elastic modulus and rupture stress of fibrin
clots prepared from Fibrin Seal-Human Immuno®. A method had to be
developed where the clot could be strained until the bulk material
ruptures. Data for a standard composition of 62.1 mg clotable
fibrinogen and 50 NIH units thrombin per ml clot in a 42 mmol CaCl
solution and a reaction time of 30 minutes at $22^{\circ}C$ were 1.48×10^5
N/m^2 for modulus and 1.11×10^5 N/m^2 for rupture stress with
reference to the unstrained section. This means an extension ratio
at rupture of 3.14. Variation of the reaction time shows that the
final mechanical strength is obtained at $22^{\circ}C$ after about 30 min.
Adequate concentrations of factor XIII are contained in the
fibrinogen solution. An increase in tensile modulus and rupture
stress could be produced by increasing fibrinogen and thrombin
concentrations. Investigation of stress relaxation was not feasible
as the main purpose was rupture of the fibrin clots.

INTRODUCTION

Biological compatibility and physiological properties determine
the desirability of clotted fibrinogen solutions as an adhesive
material. It was the objective to study some mechanical properties
of fibrin clots and to devise a method of sample preparation where
rupture of the bulk material could be attained.
Mechanical stability of the clot is produced by conversion of
fibrinogen to fibrin by thrombin succeeded by a polymerization
process with participation of Ca ions and factor XIII (fibrin
stabilizing factor). The fibrinogen molecule (m.w. 340.000)
consists of 6 peptide chains linked together by 29 disulphide bonds
(Henschen et al, 1978). The polymerization process yields 6 mol
intermolecular cross-links per mol fibrin (Pisano et al, 1972).
Clot rigidity is usually determined in a shear stress geometry but
adhesiveness is not sufficient to sustain rupture stress. We have
therefore chosen a tensile stress-strain experiment.

MATERIALS AND METHODS

The fibrinogen solutions '(Fibrin Seal-Human Immuno[®]) were obtained
from Immuno GmbH., Vienna, containing 74.5 mg clotable fibrinogen
per ml. This corresponds to an enrichment from human plasma of
about 20 while factor XIII is enriched tenfold. A standard
composition was chosen according to Lindner et al (1980), giving
final concentrations of 62.1 mg clotable fibrinogen and 50 NIH
units bovine thrombine (Topostasin[®], Hoffmann-La Roche) per ml clot
in a 42 mmol CaCl solution. Fibrin clots were cast by emptying
simultaneously two syringes into the mold (Fig. 1) from one end
until discharging from the other side. At both ends the clot
penetrates a sponge-like disk which is fixed in the holders. The
diameter of the sample is reduced to 2.5 mm between the holders.
It is thus possible to strain the clot till rupture.

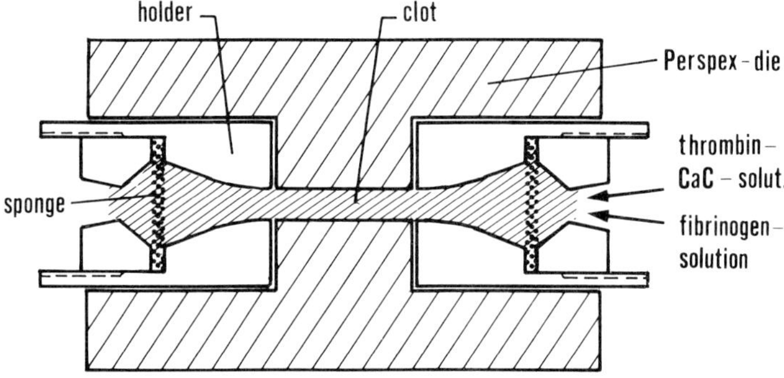

Fig. 1.   Schematic cross-section of the mold for
preparation of fibrin clot samples.

The assembly was fixed in a tensile testing machine (Instron model
1253). The Perspex dies were removed immediately before measurement. The samples were strained at a speed of 100 mm/min. The
tensile modulus of elasticity was determined from the slope of the
stress-strain curve at zero stress. Initial sample length was
taken as 22.6 mm as the length of an equivalent cylindrical
specimen assuming negligible volume change. Rupture stress is
always referred to the unstrained section of the clot. The measurements were made at 22°C.

RESULTS

A typical stress-strain curve of a clot at 30 min after preparation
is shown in Fig. 2. From 5 measurements a mean tensile modulus of
1.48×10^5 N/m^2 (1509 g/cm^2)±5.3%, a mean rupture stress of 1.11×10^5

N/m^2 (1133 g/cm^2)±22% and a mean extension ratio at rupture of
3.14±0.36 were determined. The progress of polymerization with
reaction time is given in fig. 3 for the same clot composition.

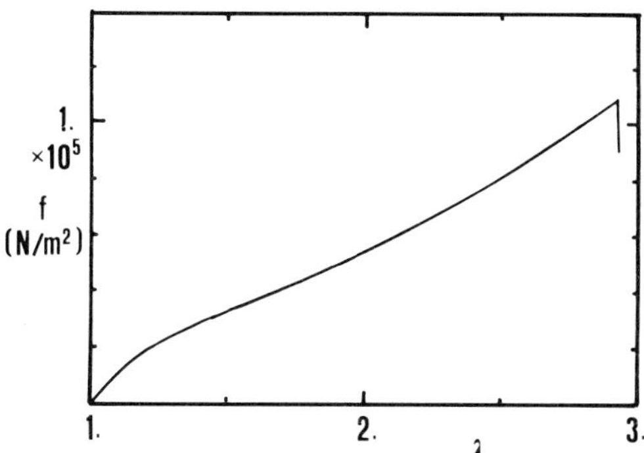

Fig. 2.   Tensile stress, f, referred to the unstrained
section of a Fibrinkleber-Human Immuno® clot against
extension ratio, λ , for a standard composition (age of
clot = 30 min).

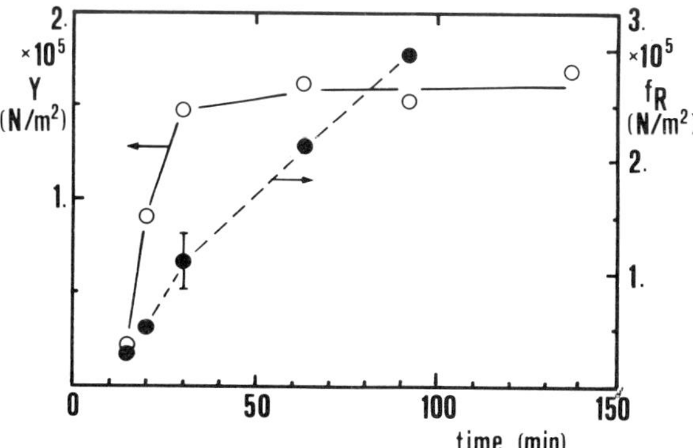

Fig. 3.   Variation of the tensile modulus, Y, and rupture
stress, f_R, with reaction time.   Open circle=Y, solid
circle=f_R.

The development of tensile modulus and rupture stress show a
different pattern. A final rupture stress was not obtained within
100 min and further experiments are required. Any measurements at
shorter reaction times than 15 min were impractical because of the
soft condition of the clot. The amount of factor XIII in the

Fibrin Seal-Human Immuno® was found to be sufficient as additional
factor XIII did not alter clot rigidity or rupture stress. For this
purpose Faktor-XIII-Konzentrat, Behringwerke AG, Marburg, was added
to the thrombin solution prior to clot preparation to give a final
concentration of 21 units/ml clot (1 unit corresponding to a
factor XIII activity of 1 ml freshly drawn citrated plasma).
The results for a variation of thrombin concentration for a
reaction time of 30 min are given in fig. 4. Modulus and rupture
stress show a similar behaviour.
The preparation of clots with higher concentrations than 500 NIH

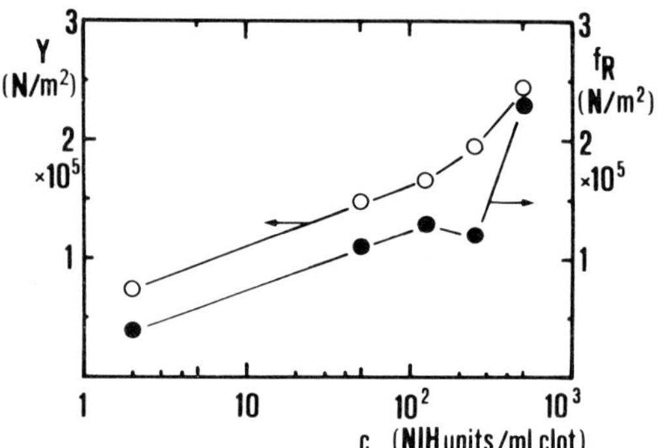

Fig. 4. Variation of the tensile modulus, Y, and rupture
stress, f_R, with thrombin concentration, c (age of clot=
30 min). Open circle=Y, solid circle=f_R.

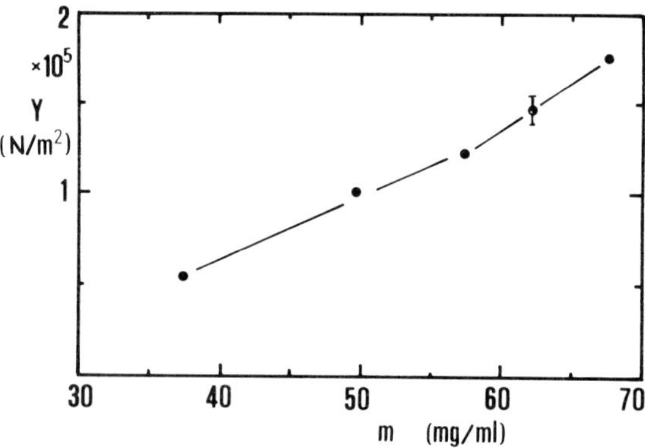

Fig. 5. Tensile modulus, Y, as a function of fibrinogen
concentration, m (age of clot=30 min).

units thrombin was not possible because the acceleration of polymerization left no time for casting. Hence no maximum in modulus and
rupture stress achievable with this material can be presented.
The variation of clot rigidity with fibrinogen concentration is
shown in fig. 5. The clots were prepared with diluted fibrinogen
solutions and strained 30 min later. The modulus increases faster
than the fibrinogen concentration. The stress relaxation data
normally could not be obtained when straining the clots till
rupture. To demonstrate the time constants which could be expected
fig. 6 shows the stress relaxation modulus for a clot of standard
composition after 2 hours reaction time.

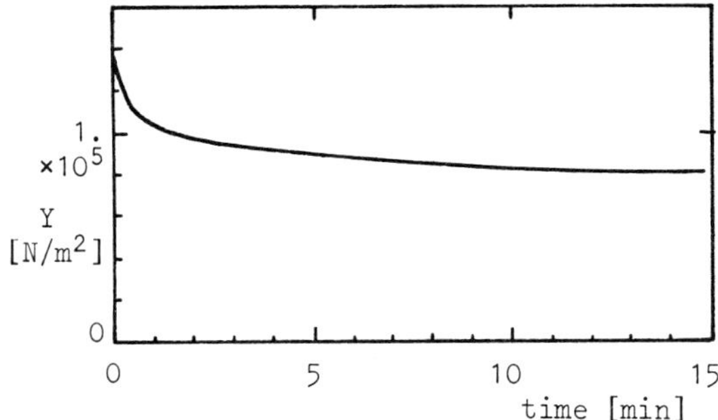

Fig. 6. Stress relaxation modulus, Y, as a function of
time (age of clot=120 min) and for an extension ratio
of 1.2.

DISCUSSION

Reproducible data for modulus and rupture stress can be obtained.
This means according to the rupture stress data that this method
yields fairly homogeneous fibrin clot samples. Direct comparison
with data for lower fibrinogen concentrations cannot be made but
the characteristics in development of modulus with time, modulus
as a function of fibrinogen concentration and stress relaxation
are similar (Carr et al, 1976, Roberts et al, 1973). Both increase
of thrombin and fibrinogen concentrations augment the tensile
strength of the clot which could mean an increased relative number
of cross-links but in the case of thrombin a time factor could be
responsible, i.e. the accelerated formation of cross-links.
The clots show viscoelastic behaviour as do fibrin clots at lower
concentration (Roberts et al, 1973) but the interrelations of the
various components in the polymerization process are not fully
determined. In the clinical situation the highest possible
concentrations of fibrinogen and thrombin and homogeneous mixing
of the liquids is advisable to achieve maximum mechanical
stability of the bulk material.

<u>REFERENCES</u>

Carr, M.E., Shen, L.L. & Hermans, J. (1976) A physical standard
of fibrinogen: Measurement of the elastic modulus of dilute fibrin
gels with a new elastometer.
Anal. Biochem., 72, 202-211.

Henschen, A., Lottspeich, F., Töpfer-Petersen, E. & Warbinek, R.
(1978) On the primary structure of fibrinogen.
Biblthca haemat., 44, 106-113.

Lindner, A., Elliott, M. & Holzer, F. (1980) Die Optimierung
des Fibrinogen-Thrombin-Klebesystems.
Wien. klin. Wschr., 92, Suppl. 109, 1-9

Pisano, J.J., Bronzert, T.J. & Peyton, M.P. (1972) ε-(γ-Glutamyl)-
lysine cross-links: Determination in fibrin from normal and
factor XIII-deficient individuals.
Annals. N.Y. Acad. Sci., 202, 98-113.

Roberts, W.W., Lorand, L. & Mockros, L.F. (1973) Viscoelastic
properties of fibrin clots.
Biorheology, 10, 29-42.

Biomaterials 1980
Edited by G. D. Winter, D. F. Gibbons, and H. Plenk, Jr.
© 1982 John Wiley and Sons Ltd.

COMPARISON OF THE STRENGTH OF CARTILAGE GLUED BY FIBRINOGEN AND CYANOACRYLATE

Claes, L., Burri, C., Helbing, G. and Lehner, E.

Department of Traumatology, University of Ulm, Oberer Eselsberg, 7900 Ulm, West-Germany

SUMMARY

In both tensile and shear tests the strength of cartilage to cartilage and cartilage to bone adhesion was proved using cyanoacrylate and fibrinogen adhesive. No significant differences were found between the strength of cartilage glued to cartilage and cartilage glued to bone. The shear and tensile strengths of the cyanoacrylate adhesive were significantly higher than those of the fibrinogen. Both adhesives show less stability in shear tests than in tensile tests. If fibrin adhesive is used in preference to cyanoacrylate, thus avoiding compatibility problems, its low strength would require immobilization of the joint or additional mechanical fixation for successful healing.

INTRODUCTION

In connection with joint trauma flake fractures of cartilage are sometimes observed in the absence of damage to the underlying bone. Stabilization of the fragments with screws, wires or sutures is difficult because of their small size. Similar problems exist in transplantation of cartilage. Therefore glueing of cartilage with tissue adhesives has been investigated and proved to be successful. In the following experiments the efficacy of a newly described fibrinogen adhesive was tested in comparison to a cyanoacrylate adhesive (Passl et al, 1976; Rupp & Stemberger, 1978).

MATERIAL AND METHODS

As test material, fresh unembalmed retropatellar joint areas were taken from 20 male one-year-old cattle (weight 500 kg). They were stored at -21° C under identical conditions prior to testing. Three cylindrical standardized

683

cartilage-bone specimens were sawn from each frozen gliding surface of the patellar joint areas. They had a diameter of 15 mm and were 20 mm long, of which 18 mm consisted of spongy bone and 2 mm of cartilage. The curva-
tures of the cartilage were cut to plane surfaces with a
microtome whereby the sectional area in one series was
localized in the cartilage and in the second series in
subchondral area. After thawing to room temperature the
plane surfaces of the specimens were glued together in
pairs. The following describes the procedures used:

1. After applying a thin layer of the commercial cyanoacrylate adhesive (Histoacryl[R]) to both surfaces, they
were fitted together and pressed for one minute.

2. Glueing of the fibrinogen adhesive was carried out as
described by the manufacturer IMMUNO, 1979. After applying a thin layer of the fibrinogen adhesive and addition
of the thrombin solution (10 National Institute of Health
thrombin/ml; 40 mmol/l $CaCl_2$; 3000 kallikrein-inactivator
-units/ml aprotinin) the specimens were pressed together
at a pressure of 1.5 N/cm².

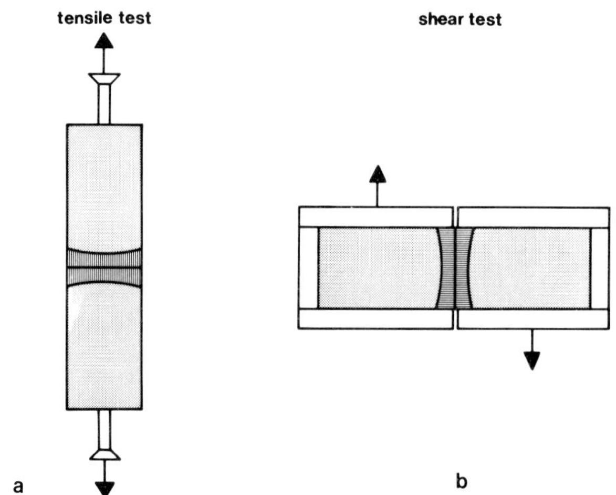

Fig. 1. Arrangement of the specimens for the
tensile (a) and shear test (b).

Specimens glued with cyanoacrylate adhesive were tested
five minutes after glueing and the others thirty minutes
later, using a material testing machine (type Zwick 1445).
The strength of the adhesion was measured by tensile and
shear tests. In tensile tests the direction of force was
vertical to the glued area (Figure 1a) and in shear tests,
tangential (Figure 1b). During tensile tests the speci-

mens were fixed by threaded screws into the spongy part
and during shear tests a special clamping device was used.
Both the tensile and the shear tests were performed with
a constant rate of deformation of 1 cm/min until tearing
occurred.During the tests the material testing machine
electronically measured and registered the forces produced.

RESULTS

The results calculated in relation to the glued area are
described in table 1 as mean values and corresponding
standard deviations.

TABLE 1. Strength of fibrinogen and cyanoacrylate glued cartilage-surfaces.

test	material	n	fibrinogen F_{max} (N/cm^2)	n	cyanoacrylate F_{max} (N/cm^2)
tensile	cartilage-cartilage	20	7.1 ± 2.8	21	85.5 ± 45.0
shear	cartilage-cartilage	17	4.6 ± 1.6	15	75.14 ± 44.7
shear	cartilage-bone	10	4.2 ± 0.6	-	-

Mean values and standard deviations.

As the results show, there were no significant differences between the strength of adhesion of the cartilage
glued to cartilage and cartilage glued to bone. Both the
shear and tensile strengths of the fibrinogen adhesive
were significantly lower than those of the cyanoacrylate.
The shear strength, which from the biomechanical point of
view is more important, was however, for both adhesives
lower than the tensile strength.

DISCUSSION

The results show the distinct superiority of the cyanoacrylate adhesive but its histological behaviour makes it

less compatible with cartilage than fibrin adhesive,
(Passl et al, 1976). Whether the relatively low strength
of the fibrinogen adhesive is sufficient in vivo can be
estimated from other authors' information on compression
and friction in joints. Frictional force on gliding materials is the product of compression and the coefficient
of friction. Under normal walking conditions, taking a
possible compression on joints of about 350 N/cm² (Brinkmann et al, 1974; Paul & Paulson, 1974) and a mean coefficient of friction of 0.02 (Freeman, 1979) a shear stress
of about 7 N/cm² would result at the cartilage surface.
The shear stress which can occur in joints is therefore
higher than the shear strength of fibrin glued cartilage
which is about 5 N/cm².

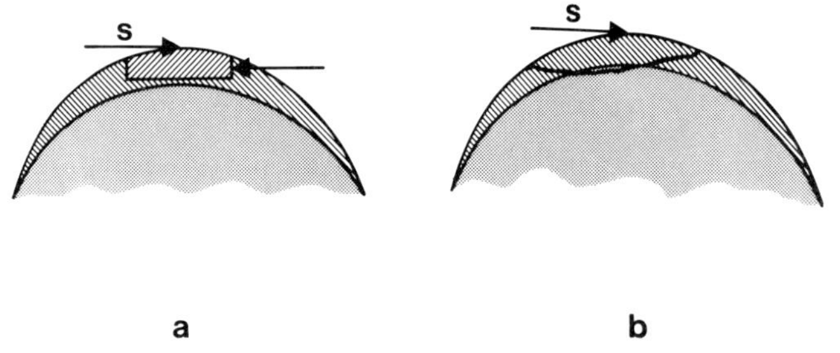

Fig. 2a. Cartilage-transplant inlaid into a hole.
The shear stress (s) at gliding surface is
apposed by the wall.
Fig. 2b. In the case of a traumatological flake
fracture the shear stress (s) is not apposed.

A flake fracture (see Figure 2b) which cannot be fixed as
an inlay, like a transplant (see Figure 2a) and which is
therefore only held by the adhesive, would in our opinion
only to be successful, if the treated joint is immobilized.

REFERENCES

Brinkmann, P., Hoefert, H., Jongen, H. Th. & Polster, J.
(1974) Biomechanik des Hüftgelenkes. Orthop., 3, 104-118.
Freeman, M.A.R. (1979) Adult Articular Cartilage, 2nd Ed.,
Tunbridge Wells: Pitmann (1979).
Passl, R., Plenk, H., Sauer, G., Spängler, H.P. &
Radaskiewicz, T. (1976) Die homologe reine Gelenkknorpel-
transplantation im Tierexperiment. Arch. orthop. Unfall-
Chir., 86, 243-256.

Paul, J.P. & Paulson, J. (1974) The analysis of forces transmitted by joints in the human body, in Experimental Stress Analysis, Conference Digest, Udine. 3.34-3.43.
Rupp, G. & Stemberger, A. (1978) Fibrinklebung in der Orthopädie, Med. Welt, 29, 766-768.

Biomaterials 1980
Edited by G. D. Winter, D. F. Gibbons, and H. Plenk, Jr.
© 1982 John Wiley and Sons Ltd.

ADHESION OF POLY(METHYL METHACRYLATE) (PMMA) ROD
ONTO HARD TISSUES

N. Nakabayashi, M. Takeyama and E. Masuhara

Institute for Medical and Dental Engineering,
Tokyo Medical and Dental University, Kanda, Tokyo 101, JAPAN

SUMMARY

Effectiveness of three functional monomers, which have both hydrophobic and hydrophilic groups, on adhesion to hard tissues was
studied. They are 4-methacryloxyethyl trimellitate anhydride (4-META)
(Takeyama 1978), 2-methacryloxyethyl phenyl hydrogen phosphate
(Phenyl-P) (Yamauchi 1979) and 2-hydroxy-3-β-naphthoxypropyl meth-
acylate (HNPM) (Nakabayashi 1978). Penetration of monomers into the
substrates was accelerated by the addition of them into MMA and
excellent adhesive strength and durability were demonstrated.

EXPERIMENTAL

Bovine or human enamel or dentine and ivory were joined with a PMMA
rod by a glue, consisting of a monomer mixture, PMMA powder and TBB-O
(Nakabayashi 1978). The monomer mixtures were 3% HNPM, 5% Phenyl-P
and 5% 4-META in MMA and MMA alone. The cemented specimens were
placed in water at 37°C for a day and their tensile adhesive strength
was measured. Some of them were further subjected to a percolation
test which emphasizes adhesive stability before the measurement. They
were alternatively introduced to two water baths for 60 sec, one maintained at 4°C and the other at 60°C, and the temperature cyclings were
repeated 60 times.

The joints were immersed in 6 N HCl for 24 hr to dissolve dentine and
in 1 N HCl for 2 hr to do enamel, and the interface of the cured adhesives was observed with an optical or a scanning electron microscope.

RESULTS AND DISCUSSION

4-META has been prepared based on the concept that monomers with
hydrophobic and hydrophilic moieties are effective in the promotion of
adhesion between dental acrylic resins and tooth substrates. Phenyl-P
and HNPM also belong to the category (Fig. 1) (Nakabayashi 1979).
The tensile adhesive strength between tooth substrates and a PMMA rod
is summarized in TABLE 1. Etching with phosphoric acid has been
necessary to adhere the resin to the enamel, but the 4-META data on
bovine enamel suggest the possibility of adherence to enamel without
prior etching. Effect of etchants, and their concentration, on the
adhesive strength and the stability of the bond between bovine enamel

689

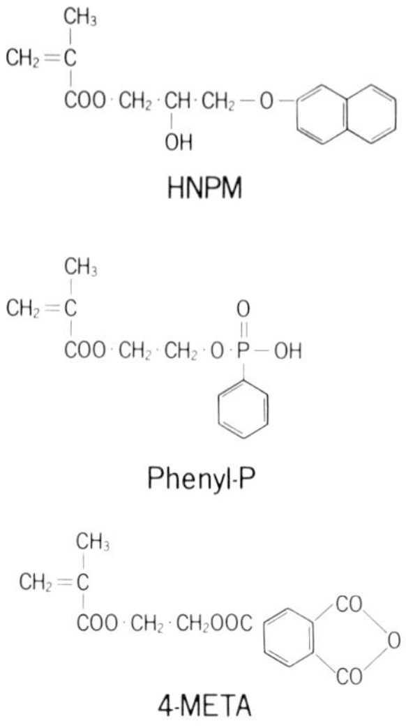

CH₃
CH₂=C
COO·CH₂·CH·CH₂—O
OH
HNPM

CH₃
CH₂=C
COO·CH₂·CH₂·O·P—OH
O
Phenyl-P

CH₃
CH₂=C
COO·CH₂·CH₂OOC
CO
O
CO
4-META

Fig. 1 Monomers with hydrophobic and hydrophilic
groups which promote adhesion of MMA
with tooth substrates

TABLE 1 Adhesive strength of PMMA rod to tooth substrates[1] (kg/cm^2)

monomer	bovine enamel		bovine dentine	ivory	human	
	brushed	ground and 2)			dentine	enamel brushed and 2)
3% HNPM	0	100	—	130	—	140
5% Pheny-P	0	100	—	125	—	135
5% 4-META	40	155	70 (179)[3]	190	140[3]	140
100% MMA	0	130	50 (110)[3]	150	110[3]	80

1) joined with new monomers in MMA, PMMA and TBB-O after a day immersion in
water at 37°

2) etched with 60% H_3PO_4 for 30 sec.

3) The dentine ground with emery paper was treated with an aqueous solution of
1% citric acid and 1% $FeCl_3$.

and a PMMA rod with the 4-META glue are illustrated in Fig. 2. Acetic acid is not as effective as citric acid. The surface morphology of the substrate has a significant effect on the adhesive strength. The bonding strength on enamel ground with emery paper and then etched with 10% citric acid is 60 kg/cm^2 after the percolation test whereas on enamel only brushed and etched with the acid it is 5 kg/cm^2. However, a 30% citric acid etch is enough to obtain significant strength (40 kg/cm^2) with brushed enamel even after the percolation. A 60% phosphoric acid etching of the enamel gave 80 kg/cm^2 for the 4-META glue and 40 kg/cm^2 for pure MMA glue. Etching with a weaker acid like citric acid is however desirable in clinical applications.

It is believed that mechanical interlocking and/or chemical reactions are important for the effective attachment of resins to tooth substrates. Fig. 3 shows that 4-META promotes penetration of monomers and suggests that the penetration into the tissues is more important for the adhesion. Initially the enamel surface etched with phosphoric acid was rougher than that etched with citric acid. However, 4-META in MMA penetrates much deeper into the enamel etched with citric acid (Fig. 3a) than MMA alone into the enamel etched with phosphoric acid (Fig. 3b). The depth of penetration into human enamel previously etched with 60% phosphoric acid was measured to show the effect of the additives on the degree of monomer penetration (Fig. 4). The rank of penetration is 5% 4-META in MMA > 5% Phenyl-P in MMA ≥ 3% HNPM in MMA > MMA. The penetration depth also alters with the position on the tooth surface. Fig. 5 shows the effect of 4-META on the penetration

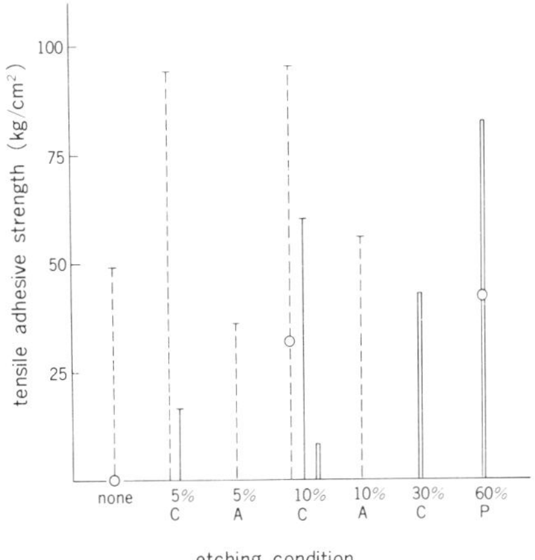

Fig. 2 Effects of etchant and region of bovine enamel on adhesive strength between PMMA rod and bovine enamel
cement: 5% 4-META in MMA, PMMA powder and TBB-O
etchant: C; citric acid, A; acetic acid, P; phosphoric acid
O MMA only, ⊢ − −⊣ ground surface, a day immersion in water at 37°C, ⊢——⊣ ground surface, a day immersion in water at 37°C+60 temperature cyclings (4°−60°), ⟺ brushed surface, a day immersion in water at 37°C+60 temperature cyclings

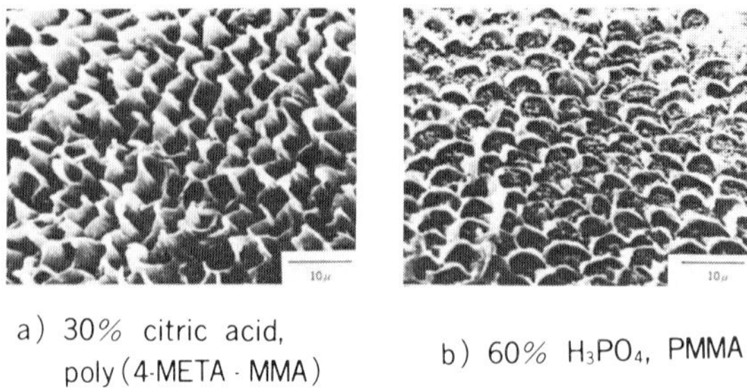

a) 30% citric acid,
poly (4-META · MMA)

b) 60% H₃PO₄, PMMA

Fig. 3 Effect of etchant and monomer on tag

Interface of adhesives cured on etched enamel
after removal of enamel by demineralization

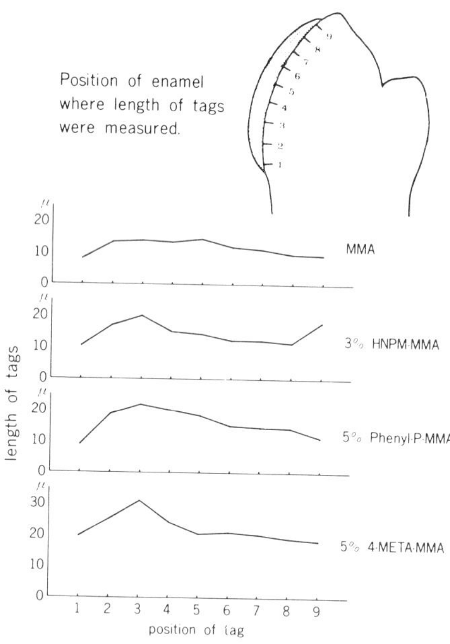

Fig. 4 Comparison of tag length with functional monomers
in MMA and PMMA cured by TBB·O

of cement into bovine dentine, after the dissolution of dentine with hydrochloric acid. Fig. 5a is a SEM picture of the dentine surface cleaned with 3% citric acid for 30 sec. Incorporation of 5% 4-META in MMA shows a greater migration into the dentinal canals (Fig. 5b), than MMA alone (Fig. 5c). Removal of the dentinal debris caused by drilling or grinding has been shown to improve adhesion. A mordant, such as ferric chloride, is also useful for the removal of debris

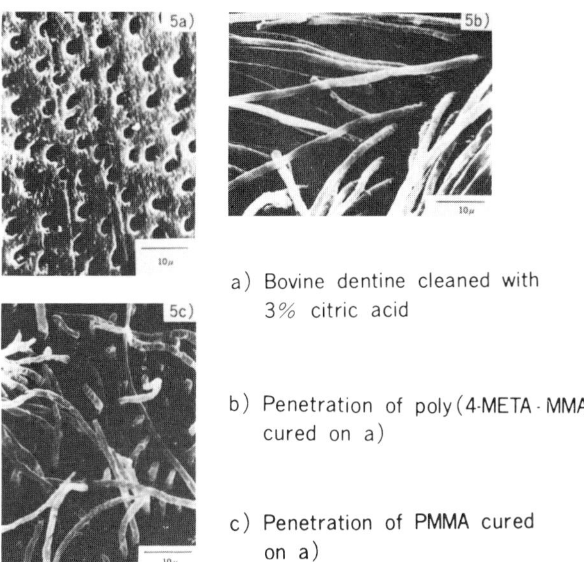

a) Bovine dentine cleaned with
3% citric acid

b) Penetration of poly(4-META-MMA)
cured on a)

c) Penetration of PMMA cured
on a)

Fig. 5 SEM pictures of adhesive interface

(Bowen 1979) (TABLE 1). Fig. 5b shows an impression of canals, with
no recognizable shrinkage due to polymerization. This suggests that
the monomers which penetrated had also been adsorbed to the substrate.
On the other hand, with MMA alone, shrinkage, presumably during polymerization, is seen in Fig. 5c and the joint fails at a lower tensile
stress of 35 kg/cm^2.

These data could be interpreted in terms of the good adhesion with the
4-META glue being due to mechanical interlocking in the canals,
however, we consider that total cross sectional area of canals is too
small to afford the large tensile strength, 145 kg/cm^2, and in addition
cohesive failure of the adhesive occurred. We thus come to the conclusion that polymerization of monomers, which penetrate into and are
adsorbed onto the tissue, must contribute to the high tensile adhesive
strength.

The tissue surface must contain hydrophobic and hydrophilic regions.
It is suggested therefore that the hydrophobic and hydrophilic groups
on monomers promote the penetration and adsorption onto these regions,
which is schematically illustrated in Fig. 6. The tooth substrates
could be said to act as template for monomer penetration and adsorption, and thus good adhesion can be obtained after polymerization due
to interlocking. Chemical reaction of the monomers with the tooth
substrate has not been confirmed however and in addition HNPM does not
have reactive group.

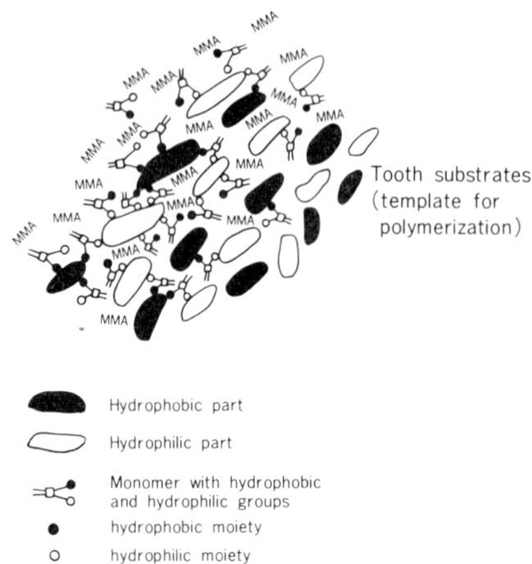

Fig. 6 Speculative illustration of penetration and adsorption
of monomers with hydrophobic and hydrophilic groups
into or onto tooth substrates

REFERENCES

Bowen, R. L. (1979) Cleaner, Mordant, and Poly SAC Effects on Composite
Adhesion to Dentine. J. Dent. Res., 58A, 260.
Nakabayashi, N. & Masuhara E. (1979) Preparation of Hard Tissue
Compatible Materials. Polymer Preprints, 20, 300-303.
Nakabayashi, N & Masuhara E. et al (1978) Development of Adhesive
Pit and Fissure Sealants Using a MMA Resin Initiated by a Tri-n-butyl
Borane Derivative. J. Biomed. Mater. Res., 12, 149-165.
Takeyama, M. & Kashibuchi N. et al (1978) Studies on Dental Self-
Curing Resins (17), Adhesion of PMMA with bovine enamel or dental
alloys. J. Japan Soc. Dent. Apparatus Mater., 19, 179-185.
Yamauchi, J. & Nakabayashi, N. et al (1979) Adhesive Agents for
Hard Tissue Containing Phosphoric Acid Monomers. Polymer Preprints,
20, 594-595.

Biomaterials in tissue and organ reconstruction

Biomaterials 1980
Edited by G. D. Winter, D. F. Gibbons, and H. Plenk, Jr.
© 1982 John Wiley and Sons Ltd.

FIBRIN CLOT SEALANTS IN MAXILLOFACIAL SURGERY

Helene Matras

Department of Maxillofacial Surgery,
University of Vienna Medical School,
Vienna, Austria

SUMMARY

Current maxillofacial applications of the fibrin clot sealing system
which was initiated by Matras et al. (1972) and is based on plasma
cryoprecipitate and specially prepared thrombin solutions are discussed. These include hemostasis, promotion of wound healing and
wound closure in macro- and microsurgery of bones and soft tissues,
replacing conventional suture materials.

INTRODUCTION

The development of the fibrin clot sealing technique as presently
used dates back to the early 197o's and was prompted by the observation of the adhesive and wound healing properties of fibrin clots
(Matras, 197o). Attempts at enhancing these properties by increasing
the fibrinogen concentration and using them in surgery were a logical
consequence. First experiences were gained in reuniting severed peripheral nerves (Matras et al., 1972).

The promising results of early animal experiments encouraged further
work designed to expand the applications and the technique was soon
introduced in other disciplines. The present report deals with the
use of fibrin clot sealants in maxillofacial surgery.

MATERIAL AND METHODS

Basically a two-component system is used for fibrin clot sealing. One
component consists of a human plasma cryoprecipitate solution which
contains 11o mg of clottable material/ml of solution, the fibrinogen
content being around 8o %. A lyophilized form is now available. The
viscous solution is applied to the desired site either alone or together with a carrier and clotted with the second component, a bovine
thrombin solution.

Clotting can be initiated by two different procedures. On consecutive
component application the two components are alternately applied to
the desired site in identical quantities. On simultaneous component
application (premixing technique) the two component solutions are
well mixed immediately before use and the mix is then applied to the
desired site. While the thrombin concentrations for consecutive

component application are high (5oo NIHU/ml), the thrombin solution
used in the premixing procedure contains just a few units of thrombin
(4 NIHU/ml). Thrombin is dissolved in distilled water enriched with
calcium ions. Aprotinin and factor XIII are added to the thrombin
solution as required for proteinase inhibition and fibrin stabilization.

APPLICATIONS OF THE FIBRIN CLOT SEALING SYSTEM (FCS)

<u>Nerve and microvascular anastomoses</u>. In humans, first clinical ex-
periences were gathered in nerve anastomoses (Kuderna and Matras,
1975). Maxillofacial applications of the system currently include
nerve anastomoses (facial - accessory, facial - hypoglossal) and
nerve grafting in selected cases involving the trigeminal, facial
and hypoglossal nerves.

For anastomosing minor vessels a combined suturing and sealing technique was developed. In animal experiments this was found to reduce
the number of sutures required for reuniting the severed common carotid of rats from an original 8 or 12 to 2 single sutures (Matras et
al., 1977). The technique was first employed clinically for extra-
intracranial anastomoses of the superficial temporal artery and a
branch of the medial cerebral artery (Kletter et al., 1978).

In the maxillofacial region proper, clot sealing is useful for
anastomosing the nutritive pedicle in free skin grafting and,
generally, for vascular repair after soft tissue injuries (e.g.
circular saw accidents).

<u>Skin graft fixation</u>. Extensive split thickness skin grafts are put in
place with just a few sutures and then firmly secured with fibrin
sealant along most of their circumference and at the undersurface.
In this application the sealant is used both for its hemostatic and
adhesive properties, thus replacing conventional suture material. As
a result, the operation time is reduced and the taking of the graft
promoted. Staindl (1977) reported the successful application of fibrin
sealant without any other conventional suturing material for the
fixation of facial skin grafts. Meanwhile we adopted an analogous
approach.

<u>Hemostasis in soft tissue defects</u>. For sealing bleeding areas in
tumors (e.g. extensive rodent ulcers) or wounds in patients prone to
develop secondary hemorrhages the fibrin clot sealant is generally
used in combination with a collagen fleece. While minor bleeding can
thus easily be controlled, the technique fails in major arterial or
venous gushes. Gastpar (1977) has employed the sealant for its hemostatic properties after tonsillectomies in patients with a hemorrhagic
diathesis.

<u>Bone sealing</u>. In bone defects involving areas which are not exposed
to mechanical stresses, minor comminuted fragments, once reduced,
are secured in place with fibrin clot sealant. The anterior frontal
sinus and the facial maxillary sinus walls can thus be reconstructed.

In combination with gelatine sponge (Spongostan[R]) or a collagen
fleece the fibrin sealant has also been used for alveolar packing
after dental extractions in cases with clotting disorders. Extensive
bony cavities left by cysts have equally been packed with the fibrin
sealant. In this application we profited from the experiences of
other workers who employed the sealing system in traumatologic and
orthopedic cases for improving bone healing (Böhler et al., 1977;
Bösch et al., 1977). Results in maxillofacial surgery were equally
satisfactory so that the system appears to have a definite place in
this application (Matras and Jesch, 1979), (Fig. 1).

Fig. 1 shows the X-rays of a female patient born 1934.

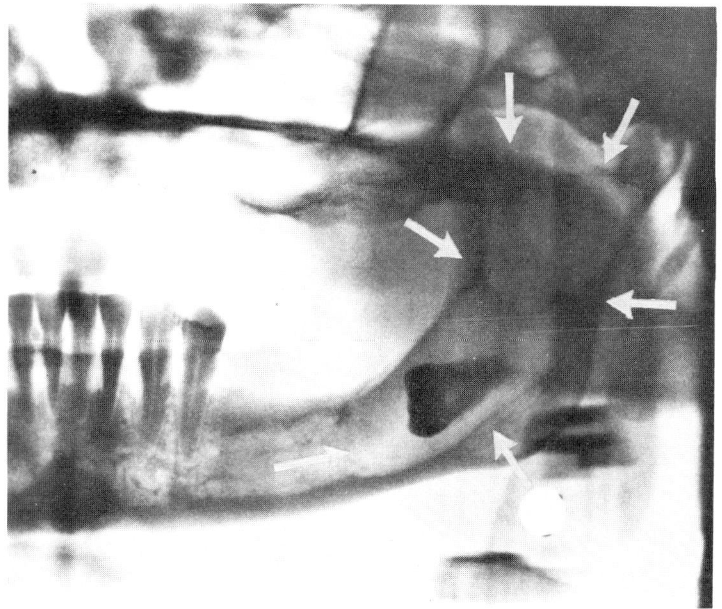

Fig. 1.a. Retained and displaced left lower wisdom tooth
with follicular cyst in corpus and ramus of mandible
extending to the notch.

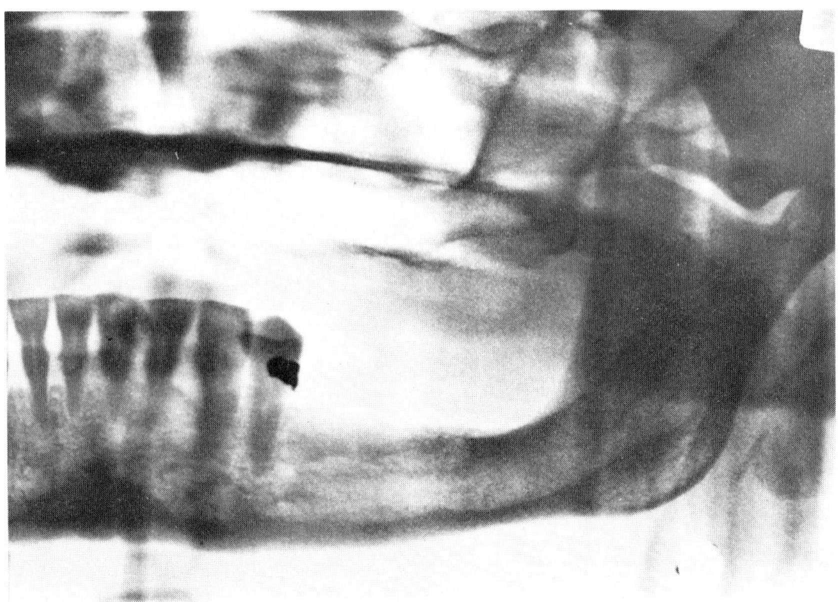

Fig. 1.b. Same patient 17 months after surgical extraction
of tooth, enucleation of cyst capsule and packing with
radiosterilized, lyophilized, homologous preserved bone
and fibrin sealant. Cancellous structure and borders of
mandibular canal restored.

Dural closure. When removing extensive malignancies in the maxillo-
ethmoidal region resections may, at times, have to be carried down
to the base of the skull and even beyond in a cranial direction. In
neoplasms infiltrating the dura, opening of the C.S.F. spaces often
is inevitable. To find out whether dural defects are eligible for
fibrin clot sealing, in vitro studies and in vivo animal experiments
were conducted which established the usefulness of the technique for
dural closure (Matras et al., 1978). Ever since, the system has been
used instead of cyanoacrylate sealants for repairing posttraumatic
and iatrogenic dural defects and reinforcing dural sutures with a
lyophilized dural patch.

DISCUSSION AND CONCLUSION

Past experience has shown fibrin clot sealing to produce a triple
effect: hemostasis, promotion of wound healing and adhesion. In
patients with clotting disorders control of bleeding from bone and
soft tissue wounds is of particular importance.

The fibrin clot sealing system is useful for alveolar packing after
dental extractions and coverage of wound surfaces.
Control of bleeding, adhesive effect and promotion of graft taking
make the sealing system particularly well suited for skin grafting.
On account of its adhesive effect, the system constitutes a valuable
alternative to conventional sutures in microsurgery and for sealing
bleeding vessels. Foreign body reactions are absent and the sealing
components are completely absorbed.
The wound healing effect of the sealant is particularly helpful in
bone defects, because it promotes and accelerates both callus formation and bony union.
Absence of neurotoxicity ensures excellent tissue tolerance in the
dural region. In addition, the sealant is completely absorbed.

In my opinion the fibrin clot sealing technique will continue to have
a definite place in the most varied maxillofacial applications.

<u>REFERENCES</u>

Böhler, N., Bösch, P., Sandbach, G., Schlag, G., Eschberger, J. &
Schmid, L. (1977) Der Einfluß von homologem Fibrinogen auf die Osteo-
tomieheilung beim Kaninchen. <u>Unfallheilk.</u>8o, 5o1-5o8
Bösch, P., Braun, F. & Spängler, H.P. (1977) Die Technik der Fibrin-
spongiosaplastik. <u>Arch.orthop.Unfall-Chir.</u>9o, 63-75
Gastpar, H. (1977) Tonsillektomie bei blutungsgefährdeten Patienten.
<u>Fortschritte d.Medizin 95</u>, 1277-128o
Kletter, G., Matras, H. & Dinges, H.P. (1978) Zur partiellen Klebung
von Mikrogefäßanastomosen im intrakraniellen Bereich. <u>Wien.klin.</u>
<u>Wschr.</u>9o, 415-419
Kuderna, H. & Matras, H. (1975) Die klinische Anwendung der Klebung
von Nervenanastomosen mit Gerinnungssubstanzen bei der Rekonstruktion
verletzter peripherer Nerven. <u>Wien.klin.Wschr.</u>87, 495-496
Matras, H. (197o) Die Wirkungen verschiedener Fibrinpräparate auf
Kontinuitätstrennungen der Rattenhaut. <u>Österr.Z.f.Stomat.</u>67, 338-359
Matras, H., Dinges, H.P., Lassmann, H. & Mamoli, B. (1972) Zur naht-
losen interfaszikulären Nerventransplantation im Tierexperiment. <u>Wien.</u>
<u>Med.Wschr.</u>122, 517-523
Matras, H., Chiari, F., Kletter, G. & Dinges, H.P. (1977) Zur Klebung
von Mikrogefäßanastomosen. Bericht d.13. Jtgg.d.Dtsch.Ges.f.plast.
und Wiederherstellungschir.Stuttgart. 1975. G.Thieme. 357-361
Matras, H., Jesch, W., Kletter, G. & Dinges, H.P. (1978) Spinale
Duraklebung mit "Fibrinkleber". Eine experimentelle Studie. <u>Wien.klin.</u>
<u>Wschr.</u>9o, 419-425
Matras, H. & Jesch, W. (1979) Die Anwendung des Fibrinklebesystems
zur Versorgung pathologischer Hohlräume im Kieferknochenbereich.
<u>Dtsch.Z.Mund-Kiefer-Gesichts-Chir.</u>3, 43-45
Staindl, O. (1977) Die Gewebeklebung mit hochkonzentriertem humanen
Fibrinogen am Beispiel der freien, autologen Hauttransplantation.
<u>Arch.Oto-Rhino-Laryng.</u>217, 219-228

Biomaterials 1980
Edited by G. D. Winter, D. F. Gibbons, and H. Plenk, Jr.
© 1982 John Wiley and Sons Ltd.

WATER-TIGHT CLOSURE OF THE SPINAL DURA
WITH A NEW FIBRIN CLOT SEALING TECHNIQUE

H.P. Dinges, Helene Matras and G. Kletter

Pathology and Bacteriology Service,
Kaiser-Franz-Josef-Spital, Vienna, Austria;
Department of Maxillofacial Surgery and
Department of Neurosurgery,
University of Vienna Medical School,
Vienna, Austria

SUMMARY

The application of a fibrin clot sealing system (FCS) in
animal experiments for water-tight dural closure is discussed. Experiments involved 6 dogs. After exposure of
the thoracic spine by laminectomy the medial spinal dura
was incised longitudinally and the cut thus produced was
sealed by alternately applying some drops of the fibrin
sealant and a thrombin solution in an identical quantity.
Early lysis of the fibrin clot was prevented by adding a
natural proteinase inhibitor to the FCS. Histologically,
wound healing was found to be complete after no more than
2 weeks with the development of a delicate scar.

The advantages of the fibrin clot sealing technique include optimum healing of the dural wound, tissue
compatibility and absence of neurotoxicity, which is
known to be associated with synthetic cyano-acrylate
tissue sealants.

Recent information on the optimum composition of the
sealing system and new application techniques are reviewed.

INTRODUCTION

To prevent the development of cerebrospinal fluid (CSF)
fistulas and its complications, a water-tight closure of
the dura is paramount in repairing dural defects. When
using conventional suturing techniques, this requires
many closely spaced single sutures. As a result, foreign
material is introduced in major amounts and wound closure
tends to be technically difficult. The use of synthetic
cyano-acrylate tissue sealants is associated with tissue

         H.P. Dinges, H. Matras and G. Kletter

intolerance and, more particularly, neurotoxicity
(Ducker, 1972).

The fibrin clot sealing system (FCS) introduced by Matras
et al in 1972 and adapted to the requirements of dural
closure in 1978 constitutes a valuable alternative (Matras
et al, 1972; Matras et al, 1978). The system imitates the
last phase of blood clotting and makes use of completely
absorbable physiologic materials which are excellently
tolerated by the tissues. Since the rate of fibrinolysis
can be controlled by adding suitable inhibitors, the
sealing system can readily be adapted to specific conditions. In attempts at repairing dural defects, it is
necessary to take into account the presence of a complete
plasminogen activator system in the dura itself (Porter
et al, 1966; Porter et al, 1969) and the existence of an
incomplete plasminogen activator system in the CSF
(Albrechtsen et al, 1958; Hemmer et al, 1970; Hindersin
and Heidrich, 1977). These tissue enzyme systems are
likely to enhance fibrinolysis during wound healing. In
the specific setting of dural repair it is desirable that
the sealant continue to be present until fibrous closure
of the wound is completed. To achieve the desired
stability, preliminary in vitro experiments were run with
the FCS to determine the efficacy of antifibrinolytic admixtures. Their outcome served as a basis for subsequent
in vivo studies.

<u>METHOD</u>

<u>In vitro studies.</u> To determine the efficacy of synthetic
or natural antifibrinolytic admixtures, 50 microliters of
the fibrin sealant were clotted with the thrombin
solutions listed in Table 1 and incubated in a CSF
solution at 37° C. The CSF solution was replaced every
3rd day and contained 1 % chloramphenicol and neomycin
sulphate to prevent bacterial growth.

TABLE 1. Fibrin clot solubility in cerebrospinal
fluid. 1 ml of the 4 thrombin solutions (in dist.
water) contained

	Thrombin 100 NIH-U[1]	E-ACA [+] 0.01 mol	Aprotinin 20000 KI-U[2]	clot solubility in CSF (in days)						
				01	03	04	08	09	18	28
1	x			−	±	+	+	+	+	+
2	x	x		−	−	−	±	+	+	+
3	x		x	−	−	−	−	−	−	−
4	x	x	x	−	−	−	−	−	−	−

[+]) epsilon-aminocaproic acid
[1] NIH-U: National Institute of Health-Units
[2] KI-U: Kallikrein Inhibitor-Units

As the results obtained showed natural antifibrinolytics
to be most satisfactory, subsequent animal experiments
were planned and executed accordingly.

<u>In vivo studies.</u> The thoracic spinal dura of 6 dogs was
exposed by a dorsal approach and incised longitudinally
for 1.5 cm (Fig. 1a). Then the cut edges were meticul-
ously coapted with 2 guy sutures and sealed with the
fibrin clot system (Figs. 1b and c).

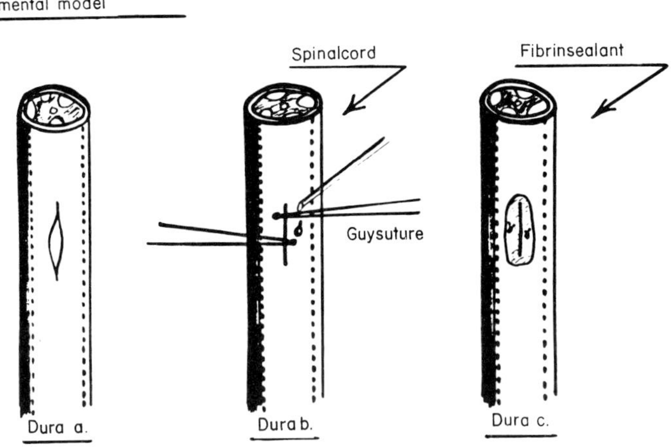

Fig. 1. Experimental technique. A 1.5 cm incision was made in the thoracic spinal dura of
the dog (a), cut edges were coapted with 2
sutures (b) and fibrin clot sealant applied (c).

Sealing solutions I and II (Table 2) were alternately and
consecutively applied in a quantity of 4 to 5 drops.

TABLE 2. Component solutions of the FCS

SOLUTION I   Fibrinkleber-Human-Immuno[R]:
                 plasma cryoprecipitate solution with 100 mp
                 protein/ml (containing 70 - 80 % fibrinogen)

SOLUTION II   To 1 ml of Ringer's solution containing
                 5.4 mequ.Ca^{++} were added:
                 thrombin (Topostasin[R])   -   100 NIH-U [1]
                 aprotinin (Trasylol[R])   -   20.000 KI-U [2]
                 F XIII (Faktor-XIII-Konzentrat[R]) - 80 U [3]

        1 see Table 1
        2 see Table 1
        3 One unit of Faktor-XIII-Konzentrat[R] represents
           the F-XIII activity of 1 ml pooled plasma.

<u>Histologic techniques.</u> Spinal blocks with the repaired
dura attached were fixed in neutral formalin and
routinely embedded in paraffin. Then sections of 4 to
6 μm thickness were prepared and stained for fibrin with
methyl violet (Gram-Weigert), phosphotungstic acid -
hematoxylin (PTAH, Mallory) and Martius scarlet blue
(MSB, Lendrum). In addition, the Sternberger immunoperoxidase reaction (Sternberger et al, 1970) in Denk's
modification (Denk et al, 1977) was used in some cases
for specific fibrin demonstration.

RESULTS

On the first and second postoperative days the coapted
dural edges were found to be covered by the fibrin clot.
In some areas there was a layer of granulocytes at the
periphery of the clot. After 7 and 8 days the dural
edges had moved apart and were bridged by rather loosely
structured fibrous tissue which was predominantly composed
of young fibrocytes and fibroblasts. This tissue was adherent to the leptomeninx in some areas. Numerous shelf-
like formations of old fibrin were still demonstrable at
the periphery of this new fibrous tissue. PTAH staining
of fibrin was found to have been partially lost by 8 days.
Fibrin formations assumed a bluish color on MSB staining
and were easily visualized with the specific immunoperoxidase reaction (Fig. 2).

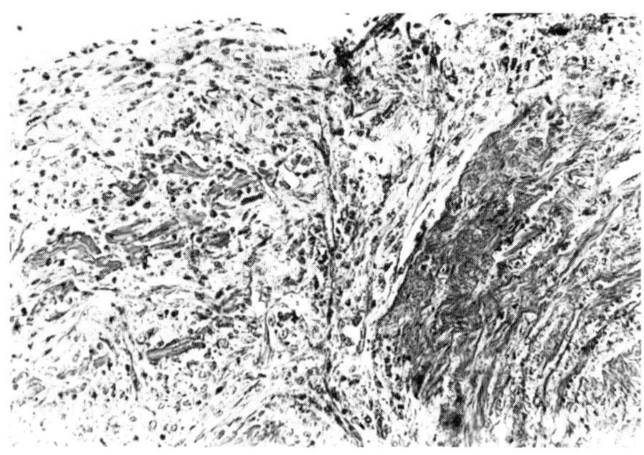

Fig. 2a. Dural closure with fibrin clot sealant,
7 days postoperatively.
Junction between dura and fibrous tissue with
fibroblasts and fibrocytes. In the periphery of
the fibrous bridge numerous shelf-like fibrin
formations can still be seen. MSB staining, x 100.

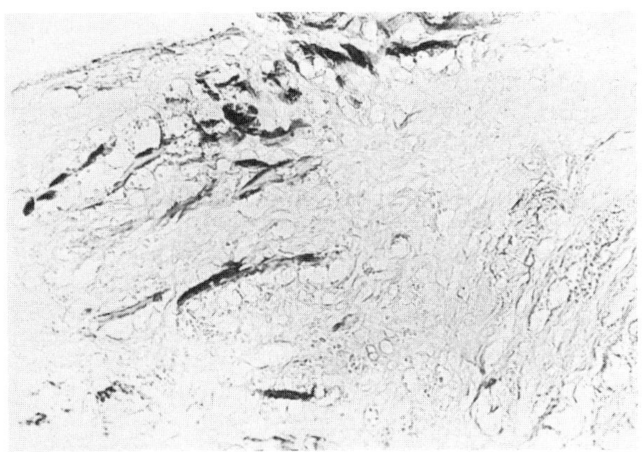

Fig. 2b. Dural closure with fibrin clot sealant,
7 days postoperatively.
Fibrin formations clearly visualized by the
immunoperoxidase reaction, x 100.

Fourteen days after dural repair the fibrous bridge was
predominantly composed of mature fibrocytes and abundant
collagen fibers and showed substantially increased
cellularity (scarring). Scar shrinkage caused the dural
edges to approach one another again. Sealant-derived
fibrin was no longer demonstrable. Conditions on day 21
were largely identical with those on day 14. In one case
the spine was found to have been injured on dural splitt-
ing.

DISCUSSION

Postoperative wound healing and histologic evaluation of
the animal experiments established that the fibrin clot
sealant alone was capable of producing a largely water-
tight closure of minor dural defects. The fibrin-
stabilizing factor XIII, contained both in the fibrin
sealant itself and in the thrombin solution, is believed
to enhance fibroblast proliferation (Beck et al, 1962;
Hörmann and Kühn, 1977).

We attempted to delay fibrinolysis until fibrous closure
of the wound in the dura was complete. As our histological investigations showed, the delay of fibrinolysis was
apparently long enough to achieve fibrous repair of the
dural wound. An exact determination of both fibrinolysis

and fibrous wound repair would require a larger material,
so that at least one animal would be available for
histologic examination on each of the first seven days.

In our preliminary studies we found that E-ACA, when added
to the FCS, produced a less pronounced antifibrinolytic
effect than the natural proteinase inhibitor aprotinin.
This might be accounted for by the binding of plasminogen-
lysine to the fibrinogen molecule during plasma
fractionation in preparing the sealant. The fibrin
binding site of the plasminogen molecule would thus no
longer be available for E-ACA so that the inhibitory
effect is lost (Castellino and Violand, 1979; Brockway
and Castellino, 1971). Aprotinin, by contrast, can
stoichiometrically bind to plasmin (Castellino and
Violand, 1979) and, consequently, suppresses its proteolytic activity. This is in agreement with our preliminary experiments and with the in vitro studies by
Seelich and Redl (1979) and by Redl et al (1979).

Recent investigations have prompted modifications to the
application technique and changes in the composition of
the sealant (Seelich and Redl, 1979). The most important
modification is the introduction of a premixing procedure
and replacement of consecutive component application by
simultaneous component application.

A reduction of the thrombin content in solution II to
4 NIH-U of thrombin slows down the clotting rate. This
allows sufficient time for the two-component sealant to
be applied to the desired site after appropriate premixing of the 2 component solutions. The most significant
advantage of premixing is the attainment of optimum fibrin
cross-linkage.

Table 3 lists the composition of Fibrinkleber-Human-
Immuno[R] (from Seelich and Redl, 1979). Since the sealant
itself has a high factor XIII content, factor XIII admixtures can be kept low, if not altogether omitted,
particularly when the premixing technique is used. Minor
aprotinin concentrations are sufficient to compensate for
the plasminogen present in the sealant.

TABLE 3.   Composition of Fibrinkleber-Human-Immuno[R]

75 - 95 %	fibrinogen
5 - 12 %	cold-insoluble-globulin (fibronectin)
15 U/ml [1]	factor XIII
1 - 3 %	albumin

The plasminogen : fibrinogen ratio is about
30 times lower than in pooled citrated plasma.

1   see Table 2

In addition, recent investigations have established the
importance of an optimum calcium ion concentration and
showed that other ions, if present in excessive quantities
interfered with fibrin cross-linkage and thus reduced the
mechanical strength of the sealing system. Table 4
illustrates what is currently thought to be the optimum
composition of solution II, the hardener of the system
(from Redl et al, 1979).

TABLE 4.   Composition of the clotting solution

40 mmol/l	$CaCl_2$ solution
4 or 500 NIH-U/ml [1]	thrombin
0 - 3000 KIU/ml [2]	aprotinin

The final $CaCl_2$ concentration should not be
below 5 mmol/l

1   see Table 1
2   see Table 1

The optimum aprotinin concentration depends on the sealing site (fibrinolytic activity of the tissue to be
sealed) and the desired sealant persistence. Whether or
not the antifibrinolytic added to the system is associated
with untoward side effects in terms of excessive fibrosis
of delicate structures, e.g. nerves, will have to be
clarified in more detailed studies.

REFERENCES

Albrechtsen, O.K. Storm, O. & Claassen, M. (1958)
Fibrinolytic activity in some human body fluids. Scand.
J. Clin. & Lab. Investigation, 10, 310-318.

Beck, E., Duckert, F., Vogel, A. & Ernst, M. (1962) Der
Einfluß des fibrinstabilisierenden Faktors (FSF) auf
Funktion und Morphologie von Fibroblasten in vitro. Zschr.
f. Zellforschung, 57, 327-346.
Brockway, W.J. & Castellino, F.J. (1971) The mechanism of
the inhibition of plasmin activity by E-Aminocaproic acid.
J. Biol. Chem., 246, 4641-4647.
Castellino, F.J. & Violand, B.N. (1979) The fibrinolytic
system - basic considerations. Progress in Cardiovascular
Diseases, 21, 241-253.
Denk, H., Radaskiewicz, T. & Weirich, E. (1977) Pronase
pretreatment of tissue sections enhances sensitivity of
the unlabelled antibody-enzyme (PAP) technique. J. Immuno-
logical Methods, 15, 163-167.
Ducker, T. (1972) Tissue adhesive in neurosurgery. In:
Tissue adhesives in surgery (Ed. T. Matsumoto), H. Huber,
Bern-Stuttgart-Wien.
Hemmer, R., Schneider, J. & Maleknasri, F. (1970) Zur
Frage der fibrinolytischen Wirksamkeit des Liquors. Ner-
venarzt, 41, 303-305.
Hindersin, P. & Heidrich, R. (1977) In-vitro-Versuche zur
Klärung der fibrinolytischen Aktivität im Normalliquor.
Psychiatr. Neurol. med. Psychol., 29, 275-284.
Hörmann, H. & Kühn, K. (1977) Das Zusammenspiel von
humoralen Faktoren, extrazellulärer Matrix und von Zellen
bei der Wundheilung. Fortschr. Med., 95, 1299-1304.
Matras, H., Dinges, H.P., Lassmann, H. & Mamoli, B. (1972)
Zur nahtlosen interfaszikulären Nerventransplantation im
Tierexperiment. Wien. med. Wschr., 122, 517-523.
Matras, H., Jesch, W., Kletter, G. & Dinges, H.P. (1978)
Spinale Duraklebung mit "Fibrinkleber". Eine experimen-
telle Studie. Wien. klin. Wschr., 90, 419-425.
Porter, J.M., Acinapura, A.J., Kapp, J.P. & Silver, D.
(1966) Fibrinolytic activity of the spinal fluid and
meninges. Surgical Forum, 17, 425-427.
Porter, J.M., Acinapura, A.J., Kapp, J.P. & Silver, D.
(1969) Fibrinolysis in the central nervous system.
Neurology, 19, 47-52.
Redl, H., Seelich, T., Guttmann, J., Dinges, H.P.,
Schlag, G., Kuderna, H. & Stachelberger, H. (1979)
Basical considerations and theoretical background of
fibrin sealing. European Surgical Research, 11, Suppl. 2,
98.
Seelich, T. & Redl, H. (1979) Theoretische Grundlagen des
Fibrinklebers. Blut, 38, 12.
Sternberger, L.A., Hardy, P.H., Cucullis, J.J. &
Meyer, H.G. (1970) The unlabelled antibody enzyme method
of immunohistochemistry: preparation and properties of
soluble antigen-antibody complex (horseradish peroxydase -
antihorseradish peroxydase) and its use in identification
of spirochets. J.Histochem.Cytochem., 18, 315-333.

Biomaterials 1980
Edited by G. D. Winter, D. F. Gibbons, and H. Plenk, Jr.
© 1982 John Wiley and Sons Ltd.

FUNCTIONAL RESTORATION OF THE TEMPORO–MANDIBULAR JOINT BY INTERPOSITION OF LYOPHILIZED DURA. CLINICAL AND EXPERIMENTAL RESULTS.

R. Timmel[1], F. Grundschober[2], K. Hollmann[1] and H. Plenk Jr.[2]

1) University Clinic of Maxillo-Facial Surgery
2) Bone Research Lab., Histological-Embryological Institute
University of Vienna, Austria

SUMMARY

This paper reports on the successful clinical application of lyophilized human dura (Lyodura®) as an interponate in ankylosis operations of the temporo-mandibular joint in man. In six of eight patients with whom movement therapy was started early, re-ankylosis could be completely prevented by this treatment. In an experimental study in domestic pigs the tissue reaction to this natural biomaterial were investigated histologically. The lyophilized dura was resorbed with a foreign-body cell reaction and substituted by the body's own tissue. It was noteworthy in this indication that formations resembling the joint were found again about five months after operation.

INTRODUCTION

Ankylosis of the temporo-mandibular joint occurs most frequently following trauma in the joint region. Such conditions can only be corrected surgically, with the objective of functional restoration of the joint. For this purpose, a modelling bone resection is performed on the condyle of mandible, but opinion is divided on the necessary extent of this resection. To prevent re-ankylosis, additional systematic functional treatment is recommended which should start as soon as possible after operation. However, since success cannot be guaranteed by these procedures alone, it was suggested over a century ago that the condyle of mandible be separated from the temporal bone by the interposition of a pediculate fascia of temporal muscle (Verneuil 1872). Thereafter a large number of alloplastic and autologous materials for this interposition were tried out: gold plate (Roser 1889), lamina of silver and celluloid (Chlumsky 1900), sheets of gutta-percha (Brophy 1914), methylmethacrylate block (Rehrmann 1960) and Proplast® (Kent et al 1975); auricular cartilage (Dufourmentel 1941) and soft tissue (Pelser 1967). In this study, the clinical and experimental results of the interposition of lyophilized dura will be presented.

MATERIAL AND METHODS

Clinical procedure: At the suggestion of Nasteff (1965), human lyophilized dura (Lyodura®, Braun-International, FRG) has been used at this clinic for the last 10 years as an interposition material in ankylosis operations of the temporo-mandibular joint (Hollmann and Timmel, 1979). The ankylosed joint (Fig. 1) is exposed by a praeauricular incision, a cleft of about 0.5 cm in width is created by bone resection of the condyle of mandible, and a sheet of gamma ray sterilized Lyodura®, 2 x 3 cm in size, is moistened in physiological saline and laid as a single or double layer into the cleft (Fig. 2a) so that a newly formed articular space becomes visible in the radiograph (Fig. 2b). On the next day, intensive movement therapy is commenced using a specially developed activator which can be adjusted to the opening distance of the mouth by a vertical expansion screw.

This study presents the results of 8 patients treated using this procedure. 4 patients were operated for unilateral ankylosis and 4 patients for bilateral ankylosis. In all patients a fracture of the condyle of mandible was the primary cause of the ankylosis. Syndesmosis was observed intraoperatively in seven joints and synostosis in five joints. The average cutting edge distance measured preoperatively was 11.8 mm (minimum 3 mm, maximum 25 mm), and increased after the operation to an average of 31 mm (minimum 25 mm, maximum 42 mm). In 1979 postoperative observation periods ranged between 1 and 9 years.

Animal experiments: The experiments were performed in 8 young domestic pigs with an average body weight of 25 kg. Under general endotracheal anaesthesia, the temporo-mandibular joint was exposed on one side in 3 animals, and on both sides in 5 animals. The articular cartilage was removed from the condyle of mandible and the temporal bone together with the articular disc and part of the capsule. Into this cleft a double layer of Lyodura® was placed on the bony stump of the condyle of mandible and fixed in position by two atraumatic Mersilen® sutures. The wound was then closed carefully. The animals were sacrificed after sequential fluorochrome labelling and observation periods of 18, 36, 50 and 140 days. The temporo-mandibular joint region was removed, fixed in Schaffer's fluid and embedded in methyl-methacrylate. Microtome and ground sections were prepared in the sagittal plane and radiomicrographs were made of selected sections.

RESULTS

Clinical observations: Postoperative wound healing ensued normally. 1 to 9 years after operation all 8 patients were completely free of subjective symptoms and pain. In no case was an open bite or malocclusion found. The cutting edge distance averaged in 6 patients 36.5 mm (minimum 29 mm, maximum 44 mm). Two of the patients, however, who had not carried out the postoperative movement therapy, showed a cutting edge distance of 4 and 14 mm respectively.

Histological Findings: The human lyophilized dura, interposed in the bare temporo-mandibular joint space, was resorbed at different rates. In some cases, only slight residues could still be detected after 18 days, whereas in others larger residues of the material were found even after 50 days. Resorption was effected by foreign-body giant cells which were always accompanied by lymphocyte and plasma cell infiltrates (Fig. 3). In many cases, there were cyst-like, small or large spaces containing material residue and accumulations of blood cells.

In only one animal were mineral deposits found within the visible lyophilized dura laminae. These deposits showed a positive calcium-salt staining reaction, fluorochrome labelling and radiodensity in the radiomicrograph (Fig. 4). In this case, the resorbing multinucleated foreign-body giant cells could not be distinguished from osteoclasts.

50 days after operation, the highly vascularized and cellular granulation tissue initially found around the implants was transformed into a more fibrous scar tissue. After 140 days, a dense fibrous connective tissue filled the entire former joint region. Within this connective tissue, there were joint-like spaces (Fig. 5a) which had a cellular lining resembling a synovial membrane (Fig. 5b). In one case two such spaces were found, leaving an articular disc-like fibre formation between them.

The condyle of mandible showed pronounced bone remodelling 18 and 36 days after operation, the bone formation proceeding distally, as indicated by fluorochrome labelling. After 50 days, fibrocartilage covered the condyle of mandible which had an almost normal shape after 140 days (Fig. 5a). In contrast, the articular surface of the temporal bone was never restored and the new bone formation at this site seemed markedly less pronounced when compared to the condyle of mandible. However, osteophytic bone formation projecting into the former implant region was found in two cases after 50 and 140 days.

DISCUSSION AND CONCLUSIONS

There remain differences of opinion regarding the extent to which the condyle of mandible should be resected and the nature of the material to be interposed. In our clinic we only remove a thin bone strip a few millimetres wide from the dorsal region of the ankylosed mandible to maintain a suitable support and to obtain a satisfactory aesthetic effect and occlusion (see Pichler & Trauner, 1948).

We regard the interposition of a material as an important advance, and have produced satisfactory results with the use of lyophilized dura. Lyodura® is a well tolerated biological implant material that does not require a second operation which frequently causes more pain to the patient than the ankylosis operation itself (Eschler & Schilli, 1967). The lyophilized material apparently withstands mechanical impact until replaced by the body's own fibrous tissue (Seiffert 1967, Jäger 1971). In addition to these clinical findings, our experimental studies have shown that tissue formation resembling the natural joint occurs by five months after implantation of Lyodura®. The importance of starting postoperative exercise therapy early to prevent re-ankylosis is generally emphasized and is demonstrated by our clinical results.

Pigs were chosen as experimental animals because as omnivores they have a temporo-mandibular joint most similar to that of man, second only to primates. However, the heterologous origin of the implant material may have caused the pronounced foreign body reaction and the ectopic mineralisation in one case, but did not seem to hinder the functional and structural restoration of the joint.

REFERENCES

Brophy, N. (1914) cited after Pichler and Trauner (1948) p. 589.

Chlumsky, V. (1900) Über die Wiederherstellung der Beweglichkeit des Gelenkes by Ankylose. Zbl. f. Chir. 27, 921-925.

Dufourmentel, L. (1941) Ankylosen (Knorpelverpflanzung) Med.acad.Chir. 67, p. 370.

Eschler, J. & Schilli, W. (1967) Die Verwendung von Knorpel bei der Bildung von Neoarthrosen des Kiefergelenkes Fortschr. Kiefer- Gesichtschir. 12, (Ed., K. Schuchardt) pp 95-97. Georg Thieme - Stuttgart.

Hollmann, K. & Timmel, R. (1979) Interposition von Lyo-Dura im Kiefergelenkbereich. Fortschr. Kiefer-Gesichtschir. 25 (Ed., K. Schuchardt) in press Georg Thieme - Stuttgart.

(Jäger, M. (1971) Experimentelle Untersuchungen zur Verwendung der lyophilisierten Dura im Bereich der Wiederherstellungschirurgie.Chirurg,42, 266-269.

Kent, J.N., Homsy, C.A. & Hinds, E.C. (1975) Proplast® in Dental Facial Reconstruction. Oral Surg. 39, 347-355.

Nasteff, D. (1965) Verwendung von lyophilisiertem Gewebe (Knochen, Knorpel, Dura) in der Kiefer- Gesichtschirurgie (Eds., Kettler & Serfling) Gewebskonserven,Herstellung und Anwendung II, pp 188-190. Volk und Gesundheit, Berlin.

Pelser, M. (1967) Die Therapie der Spätfolgen nach Traumen im Kiefer- und Gesichtsbereich. Fortschr. Kiefer- Gesichtschir. 12, (Ed., K. Schuchardt), pp 57-63. Georg Thieme - Stuttgart.

Pichler, H. & Trauner, R. (1948) Mund- und Kieferchirurgie Vol. II/2, pp 584-597. Urban Schwarzenberg, Wien.

Rehrmann, A. (1967) Eine Methode zur operativen Beseitigung der doppelseitigen Ankylose der Kiefergelenke durch breite Knochenresektion, temporäre Implantation von Palavitkörpern und autologe Knochentransplantationen. Fortschr. Kiefer- Gesichtschir. 12, (Ed., K. Schuchardt), pp 64-71. Georg Thieme - Stuttgart.

Roser, K.(1898) Behandlung der Kiefergelenksankylose. Zbl.f.Chir.25, 122-125.

Seiffert, K.E. (1966) Biologische Grundlagen der homologen Transplantation konservierter Bindegewebe. Langenbecks Arch. klin. Chir. 316, 526-531.

Verneuil, A.A.S. (1872) De la création d'une fausse articulation par section ou résection partielle de l'os maxillaire inférieur. Arch.Gen.de Medic.15, 284-296.

FIGURES

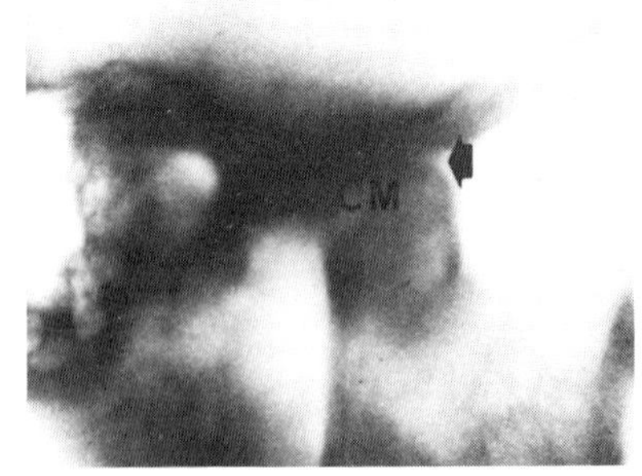

Fig. 1 Pre-operative tomograph of an ankylosed human temporomandibular joint (CM = condyle of mandible).

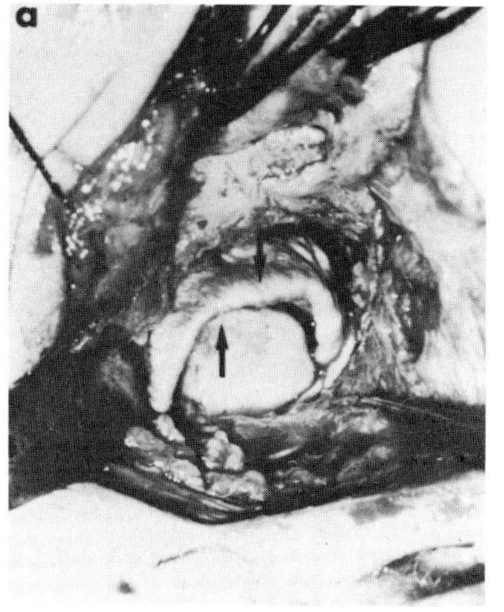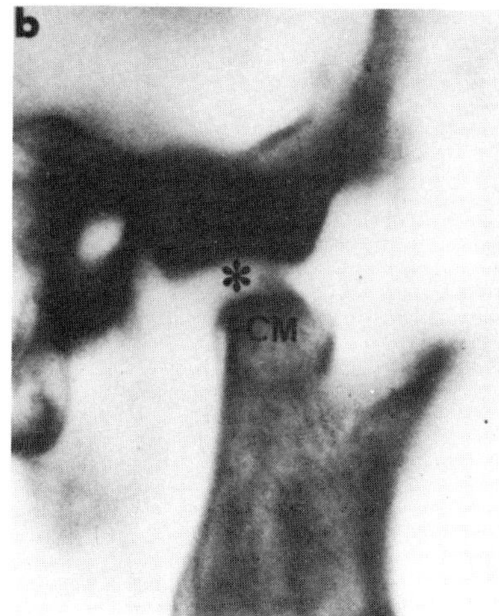

Fig. 2: a) The human temporo-mandibular joint after resection of the ankylosis and interposition of a two-fold layer of Lyodura® (arrows). b) Post-operative tomograph, showing a newly created joint space (asterisk).

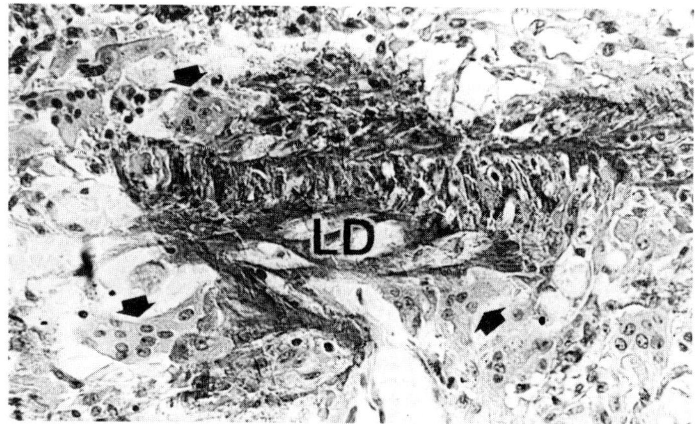

Fig. 3: Microtome section of the temporo-mandibular joint region of a pig 18 days after implantation (Trichrome Goldner, 166 x). Remnants of Lyodura (LD) are being resorbed by multinucleated giant cells (arrows).

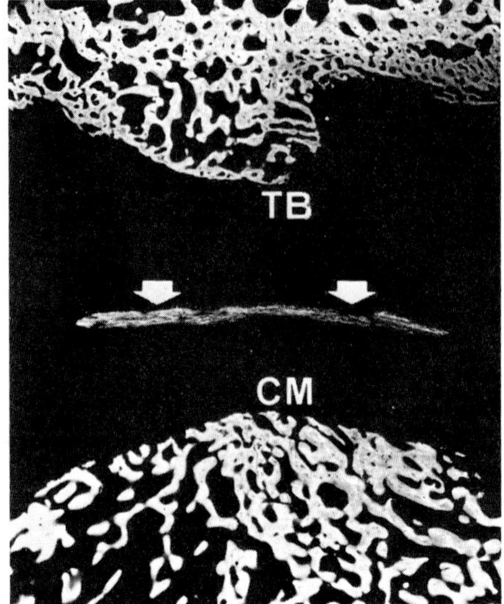

Fig. 4: Radiomicrograph of a sagittal ground section of the temporo-mandibular joint of a pig 36 days after implantation (10 x).   Radiodense deposits within the Lyodura (arrows). (TB = temporal bone, CM = condyle of mandible).

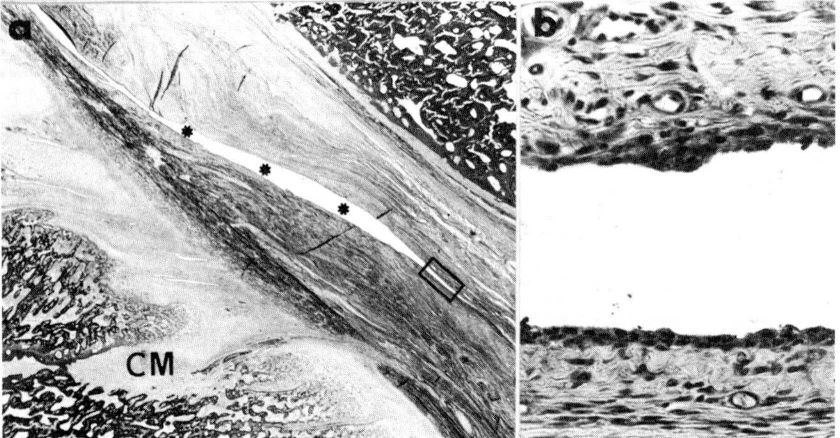

Fig. 5 a-b: Sagittal section of the temporo-mandibular joint region of a pig 140 days after implantation (a: Trichrome Goldner, 9 x; b: Toluidine-blue, 250 x).
The Lyodura has been completely replaced by fibrous connective tissue, the fibres of which run parallel to the articular surface. The joint-like space (asterisks) is lined by synovial cells (b = enlargement of a). Note the fibrocartilage on the surface of the condyle of mandible (CM).

Biomaterials 1980
Edited by G. D. Winter, D. F. Gibbons, and H. Plenk, Jr.
© 1982 John Wiley and Sons Ltd.

ELECTRON MICROSCOPE OBSERVATIONS OF AL_2O_3
CERAMIC IMPLANTS IN MIDDLE EAR SURGERY

K. Jahnke, M. Galic, W. Eitel and H. Heumann

Department of Otorhinolaryngology,
University of Tubingen, Germany.

SUMMARY

Scanning and transmission electron microscope investigations were
performed in order to study the biocompatibility of Al2O3 ceramic
in the middle ear. Within three weeks the implants were already
covered with a delicate mucous membrane. Usually one could find
a cuboidal epithelium with microvilli, occasionally some ciliated
cells, both having an intact basement membrane. There was a normal
subepithelial cell layer with active fibroblasts, blood vessels and
nerve fibres. Signs of incompatibility were not observed. The
results are in accordance with our preliminary clinical experiences.

INTRODUCTION

The outstanding biocompatibility of aluminium oxide ceramic has
already been proved by several years of use in orthopaedics and
dentistry (Griss et al.,1973; Heimke et al.,1977). Nevertheless
before the introduction of this ceramic into middle ear surgery,
animal experiments were thought to be necessary because this was a
new application.

MATERIALS AND METHODS

Al_2O_3 ceramic prostheses were implanted into the middle ear of 24
healthy rabbits (body weight 2.1 – 3.4 kg, both sexes). The
prostheses were positioned between the eardrum or handle of the
malleus and the head of the stapes or footplate. The animals were
not given any antibiotics. They were killed at intervals of three
weeks, 1, 3, 5, 8 and 10 months. The middle ears were fixed with
2 % paraformaldehyde + 2.5 % glutaradehyde in 0.1 M cacodylate
buffer (pH 7.4) for 1 h at $0 - 4^0C$. After washing in the buffer
the specimens were fixed with 1 % osmium tetroxide in 0.1 M
cacodylate buffer (pH 7.4) for 1 h at $0 - 4^0C$ and washed again.
Following graded acetone dehydration and critical point drying using
carbon dioxide the specimens for scanning electron microscopy were
double coated with carbon and gold. For transmission electron microscopy the specimens were embedded in araldite. Thin sections were
briefly stained with lead citrate and studied on a Philips 301 electron
microscope.

RESULTS

Within 3 weeks the implant was completely covered with a thin
delicate middle ear mucosa, the contour and colour of the
prosthesis could be clearly recognised. In electron scanning two
kinds of epithelium could be differentiated. Usually one could find
a cuboidal epithelium with microville which were seen more
concentrated near the cell borders. Occasionally some ciliated
epithelial cells with evenly distributed kinocilia were identified.
The mucosa of the undersurface of the eardrum was found to continue
as the mucosa covering the implant. Where the prosthesis was
separated from the head of the stapes a layer of connective tissue
was visible. Findings after 10 months interval were analogous.
These results were confirmed by our transmission electron microscopic studies. The epithelial cells of the mucosa presented a
normal appearance, with an intact basement membrane (Figs. 1, 2).
There were one or two rows of cuboidal cells with microville at the
surface, normal intercellular junctions and a well organised cytoplasm containing many cell organelles. In animals which were killed
after a 3 week interval we found signs of a wound healing reaction
or of a slight inflammation, i.e. some granulocytes, but the mucosa
of animals which were killed after long implantation times (5 or 10
months) had no signs of inflammation. No macrophages or giant cells
were detected in any of the specimens. The thin subepithelial cell
layer (Figs. 1, 3) consists of (a) active fibroblasts in different
stages, which exhibit a prominent endoplasmic reticulum with many
ribosomes, (b) a smooth ground substance and (c) mature parallel-
running collagen fibres, and after short intervals procollagen.
There are many blood vessels whose endothelial cells contain a high
amount of micropinocytotic vesicles, and some nerve fibres. No
thick fibrous layer was seen.

DISCUSSION AND CONCLUSIONS

The electron microscopic study has shown that a normal healthy
mucous membrane covers aluminium oxide ceramic implants after
implantation into the middle ear. Signs of incompatibility
(macrophages, giant cells, a thick fibrous tissue layer, necrotic
tissue) were not observed. A few granulocytes were seen after short
implantation times as in normal wound healing. A fibrous connection
with the head of the stapes is interpreted to be the result of
shearing motions (Heimke et al., 1977). To date we have implanted
more than 200 aluminium oxide ceramic prostheses. The outstanding
biocompatibility of this material was confirmed (Jahnke et al.,
1979; Jahnke & Plester, 1980). The ease and precision with which
this ceramic can be shaped during the operation has proven
especially advantageous in clinical practice. Thus precision
positioning can be achieved. There is no fixation to the surrounding
bone, and of course no partial resorption occurs. Further advantages
are the rigidity of the material and that a joint-like connection
with the rest of the auditory ossicular chain is formed. Our
preliminary results, covering a period of over 2 years, are very
encouraging as far as compatibility and function are concerned.

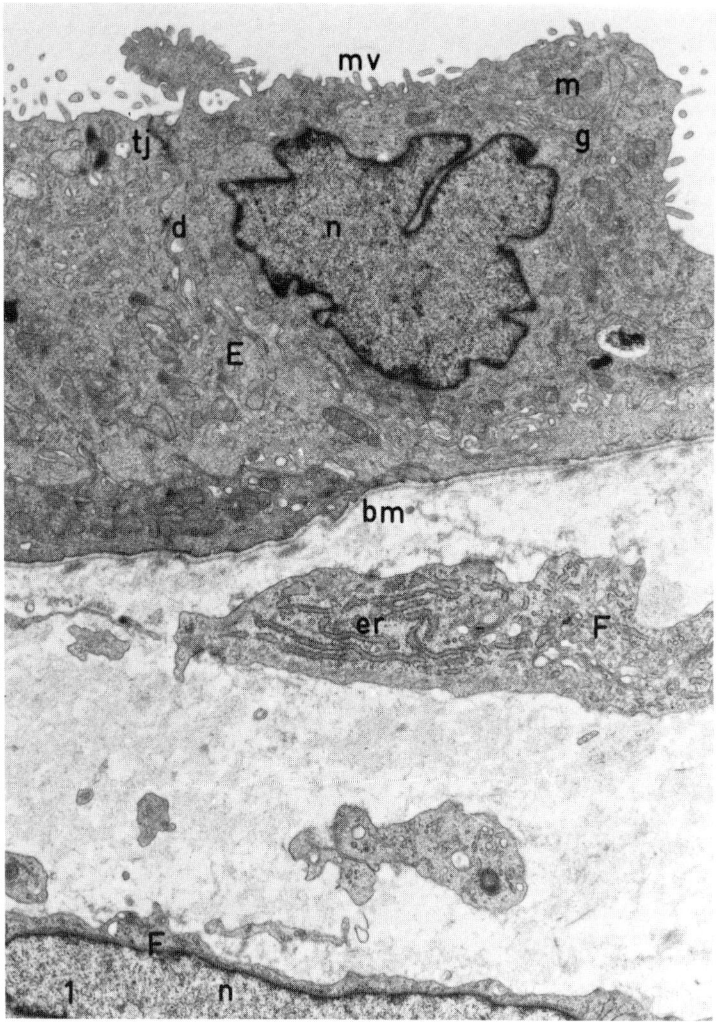

Fig. 1. Transmission electron micrograph (TEM) of middle
ear mucosa (rabbit) on the Al_2O_3 ceramic prosthesis, 3
weeks after implantation. The normal epithelial cell
layer (E) can be seen with microville (mv), mitochondria
(m), Golgi membranes (g) and a continuous basement membrane
(bm). The cells are connected by tight junctions (tj) and
desmosomes (d). The young fibroblasts (F) exhibit a
prominent rough endoplasmic reticulum (er). n - nucleus.
x 10400

  K. Jahnke et al.

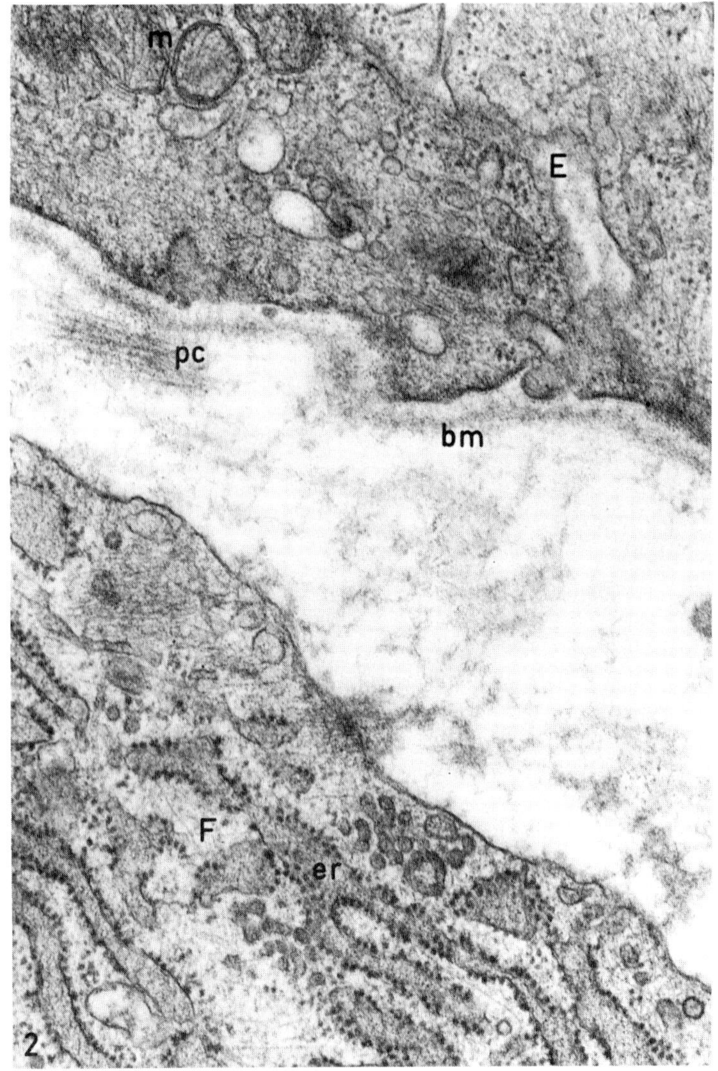

Fig. 2. Higher magnification of Fig. 1. A normal epithelial cell (E) with mitochondria (m) and a continuous basement membrane (bm). The fibroblast (F) contains an endoplasmic reticulum with many ribosomes (er). Some procollagen fibres (pc) are in the interstitial space. x 5800

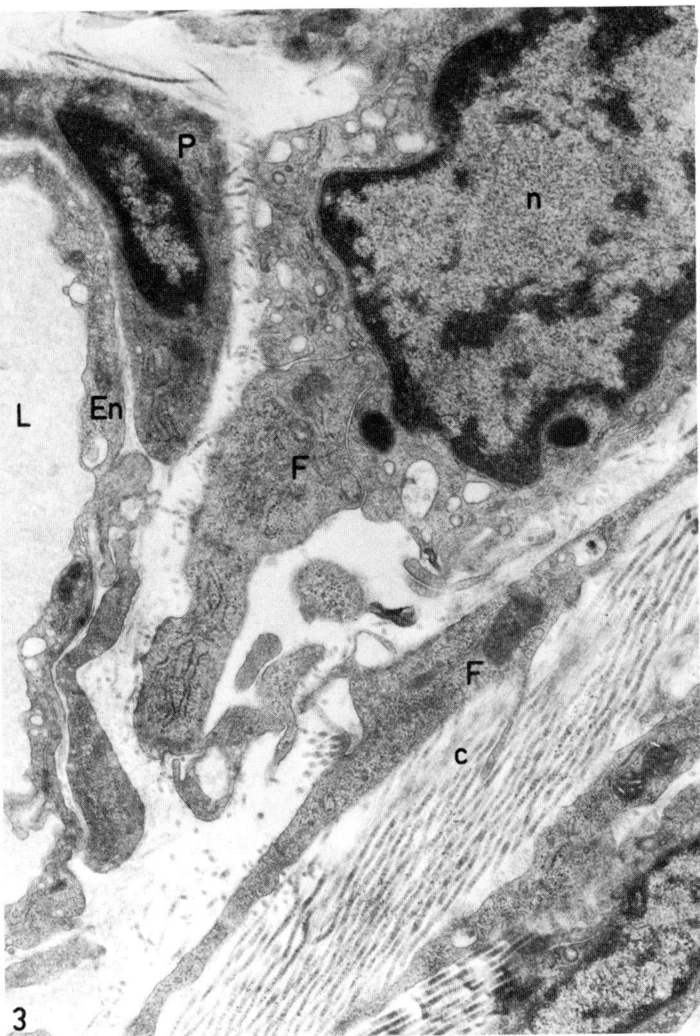

Fig. 3. Middle ear mucosa (rabbit) on the ceramic prosthesis, 5 months after implantation, subepithelial region (TEM). A capillary (L = lumen) with micropinocytotic vesicles containing endothelial cells (En) and pericytes (P) can be seen. F = Fibroblasts, C = mature collagen fibres, n = nucleus. x 16000

<u>REFERENCES</u>

Griss, P., v.Andrian-Werburg, H., Krempien, B. & Heimke, G. (1973)
Biological activity and histocompatibility of dense Al_2O_3/MgO
ceramic implants in rats. <u>J. Biomed. Mater. Res.</u>, 4, 453-462.
Heimke, G., Griss. P., Jentschura, G., Krempien, B., Gugel, E.,
Petzenhauser, I. & Hennicke, H.W. (1977) Keramische und keramic-
beschitchtete Knochenersatzwerkstoffe. <u>BMFT, T 77-70</u>, 1-190.
Jahnke, K., Plester, D. & Heimke, G. (1979) Aluminiumoxide-Keramik,
ein bioinertes material fur die mittelohrchirurgie. <u>Arch. Oto-
rhinolaryngol, 223</u>, 373-376.
Jahnke, K. & Plester, D. (1980a) Keramik-implantate in der
mittelohrchirurgie. <u>HNO, 28</u>, 109-114.
Jahnke, K. & Plester, D. (1980b) Praktische hinweise zur
anwendung von mittelohr-implantaten aus aluminiumoxide-keramik.
<u>HNO, 28</u>, 115-118.

Biomaterials 1980
Edited by G. D. Winter, D. F. Gibbons, and H. Plenk, Jr.
© 1982 John Wiley and Sons Ltd.

AN IMPLANTABLE AUDITORY PROSTHESIS AND ITS PACKAGING

I. Hochmair-Desoyer, E. Hochmair, K. Burian[1]

Technical University of Vienna, Gusshausstr. 27,
A-1040 Vienna, Austria
[1]II. ENT-Dept., University of Vienna, Austria

SUMMARY

Despite the long experience with pacemakers the application of new implantable electronic circuits presents new packaging problems necessitating further development of packaging technology. A glass package has been developed for a multichannel auditory prosthesis. This package consumes very little additional volume. Due to the use of a nonconducting material it allows placement of a receiving antenna coil inside the package. Hermeticity tests confirm that this package is suitable for long term implantable electronic devices. The glass package being designed for the encapsulation of hybrid circuits is contrasted to the epoxy moulding technique for a simpler stimulator version using discrete components.

INTRODUCTION

In the majority of cases with total deafness, auditory sensations can still be elicited by means of direct electrical stimulation of the auditory nerve. In order to achieve an auditory prosthesis which can deliver stimulus pulse trains to several restricted sites within the acoustic nerve a partly implantable stimulation system has been developed. This system comprises a flexible eight-channel electrode which can be inserted into the cochlea via the round window, an implantable receiver-driver circuit, and an external sound processor including a transmitter. Through the help of this prosthesis sound recognition and limited speech understanding for completely deaf persons can be provided (Hochmair-Desoyer et al, 1980).

Two different types of implantable receivers have been developed, an eight-channel thin film hybrid version and a four-channel circuit using discrete components. In both cases the package has to prevent adverse effects of the implant on the biological system and vice versa. The completely different packaging requirements for these two types of implants will be discussed in the following. The use of implantable electronic circuits is relatively new. The only widely used implantable circuit is the pacemaker. Problems encountered in providing a package for the auditory stimulator are different from pacemaker packaging. Firstly, only very little space is available, and

721

    I. Hochmair-Desoyer, E. Hochmair, and K. Burian

secondly, hermetic packages with up to 10 feed throughs are necessary
since usually several sites of the cochlea are to be stimulated.
For these reasons pacemaker cases cannot be used. Commercially available gold plated Kovar hybrid cases show corrosion and are not biocompatible. Also, all packages containing feed throughs in the form
of rods surrounded by sealing glass are sensitive to cracks formed
through stress excerted on the rods leading to an increase in leak
rate. Therefore, a new packaging technology had to be developed.

MATERIALS AND METHODS

Packaging of thin film hybrid circuits. In order to obtain a sufficiently long life time in the order of 20 years the package must be
hermetic. Only metals, ceramics or glasses are possible candidates for
this package. Glass has been chosen as the package material for the
following reasons:
>   nontoxicity,
>   no inflammatory responses,
>   not carcinogenic,
>   small size since only little additional volume is needed for en-
>   capsulation,
>   many different shapes can be realized by simply changing the
>   grinding tool,
>   the receiver coil can be placed inside the nonconducting package,
>   transparency enables visual control of the circuit.

The package consists of the substrate for the circuit serving as the
bottom, a glass frame, and a glass lid (Fig. 1). These three parts
are produced by ultrasonically cutting them from Corning Glass 7059.
After the resistor and conductor patterns on the substrate are generated by vacuum deposition and etching, a solderable layer (NiCr - Ti-
Pd-Au) is deposited on the lid and frame. The glass frame is soldered
to the substrate by means of low-melting (450°C) solder glass powder
having a thermal expansion coefficient which matches that of Corning
7059 (Fig. 2). Chromium paths of 0.2 μm passing beneath the glass
frame serve as feed throughs. The solder process has to be carried out

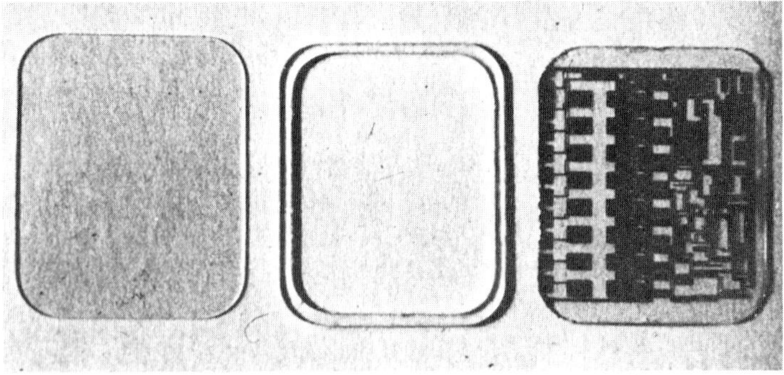

Fig. 1. Bottom (substrate), frame and lid of the glass
package ultrasonically cut from Corning Glass 7059

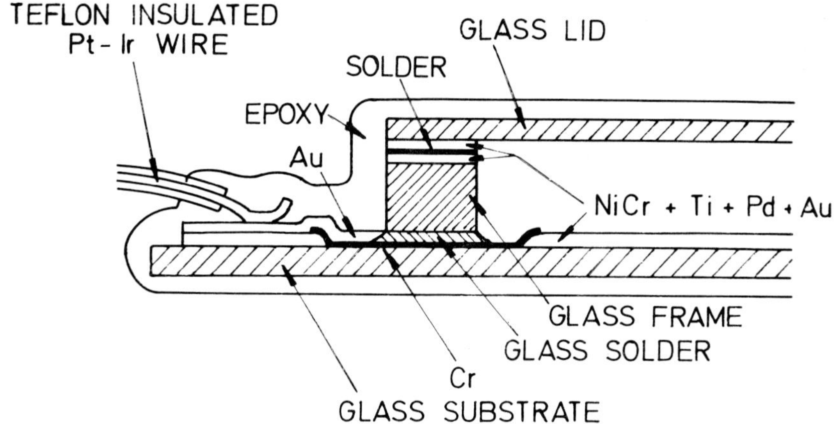

Fig. 2.   Schematic of assembled package

quickly (5 min) and under nitrogen atmospere in order to avoid resistance changes. After mounting and bonding of the chip components, followed by testing and cleaning, the package parts are vacuum baked at 150°C for 72 hours. Then the lid is preform soldered to the frame under low humidity conditions.

Encapsulation of discrete stimulation circuit. For the implant using discrete components no overall hermetic encapsulation is necessary. Moisture sensitive components, like diodes, are already contained in a hermetic case. For these implants pacemaker epoxy encapsulation (HY C8-W795, HY H-W796) is used. Due to the inevitable moisture penetration of epoxy the circuit has to be designed to operate in a wet environment. Components are not mounted on a substrate in order to avoid shunting due to a water film on the substrate surface.

RESULTS

For the glass package helium leak rates have been determined to be better than 10^{-9} atm cm^3/s. In vitro life tests still under way were started two and a half years ago. For a total of four circuits no failure has occurred yet. At the external connections to the eight wires leading to the multichannel electrode minor shunts can occur, but they do not represent a problem since their impedance is high compared to the electrode impedance. One circuit has been implanted in a deaf human volunteer for a period of six months. During this time the circuit was functioning properly before it had to be explanted for medical reasons not connected with the implant.

In vitro testing of the epoxy-moulded discrete prosthesis in 37°C saline solution under the comparatively high intensity of 500nC/pulse (this level is much higher than the maximum used for actual stimulation) has been performed over a period of now 12.500 hours accumulating a total charge of ± 6.700 Coulomb per electrode without any degradation or changes in performance. Considering an on-time of 12 hours per day a minimum lifetime of three years could be expected from the in vitro tests. In six humans equipped with this auditory prosthesis for different periods of time (the longest now being two and a half years) there has been no failure so far.

DISCUSSION

Since the problem of hermetic packages for implantable electronic circuits other than pacemakers arose, a number of solutions have been proposed: Parylene-coated gold-plated Kovar packages (Knutti et al, 1979) or Ceramic cases with gold caps (Donaldson 1979). For a number of applications the described glass package represents an advantageous solution because of its small volume, nonconductivity, transparency and the use of thin film feed throughs instead of stress-sensitive rods.

ACKNOWLEDGEMENTS

This work is supported by the Austrian Research Counsil.

REFERENCES

Donaldson, P.E.K. (1979) Helium leak measurements as a predictor of hermetic package life in surgically-implanted microelectronic devices. Proc. European Hybrid Microelectronics Conference 1979, Ghent, Belgium, May, 479-484.

Hochmair-Desoyer, I.J., Hochmair, E.S., Fischer, R.E., and Burian, K. (1980) Cochlear prostheses in use: Recent speech comprehension results. Arch. ORL (in press).

Knutti, J.W., Gschwend, S.J., Allen, H.V., and Meindl, J.D. (1979) Implantable system assembly and encapsulation. Digest of technical papers, Workshop on implantable transducers and systems: Packaging methods and testing criteria, Stanford University, California, June 1979, 17-25.

Biomaterials 1980
Edited by G. D. Winter, D. F. Gibbons, and H. Plenk, Jr.
© 1982 John Wiley and Sons Ltd.

BREAK UP TIME AND KINETICS OF DRY SPOT FORMATION OF
TEAR FILM ON MODIFIED SILICONE CONTACT LENSES

J.E. Proust, A. Baszkin, L. Ter-Minassian-Saraga

Physico-Chimie des Surfaces et des Membranes,
45, rue des Saints-Pères, 75270 Paris cedex, France

G. Wajs

Essilor International,
2 bis, rue des 2 communes, 94300 Vincennes, France

S. Tchaliovska,

Faculty of Chemistry,
University of Sofia, 1 Anton Ivanov, Sofia, Bulgaria

<u>SUMMARY</u>

During recent years, silicones found use as a material for contact
lenses. Their high permeability to oxygen is the main reason for
this application. However silicones are highly hydrophobic and need
surface modification to fulfil the ocular requirements. One possibility would be to graft a polar monomer on the silicone substrate.

The goal of this work was to gain an understanding of the role of
grafting on stability of tear films on these polymers. Two methods
were used to investigate this property : wettability of the lenses
measured by contact angles and stability of tear films obtained by
means of a specially constructed instrument and recorded on 16 mm
size film.

The stability and wettability of silicone grafted (poly vinyl pyrrolidone) were studied as a function of the degree of grafting,
hydration of silicone and the concentration of proteins in the
lacrymal film.

<u>INTRODUCTION</u>

The knowledge of surface properties of contact lenses is essential
to understand the mechanism of their wettability by the tear film.
Lenses manufactured out of the poly(methacrylate) hydrogels, with
water a content ranging from 37% to 40%, are not permeable enough
for oxygen to allow a sufficiently long contact with the corneal
epithelium. This is the reason why, during the recent years, silicones which exibit good oxygen permeability have found their use as
materials for contact lenses. The highly hydrophobic character of
silicones is, however, a major obstacle for their immediate application for contact lenses. Good wettability by a tear film is

essential for physiological reasons and also to obtain perfect
vision.

Recently, many studies have been carried out to find an appropriate
method of modification of the surface properties of silicones to
improve their use as a material for contact lenses. Grafting of a
hydrophilic monomer such as vinyl pyrrolidone on the silicone
substrate is expected to modify the surface of the polymer and thus
to improve the conditions for the stability of the lacrymal film.

MATERIALS AND METHODS

Silicones. The samples of silicones, poly(dimethyl siloxane), used
in this study were of the dimensions (1cm x 1cm x 0.05cm).

Grafting. Silicones were grafted with poly(vinyl pyrrolidone) (PVP)
by a radiochemical procedure described by Laizer (1969). The degree
of grafting ranges from 3 to 10% (weight percentage).

Water. Water was triple-distilled from a permanganate solution using
Pyrex apparatus. Its surface tension was 72.75 dynes/cm at room
temperature.

Artificial tear solution (standard solution). This solution was
prepared according to the formula proposed by Holly (1974) : 0.22%
w/w mucin (bovine submaxillary mucin), 0.2% w/w albumin (BSA purity
96-99%), 0.1% w/w γ-globulin (purity 99%), and 0.08% w/w lysozyme
(egg lysozyme). All products were from Sigma. The proteins were
dissolved in NaOH 10^{-4} M and then introduced to the phosphate buffer
solution (pH = 7.5) containing NaCl (0.15 M). Pure nitrogen was
bubbled through all inorganic aqueous solutions to remove greasy
impurities.

Cleaning of polymer samples. All polymer samples, before contact
angle and film stability measurements, were cleaned with sodium
oleate solution by rubbing their surfaces with soft cotton pads.
After cleaning the samples were rinsed several times with hot water
and then with distilled water. This rigorous cleaning and the choice
of the soap have an important effect on the values of measured parameters (Tchaliovska, 1978).

Wettability measurements. Wettability of silicone grafted PVP
samples was determined by contact angles of sessile drops of artificial tear liquid (standard solution) in a thermostatically controlled
closed chamber. Both the advancing (θ_A) and the receding (θ_R) contact
angles were measured with an accuracy of ± 2°. We have also measured
the readvancing contact angles. In this case the drop of the tear
solution is redeposited in the same place on the silicone surface
where the advancing contact angle was measured. Fig.1 shows the
techniques used for contact angle measurements.

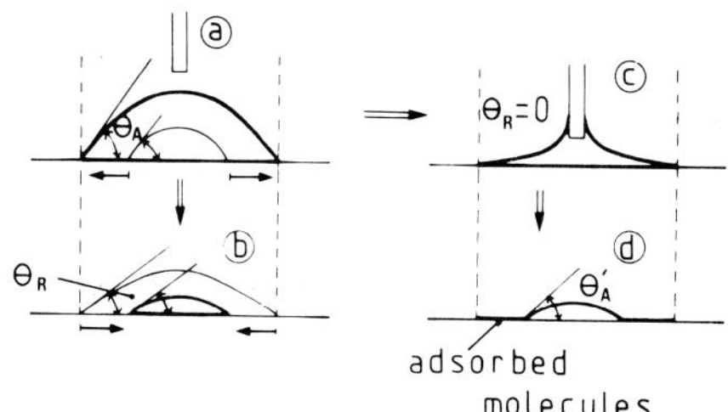

Fig.1. Contact angle measurements.
a) advancing Θ_A : drop increase. b) receding Θ_R : drop
decrease. c) the receding Θ_R is zero : the diameter of
the drop remains constant. d) readvancing Θ_A : the drop
is deposited on the same place on which previous drop
was placed.

Stability of tear films on silicone samples. The diagram of the
instrument used for these measurements is shown in Fig.2. It is
similar to that which we have used for thin liquid crystal films
(Proust, 1979) and which was initially developed by Scheludko (1970).

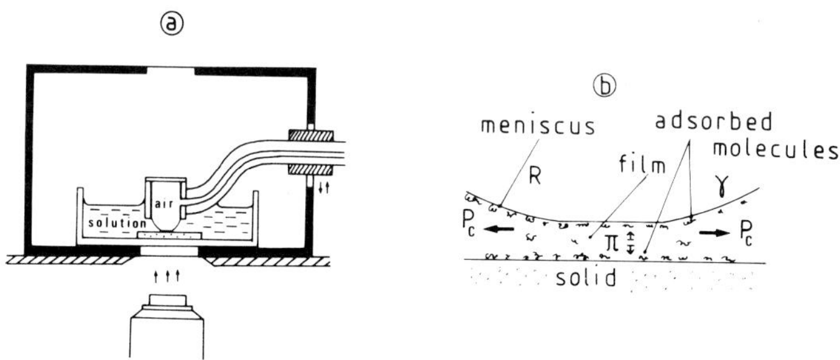

Fig.2. Thin film on solid substrate.
a) diagram of the instrument. b) thin film : capillary
pressure $P_C \propto \gamma/R$ equilibrates the disjoining pressure π.

The sample is placed at the bottom of the cell made of the optical
quality glass which is filled with a tear solution of a given
concentration. An air bubble is formed in the solution by means of
a capillary tube. The pressure of the air bubble is maintained
constant using a mercury pump and is adjusted with a manometer. The
distance between the capillary tube and the sample may be adjusted
so as to obtain a thin film of the solution between the air and the
sample. The cell is fixed on a table of a metallographic microscope

and the kinetics of the failure or of the formation of the liquid
film may be photographed by means of a camera.

When a thin liquid film is obtained on the solid surface, a meniscus
forms in which capillary pressure is directly proportional to the
surface tension of the solution and inversely proportional to the
radius of curvature of the meniscus ($P_C = \propto \gamma/R$). The capillary
pressure induces the thinning of the liquid film (see Fig.2). The
stability limit of the film is achieved when the pressure inside
the film (known as the disjoining pressure π) precisely opposes the
capillary pressure. The disjoining pressure, defined by Derjaguin
(1939) is equal to $\pi(h) = - 1/A\ (\delta F/\delta h)_{A,V,T}$ where h is the
thickness, F the free energy, A the area, T the temperature and V
the volume of the film. This disjoining pressure is the resultant
of many forces (Van der Waals, electrostatic and structural) opera-
ting at the interfaces.

The described method requires precise control. The presence of any
impurities at the surface under study must be avoided. Two parameters of the tear films were measured : the break-up time and the
kinetics of dry spot formation. The break-up time may be defined as
a time which elapses from the moment when the liquid film attains
its constant radius ($R \simeq 100\ \mu m$) and the appearance of the first
hole (Proust, 1979b). The kinetics of dry spot formation is measured
as $d\phi/dt$ the change with time of the mean diameter (ϕ) of a hole
formed in the liquid film. These kinetics have been systematically
measured for 15 minutes after equilibrium. The kinetics of failure
becomes slower if the film is formed at the same place on the
sample which had already been used for a previous measurement.
Consequently the measurements were always made at new locations.

RESULTS AND DISCUSSION

<u>Wettability of silicone grafted PVP surfaces</u>. The wettability of
silicone grafted PVP was studied as function of the degree of
grafting, hydration of silicone and the nature of the wetting
liquid.

From the results obtained with water, it appears that the degree of
grafting enhances wettability both on the hydrated and on the non-
hydrated surfaces. The increase of the wettability of hydrated
samples may be attributed to the reorientation of the hydrophilic
groups of the PVP towards the surface of polymer.

Wetting of silicone samples by artificial tear solutions shows the
decrease, as compared with water, of the contact angle due to the
lower surface tension of these solutions and the adsorption of the
film constituents on silicones. The hydration of samples decreases
their wettability which is contrary to the results obtained with
water. This may be due to the decrease of the solid-liquid interfacial tension. The decrease makes adsorption of tear constituents
on the surface less likely and could explain the increase in contact

angle. Details of these measurements were described by Baszkin (1978).

An interesting observation was also made from the readvancing contact angles which always have different values to Θ_A. This angle becomes zero for grafted silicones with dilutions of the standard solution lower than 300 x and for the ungrafted surfaces with dilutions lower than 40 x (see Table 1). We think that this is due to protein adsorption on silicone samples. An analogous effect has been found by Guastalla (1952) for paraffin which becomes wettable when subjected to the reversible adsorption of fatty acid molecules. In the case of protein adsorption on silicone samples, the process seems to be irreversible at high concentrations but reversible for diluted standard solution concentrations. Indeed the amounts of irreversibly adsorbed protein on a hydrophobic surface depend upon the effective number of adsorption sites (Brynda, 1978).

Stability of tear films on silicones and silicones grafted with PVP.

TABLE 1. Break-up time, kinetics of dry spot formation and contact angles of artificial tear solutions on silicone and silicone grafted with PVP.

dilution of the standard solution	substrate	break-up time	kinetics of dry spot formation	$\Theta_A.$	$\Theta_R.$	readvancing
standard solution	silicone PVP	stable	stable	80°	0°	0°
	silicone	5.5 sec	18 µ/sec	90°	0°	0°
4 x*	silicone PVP	stable	stable	80°	0°	0°
	silicone	stable	stable	90°	0°	0°
40 x	silicone PVP	0.75 sec	110 µ/sec	82°	0°	0°
	silicone	0.25 sec	500 µ/sec	90°	0°	0°
100 x	silicone PVP	stable**	stable**	92°	0°	0°
	silicone	0.3 sec	600 µ/sec	90°	30°	90°
200 x	silicone PVP	stable**	stable**	80°	0°	0°
	silicone	0.7 sec	70 µ/sec	90°	30°	90°
300 x	silicone PVP	0.75 sec	45 µ/sec	86°	0°	0°
	silicone	0.22 sec	1000 µ/sec	90°	30°	90°
500 x	silicone PVP	0.7 sec	55 µ/sec	96°	10°	75°
	silicone	0.1 sec	3000 µ/sec	108°	55°	108°
1000 x	silicone PVP	< 0.1 sec	explosive	96°	10°	96°
	silicone	< 0.1 sec	explosive	118°	80°	118°

* The most stable films are obtained for this concentration.
** The film is formed of the "dried" layer of proteins.

The results summarized in the Table 1 reveal the correlation between
the break-up time and the kinetics of dry spot formation. This
relationship is valid for the grafted as well as for ungrafted
samples. With diluted standard solutions (dilutions higher than
1000 x), the kinetics of dry spot formation is very rapid (instantaneous). For the dilution range (100 x - 200 x) the films are
very thin (< 200 Å) giving almost a dry surface, while for the
dilution range (< 40 x) the films are thick (> 1000 Å) and heterogeneous. Other experiments with a solution containing only albumin
have shown that the thin film has the same dimensions as that
obtained for (100 x - 200 x) dilutions of the standard solution.
With only mucin present in the solution, the films are heterogeneous
and similar to those found with concentrated standard solutions. It
appears therefore that each protein in the standard solution has
a specific effect upon the thinning of the film. It seems likely
also that these proteins behave competitively in controlling the
stability and the structure of the films.

A concentrated effort is now underway in our laboratory to define
the specific role of the proteins to explain the behaviour of the
lacrymal film. This work will be reported in later papers.

ACKNOWLEDGEMENT

We thank J.C. Meslard (Essilor) for his technical assistance and
V. Malet for typing this paper.

This work was supported by DGRST grant n°78 7 0159.

REFERENCES

Baszkin, A., Boissonnade, M.M., Proust, J.E., Tchaliovska, S., Ter-
Minassian-Saraga, L. & Wajs, G. (1978) Silicone grafted with poly
(vinyl pyrrolidone) for contact lenses. Surface properties and
stability of thin tear film. J. of Bioengineering, 2, 527-537.
Brynda, E., Houska, M., Pokorna, Z., Cepalova, N.A., Moiseev Yu, V.
& Kalal, J. (1978) Irreversible adsorption of human serum albumin
onto polyethylene film. J. of Bioengineering, 2, 411-418.
Derjaguin, B.V. & Kussakov, M.M. (1939) Theory of interaction of
particles in presence of electric double layers and the stability
of lyophobe colloids and disperse systems. Acta Physiochim. USSR, 10
25, 153-161.
Guastalla, L.P. (1952) Adsorption de l'acide palmitique sur la
paraffine. C.R. Acad. Sci. Paris, 234, 2051-2053.
Holly, F.J. (1974) Surface chemistry of tear film component analogs.
J. Colloid Interface Sci., 49, 221-231.
Laizer, J. & Wajs, G. (1969) Large radioactive sources for industrial
processes. Proceedings of the Conference in Munich, (Eds. Int. Atom
Energy Agency), pp.205-212, Vienna.
Proust, J.E. & Ter-Minassian-Saraga, L. (1979a) Films minces de
cristaux liquides. J. de Physique, 40 (4), C3, 490-496.

Proust, J.E. & Tchaliovska, S. (1979b) Etude de la stabilité des films de larme sur le silicone. Film 16 mm, Edited by SERDDAV-CNRS, 27 rue Paul Bert, 94204 Ivry cedex, France.

Scheludko, A., Tchaliovska, S. & Fabrikant, S. (1970) Contact between a gas bubble and a solid surface and a froth flotation. Spec. Discuss. Faraday Soc., 1, 112–117.

Tchaliovska, S. & Alexander, L.B. (1978) Determination of distribution function of contact angles method for evaluating regeneration of a spherical solid surface during wetting action. Chem. Tech., 30 (6), 301–303.

Biomaterials 1980
Edited by G. D. Winter, D. F. Gibbons, and H. Plenk, Jr.
© 1982 John Wiley and Sons Ltd.

VISUAL REHABILITATION WITH ALUMINUM OXIDE CERAMIC CORNEAL PROSTHESIS

Frank M. Polack, M.D.

Department of Ophthalmology, University of Florida
Gainesville, Florida, 32610, USA

SUMMARY

Keratoprostheses are indicated in cases of severe corneal disease not amenable to keratoplasty. For many years an ideal material has been looked for to prolong the tolerance of these implants. This paper describes the various problems encountered with acrylic implants mostly due to lack of biocompatibility. Ceramics have shown excellent tissue tolerance and bioadhesion. For this reason they are now considered as ideal materials for corneal prostheses.

INTRODUCTION

The replacement of an opaque cornea with glass was attempted as early as 1771, by Pellier de Quingsy (Cardona, et. al., 1972). His and subsequent attempts by others failed because of lack of instrumentation, poor understanding of corneal physiology, infection and poor mechanical design of the implant. During World War II, it was observed that methylmethacrylate particles embedded in the corneas of airplane pilots were well tolerated for many years. In the 50's, with further development of plastics and with this background information, investigators tried different designs of acrylic implants (Stone, 1955; Barraquer, 1960; Cardona, 1962; Strampelli, 1963; Brown & Dohlman, 1963; Alamillo & Alamillo, 1963; Choyce, 1967; Girard, et. al., 1969). Numerous corneal optical devices have been designed, but tolerance and retention varied because of differences in material quality, configuration, surgical technique, and the status of the recipient cornea.

MATERIALS AND METHODS

Plastic Corneal Prosthesis

It has been observed that methylmethacrylate of good quality with minimal amount of residual monomers are well tolerated by ocular tissues (Cardona, 1970). Plastic impurities, residual monomers, and residual sterilization gas (ETOH), are all causes of persistent ocular inflammation, tissue destruction and eventual expulsion of the implant. The design of the corneal implant requires an optical element and a supporting flange or skirt. Solid supporting plates larger than 5 mm cause thinning and disintegration of corneal tissue covering this portion of the prosthesis; this problem is apparently caused by poor fluid transport across the cornea and dryness of the superficial layers. Fenestrations or holes made in the supporting plate reduce the chances of breakdown of the recipient cornea (Knowles, 1961); however, disintegration of corneal tissue around the optical prosthesis has also been a persistent problem with acrylic prostheses (Cardone,

                                    F.M. Polack

1970). Lack of biocompatibility of connective tissue with the surface of
the implant facilitated the ingrowth of surface epithelium along the surface
of the implant causing its eventual extrusion and dispersion of epithelial
cells inside the eye. To improve the stability of this implant, the retaining plate has been made of teflon (Castroviejo & Cardona & DeVoe, 1969),
dacron mesh (Girard, et. al., 1969), silicone (Brown & Dohlman, 1963),
platinum or gold (Alamillo & Alamillo, 1963). Figure 1 shows the various
designs of keratoprostheses, all of which attempt to solve these problems
of extrusion. The nut and bolt concept of Cardona's prosthesis (1970)
answers in part the problem of leveling the optical surface with the surface
of the globe. However, the incorporation of the supporting plate or the
optical cylinder to the connective tissue was not obtained with plastic
materials.

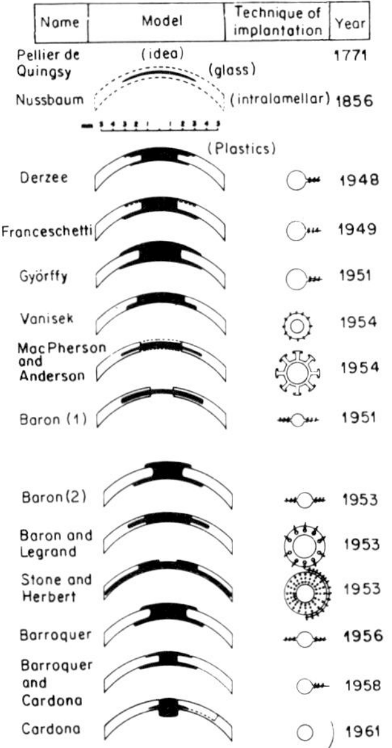

Corneal Optical Prosthesis wth Autologous Bone Supporting Plate

Strampelli (1963) designed a corneal prosthesis
where the supporting plate was a disc of autologous bone obtained from the mandible of the
patient, incorporating the enamel and the root
canal of a tooth. The optical cylinder, made of
methylmethacrylate, was inlaid in the root canal
of the dental piece. The autologous bone was
sutured to the surface of the globe and covered
with soft tissue or the eyelids; eventually the
bone was firmly incorporated to the surrounding
ocular tissue. The extrusion of this implant was
not possible, however, erosion of surface tissue
and ulceration was still seen around the plastic
optical portion. Strampelli's concept of a
biocompatible material, so it could be well incorporated to the ocular tissues, was the basis
for our design of a keratoprosthesis with a material which would be tolerated by human tissue
almost as well as autologous bone. Ceramics seem
to provide the answer for this biocompatible
material which has been used in orthopedic and
dental surgery with satisfactory results.

Fig. 1 – Evolution of principal keratoprosthesis (Cardona, 1962)

Based on our experience and that of others, it appears that the ideal keratoprosthesis should be made of one single material and that this material
should be entirely biocompatible. The optical element should be adjustable
to the surface of the globe and the surgical technique should be simple.

Ceramic Materials

The two types of ceramics explored as potential material for corneal prostheses were the silica (SiO_2) (Polack & Hench, 1975; Bigar, 1978; Hoffman
& Harnisch & Strunz, 1978) and the aluminum oxide (Al_2O_3) (Heimke & Polack,
1977; Polack & Heimke, 1978, 1980) ceramics. A comparative investigation of
silica and the aluminum oxide material in our laboratory revealed that the
latter was better tolerated. Therefore, Al_2O_3 ceramic was selected for our

corneal prosthesis. It is possible that the intolerance to the silica ceramic was caused by contamination of the material with metallic powders since
the method of grinding and polishing were entirely different. Diamond tools
were used for the manufacture and tooling of the aluminum oxide material and
handling was always done under sterile techniques.

Aluminum Oxide or Corundum

The polycrystalline without pores can be finished with a rough or smooth surface (Heimke & Polack, 1977; Heimke, 1978). The randomly dispersed crystals
produce an opaque material, but if a single crystal is properly cut, it is
transparent with a refractive index of 1.767.

The corneal prosthesis consists of an opaque 6 mm ceramic retaining disc
with a threaded central perforation to accommodate a 3 mm diameter aluminum

oxide optical cylinder (Fig. 2). The
disc has a rough surface, smooth edges,
and a posterior curvature of 8 mm radius.
It is 1 mm thick centrally, with tapering edges. There are several sets of
small holes for the placement of sutures.
The optical cylinder has a power of 60
diopters and is 9 mm long. Prior to
use, implants are cleaned with ultrasound and steam sterilized. The implant
is either fixed directly to the patient's corneal or fixed to an Eye Bank
Cornea.

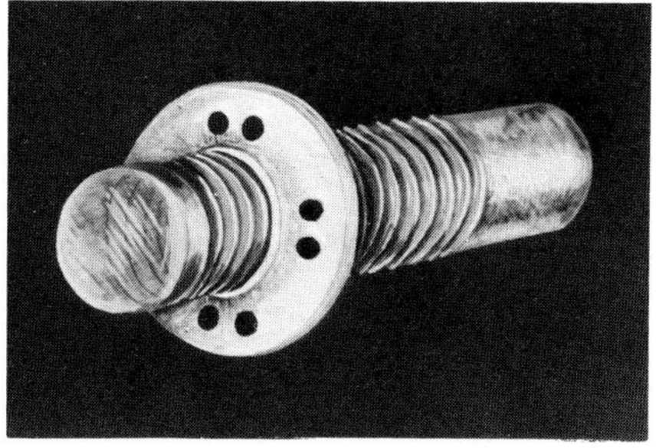

Fig. 2 - The ceramic
keratoprosthesis

Surgical Technique

The surgical techniques have been described in detail in other publications
(Heimke & Polack, 1977; Heimke, 1978; Polack & Heimke, 1980). Basically it
consists of one technique for patients with good conjunctiva and another
for patients with dry eye (Figs. 3 & 4). In the first case the prosthesis

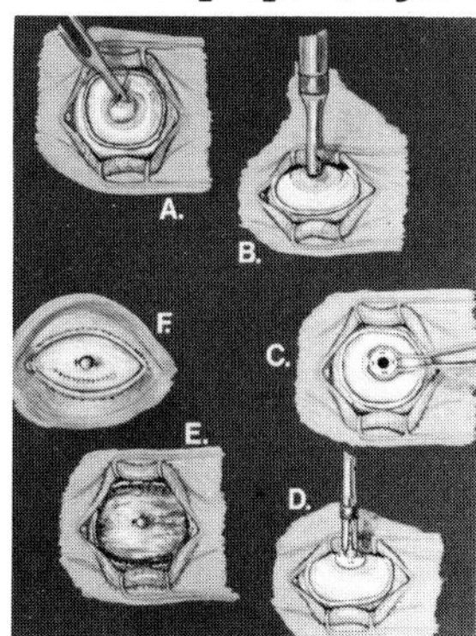

Fig. 3 - A-F Steps showing the
insertion of the Keratoprosthesis through the conjunctiva.

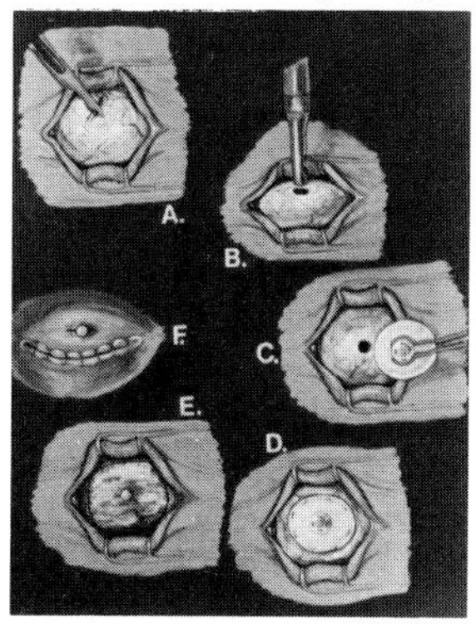

Fig. 4 - A-F Steps showing the
insertion of the keratoprosthesis through the lid.

can be exteriorized to the corneal and covered with conjunctiva after the insertion of a layer of periosteal tissue. In patients with very dry eyes and
without normal conjunctiva, the prosthesis has to be exteriorized through
the skin of the lid. The optical device requires that these recipient eyes
be aphakic, therefore, if the lens is present, whether it is clear or not,
it has to be removed by means of a standard intracapsular cataract extraction

If the technique used is exteriorization through the conjunctiva, the patient
will need little care following surgery. However, when the prosthesis is
brought through the skin, it requires permanent and daily care because of
the risk of infection of the skin border through which the prosthesis is
exteriorized. The visual results depend on the status of the retina.
Additional optical correction can be obtained with spectacles.

RESULTS

Table 1 describes seven patients who have received a ceramic corneal prosthesis and the length of follow-up.

Table I

Case	Age	Diagnosis	VA	Date	Operation	VA
1	56	Pemphigoid	HM	03/31/78	Through lid Sector Iridec-tomy, ICCE	20/30 1½ year
2	50	Failed Grafts (10) Interstitial Keratitis	LP	10/31/78	Transconjunc-tival	HM 3' 8 mos.
3	62	Pemphigoid, Failed Grafts	LP	03/06/79	Through lid	NLP 1 year
4	51	Pemphigoid	LP	09/25/79	Through lid Peripheral Ir-idectomy, ICCE	20/50 3 wks.
5	67	Stevens-Johnson Syndrome	LP	10/16/79	Through lid Total Iridec-tomy, ICCE	20/40 1 mo.
6	79	Basal Cell Carcinoma (lids)	LP	05/08/79	Through lid	20/80 10 mos.
7	15	Corneal Scarring	LP	06/01/78	Transconjunc-tival	FC 18 mos

DISCUSSION

This paper presents the results on seven patients who received a ceramic
corneal prosthesis device. At the time of this writing, the oldest patient
has a keratoprosthesis for over a year and a half retaining a vision of
better than 20/30. Five of these patients had the prosthesis placed throug
the lid because of the lack of conjunctival tissue to cover the prosthetic
implant. The through the lid implantation of this ceramic implant has been

the method of choice in patients with dry eyes due to Stevens-Johnson syn-
drome, ocular pemphigoid, or chemical burns. Since the first two inflammatory processes compromise only the anterior segment of the eye, the retina
is usually spared and the visual acuity has been excellent in most of these
patients. In those who had chemical injuries, the retina often had suffered
some degree of inflammatory reaction and the visual acuity was not always
satisfactory. Firm adhesion of fibroblastic and epithelial tissue was expected to occur, however, in most cases the adhesion is only observed in
the portions of the optical cylinder but not on the surface. This opens
a potential problem which is that of infection of the skin around the glass
implant, a problem that occurred in two of our patients between six and
eight months after surgery. Patients are instructed to carefully clean the
skin around the prosthesis with a mild soap and apply an antibiotic ointment
daily. The hardness of the ceramic material eliminates the possibility of
scratching or breakdown of the implant's surface and preserves the optical
surface intact. Following this study, five additional prostheses have been
implanted with satisfactory results. The long-term acceptance of these
materials by ocular tissues is still under study.

REFERENCES

Alamillo, M. & Alamillo, R. (1963). Implantation of an artificial cornea.
Amer. J. Ophthalmol. 56:937-941.
Barraquer, J. (1960). Inclusion de protesis opticas corneanas, corneas
acrilicas o queratoprotesis. Ann. Inst. Barraquer 1:243-247.
Bigar, F., Krahenmann, A., Landolt, E. & Witner, R. (1977). Die Gewebever-
traglichkeit bioaktiver glaskeramik in der hornhaut und bindehaut. Deutsche
Ophthalmologische Gesellschaft, Bericht uber die, Kunststoffimplantate in
der Ophthalmologie.
Blencke, A., Hagen, Pl, Bromer, H. & Deutscher, K. (1978). Untersuchungen
uber die verwendarkeit von glaskeramiken zur osteo-odonto-keratoplastik.
Ophthalmologica,(Basel) 176:105-112.
Brown, S.I. & Dohnman, C.H. (1963). A buried corneal prosthesis. Arch.
Ophthalmol. 70:736.
Cardona, H. (1962). Keratoprosthesis: Acrylic optical cylinder with sup-
porting intralamellar plate. Amer. J. Ophthalmol. 54:284-294.
Cardona, H. (1970). Keratoprosthesis, Round Table. In Corneal and Exter-
nal Diseases of the Eye, Polack, F.M. (Editor), Charles B. Thomas, Spring-
field, Illinois, p. 328.
Cardona, H. (1970). Personal communication.
Cardona, H., Castroviejo, R. & DeVoe, A.G. (1972). Advances in prostho-
keratoplasty. In Casey, T.A., Corneal Grafting, Butterworths, London,
p. 313.
Castroviejo, R., Cardona, H. & DeVoe, A.G. (1969). Present status of pros-
thokeratoplasty. Amer. J. Ophthalmol. 68:613-625.
Choyce, D.P. (1967). The treatment of bullous keratopathy with acrylic
inlays: Experience with Choyce two-piece acrylic keratoprosthesis. In
Corneo-Plastic Surgery, Proceedings of the II International Corneo-Plastic
Conference, Rycroft, P.V. (Editor), Lond., Pergamon Press, p. 399.
Girard, L.J., Moore, C.D., Soper, J.W. & O'Bannon, W. (1969). Prostheto-
sclerokeratoplasty - Implantation of a keratoprosthesis using full thickness onlay sclera and sliding conjunctival flap. Trans. Amer. Acad. Ophth.
73:936-961.

Griss, P., Siber, R., Merkle, B., Haehner, K., Heimke, G. & Krempien, B. (1976). Biomechanically induced tissue reactions after Al_2O_3 ceramic hip joint replacement. Experimental and early clinical results.[3] J. Biomed. Mater. Res. Symp. 7:519-528.

Hoffman, F., Harnisch, J.P., Strunz, V., Bunte, M., Gross, U.M., Manner, K., Bromer, H. & Deutscher, K. (1978). Osteo-Keramo-Keratoprosthese. Ein Modifikation der Oster-Odonot-Keratoprosthese nach Strampelli. Klin. Mbl. Augenheilk. 173:747-755.

Krempien, V.B., Schulte, W., Kleineikenscheidt, H., Linder, K., Schareyka, R. & Heimke, G. (1978). Lichtoptische und rasterelektronen-mikroskopische untersuchungen an der grenzflache von implantaten aus aluminiumoxid-keramik im unterkieferknochen von hunden. Dtsch. zahnarztel. Z. 33.

Polack, F.M. (1972). Visual restoration with plastic corneal implants. S. Med. J. 65:1118.

Polack, F M. & Heimke, G. (1980). Ceramic keratoprostheses. Ophthalmology, AAO, 87:7.

Polack, F.M. & Heimke, G. (1978). Keramische keratoprosthesen (II). Proc. German Congress Ophthal. (Heidelberg), Bergmann, Verlag, Munich.

Polack, F.M. & Hench, L.L. (1975). Bioceramics in progress report to National Institute of General Medical Sciences (GM-21056), National Institutes of Health.

Stone W., Jr. (1955). Study of patency of openings in corneas anterior to interlamellar plastic artificial discs. Amer. J. Ophthalmol. 39:185.

Strampelli, B. (1963). Osteo-odontocheratoprotesi. Ospedali Riuniti di Roma, Report Oculistico, Ospedale di S. Geovanni, P. 1039-1044.

Biomaterials 1980
Edited by G. D. Winter, D. F. Gibbons, and H. Plenk, Jr.
© 1982 John Wiley and Sons Ltd.

EVALUATION OF VARIOUSLY MODIFIED MICROPOROUS POLYTETRA-
FLUOROETHYLENE TRACHEAL PROSTHESES

J.R. Bottema[*], I. Molenaar[*], Ch.R.H. Wildevuur[*]
H.W.M. ten Hoopen[**] and J. Feijen[**]

[*]Department of Experimental Surgery and Centre for
Electron Microscopy, University of Groningen,
Groningen, The Netherlands.
[**]Department of Chemical Technology, Twente University
of Technology, Enschede, The Netherlands.

<u>SUMMARY</u>

Variously modified microporous polytetrafluoroethylene tracheal
prostheses (0.5 cm) were implanted in rabbits for periods of three
weeks. Prostheses of group I (non-modified) showed a complete overgrowth with connective tissue covered by a mucous membrane. In
group II (treatment with a sodium-naftalene-tetrahydrofuran solution)
the prostheses showed a thicker layer of connective tissue and sometimes obstruction. Prostheses coated with poly-dl-lactic acid (group
III) were covered with a thinner layer of connective tissue than the
prostheses of group I. Some cases of infection were observed in all
groups, and may have been caused by the insufficiently controlled
dosage of antibiotics. Release of antibiotics from porous teflon
prostheses (group IV) retarded the coverage of the prostheses with a
mucosa layer and did not prevent the occurrence of infection.

<u>INTRODUCTION</u>

Several types of materials, including ceramics (Hulbert et al, 1971),
porous polymers (Thomas, 1973; Pizzoferrato et al, 1979; Nelson
et al, 1979) and non-porous polymers (Wykoff, 1973; Moritz et al,
1975) have been applied in tracheal prostheses. These materials have
not met the qualifications which are necessary for this application.
These qualifications are: (a) the material should not stimulate
hypergranulation, which causes luminal obstruction, (b) the materials
should permit overgrowth of a mucous membrane on the inside of the
prostheses and (c) the materials should offer resistance to the
occurrence of infection. The first two requirements have been met by
using microporous polytetrafluoroethylene (PTFE), (Bottema and Wildevuur, 1978; Bottema et al, 1980) but resistance to infection has
not as yet been realized. The occurrence of infection can be decreased by proper treatment with antibiotics or by using materials which
induce rapid overgrowth of tissue. This last feature protects the
materials from the contaminating air.

The purpose of this investigation was to evaluate various treatments
of the microporous PTFE with respect to stimulation of overgrowth of
tissue and to study the effects of release of antibiotics from the
prostheses.

MATERIALS AND METHODS

Four groups of differently treated tracheal prostheses (length 0.5 cm,
internal diameter 0.6 cm) were tested in rabbits by methods described
in detail elsewhere (Bottema, et al, 1980). The prostheses were
either reinforced by stainless steel springs (1 USP, Ethicon [R])
fixed to the prostheses by Vicryl [R] (6-0) sutures or by using a
teflon spiral wrap (Impra, Phoenix, Arizona).

Group I: The prostheses were made of microporous polytetrafluorethylene (PTFE), pore size 30 μm (kindly supplied by Impra, Phoenix,
Arizona). Before implantation the prostheses were sterilized by steam
sterilization.

Group II: PTFE prostheses of group I were treated for 15-16 minutes
with a sodium-naphtalene-tetrahydrofuran solution (SNT), containing
0.14 g sodium, 0.84 g naphtalene and 50 ml tetrahydrofuran. After
treatment the prostheses were immersed for 3 hours in tetrahydrofuran followed by immersion in refluxing tetrahydrofuran for 2.5
hours. The prostheses were then dried in air and treated with water
for 3 hours followed by drying in vacuo for at least 24 hours. Non-
porous PTFE films were treated in an identical manner to study the
chemical characteristics after treatment.

Group III: PTFE prostheses of group I were coated with poly-dl-lactic
acid, Mn 59000, by dipping the prostheses in a solution of poly-dl-
lactic acid, (PDLA) in chloroform (35 g L^{-1}) for 30 seconds and air
drying for 5 minutes. The procedure was repeated six times and after
the last dipcoat the prostheses were dried for 20 hours in air and
in vacuo. The prostheses were sterilized with ethylene oxide (6 h,
$23^{o}C$, humidity 100%).

Group IV: PTFE prostheses of group I were treated with a warm ($60^{o}C$)
solution of trimethoprim in ethanol (25 g L^{-1}) and a solution of
sulfamethoxazole in acetone (100 g L^{-1}) in such a way that the upper
part of each prosthesis contained one compound and the lower part of
the same prosthesis contained the other compound. After each treatment the prostheses were dried for 30 minutes in vacuo. Finally each
prosthesis contained about 10 mg sulfamethoxazole and 2 mg trimethoprim.

Prostheses of groups III and IV were sterilized with ethylene oxide
(2 h, $50^{o}C$, humidity 70%). All animals received antibiotics (Eusa-
prim [R], 160 mg trimethoprim and 800 mg sulfamethoxazole in 0.5 L
drinking water daily) for 3 weeks, except group IV. The animals
were killed after 3 weeks of implantation, the grafts inspected,
biologically cultured and processed for ligth microscopy (Bottema
and Wildevuur, 1980).

RESULTS

A summary of the results is presented in Tables 1 and 2.

Group I: The PTFE prostheses showed obstructions in 20% of the cases.
These were located in the central section of the grafts. No hypergranulation at the anastomosis side was observed. The ingrowth of

Table 1 Tissue growth on different tracheal prostheses,
3 weeks after implantation.

Group	1 Obstruction %	2 Ingrowth %	3 Overgrowth %	4 Overgrowth % a	b
I (PTFE n = 10	20	50	80	30	50
II (SNT) n = 10	60	0	70	0	70
III (PDLA) n = 10	10	0	60	50	10
IV (antibiotics) n = 10	10	20	20	20	0

1. Proportion in which the internal diameter of the lumen was decreased by more than three times the wall thickness of the prosthesis.
2. Proportion where more than 50% of the void volume was penetrated
   by tissue.
3. Proportion where overgrowth of connective tissue was complete.
4. Thickness of overgrowing layer less than (a) or more than (b)
   twice the wall thickness of prosthesis. PTFE; polytetrafluorethylene, SNT; sodium-naphtalene-tetrahydrofuran, PDLA; poly-
   dl-lactic acid.

Table 2 Infection in rabbits after implantation of
tracheal prostheses.

Group	Trachea Culture %	Histology %	Lung Culture %
I (PTFE) n = 10	30	20	40
II (SNT) n = 10	40	10	50
III (PDLA) n = 10	30	20	20
IV (antibiotics) n = 10	60	60	100

PTFE; polytetrafluorethylene, SNT; sodium-naphta--
lene-tetrahydrofuran, PDLA; poly-dl-lactic acid.
Animals in groups I, II and III received Eusaprim^R
for 3 weeks following implantation of the prostheses.
The following microorganisms were detected: Bacillus
species (14x), Staph. epidermidis (13x), E.coli (4x),
Pseudomonas species (3x), Staph. aureus (2x), Strept.
viridans (2x), Strept. faecalis (1x)

cells from the peritracheal area was moderate. Overgrowth of tissue,
covering the prostheses on the inside was complete in 80% of the
animals and the other 20% were nearly complete. The thickness of the
connective tissue layer varied from one to four times the wall
thickness of the prosthesis (0.7 mm). A mucous membrane was observed
in every case where the grafts were completely covered on the inside.
Group II: Studies with PTFE films showed that after treatment with

SNT, the contact angle θ (PTFE-water-air) changed from 100-109° to
51-77° (Meier and Petrie, 1973). The treatment causes a brownish
colour caused by the formation of a carbonaceous surface (Janstra
et al, 1975). Scanning electron microscopy (SEM) shows that the surface structure of the prosthesis has changed after treatment (Figs.
1a and 1b). Interconnecting PTFE threads become loose and disinte-
grate. The number of obstructions of the implanted grafts was considerably increased (60%). The ingrowth of tissue was minimal.
However the overgrowing connective tissue layer on the inside of the
prosthesis was 3 - 4 times the thickness of the prosthetic wall. The
development of the mucous membrane was seriously inhibited.

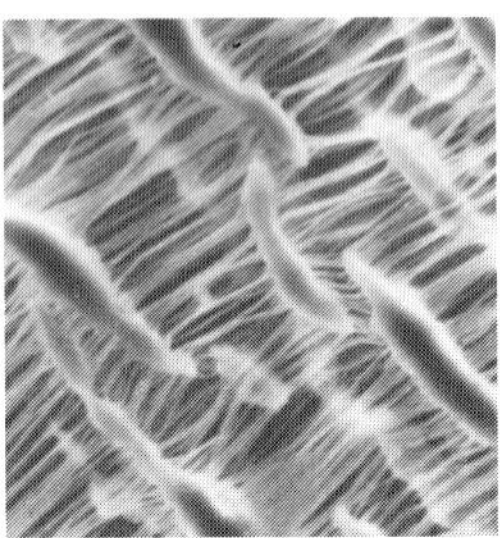 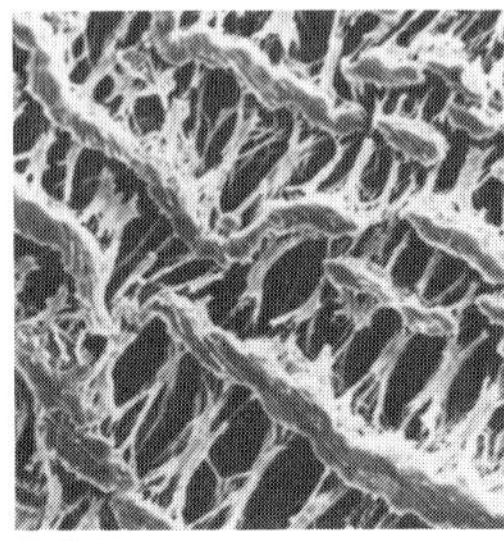 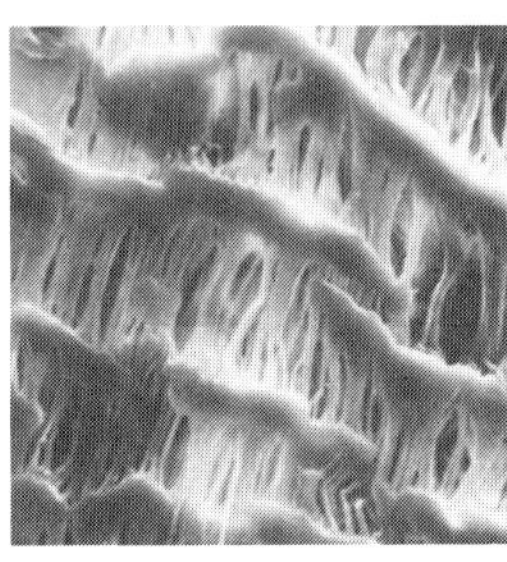

a   b   c

Fig. 1 Scanning electron micrograph to show (a) the
structure of the microporous polytetrafluoroethylene
used to construct tracheal psotheses (500x); (b) the
structure of the microporous polytetrafluoroethylene
treated with sodium-naphtalene-tetrahydrofuran (500x);
(c) the structure of the microporous polytetrafluoroethylene coated with poly-dl-lactic acid (500x).

<u>Group III</u>: SEM of the treated prostheses revealed that the porous
surface structure has slightly changed (Fig. 1c). Only one obstruction was seen in the implanted grafts, which was located at the
anastomosis. This graft was infected and showed no overgrowth of
tissue. Ingrowth of tissue was minimal in all cases. Only 60% of the
grafts were completely overgrown with a very thin layer of connective
tissue..
<u>Group IV</u>: There was only one obstruction and this was located at the
anastomosis. The graft was infected and there was minimal tissue
overgrowth. In- and overgrowth of tissue was minimal for the other
9 prostheses. The occurrence of infection was high when no systemic
antibiotic was given (group IV). Locally applied antibiotics could
not prevent infection. It seems that coating with PDLA (group III)
afforded protection against infection, especcially for the lungs.

DISCUSSION

An ideal tracheal prosthesis shows no airway obstruction and will have
a mucous membrane with a restored ciliar activity to maintain a physiological clearing mechanism in the airway. Growth of tissue into

porous prostheses stabilises the implant without hypergranulation.
Nutrition can be provided through a porous prosthesis for the epithelial layer on the air side of the prosthesis. Overgrowth with a
thin connective tissue layer is desirable to obtain a well differentiated epithelial layer (Botteman et al, 1980). A problem very often
encountered with porous prostheses is the occurrence of infections.
The purpose of this study was to investigate whether this problem
could be solved by either a rapid overgrowth of connective tissue
or the local application of antibiotics.

PTFE was modified in three different ways. Treatment with the SNT
method (group II) was intended to cause a rapid attachment to surrounding cells, which in turn prevents infection (Schneider et al,
1978). Coating with PDLA (group III) modifies the surface (decrease
of pore size) and decreases the local pH after degradation, which
possibly reduces infection. Local release of antibiotics (group IV)
might give more effective local prevention of infection.

In group II overgrowth of tissue was highly stimulated and the
tissue layer became too thick. This must be caused by the change
in surface chemistry of the prosthesis, which had a carbonaceous
surface and possibly increased hydrophilicity and/or the change in
surface morphology.

In group III the quality of the overgrowing connective tissue layer
was excellent. Ingrowth was negligible which indicates that the
coating should not be applied on the outside of the prosthesis. Only
one prosthesis became obstructed and the rate of infection, especially of the lungs, was low.

The use of local antibiotics did not prevent the occurrence of infection. Possible reasons are:
(a) the release rate of the antibiotics was too fast
(b) the antibiotic inhibited cellular growth and the prosthesis was
     exposed for a longer time to contaminated air.
We conclude that coating of the inner side of PTFE prostheses with
poly-dl-lactic acid seems to provide the best treatment for microporous tracheal prostheses. Specific systemic antibiotic prophylaxis
is still needed to minimize infection during the period that the
prosthesis is not completely incorporated.

ACKNOWLEDGEMENT

This study was supported by a grant from the Koningin Wilhelmina
Fonds, Amsterdam, the Netherlands.

REFERENCES

Bottema, J.R. & Wildevuur, Ch.R.H. (1978). Tracheal prosthesis:
evaluation of microporous material, Proceedings ESAO, V, 206-209.
Bottema, J.R. Feijen, J., Molenaar, I., ten Hoopen, H.W.M. & Wildevuur, Ch.R.H., (1980), Microporous tracheal prosthesis, TASAIO,
XXVI, 413-417.
Hulbert, S.F., Morrison, S.J., & Klawitter, J.J. (1971). Compatibility of porous ceramics with soft tissue; Application to tracheal

prostheses, J. Biomed. Mater. Res. Symp., 2, 269-279.
Janstra, J., Dousek, F.P., & Riha, J. (1975). Quantitative explana-
tion of the mechanism of corrosion of poly(tetrafluoroethylene)
caused by active alkali metals, J. Appl. Polymer Sci., 19, 3201-3210.
Meier, J.F. & Petrie, E.M. (1973). The effect of ultraviolet radia-
tion on sodium etched poly(tetrafluoroethylene) bonded to polyure-
thane elastomer, J. Appl. Polymer Sci., 17, 1007-1017.
Moritz, E., Braun, F., Fasol, P., Losert, U., Schlick, W., &
Sprängler, P., (1975). Prosthetic tracheal replacement, Proceedings
ESAO, II, 188-192.
Nelson, R.J., White, R.A. Lawrence, R.S., Walkinshaw, M.D.,
Fiaschetti, F.L., White, E.W., & Hirose, F.M. (1979). Development of
a microporous tracheal prosthesis, TASAIO, XXV, 8-13.
Pizzoferrato, A., Leake, D., Michieli, S., Haubold, A., & Freeman, S.,
(1979). Preliminary histologic evaluation of a biocompatible mesh
for tracheal reconstruction, Biomat. Med. Dev. Art. Org., 7, 321-331.
Schneider, U.A., Haussener, V., & Geret, V., (1978). New teflon
surface allowing surrounding tissue direct attachment, abstracts of
BES 71st scientific meeting, third conference on materials for use in
medicine and biology, Mechanical properties of Biomaterials, session
four, 13-15 Sept. 1978, University of Keele. (U.K.).
Thomas, P.A. (1973), Experimental evaluation of woven poly(lactic
acid), polyester tubes as tracheal prostheses, Annual summary report,
USAMRDC, contract no. DADA17-72-C-2009.
Wykoff, T.W., (1973), A preliminary report on segmental tracheal
prosthetic replacement in dogs. Laryngoscope, 83, 1072-1077.

Biomaterials 1980
Edited by G. D. Winter, D. F. Gibbons, and H. Plenk, Jr.
© 1982 John Wiley and Sons Ltd.

COLLAGEN COATED POLYPROPYLENE MESHES
FOR RECONSTRUCTIVE SURGERY OF THE TRACHEA

Y. Shimizu, Y. Miyamoto, T. Teramatsu*, T. Hino**,
U. Shibata***, and S. Okamura****

* Dept. of Thoracic Surgery, Chest Disease Research
Institute, Kyoto University, Sakyo-ku (606), Kyoto Japan
** Research Institute for Production Development
*** Central Research Laboratories, Meiji Seika
****Kyoto Industrial University

SUMMARY

We tried to reconstruct cervical trachea of dogs by means of patch
graft using composite of collagen and plastics. In this study, we
prepared two types of composite meshes. One is collagen coated fine
Marlex mesh. Another one is collagen coated heavy Marlex mesh. In
the 5 dogs with non coated simple plastic meshes, 3 dogs died because
of air leakage or excessive granulation. In the 6 dogs with collagen
coated fine mesh, the results in 5 dogs were satisfactory up to 19
months. In the 5 dogs with collagen coated heavy mesh, all dogs had
ulcer formation or overgrowth of granulation. From these results, we
consider that collagen coating effectively prevents air leakage and
that highly porous, elastic, fine mesh is better than rigid, heavy
mesh for the repair of tracheal defects.

INTRODUCTION

Although there have been many efforts to reconstruct trachea using
artificial materials, many problems remain to solved. Ideally,
artificial trachea should be airtight, be rigid enough to prevent
airway collapse, be well accepted by the host, and finally, be covered
by respiratory epithelium. In order to fulfill these prerequisites,
we have been developing composite meshes of collagen and plastics.
We have previously reported that films of a polymer-collagen composite
implanted into the dorsal subcutaneous tissue or rabbits appear to
have higher tissue affinity and to be more quickly incorporated into
the tissue than non-treated plastics. A collagen coating seems to
have an ability to stimulate tissue regeneration by promoting cell
growth (Shimizu et al. 1977; Shimizu et al. 1978). Currently, we are
trying to reconstruct the trachea with our newly developed materials.
In this report, we present the results of our experiments to date,
especially the results of reconstruction by means of patch grafts and
discuss the influences of the chemical and physical properties of the
implanted materials on the tissue response.

MATERIALS AND METHODS

Fabrication of the composite comprises three processes. Active
radicals are generated on the surface of plastics by means of plasma
treatment. Proctase treated bovine collagen is coated onto the
plastics. Co-polymerization is effected by ultraviolet irradiation.
In this study, we prepared two types of composite meshes having
different porosity, rigidity, and elasticity. One is composed of
collagen and fine polypropylene mesh, which is called Marlex mesh and
which is generally used for repair of abdominal wall defects or
inguinal hernias. This mesh is knitted with fine fibers to have high
porosity and elasticity. Another one is composed of collagen and high
density polyethylene mesh, which is called heavy Marlex mesh or
tracheal Marlex mesh and generally used for tracheal reconstruction.
This mesh is woven with thick fibers to have rigidity. Using these
meshes, we replaced the cervical trachea of dogs with patchgraft.
The operation were performed under intravenous anesthesia. The
cervical trachea was exposed and a window-shaped defect of about half
of the circumference, containing 6 to 8 cartilagenous rings was
created on the anterior wall of the trachea. The patch graft was
sutured on the outer surface of the trachea with 3 - 0 Tevdek. To
evaluated the wound healing of the inner surface of the reconstructed
trachea, endoscopic observation was performed at various intervals
after operation and some dogs were killed to observe the microscopic
findings of the implanted patch grafts.

RESULTS

In 5 of the 6 dogs whose trachea were reconstructed with the composite
of collagen and fine Marlex mesh, the endoluminar surface was found to
be covered with a white, thin epithelium-like layer 3 or 4 weeks after
operation. In one dog only, an overgrowth of granulation was found.
Fig. 1 is the endoscopic findings of this type of composite mesh one
and a half year after operation. The implanted mesh is completely
covered with a thin epithelium-like layer. Fig. 2 is the microscopic
findings of the specimen which was obtained from the dog killed for
histological study after 5 months. The section was obtained from the
center of the inner surface of the patch graft. The inner surface is
completely covered with ciliated epithelium and the underlying
fibrous tissue is thin and inflamed.
Similar operations were performed using the composite meshes of
collagen and heavy Marlex mesh in the other 5 dogs. Endoscopy
revealed that 3 dogs had ulcer formation (Fig. 3) and 2 dogs had
excessive granulation in the proximal portion. Microscopic examination
revealed ciliated epithelium only in the distal protion in this group.
In the proximal portion a squamous epithelial lining is present and
the underlying fibrous tissue is thicker and more inflameded than in
the case of fine composite mesh (Fig. 4)
The experimental results are summarized in Table 1. In the 5 dogs
with non coated simple plastic meshes, 2 dogs died in the early post-
operative stage because of air leakage or excessive granulation.
In the 6 dogs with collagen coated fine mesh, one dog, killed after
19 months had developed excessive granulations, 3 animals were still
satisfactory after 17 - 19 months.

TABLE 1. Experimental results of tracheal patchgrafts

Materials	Time (months)	Result
fine Marlex mesh	19	alive, good
"	17	alive, good
"	17	alive, granulation (+)
heavy Marlex mesh	10 days	died, air leakage
"	2 days	died air leakage
collagen coated fine Marlex mesh	5	sacrificed, good
"	19	sacrificed, granulation (+)
"	19	alive, good
"	19	alive, good
"	6	sacrificed, good
"	17	alive, good
collagen coated heavy Marlex mesh	6	sacrificed, ulcer (+)
"	11	sacrificed, ulcer (+)
"	7	sacrificed, ulcer (+)
"	22	died, granulation (+)
"	6	died, granulation (+)

DISCUSSION AND CONCLUSION

On the basis of these results, we consider that collagen coating is
effective in preventing air leakage from the pores of the meshes.
Differences in the results between fine composite mesh and heavy
composite mesh are mainly caused by their physical properties because
they were both coated with collagen and hence their chemical
properties are probably the same. This suggests that the physical
properties of meshes are as significant as their chemical properties
for the success of this procedure. We believe that highly porous,
elastic, fine mesh is better than heavy, rigid mesh for the repair of
tracheal defects, especially for the cervical trachea which is very
mobile. We are therefore trying to develop tubular prostheses composed
of collagen coated fine mesh and supporting rings.

REFERENCES

Shimizu, Y., Abe, R., Teramatsu, T., Okamura, S. & Hino, T. (1977)
Studies on copolymers of collagen and a synthetic polymer. Biomat.
Med. Dev. Art. Org., 5, 49-66.
Shimizu, Y., Miyamoto, Y., Teramatsu, T., Okamura, S. & Hino, T. (1978)
Studies on composites of collagen and a synthetic polymer, Biomat.
Med. Dev. Art. Org., 6, 375-391.

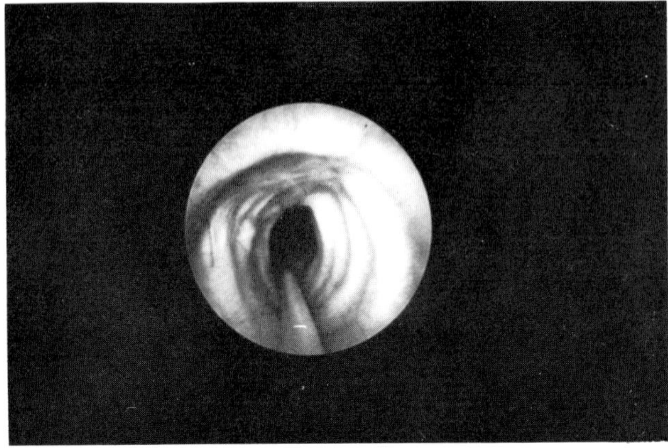

Fig. 1. Photograph, through the endoscope of collagen and
fine Marlex mesh. The implanted mesh is completely
covered with a thin epithelium-like layer.

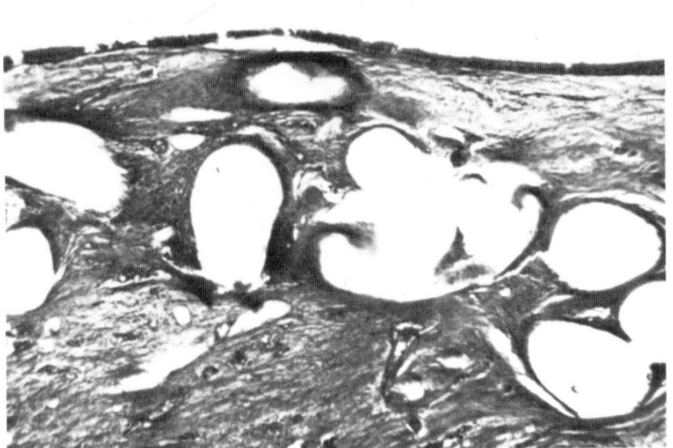

Fig. 2. Photomicrograph of a specimen obtained from the
sacrificed dog of the group using composite of collagen
and fine Marlex mesh. The inner surface is covered with
ciliated epithelium and the underlying fibrous tissue is
thin and inflamed.

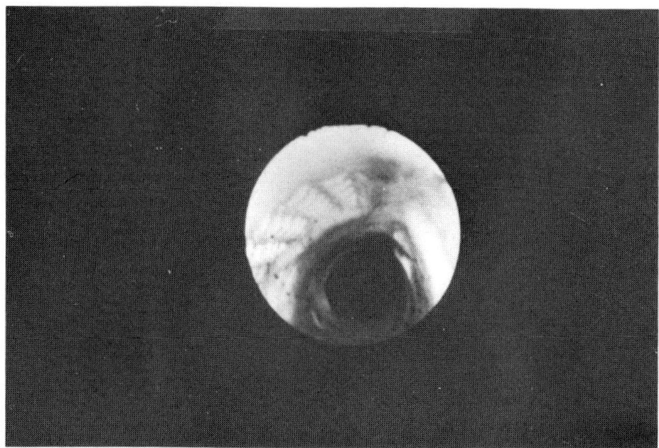

Fig. 3. Photograph, through the endoscope of the proximal portion of the composite of collagen and heavy Marlex mesh. Ulcer formation can be observed.

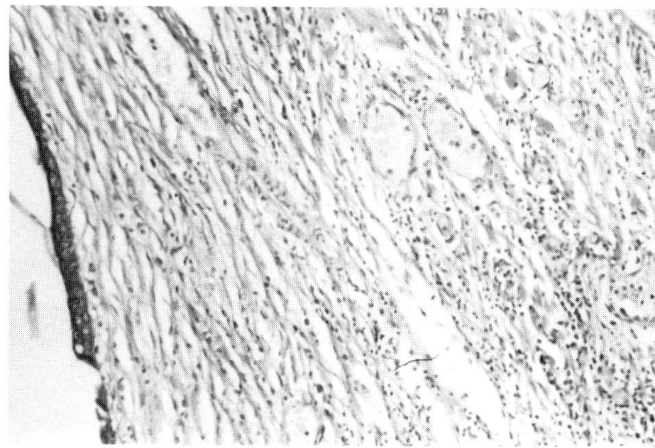

Fig. 4. Photomicrograph of the specimen which was obtained from the proximal portion of composite of collagen and Heavy Marlex mesh. Squamous epithelium lines over thick and inflamed vascular connective tissue.

Biomaterials 1980
Edited by G. D. Winter, D. F. Gibbons, and H. Plenk, Jr.
© 1982 John Wiley and Sons Ltd.

BIOLOGICAL BEHAVIOUR OF AUTOLOGOUS VEIN OR BILE DUCT USED FOR BILIARY TRACT REPLACEMENT.

C. Doillon, E. Chignier, G. Dureau and R. Eloy.

Unit 37 - INSERM - Cardiovascular surgery and organ transplantation laboratory.
18 av. Doyen Lépine - 69500 Bron - France.

SUMMARY

Bile duct replacement with autologous vein or bile duct was studied using rats. Initial complete epithelial or endothelial cell loss resulted in a biliary sludge which irritated the tissues and induced a fibrotic reaction. Pretreatment of the graft by immersion in concentrated glycerol removed the epithelial cells before implantation and this improved the long-term results.

INTRODUCTION

Despite many attempts to replace the common bile duct by biological materials (Pearce et al., 1951 ; Belzer et al., 1965 ; Wittrin et al., 1978) fibrosclerosis and chronic inflammation were generally observed within 3 weeks of surgery. Epithelialization of the common bile duct was irregularly noted. A lack of vascularity was considered to be responsible for these bad results. Ulin et al., (1955) and Lindenauer et al., (1966) using vascularized vein grafts showed that the irritative effect of bile was also involved. Disturbances of bile duct motility (Dunphy et al., 1962) or lack nutrition of the graft via the luminal pathway (Myers et al., 1960) were also implicated.
The aim of the present study was to evaluate the histological and ultrastructural fate of autologous bile duct or femoral vein when used as substitutes for the biliary tract in rats and to analyze the role of different etiopathogenic factors.

MATERIALS AND METHODS

The experiments were carried out under general anesthesia (intraperitoneal sodium pentobarbital 0.15 %) on female Wister rats, weighing about 250 g. Through an abdominal midline incision the common bile duct was identified and carefully isolated. A segment of the duct of 0.5 cm length was resected below the portal bifurcation and above the pancreatic duct junction . Microsurgical techniques were used (Zeiss operator microscope - magnification 5 to 25) and reimplantation and

anastomosis of duct or vein was performed with interupted 10/0 nylon
microsutures (Spingler & Tritt : Chirurgische Nadein Supramid Perlon)
The biliary implants consisted of autologous femoral vein or bile duct
immersed before implantation either in Hank'solution at 4°C for 10 minutes or in 87 % glycerol solution for 10 minutes at 40°C and rehydrated. The animals were killed after 24 and 72 hours and on the 7th and
15th day and after 2 and 3 months post-operatively. Each group comprised at least three animals. One part of the transplant was fixed in
Bouin's solution and stained with hematoxylin eosin for histological
examination.
The other part was immersed into a 2 % glutaraldehyde solution buffered with 0.2 M cacodylate. The specimen was dehydrated in acetone,
dried by the critical point method using CO2 and then coated with gold.
This second specimen was studied by scanning electron microscopy
(SEM) using the Cambridge steroscan microscope.

RESULTS

1°) <u>Non treated grafts</u> : The SEM specimens revealed that, in non treated implants, the normal bile epithelium, consisting of epithelial microvillous cells with regularly interposed goblet cells, was lost within 24 hours (Figure 1) leading to the early exposure of the underlying connective tissue to the bile components. Similarly the endothelial cells were desquamated from the autologous non treated vein in
the 24 hour specimen (Figure 2). After 72 hours a fibrinous acellular
material recovered the surface of the graft. The histological study
confirmed these observations and showed the initiation of an inflammatory reaction. This shedding of the superficial epithelium or endothelium led to the early accumulation of a sludge of dead cells in non
treated grafts of either bile or vein origin.

Between the 7th and 15th post-operative day epithelialization of the
grafted tissue occurred (Figure 3) and after one month epithelial cells
completely covered the bile or vein grafts. Even globets cells were
present. Histological examination of the non treated transplants demonstrated an intense fibrosclerosis in the walls of both bile and
vein grafts by the end of the first post-operative month (Figure 4).
The degree of fibrosis was similar in bile and vein grafts.

2°) <u>Glycerol-treated grafts</u> : The pretreatment of the vein or bile
grafts by immersion in concentrated glycerol resulted in extensive
surface cell desquamation (Figures 5 and 6). Thus the initial cell shedding observed during the first 24 post-operative hours after implantation of non-treated tissue was induced in vitro prior to surgical implantation. No biliary sludge was observed in these animals. Epithelialization of the bile or vein graft took place as on the non treated
grafts after the 7th post-operative day. Histologically there was less
inflammation than was seen with non-treated implants. After the 2nd and

3rd post-operative months the fibrotic reaction was still reduced (Figure 7).

DISCUSSION

We have found that superficial cell shedding is the initial feature of either non treated bile or vein grafting procedures. This results in accumulation of sludge in the lumen of the grafts which may bring about the formation of stasis gallstones (Doillon et al., 1980). Nevertheless epithelialization and glandular structures are present several weeks after implantation. The long term fate of these procedures is limited by the intense fibrosclerosis of the connective tissue within the graft. Therefore glycerol pretreatment of the tissue appears advantageous because the cell shedding occurs before grafting, biliary sludge is reduced or absent and epithelialization still takes place. Moreover the long term results are improved because of the reduced fibrotic reaction in the graft wall. We deduce that the initial biliary sludge, in the absence of adequate drainage may induce a dense connective tissue reaction by irritating the exposed connective tissues in the graft wall. The glycerol pretreatment decreases bile stasis and allows recovery of cellularity within the grafted tissue. This rare phenomenon of cell proliferation within preserved tissue was not seen when glutaraldehyde-treated cardiac valves were used (Barratt-Boyes, 1979).

REFERENCES

Barratt-Boyes, B.G. (1979) Cardiothoracic surgery in the antipodes. J. Thorac. Cardiovasc. Surg., 78, 804-822.
Belzer, F.O., Watts, J.Mc.K., Ross, H.B. & Dunphy, J.E. (1965) Auto-reconstruction of the common bile duct after venous patch graft. Ann. Surg., 102, 346-355
Doillon, C., Dureau, G., Chignier, E., & Eloy, R.(1980) Course of the initial epithelial lesions associated with autologous bile duct replacement. Amer. J. Surg. (in press)
Dunphy, J.E. & Stephens, F.O. (1962) Experimental study of the effect of grafts in the common duct on biliary and hepatic function. Ann. Surg., 155, 906-923.
Lindenauer, S.M. & Child, C.G. (1966) Vascularized venous autografts in common bile duct reconstruction. Arch. Surg., 92, 749-751
Myers, R.T. Meredith, J.H. Rhodes, J. & Gilbert, J.W. (1960). The fate of free grafts in the common bile duct. Ann. Surg., 151, 776-780
Pearce, E.E. Ulin, A.W. Entine, J.H. & Froio, G. (1951) Experimental reconstruction of the extrahepatic biliary system using free venous grafts. Ann. Surg., 134, 808-814

Ulin, A.W., Shoemaker, W.C. & Entine, J.H. (1955) Vascularized venous grafts in the experimental reconstruction of the common bile duct.
Ann. Surg.142, 279-282.
Wittrin, G., Clemens M., Arndt, M. & Rhuland D. (1978) Choledechuser-
satz durch ein autologes venentransplantat. Res. Exp. Med. 173, 95-103

FIGURES

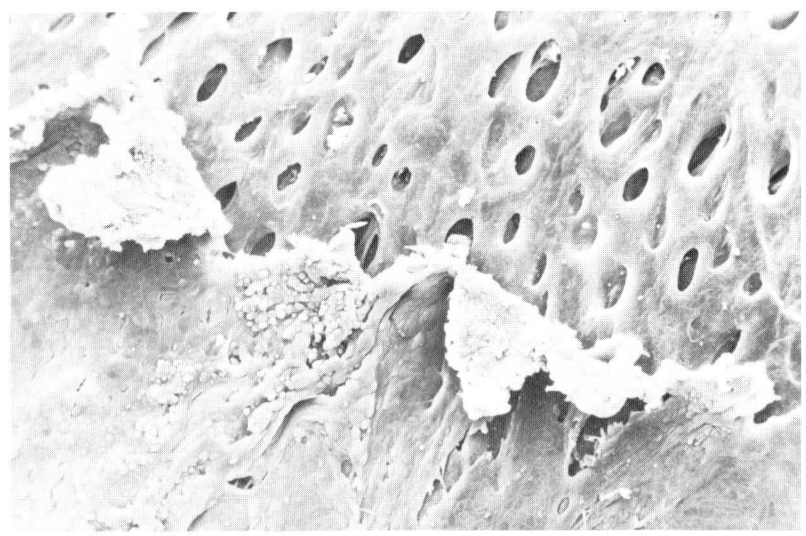

Fig. 1 Complete epithelial cell sheding on the
grafted autologous bile duct 24 hours after surgery.
X 250.

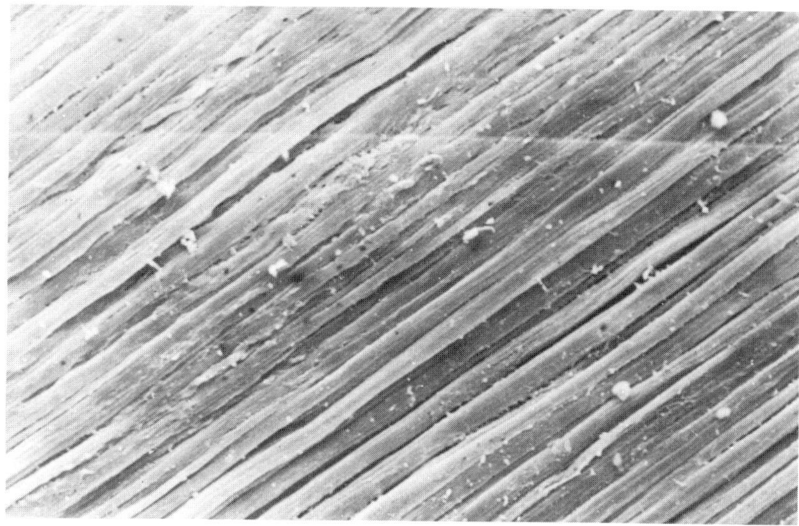

Fig. 2 Complete endothelial cell loss of the autologous
vein graft used as biliary substitute 72 hours after surgery leading to exposure of the collagen fibers. X 2,000.

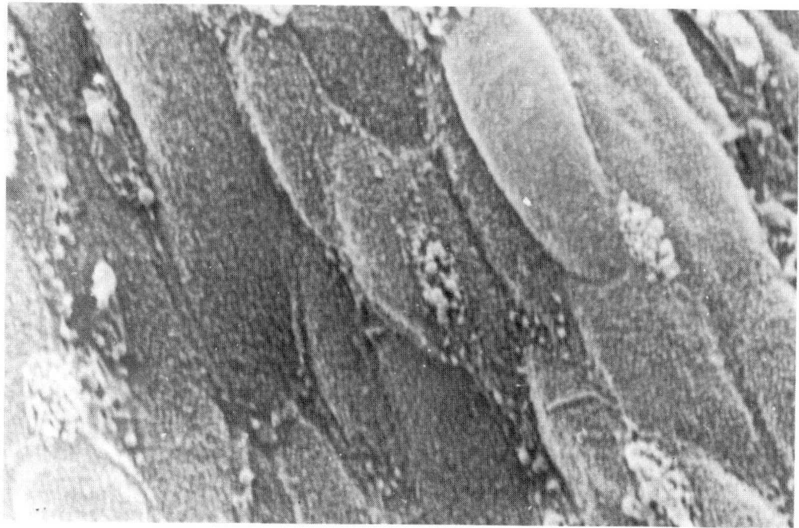

Fig. 3 Epithelialization of a venous implant 8-15 days
after being grafted as bile duct substitute. X 5,000.

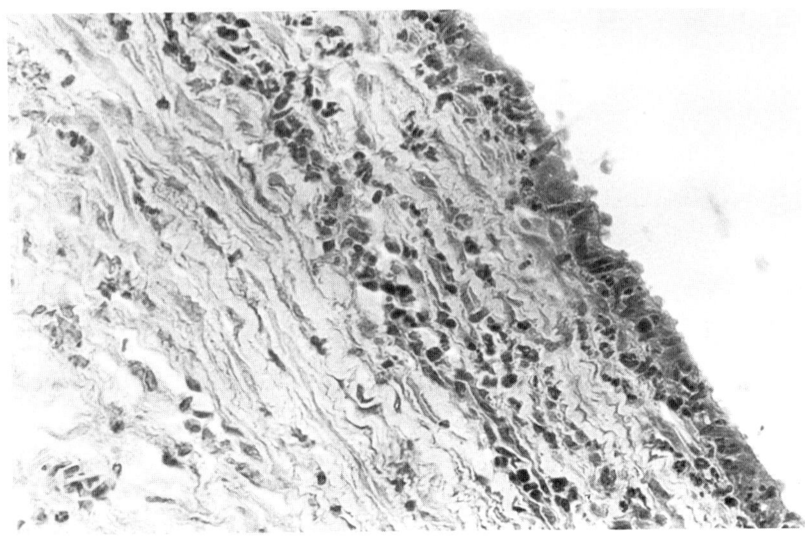

Fig. 4 Epithelialization, glandular formation and fibrosis of an autologous biliary graft. X 437.

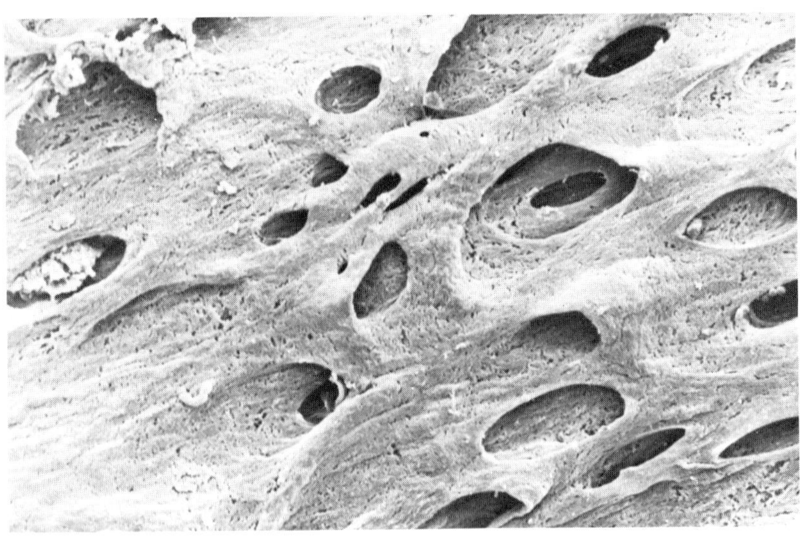

Fig. 5 Effect of glycerol treatment on the bile duct epithelium showing complete epithelial cell loss. X 500.

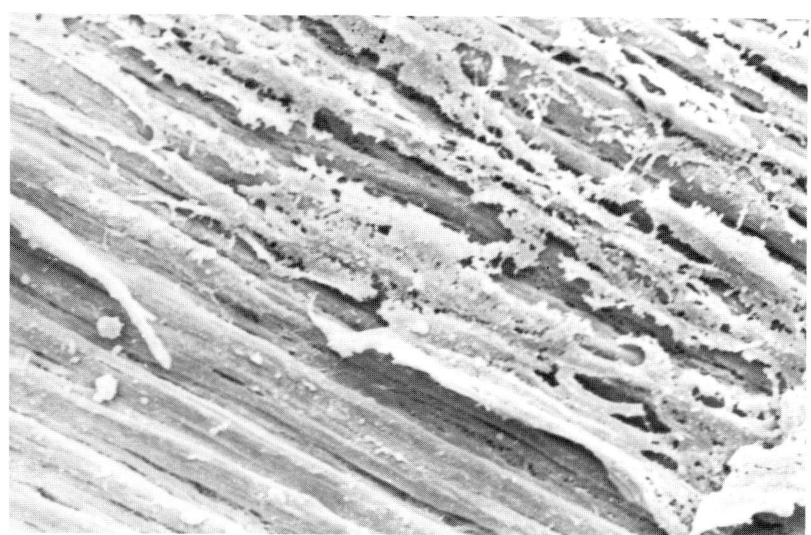

Fig. 6 Effect of glycerol treatment on the rat femoral vein and loss of endothelial cell layer. X 2,000.

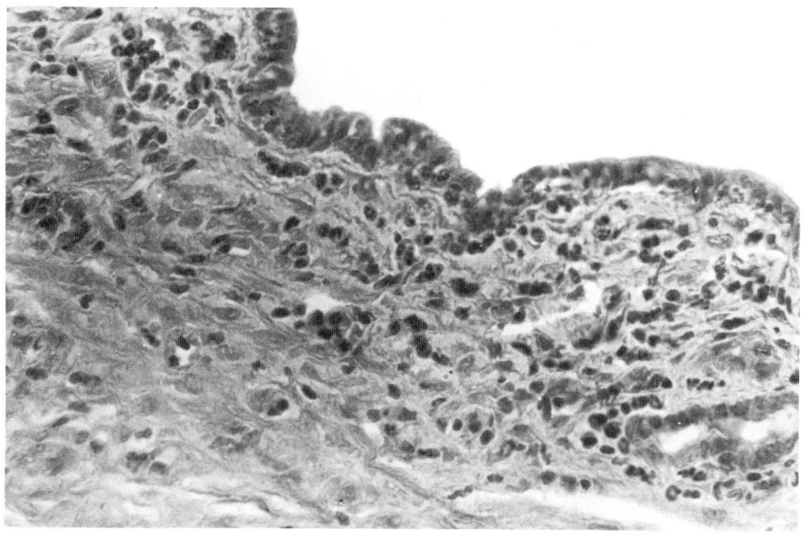

Fig. 7 Appearance of a glucerol pretreated venous graft used as bile duct substitute for 3 months. Note epithelial layer, glandular structures and limited fibrosis. X 437.

Biomaterials 1980
Edited by G. D. Winter, D. F. Gibbons, and H. Plenk, Jr.
© 1982 John. Wiley and Sons Ltd.

EXPERIMENTAL PANCREATIC DUCT OBSTRUCTION
WITH AN ALCOHOLIC PROLAMINE SOLUTION[R]
PRODUCING A PANCREATIC EXOCRINE ATROPHY

H.Dahlke, N.Dociu, H.Muxfeldt,
K.Thurau, M.-E.Treppl

ETHICON GmbH., Department of Development and
Research, Hamburg, Federal Republic of Germany

SUMMARY

A simple method for retrogard transduodenal occlusion of
the pancreatic duct is presented.
The substance used for this procedure, ETHIBLOC[R]
OCCLUSION GEL*, is an alcoholic prolamine solution
containing a radiopaque medium which precipitates in
contact with aqueous fluids. When applied with continuous
manual pressure it possesses the capability of filling
the entire duct system down to the most peripheral areas.
Biochemical results demonstrate a distinct exocrine
hypofunction of the pancreas, and also show that the
development of an acute inflammatory reaction is not
produced, except in the immediate post-operative period.
In contrast, the endocrine function of the pancreas
remains unaffected; normoglycemia is demonstrated
throughout the entire period of observation. Histological
findings corroborate the biochemical results. The
glandular acini underwent a progressive atrophy, while
the endocrine elements continue to function at a
satisfactory level. It appears that the obstruction of
the pancreatic duct with ETHIBLOC[R] OCCLUSION GEL could
be a recommendable conservative method for the treatment
of chronic relapsing pancreatitis.

INTRODUCTION

Chronic relapsing pancreatitis has become one of the
accompanying pathological " achievements" of our modern
style of life. A resection of the gland or a total
pancreatectomy bring the risk of a generally high
morbidity and mortality rate. Moreover, social and
psychological aspects of the patient's background make
the recommendation for such surgical interventions even
more difficult. For just these reasons it was attempted
to treat chronic relapsing pancreatitis by a ligation of
the pancreatic duct. Because of severe

*ETHICON GmbH.

technical difficulties with this method newer procedures are being sought. The attempt was made to seek a substance to occlude the pancreatic duct and thus to accelerate the atrophy of the exocrine pancreas, while preserving the endocrine function. In contrast to a partial obstruction of the pancreatic duct, which can trigger a chronic inflammatory condition of the pancreas, a total occlusion of the duct results in a quiet atrophy of the exocrine elements, while the endocrine part remains functional.

Favourable results have been achieved using ETHIBLOC[(R)] OCCLUSION GEL, a compound which fills the entire duct systems down to even the most peripheral areas. It is an alcoholic prolamine solution with an additional radiopaque medium which precipitates in contact with aqueous fluids. Promising experimental and clinical findings were reported by GEBHARDT et al.(1978a,b), GALL et al.(1979), RÖSCH et al.(1979) and WAYAND et al. (1979), using ETHIBLOC[(R)] OCCLUSION GEL for a total obstruction of the pancreatic duct and by BÜCHELER et al.(1978) and HUPE et al.(1978, 1979) in a palliative arterial embolisation of kidney tumours prior to nephrectomy. The present investigation was designed to assess the pathophysiological modifications following a total pancreatic duct obstruction with ETHIBLOC[(R)] OCCLUSION GEL in minipigs.

MATERIALS AND METHODS

6 adult minipigs of the Göttingen strain ranging in weight from 25 to 35 kg were used. The animals were anesthetized with STRESNIL[(R)]* and HYPNODIL[(R)]* and prepared for laparotomy. The abdomen was entered through a midline incision, and a loop of duodenum was laid out and opened longitudinally for 5 cms along the antimesenteric border. After location of the opening of the pancreatic duct, approx. 5 cc ETHIBLOC[(R)] was injected into it under continuous manual pressure. The duodenum was sutured and the abdominal wall was closed in two layers, using VICRYL**suture material throughout. In the postoperative period the animals were given water ad lib. and were placed on a soft diet for the first week. Thereafter, they were maintained on a standard diet with no supplements.

During the follow-up the exocrine pancreatic function was tested using two methods: serum amylase, assessed spectrophotometrically by the method of STREET&CLOSE (1956). Also the "PABA" test, the method described by GYR et al.(1974) and modified by FREUDIGER et al. (1976), was used. The endocrine function was determined by the tolbutamide tolerance test(capillary blood

*JANSSEN GmbH.   **ETHICON GmbH.

analysis after i.v.administration of RASTINON*), and
through the measurement of the fasting blood sugar level
(o-toluidine-method).

4 healthy animals of the same age, weight and strain were
used as a control group. The pigs were sacrificed 10, 20,
28, 35, 70 and 230 days after occlusion.

RESULTS

<u>Serum Amylase:</u>   Fig. 1 depicts the level of serum amylase.
Note the rapid transient increase immediately after the
surgical trauma, which reached a maximum value of
75o3,12 u/l - a 4,67 fold increase over the basal level
of 16o8,32 u/l. The serum amylase fell promptly thereafter
and remained at approximately the same level as prior
to the operation - excluding an accute pancreatitis but
not ruling out a possible chronic process.

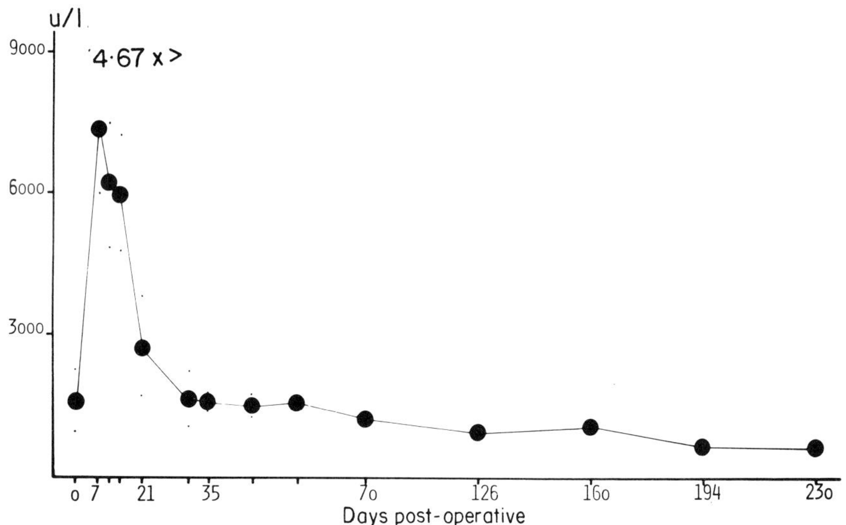

<u>Fig. 1</u>   Post-operative Variation of the Serum Amylase Level

A better indicator of an accute pancreatitis is the serum
lipase increase. Measuring of the serum lipase was done
during this study using a calibrated colour chart as
described by HÄRTEL et al.(1971); however, this serum
quantitative screening test did not provide the required
accuracy.

<u>PABA-Test:</u> The level of the tracer in the plasma of the
occluded animals remained low throughout the entire
observation period of 210 minutes(Fig. 2). In contrast,
* HOECHST AG.

the PABA-level in the control group rose rapidly over
the first 90 minutes and gradually decreased thereafter.

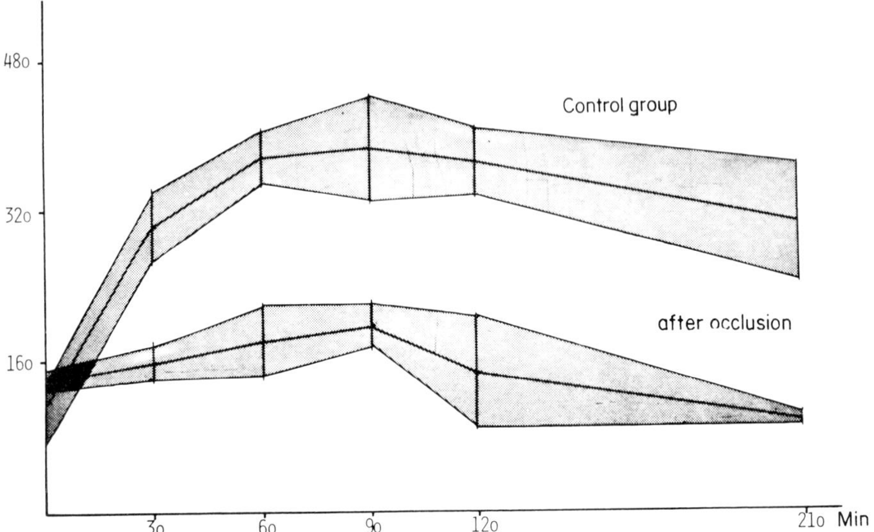

Fig. 2   The Exocrine Pancreatic Function after Oral
         Administration of P-Aminobenzoic Acid

This test has proven to be a very convenient index
of exocrine pancreatic function and compared with the
usual PABA evaluations in feces or urine to be much
easier and safer.

Tolbutamide Test: After the i.v.administration of
RASTINON the blood glucose level decreased during
the first 30 minutes reaching a mean value of 63,14
mg%(Fig. 3). 120 minutes post administration, it
began to rise constantly, returning to a normal
level of 85,86 mg%, thus proving a preservation of
the endocrine function.

Blood glucose in the occluded animals remained at
a normoglycemic level (between 60 and 102 mg %)
through the entire length of the study (Fig. 4).

Gross examination revealed variations in the post-
operative shape and weight of the pancreas. The first
three pigs were killed at 10, 20 and 28 days after
occlusion. Each pig exhibited an increase in the
weight of the pancreas, as well as moderate congestion
and swelling. The presence of small peri-pancreatic
foci of necrosis was also noted. These findings were
obviously due to the recent surgical manipulations.

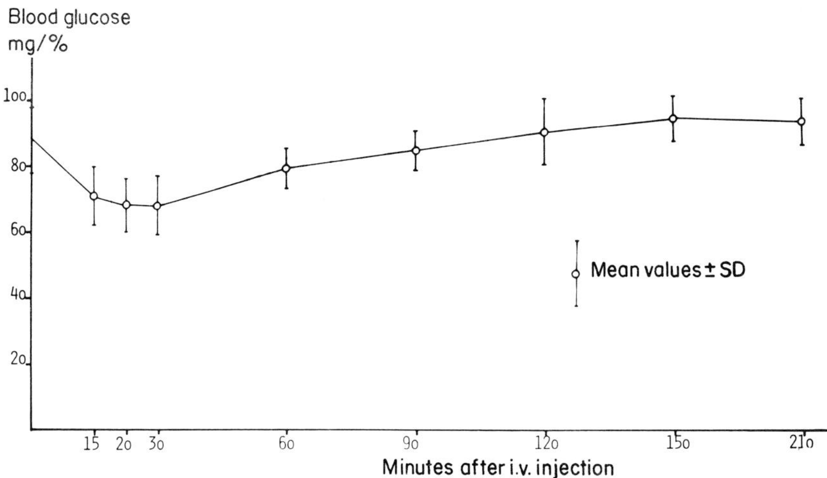

<u>Fig. 3</u>   Effect of Tolbutamide (RASTINON^(R) - 25 mg/kg
Body Weight) on the Blood Sugar Level

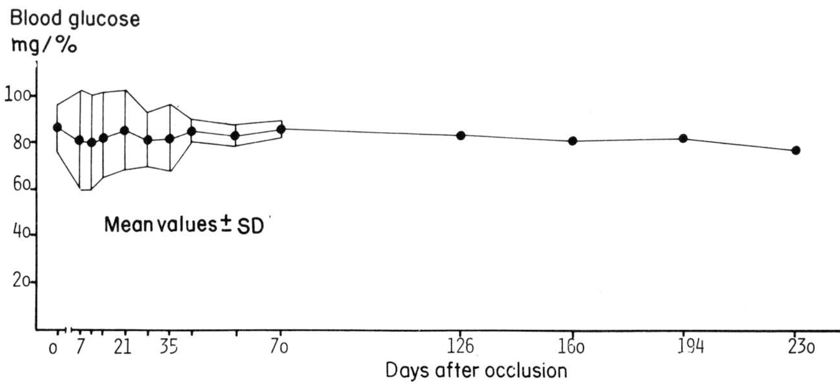

<u>Fig. 4</u> Fasting Blood Glucose Levels

Noteworthy in the second and third animal was the presence
of a large quantity of occluding compound in the area
between the head and the body of the pancreas; this is
assumed to be the result of a delated application of
ETHIBLOC^(R) . Behind this area the ductuls were slightly
dilatated. A progressive decrease in the weight of the

pancreas of the remaining three pigs was visible. 230
days after occlusion the severely scarred pancreas was
reduced to 35% of the mean weight of the pancreas in the
control group.

As depicted in the following two micrographs, the exocrine
elements of the pancreas underwent a progressive atrophy
over the 230-day observation period after occlusion,
while, at the same time, the endocrine part remained
largely unaffected.

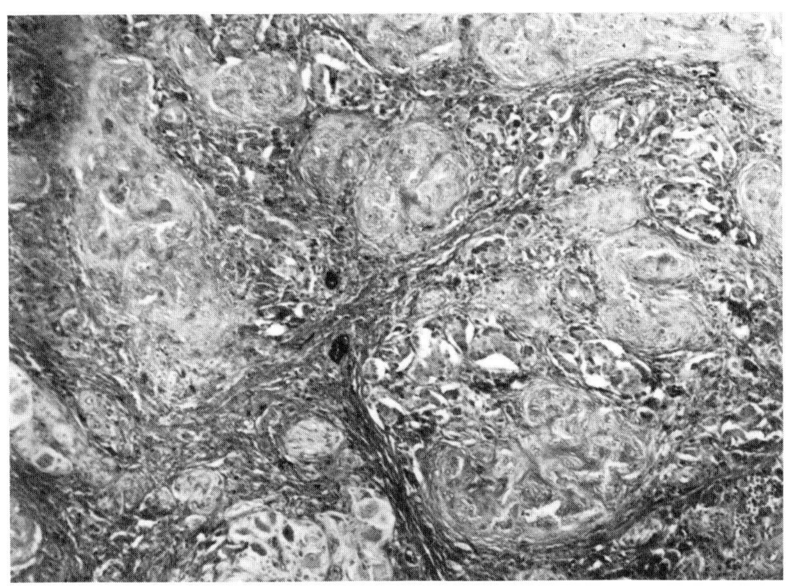

Fig. 5   Section taken 70 days after occlusion, showing
          an increase of the interlobular and interacinar
          tissue compressing the secretory elements, also
          a ribbon-like arrangement of some islet-cells.
          Masson-Goldner, Magnification x 25

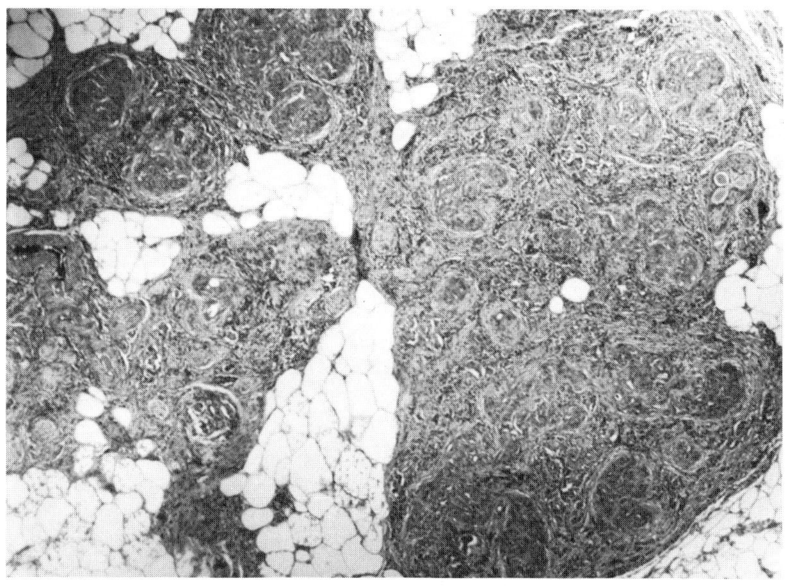

<u>Fig. 6</u>   Low power view of the Pancreas 230 Days
         following Duct Obstruction depicting an
         advanced Atrophy of the Pancreatic Tissue.
         Among the incapsulated Exocrine Remnants are
         scattered, deformed, but apparently still
         functional Islets of Langerhans.
         Hematoxylin&Eosin, Magnification x 12,5

Long term studies are still being conducted to prove the
resorption of ETHIBLOC[R], the possible regeneration
ability of the exocrine pancreas as well as the continuous
functioning of the islets of Langerhans over an extended
period of time.

<u>REFERENCES</u>

Bücheler, E., Hupe, W., Klosterhalfen, H., Altenähr, E.&
Erbe, W.(1978) Neue Substanz zur therapeutischen Emboli-
sation von Nierentumoren. <u>Fortschr.Röntgenstr.</u>, <u>128</u>, 599-6o3.
Freudiger, U.& Bigler, B.(1976) Die Diagnose der chro-
nischen exokrinen Pankreasinsuffizienz mit dem PABA-Test.
<u>Kleintier-Praxis 22</u>, 45-84.
Gall, F.P.& Gebhardt, Ch.(1979) Ein neues Konzept in der
Chirurgie der chronischen Pankreatitis. <u>Dtsch.med.Wschr.</u>
<u>28</u>, 1oo3-1006.

 H.Dahlke, N.Dociu, H.Muxfeldt, K.Thurau, M.-E.Treppl

Gebhardt, Ch.& Stolte, M.(1978 a) Pankreasgang-Okklusion durch Injektion einer schnellhärtenden Aminosäurelösung. Langenbecks Arch.Chir., 346, 149-166.
Gebhardt, Ch.& Stolte, M.(1978 b) Die Ausschaltung des exkretorischen Pankreasparenchyms durch intraductale Injektion einer schnellhärtenden Aminosäurelösung. Chirurg, 49, 428-430
Gyr, K., Wolf, R.H., Imondi, A.R. & Felsenfeld, O. (1974) Experiences with a new test of exocrine pancreatic function in protein deficient patas monkeys. Schweiz. med. Wschr., 104, 1888-1889
Härtel, A., Banauch, D. & Helger, R.(1971) Z.Klin.Chem. u.Klin.Biochem., 9, 396-398.
Hupe, W., Bücheler, E. & Altenähr, E. (1978). Eine Substanz zur Gefäßembolisierung von Hypernephromen. 4.Symp.Exp. Urol., Kassel
Hupe, W., Klosterhalfen, H., Bücheler, E. & Altenähr, E. (1979) Eine neue Technologie zur Embolisation des Hypernephroms. XVIII. Congr. Soc. Intn. d'Urol., Paris
Rösch, W., Phillip, J. & Gebhardt, Ch. (1979) Endoscopic duct obstruction in chronic pancreatitis. Endoscopy, 1, 43-46.
Street, H.V. & Close, J.R. (1956) Clin.Chim.Acta 1, 256-258.
Wayand, W. & Umlauft, M.(1979) Vorläufige Ergebnisse zur Ausschaltung des exokrinen Pankreasanteiles. 2o.Tagung d.Österr.Ges.f.Chirurgie, Innsbruck

Biomaterials 1980 .
Edited by G. D. Winter, D. F. Gibbons, and H. Plenk, Jr.
© 1982 John Wiley and Sons Ltd.

SHAPE MEMORY EFFECT IN BIOMEDICAL DEVICES

R. Kousbroek, G. Van der Perre, E. Aernoudt and J.C. Mulier

ICOBI - Biomaterials and Biomechanics section
Katholieke Universiteit Leuven, Belgium

SUMMARY

The phenomenon by which, after an apparent plastic deformation, a
metal alloy remembers its preceding shape when the temperature is
changed is known as the shape memory effect. Many interesting applications of this shape memory effect for both internal and external
applications in the field of biomedical engineering remain unexplored.
As a first result of our research on the possible use of the shape
memory effect in biomedical devices two applications have been
developed : an intramedullary fixation nail and a dynamic handsplint.

INTRODUCTION

When a metal alloy is plastically deformed, a permanent deformation is
left after unloading. A new force with opposite sign is needed to
bring the alloy back to its original shape. The shape memory alloys
distinguish themselves from the "usual" alloys by the fact that after
an apparent plastic deformation they return to their preceding shape
when the temperature is changed. This phenomenon is caused by the reverse transformation of the deformed, low temperature, martensitic
phase into the high temperature parent phase; this reversal may, totally or partially, recover the original shape. If subsequent changes
in temperature don't continue to influence the macroscopic shape the
effect is called the one-way shape memory effect (SME). If, in contrast with the one-way SME, a subsequent cooling again influences
the macroscopic shape, the effect is called the two-way SME, i.e. at
a certain lower temperature the alloy remembers again the deformed
low temperature shape. Initially, the shape recovery on cooling is
considerably less than on heating, but after a number of strain-
temperature cycles the macroscopic shape will vary between the "high-
temperature" and "low-temperature" shape without any applied forces.
A remarkable effect concommitant with the change in shape on heating
is the appearance of an external force, which can perform work.

Although the SME was recognized more than 40 years ago (Greninger and
Mooradian, 1938) its usefulness was only recognized about 10 years
ago (Wagner and Jackson, 1969). Since that time many potential applications have been suggested which fall into the industrial, mechanical, energy and medical fields. The SME has been proposed for different disciplines of medicine, especially in orthopaedics and dentistry. The dynamic compression bone plate is one of the most frequently

described orthopaedic applications (Johnson and Alicandri, 1974; Hughes, 1977; Baumgart et al., 1977), followed by the intramedullary fixation nail (Hughes, 1977; Bensmann et al., 1979). Other potential applications in orthopaedics are a total hip prosthesis fixation system (Hughes, 1977), a total surface replacement arthroplasty (Bensmann et al., 1979), and devices for treatment of scoliosis (Schmerling et al., 1976; Baumgart et al., 1978).
In dentistry, attention is focussed on orthodontic devices (Civjan et al., 1975; Andreasen and Morrow, 1978) and osteosynthetic jaw material (Civjan et al., 1975, Bensmann et al., 1979). Andreasen and Morrow, however, don't use the SME, but the relatively low Young-modulus of an SME alloy (Nitinol) in the martensitic condition (30 GPa) in comparison with the Young-modulus of stainless steel (200 GPa). In combination with a cold work process, when the Nitinol has been drawn into a high-strength orthodontic wire, the alloy exhibits an outstanding elasticity.
Other promising applications are a vena cava filter (Simon et al., 1977) and an artifical heart muscle (Page and Sawyer, 1974).

The advantage of internal application of the SME-alloy is that the devices can be implanted in a shape which is optimal for surgery, after which it takes the desired functional shape in situ in the body.

SME-MATERIALS

Although the SME has been observed in a number of nickel and copper based alloys, the effect appears most efficiently in Nitinol and Cu-Zn-Al. Nitinol is an equiatomic alloy of nickel and titanium. Because of its excellent biocompatibility (Cutright et al., 1973; Castleman et al, 1976; Hughes, 1977) Nitinol is the most obvious SME-alloy for internal applications. Because Nitinol is difficult and expensive to manufacture the attention for the external applications has focussed on Cu-Zn-Al, a ternary alloy of copper, zinc, and aluminium. In the field of orthotic applications the SME of Cu-Zn-Al can be used to simplify the moving parts of dynamic rehabilitation devices.

The transition temperature range (TTR) for both of these SME alloys is strongly dependent on the composition. Slight alterations in composition can markedly alter the TTR. For internal applications, the TTR has to be far enough below body temperature to assure a complete SME at body temperature. For external applications the TTR is less critical and mainly dependent on the applied heating- and cooling system. As a first result of our research on possible uses of the SME in biomedical devices two applications have been developed : an intramedullary fixation nail and a dynamic handsplint.

Intramedullary Fixation Nail. In the design of the intramedullary fixation nail with SME-elements the following conditions were considered :
a) at low temperature (T < TTR) the nail should possess a suitable shape making insertion and, if necessary, extraction of the nail easy;
b) at high temperature (TTR < T ≤ 37°C) the nail should fit strongly in the fractured bone without causing damage to the bone structure, e.g. bone necrosis and bone resorption;

c) in addition to a tight diametral fit of the nail at "high" temperature, the nail must also apply a certain amount of compression in order to press the fractured surfaces together.

The proposed intramedullary nail is depicted in Figure 1. The nail consists of two polymer profiled rods interconnected by an SME-compression
rod. The outer diameter of these rods is equal to or slightly less than
the inside diameter of the reamed medular canal.

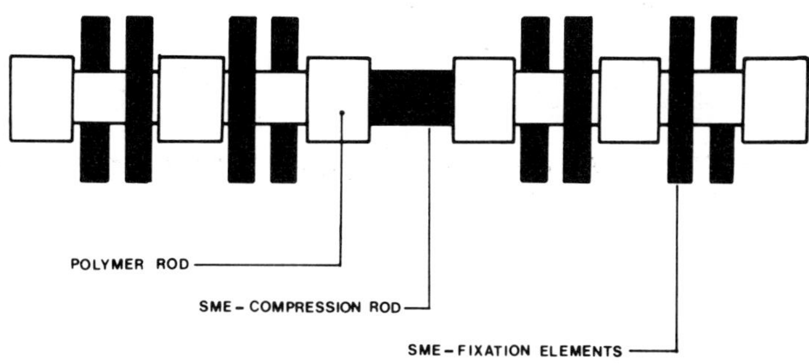

Fig. 1   SME-intramedullary fixation nail

Attached to the profiled rods are independently movable SME-fixation
elements. The SME-fixation elements are strips which "remember"
(T > TTR) their undeformed straight shape. Transformation to their
undeformed shape allows the fixation elements to contact the wall of
the reamed medullar canal, resulting in a firm union between the
bone and the nail (Fig. 2).

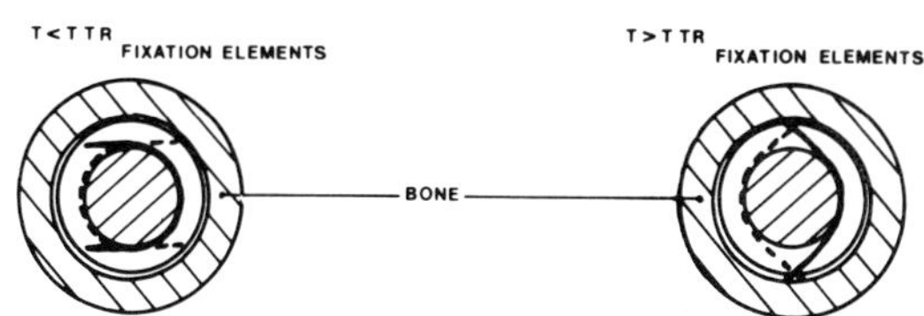

Fig. 2   Fixation elements in martensitic and parent phase

For optimal compression, the SME-fixation elements and the SME-compression rod should possess different TTR's, e.g. :

$$(A_f)_{\text{FIXATION ELEMENTS}} \leqslant (A_s)_{\text{COMPRESSION ROD}}$$

with A_s = start transformation on heating

A_f = end transformation on heating

and $(A_f)_{\text{COMPRESSION ROD}}$ = max. 20°C

This assures that axial compression will start only after the fixation elements are firmly fitted to the bone. Full compression will
be accomplished before body temperature has been reached, as is

depicted in Figure 3. The compression-rod displays one-way SME, while
the fixation elements possess two-way SME.

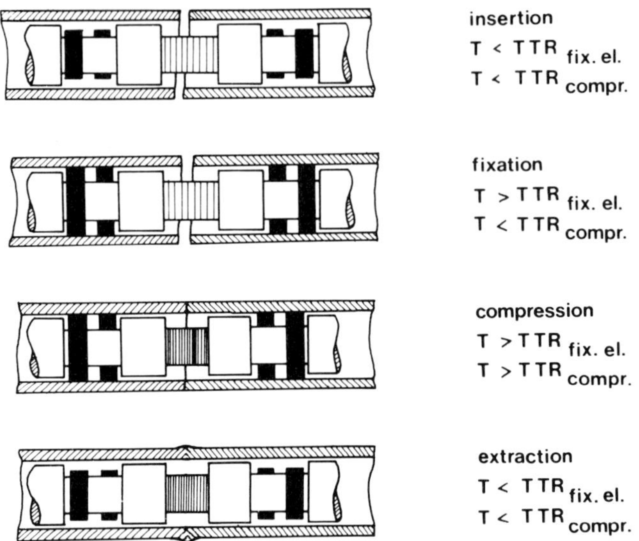

Fig. 3   Sequence of SME-transformation

An important advantage of this SME-fixation system is that in the
case of an irregular shaped medullary canal or after bone resorption
a tight fit of the nail in the medullary canal still exists due to
the independent SME-elements.

Dynamic Handsplint. A dynamic handsplint has been designed in the
shape of a glove on which a flexion or an extension motion can be
imposed by means of fixed strips of Cu-Zn-Al. The dynamic handsplint
is intended to be used for the rehabilitation of certain groups of
muscles of a partially functionally paralyzed hand in order to re-
gain natural function and to prevent further disfigurement. The
change in shape can be obtained by spanning each finger (except the
thumb) of the glove with a number of strips, which are interconnected
by rigid 90° joints. To impose flexion one starts with straight
strips. After deformation of the low temperature, martensitic phase
over a certain radius of curvature the hand reaches an extension
phase (Fig. 4a).

On raising the temperature above the transition temperature A_s the
deformed strips remember their undeformed, straight shape to which
they return, the inherent force moving the hand. Because of the rigid,
90° connection between the SME-strips a flexion phase will be
reached (Fig. 4b).

On subsequent cooling below the transition temperature (M_s) the patient can straighten the hand without any resistance from the metal
strips, which are again deformed (M_s = start transformation on cooling).

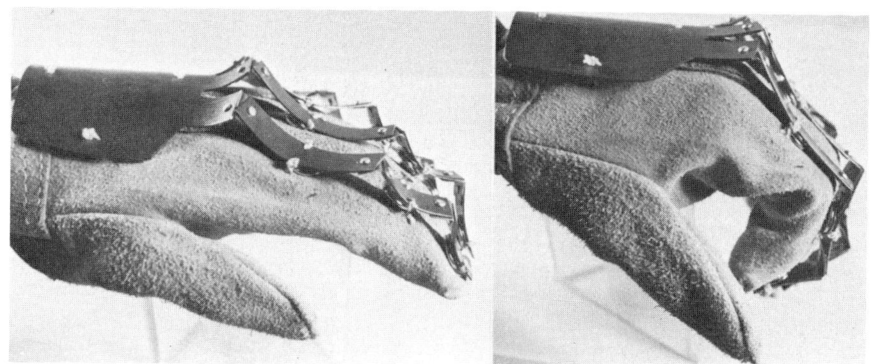

Fig. 4 a) extension phase   b) flexion phase

A new cycle can then be started. To obtain an imposed extension motion one starts with bent strips which are initially deformed to
straight strips.

DISCUSSION

The two proposed devices are intended to improve existing devices and
methods in their own domain of application. Only the principle of the
designs is depicted and a number of adaptions are still desirable.
Work is in progress, but it is already clear that the final devices
promise many advantages in comparison to existing devices. The SME-
fixation elements assure a tight fit between the intramedullary nail
and the bone, thus preventing rotation of the two bone fragments.
The addition of the compression rod should improve the healing process of the fracture in a similar way to that described for the ex-
tramedullary dynamic compression bone plates. The use of a polymer
for the profiled rods is based on the following factors :

1) in contrast with a metal, a polymer doesn't cause electrochemical
corrosion reactions with the SME-alloy;
2) recently it has been shown, that a flexible intramedullary rod may
have advantages in comparison with a rigid rod (Klopper, 1979; Wang
et al., 1980). These advantages are a) no removal of the fixation
device is required after the fracture is healed. In fact, due to a
reduced rigidity of the fixation device no stress protection, secondary to the forces transmitted through the device and under conventional circumstances followed by osteoporosis, is to be expected;
b) due to a limited degree of motion at the fracture site the formation of an external callus will be stimulated, resulting in a more
rapid and stronger healing of the fracture.

In vitro and in vivo experiments are needed to prove the potential
advantages of the SME-intramedullary fixation nail.
The most important reason for the development of the dynamic handsplint is its simplicity. The main problem remaining is to find a
suitable heating and cooling system. If such a system, together with
the SME-strips, can be fixed in a compact way to the glove, this
dynamic handsplint offers important practical, aesthetical and psycho-

logical advantages for the patient when compared with existing, often ugly looking devices.

<u>REFERENCES</u>

Andreasen, G.F. & Morrow, R.E. (1978) Laboratory and clinical analyses of Nitinol wire. Am. J. Orthond., 73, 142-151.

Baumgart, F., Bensmann, G. & Hartwig, J. (1977) Mechanische Probleme bei der Nutzung des Memory Effektes für Osteosyntheseplatten. Techn. Mitt. Krupp; Forsch.-Ber., 35, 157-172.

Baumgart, F., Bensmann, G., Haasters, J., Nölker, A. & Schlegel, K.F. (1978) Zur Dwyerschen Skoliosenoperation mittels Drähten aus Memory-Legierungen; Eine Experimentelle Studie. Arch. Orth. Traum. Surg., 91, 67-75.

Bensmann, G., Baumgart, F., Hartwig, J. & Haasters, J. (1979) Untersuchungen der Memory-Legierung Nickel-Titan und Überlegungen zu ihrer Anwendung im Bereich der Medizin. Techn. Mitt. Krupp; Forsch.-Ber.,37, 21-33.

Castleman, L.S., Motzkin, S.M., Alicandri, F.P., Bonawit, V.L. & Johnson, A.A. (1976) Biocompatibility of Nitinol alloy as an implant material. J. Biomed. Mater. Res., 10, 695-731.

Civjan, S., Huget, E.F. & DeSimon, L.B. (1975) Potential applications of certain nickel-titanium (Nitinol) alloys. J. Dent. Res., 54, 89-96.

Cutright, D.E., Bhaskar, S.N., Perez, B., Johnson, R.M. & Cowan, G.S.M. (1973) Tissue reaction to Nitinol wire alloy. Oral Surg., 35, 578-584.

Greninger, A.B. & Mooradian, V.G. (1938) Strain transformation in metastable beta copper-zinc and beta copper-tin alloys. Trans. AIME, 128, 337-355.

Hughes, J.L. (1977) Evaluation of Nitinol for use as a material in the construction of orthopaedic implants. Final Report DAMD 17-74-C-4041, US Army Medical Research and Development Command, Frederick, Md.

Johnson, A.A. & Alicandri, F.P. (1974) Thermoconstrictive surgical appliance; U.S. Patent 3,786,806.

Klopper, P.J. (1979) Intramedullary fixation with polymers, in Proc. 3rd Int. Conf. Plastics in Medicine and Surgery, 17.1.

Page, M. & Sawyer, P.N. (1974) Prosthetic pump; U.S. Patent 3,827,426.

Schmerling, M.A., Wilkov, M.A., Sanders, A.E. & Woosley, J.E. (1976) Using the shape recovery of Nitinol in the Harrington rod treatment of scoliosis. J. Biomed. Mater. Res., 10, 879-892.

Simon, M., Kaplow, R., Salzman, E. & Freiman, D. (1977) A vena cava filter using thermal shape memory alloy. Radiology, 125, 89-94.

Wagner, H.J. & Jackson, C.M. (1969) What you can do with that memory alloy. Materials Engineering, 70, 28-31.

Wang, G.J., Dunstan, J.C., Reger, S.I., Schildwachter, T.L., Stamp, W.G. & Hubbard, S. (1980) Treatment of femoral fracture with rigid and flexible rod, in Proc. 26th Ann. Meeting ORS, 5, 172.

PART 4

CHARACTERISATION AND SPECIFIC TISSUE RESPONSES TO POLYMERS

Biomaterials 1980
Edited by G. D. Winter, D. F. Gibbons, and H. Plenk, Jr.
© 1982 John Wiley and Sons Ltd.

THE DEGRADATION OF POLY(2-VINYLPYRIDINE 1-OXIDE)

V. N. Hasırcı

Department of Biological Sciences,
Middle East Technical University,
Ankara, TURKEY

SUMMARY

Poly(2-vinylpyridine 1-oxide), PVNO, a water soluble
polymer used in the chemotherapy of experimental silicosis
in vitro and in vivo, was subjected to conditions simulating long term contact with biological media and signs
of degradation were searched using UV and IR spectroscopy,
viscometry, gel permeation chromatography and a hemolytic
activity test. Deoxygenation of the pyridine ring was
observed to a small extent with no decrease in the capacity of PVNO to prevent the hemolytic activity of quartz.

INTRODUCTION

Poly(2-vinylpyridine 1-oxide), PVNO, was first reported as
a chemotherapeutic agent against silicosis, a disease
caused by the inhalation of quartz dust, in 1960
(Schlipköter and Brockhaus, 1960). An intensive research
was then started to investigate the action of PVNO in cell
culture, in experimental animals and in chemical medium
(Allison, 1970; Holt, 1971). In these short duration experiments, it was generally assumed that PVNO is stable and
non-toxic. Clinical use of PVNO would, however, be of long
duration and the stability of PVNO after a long-term contact with the biological medium has to be investigated.
Degradation of PVNO could take place by any one or any
combination of the following mechanisms:

a.   Degradation by depropagation, which would produce
monomers of PVNO which have been shown to be quite toxic
(Hasırcı and Holt, 1977).

b.   Degradation by random scission of the polymer backbone which would lead to the formation of low molecular
weight fragments like dimers and oligomers of which the
dimers are toxic (Hasırcı and Holt, 1977).

c.   Degradation of the side chain, which would lead to
altered monomeric units whose effect on the biological
medium can not be foreseen.

773

d.   Degradation by crosslinking, which would lead to formation of gels the removal of which by excretion would not
be possible and the therapeutic action would most probably
be impaired.

The determination of the mode of degradation of PVNO is
not only important for its chemotherapeutic use but also
for its possible use as a biomaterial in membranes and in
drug release supports. In this study PVNO was subjected to
conditions simulating long term contact with biological
media and signs of degradation were detected using UV and
IR spectroscopy, viscometry, gel permeation chromatography
and hemolytical activity test.

MATERIALS AND METHODS

Degradation.   The degradation procedure is a modification
of a method developed to simulate the effects of long term
implantation of polymers and employs a pseudo-extra--
cellular fluid, PECF, as a substitute for the biological
medium, (Homsy, 1970). A 10% PVNO solution was prepared by
dissolving a high molecular weight stock PVNO (MW:200,000)
in PECF, a litre of which contained Na^+, 145 mmol; K^+,
5 mmol; Cl^-, 118 mmol; HCO_3^-, 30 mmol; HPO_4^-, 2 mmol, and
2 ml of this solution was transferred into an ampoule. The
ampoule was heat sealed and kept in an oven at 115°C for
64 h. Two other modifications of the procedure involving
degradation at 70°C for 64 h. and at 37°C for 1 month were
also applied.

Gel Permeation Chromatography.   Gel permeation chromatographs of the samples were obtained by using two columns
connected in series (29 cm, Ø1.3 cm and 27 cm, Ø2.5 cm)
packed with Sephadex G-15. The applied pressure was 70 cm,
the void volume was 696 drops and the flow rate was 2
drops per minute. The absorptions of the solutions at
254 nm were measured and the results are shown in Figure 1.

Viscometry.   A dust free PECF was obtained by filtration
through a sintered funnel. The determinations were made
using an Ubbelohde type viscometer at 34.5°C. The flow
time for PECF was 150.53 ± 0.17 seconds.

Infrared and Ultraviolet Spectroscopy.   The PVNO solution
that had undergone degradation was extracted with chloroform (1:3) and dried over calcium chloride. For IR measurements Perkin-Elmer and for UV measurements GCA Mc
Pherson double beam spectrophotometers were used, and the
results are shown in Figures 2 and 3, respectively.

Hemolytic Activity of Quartz.   Quartz (50 mg) was weighed
in 10 ml graduated cylinders, and then, PECF, PVNO and 3%
fresh sheep erythrocyte solutions were added according to
Table 1. The mixtures were shaken in a waterbath at 37°C

for 2 h. and centrifuged (2000 rpm, 10 min.). The hemo-globin concentration in the supernatants were measured spectrophotometrically at 541.5 nm.

TABLE 1.   Contents of tubes in the hemolytical activity test

Sample No	1	2	3	4	5	6	7	8	9
Quartz (50 mg)	X	X		X					
PVNO stock 10.08%, ml		0.5	0.5				0.5		
PVNO-D (115) 10.08%, ml				0.5	0.5	0.5			
Erythrocyte 3%, ml	4	4	4	4	4			4	1
PECF, ml	4	3.5	3.5	3.5	3.5	7.5	7.5	4	
Dist. water, ml									4

Numbers 7 and 8 combined are the blanks for numbers 2 and 3, numbers 6 and 8 combined are the blanks for numbers 4 and 5, number 4 is the blank for number 1, and number 9 is the 100% hemolysis sample.

RESULTS

Gel Permeation Chromatography. Sephadex G-15 is known to exclude molecules with molecular weights higher than about 1000. Figure 1 shows that stock PVNO (MW: 200,000) and PVNO-1000 were completely excluded without entering the beads (elution volume, Ve: 696 drops). PVNO-2, a PVNO dimer analogue, was not excluded at all and yielded Ve: 1300 drops. PVNO-D (115), the polymer that underwent degradation at 115°C, was completely excluded and its chromatograph fitted the chromatograph for stock PVNO completely.

Viscometry. The viscosity data was plotted according to Huggins equation, $\eta_{sp}/c = [\eta] + k'[\eta]^2 c$, (Huggins, 1942). The values of the limiting viscosity number, $[\eta]$, for stock PVNO, PVNO-D (70) and PVNO-D (115) were determined from the intercepts to be 0.1194, 0.1164 and 0.1213, respectively. The slopes on the other hand yielded $k'[\eta]^2$ values of 0.0087, 0.0055 and 0.0036 for the above mention-ed compounds.

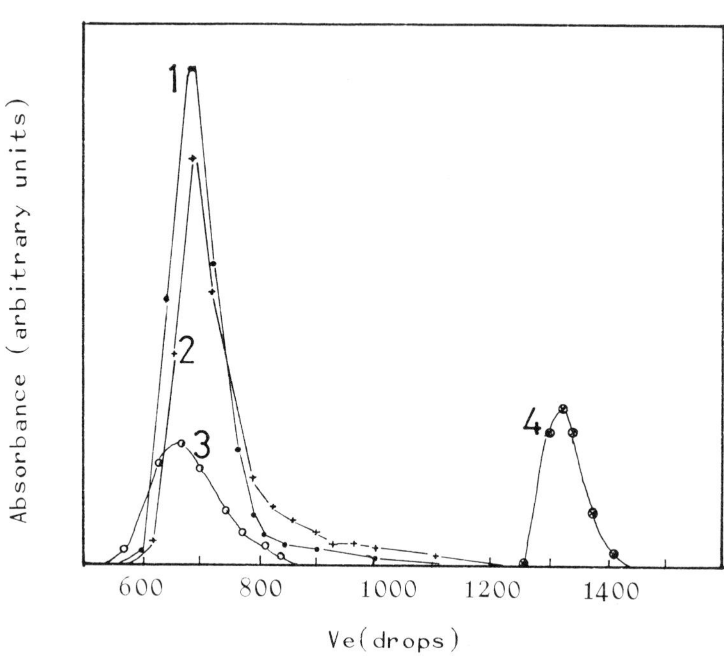

Fig. 1. Gel permeation chromatographs of PVNO-D
(115) (1) stock PVNO (2), PVNO-1000 (3) and
PVNO-2 (4) using columns packed with Sephadex G-15.

<u>IR Spectra</u>. In the IR spectrum of PVNO the peak at around
1220 cm^{-1} indicates the stretching vibration of the N-O
group. The inspection of the IR spectra for stock PVNO,
PVNO-D (115) and PVN (unoxidized form of PVNO) reveals
that the degraded product resembles PVN rather than PVNO
because the peak at 1220 cm^{-1} does not appear in PVNO-D
(115) (Fig. 2).

<u>UV Spectra</u>. Undegraded PVNO and PVN when in chloroform
solution absorb at 273 nm and 263 nm, respectively.
Figure 3 shows that upon degradation at 37°C λ_{max} of PVNO
was unchanged, at 70°C λ_{max} was still unchanged but a
shoulder at a lower wavelength appeared, and at 115°C
λ_{max} shifted to 263 nm.

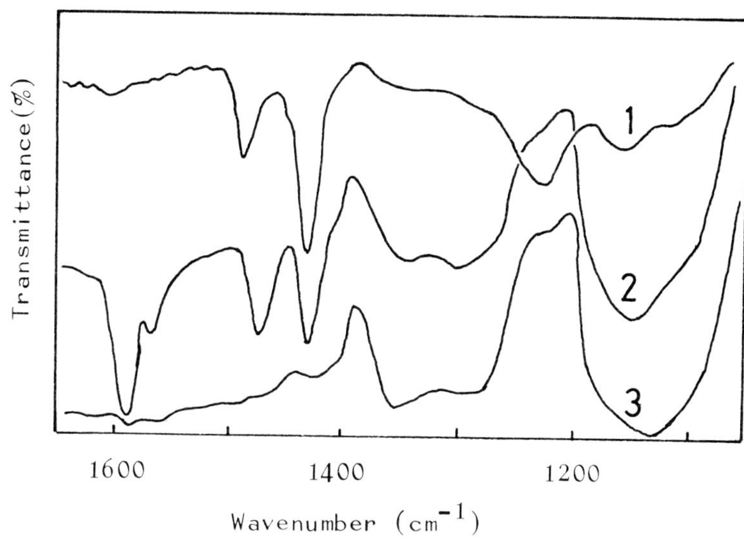

Fig. 2.   Infrared spectra of stock PVNO (1), PVN
(2) and PVNO-D (115) (3) (in chloroform).

<u>Hemolytic Activity Test</u>.   Only the contents of tube
number 1 was found to cause hemolysis to a degree of 5.66%
compared to the 100% hemolysis sample (Tube No: 9) after
taking the absorptions due to the blanks into account. In
the PVNO containing tubes the hemolytic activity of quartz
was completely suppressed even when the polymer was degraded.

DISCUSSIONS AND CONCLUSIONS

The results of gel permeation chromatography indicated
that degradation at 115°C for 64 h. does not cause the
formation of any low molecular fragments because no peaks
with elution volume higher than the void volume (Ve: 696
drops) appeared. Viscometry results implied that upon
degradation a change in the polymer-solvent interaction
has taken place. Since it was observed that $[\eta]$ values
were constant within the limits of experimental error but
$k'[\eta]^2$ were quite different for stock PVNO, PVNO-D (70)
and PVNO-D (115) it can be concluded that the polymer
chemical structure has changed but the chain length has
not been altered. k' is a constant for a specific polymer
in a specific solvent, independent of molecular weight.
The UV and IR spectra indicated that the N-O bond is
broken upon degradation when the degradation temperature
was 70°C or 115°C. All these results suggest that the only
type of degradation that takes place on PVNO is the

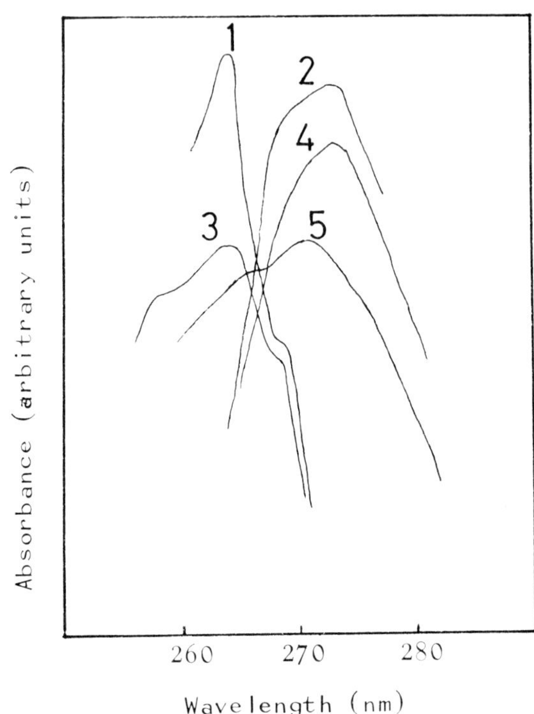

Fig. 3. Ultraviolet spectra of PVN (1), stock PVNO (2), PVNO-D (115) (3), PVNO-D (37) (4) and PVNO-D (70) (5) (in chloroform).

degradation of the side chain leading to deoxygenation of the pyridine ring. It is known that deoxygenation of pyridine N-oxide takes place at high temperatures (Katritzky and Lagowski, 1971) and in this study this was shown to be true when pyridine 1-oxide is the side chain of a polymer molecule. This casts some doubts on the validity of the widely accepted assumption that high temperature simulates long term implantation because PVNO does not undergo degradation at body temperature even after one month storage in PECF.

The hemolytic activity test indicated that deoxygenation does not impair the therapeutic activity of PVNO because it was observed that both the stock and the degraded polymer completely prevented the hemolytic activity of quartz. One can also conclude that the degraded polymer itself does not have hemolytic activity.

Thus, it seems that PVNO is quite bioresistant under normal physiological conditions and its prolonged use as a chemotherapeutic agent or as a biomaterial should not cause any toxic effects because of degradation in the body.

REFERENCES

Allison, A. C. (1970) Effects of silica and asbestos on cells in culture, in Inhaled Particles (Ed., C. N. Davies), p. 347. Pergamon Press, Oxford.
Hasirci, V. N. & Holt, P. F. (1977) Poly(2-vinylpyridine 1-oxide) in silicosis therapy: Effective molecular weight, Int. Arch. Occup. Environ. Hlth., 38, 177-188.
Holt, P. F. (1971) Poly(vinylpyridine oxides) in pneumoconiosis research, Brit. J. Industr. Med., 28, 72-77.
Homsy, C. A. (1970) Biocompatibility in selection of materials for implantation, J. Biomed. Mater. Res., 4, 341-356.
Huggins, M. L. (1942) J. Amer. Chem. Soc., 64, 2716
Katritzky, A. R. & Lagowski, J. M. (1971) Reactions at N-oxide rings, in Chemistry of the heterocyclic N-oxides, p. 229, Academic Press, London, New York.
Schlipköter, H. W. & Brockhaus, A. (1960) The action of Polyvinylpyridine on experimental silicosis, Dtsch. Med. Wschr., 85, 920-933.

Biomaterials 1980
Edited by G. D. Winter, D. F. Gibbons, and H. Plenk, Jr.
© 1982 John Wiley and Sons Ltd.

THE CRYSTALLIZATION PHENOMENON OF THE POLYGLYCOLIC ACID SUTURE

C. C. Chu

Department of Design and Environmental Analysis
Martha Van Rensselaer Hall
Cornell University, Ithaca, NY 14853 USA

SUMMARY

Because of the simple chemical structure and stereoregularity of polyglycolic acid suture (PGA), it usually occurs in the semi-crystalline form. The properties of a semi-crystalline polymer can be controlled by crystallization conditions. Thus, an understanding of the functional dependence of PGA properties on crystallization provides a means to study the biodegradation phenomenon of PGA sutures. In this report, the dependence of crystallinity of PGA on temperature was examined by using differential scanning calorimetric (DSC) technique. The temperature used for isothermal crystallization were 27°C, 167°C, 177°C, 187°C, 197°C, 202°C, 208°C, 210°C and 212°C. The degree of crystallinity was calculated from the heat of fusion data. It was found that the level of crystallinity changed from 33% at Tc = 27°C to 64% at Tc = 212°C. The increase, however, is not linear over the entire temperature range. There were very small changes in the level of crystallinity in PGA crystallized below 167°C. As the temperature increased, however, there was a sharp increase in the level of crystallinity. An extrapolation of the crystallinity-temperature curve toward even higher Tc suggests that still higher levels of crystallinity could be achieved even though it is practically impossible. Since a wide range of crystallinity of PGA can be achieved, this polymer provides an ideal model for the study of the biodegradation phenomenon.

INTRODUCTION

Specific surgical applications necessitate various types of suture materials. The use of absorbable sutures provides certain advantages, such as obviating the removal of sutures after surgery. The recent development of synthetic absorbable sutures has improved the efficacy of absorbable sutures in wound closure. The two synthetic absorbable sutures, i.e. polyglycolic acid (Dexon[R]) from the American Cyanamid Co. and i.e. poly(glycolide-lactide) copolymer (Vicryl[R]) from Ethicon, overcome some of the disadvantages of catgut and reconstituted collagens. These synthetic absorbable sutures show generally better mechanical strength, slower rate of reduction of tensile strength, and minimum tissue response (Frazza & Schmidt, 1971; Katz & Turner, 1970; Pavan et.al., 1979; Salthouse & Matlaga, 1977). The successful

use of these suture materials in wound closure has also generated
considerable interest in other possible applications for these
polymers in medicine.

Because their ability to degrade involves a loss of tensile strength
during degradation, the phenomenon of biodegradation of PGA and its
copolymers has been the subject of extensive research for the past
decade in order to achieve a better understanding of the phenomenon.

The chemical, physical and mechanical properties of polyglycolic acid
(PGA) have been much investigated (Chujo et.al., 1967a, b; Gilding
and Reed, 1979). PGA is the simplest aliphatic polyester. It has a
melting point ranging from 224-227°C, and, because of its simple
chemical structure and stereoregularity, it usually occurs in the
semi-crystalline form. Published information on the crystallization phenomenon is surprisingly sparse. The only available crystallization data in the literature are from X-ray diffraction studies of
the crystal structure in which the dimensions of the orthorhombic
unit cell were measured. These dimensions are: a = 5.22 Å, b = 6.19
Å and c (the fiber axis) = 7.02 Å (Chatani et.al., 1968). Since it
is a semi-crystalline polymer, it should possess one of the most
important characteristics of a semi-crystalline polymer--the dependence of crystalline structure on crystallization conditions (Mandelkern, 1964). It is the objective of this paper to report the dependence of crystallinity on temperature. The choice of crystallinity
as the parameter for this investigation is due to the well-established fact that virtually all properties (thermodynamic, physical, mechanical and optical) of semi-crystalline polymers depend on their
degree of crystallinity (Mandelkern, 1975; Sharpe, 1966). Thus, the
properties of a semi-crystalline polymer can be controlled by crystallization conditions. An understanding of the functional dependence of crystallinity on temperature provides a means to demonstrate
the control of the properties of a semi-crystalline polymer. Such an
understanding is particularly important in the study of the biodegradation phenomenon of PGA sutures because it provides a feasible and
experimentally sound alternative to the methods currently used to
examine this phenomenon.

MATERIALS AND METHODS

Size 1-0 Dexon[R] from the American Cyanamid Co. was used. These sutures are sterilized with ethylene oxide and packed in sealed plastic
bags. They were chopped into segments ranging from 3 to 5 mm long,
and stored dry with P_2O_5 and anhydrous $CaSO_4$ in a desiccator before
use. Ten milligrams of chopped PGA sutures were accurately measured
with a Cahn microbalance and then packed in an aluminum sample pan;
the pan was then crimped. A Perkin-Elmer differential scanning calo-
rimeter (DSC) model 1B was used, calibrated with the standard Indium
supplied by the manufacturer. The sample was heated to 245°C for 20
minutes and then rapidly undercooled to the desired crystallization
temperature. The sample holder took less than about 30 seconds to
reach the new thermal equilibrium. The time for isothermal crystal-

lization depended on the temperature and ranged from less than one hour to as long as 3 weeks. The temperatures used for isothermal crystallization, T_c, were 27°C (room temperature), 167°C, 177°C, 187°C, 197°C, 202°C, 208°C, 210°C, and 212°C.

The crystallized specimens were reweighed and repacked in new aluminum sample pans for crystallinity determination. They were placed inside the sample holder of the DSC and kept at 167°C for 3 minutes to reach thermal equilibrium. The DSC was programmed to increase the temperature at a scan speed 10°/min. and range 16. A melting curve would be produced during the crystallization-melting transition. After the baseline had been attained, the heat of fusion (ΔH) and the percentage of crystallinity were calculated in the usual manner. A value of 49.34 cal/g for ΔH of 100% crystallized PGA was used to calculate the level of crystallinity (Brandrup and Immergut, 1975).

RESULTS AND DISCUSSIONS

The results of the DSC study of PGA crystallized at different temperatures are summarized in Figure 1. It shows that the level of crystallinity, as it changed from 33% at T_c = 27°C to 64% at T_c = 212°C, depended largely on the crystallization temperature. The degree of crystallinity, however, did not increase linearly over the entire temperature range. There were very small changes in the level of crystallinity in PGA crystallized below 167°C. As the temperature of crystallization increased, however, there was a sharp increase in the level of crystallinity and in the sensitivity of crystallinity to small changes in temperature. For example, as T_c increased from 27°C to 167°C, crystallinity increased by an almost insignificant 4% over a temperature range of 140 degrees. As T_c increased further to 197°C, the level of crystallinity increased from 37% to 47%. For T_c above 197°C, an even more profound increase in crystallinity occurred. In this higher temperature range, a change of temperature of 5°C - say from 207°C to 212°C - resulted in 6% increase in crystallinity.

An extrapolation of the crystallinity - temperature curve toward even higher T_c suggests that still higher levels of crystallinity could be achieved: 100% crystallinity is theoretically possible at T_c of 225°C, which is exactly within the reported range of temperatures at which PGA melts, 224°C - 227°C (Frazza, 1971; Chujo, 1967a). This clearly illustrates the well-established fact that a completely crystalline polymer can only be achieved when its crystallization temperature is also its melting temperature (Mandelkern, 1964). However, the time required to achieve 100% crystallization of PGA would be intolerably long, making 100% crystallized PGA a practical impossibility. This temperature dependence of the level of crystallinity has also been found in linear polyethylene (Mandelkern et.al., 1961).

From the point of view of thermodynamic equilibrium, polymers of high molecular weight and stereoregularity should achieve very high levels of crystallinity. However, this is not what we observe in PGA or in other polymers, because Tc must be well below the polymer's melting temperature (a condition far removed from equilibrium) if the polymer is to crystallize at a practicable rate. This undercooling has been reported to be a function of the molecular weight, type of solvent, concentration, and of the chemical structure of the repeating unit (Chu, 1976; Mandelkern, 1964).

Because of the difficulty of achieving 100% crystallinity in polymers, they are usually produced in a polycrystalline state with a complex crystalline morphology, which is responsible for the wide range of properties observed in semi-crystalline polymers (Mandelkern, 1975). What is of interest is how the observed crystalline morphology affects the biodegradation phenomena of absorbable polymers. Several investigators have suggested that degradation starts in the amorphous region of the crystallites and then gradually attacks the remaining crystalline regions, (Pavan, 1979; Atlas and Mark, 1964; Moiseer et. al., 1979). Since we have demonstrated the possiblity of achieving a wide range of levels of crystallinity in PGA, this polymer provides an ideal model for the study of the biodegradation phenomenon.

ACKNOWLEDGMENT

This work is sponsored by the College of Human Ecology, Cornell University. We would also like to thank the American Cyanamid Co. for their kind supply of the materials.

REFERENCES

Atlas, S.M. and Mark, H.F. (1964). 'Resistance of polymers to degradation' Symposium in Plastics in Surgical Implants, <u>ASTM Publication # 386</u>, p.63, Indianapolis, Indiana, Nov. 5-6.

Brandrup, J., Immergut, E.H. (Editors) (1975). <u>Polymer Handbook</u>, 2nd ed. P.III-33, Wiley, New York.

Chatani, Y., Suehiro, K., Okita, Y., Tadokoro, H., and Chujo, K., (1968). 'Structural Studies of Polyesters. I. Crystal structure of polyglycolide', <u>Die Makromole, Chemie, 113</u>, 215.

Chu, C. (1976). 'The effects of molecular weight and concentration on the crystallization kinetics of polyethylene n-hexadecane system', Ph.D. thesis, Florida State University, Tallahassee, Florida.

Chujo, K., Kobayashi, H., Suzuki, J., and Tokuhara, S. (1967a). 'Physical and Chemical Characteristics of Polyglycolide', <u>Die Makromole. Chemie, 100</u>, 262.

Chujo, K., Kobayashi, H., Suzuki, J., Tokuhara, S., and Tanabe, M. (1967b). 'Ring-opening polymerization of glycolide', <u>Die Makromole. Chemie, 100</u>, 267.

Frazza, E.J., and Schmitt, E.E. (1971). 'A new absorbable suture', <u>J. Biomed. Mater. Res., Symp. #1</u>, p.43.

Gilding, D.K., and Reed, A.M. (1979). 'Biodegradable polymers for use in surgery - polyglycolic/polylactic acid homo- and copolymers: 1 , Polymer, 20, 1459.

Katz, A.R., and Turner, R.J. (1970). 'Evaluation of tensile and absorption properties of polyglycolic acid sutures', Surg. Gynecol. & Obst. 131, 701.

Mandelkern, L. (1975). 'Morphology of Semi-Crystalline Polymers' in Characterization of Materials in Research, Ceramics and Polymers, Chapter 13, Syracuse University Press, New York.

Mandelkern, L. (1964). Crystallization of Polymers, McGraw Hill, New York.

Mandelkern, L., Posner, A.S., Diori, A.F., and Roberts, D.E. (1961). 'Low-angle X-ray diffraction of Crystalline Nonoriented Polyethylene and its Relation to Crystallization Mechanisms', J. Appl. Phys., 32 1509.

Mandelkern, L. (1964). 'Crystallization kinetics of polymer-diluent mixtures; temperature coefficient of the process', Polymer, 5, 637.

Moiseer, Yu., Daurava, T.T., Voronkova, O.S., Gumargalieva, K.A., and Privalora, L.G. (1979). 'The specificity of polymer degradation in the living body', J. Polym. Sci., Polym. Symp. #66, p.269.

Pavan, A., Bosio, M., Longo, T. (1979). 'A comparative study of poly(glycolic acid) and catgut as suture materials. Histomorphology and Mechanical Properties', J. Biomed. Mater. Res., 13, 447.

Salthouse, T.N. and Matlaga, B.F. (1977). 'Comparative tissue response to six suture materials in rabbit cornea, sclera, and ocular muscle', Am. J. Ophthalm., 84(2), 224.

Sharpe, A. (1966). Introduction to Polymer Crystallization, Edward Arnold, London.

C. C. Chu

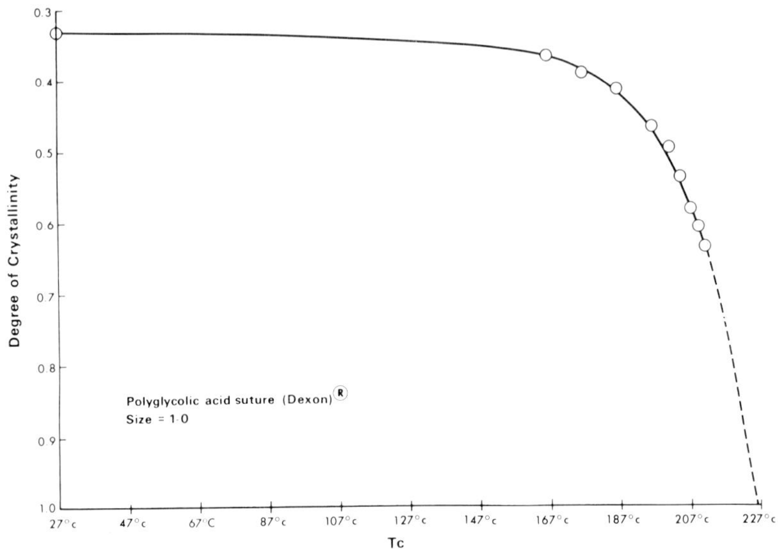

Figure 1. Effect of Crystallization Temperature on the Level of Crystallinity of Polyglycolic Acid Suture.

Biomaterials 1980
Edited by G. D. Winter, D. F. Gibbons, and H. Plenk, Jr.
© 1982 John Wiley and Sons Ltd.

EFFECT OF MOTION ON POLYMER IMPLANT CAPSULE FORMATION IN MUSCLE

T. Kupp[*], P. Hochman[**], J. Hale[*,***], and
J. Black[*,****]

[*]   Dept. of Bioengineering, U. of Pa.,
         Phila., Pa. USA

[**]   Extracorporeal Medical Specialties Inc.,
         King of Prussia, Pa. USA

[***]   Dept. of Radiology, U. of Pa., Hospital of the
         U. of Pa., Phila., Pa. USA

[****]   Dept. of Orthopaedic Surgery, U. of Pa.,
         Phila., Pa. USA

SUMMARY

This study examines the widely held view that implant-tissue
motion increases fibrosis. Two implant materials, polyester and
polyacetal, were placed at minimal and maximal motion sites in
rat muscle, verified by a stereo-radiographic study with metallic
markers. These sites were within the belly of the vastus lateralis,
and between the biceps femoris and fasciae latae respectively.
Twenty-one days after implantation the animals were sacrificed and
mean capsule thicknesses about the implant were measured. The results
indicate that the fibrous capsule thickness depends upon both a
chemical (intrinsic) and a mechanical (extrinsic) effect.

INTRODUCTION

When an implant is placed in tissue, a general or specific response
will occur, resulting either in catabolic degradation or neutralization of the implant, or in its isolation to the smallest volume
possible (Coleman *et al.*, 1974b, Vistnes *et al.*, 1978). For an
implant which is not susceptible to specific degradation or neutralization, the general response is one of inflammation leading to
fibrous encapsulation.

Following the successful response to an inflammatory challenge, a
locally decreased tissue mass results (Black, 1981). Neutrophils,

787

monocytes, and macrophages will have phagocytized the dead cells, and new cells will replace them through mitosis of the cell types present. In conjunction with this, muccopolysaccharides and collagen are synthesized, which together, form the scaffold for cellular reconstruction and remodeling. This "scar" is a thin wall of dense non-adherent collagenous material, the fibers of which allign themselves parallel to the implant surface (Bagnall, 1977).

The size of the scar is believed to be dependent upon three major factors (Coleman *et al.*, 1974a): geometrical, chemical and mechanical.

The most common of these in capsule formation is the chemical nature of the implant. Most implants are not truly inert, thus providing many chemical stimuli for inflammation. These stimuli include the corrosion products of metals, and the residues of polymers. Homsy (1970) quantitated these effects. Twenty-five materials were tested by elution in a pseudo-extracellular fluid (62 hours at 115°C). The low molecular weight degradation products in the elutant were quantitated and their concentration was related to the tissue culture response observed when the elutant was incorporated in the nutrient medium for newborn mouse heart cells. A high degree of correlation between low molecular weight moiety concentration in the medium and adverse tissue response was found.

Matlaga *et al.*, (1976) examined the geometrical factor through the use of triangular, pentagonal, and circular rod shaped implants placed in rat gluteal muscle. Using microspectrophotometric quantitation of acid phosphatase activity as the critical parameter, they were able to show differences in the tissue response between cross sections of the three configurations. The greatest reaction was found with the triangular shaped implants, both in the number of inflammatory cells present and in the amount of enzyme activity.

The third and usually neglected major factor affecting soft tissue reaction to implants is mechanical. It is widely believed that implant-tissue motion increases fibrosis proportionately. Kaminski *et al.*, (1968) compared several different implantation sites, and found muscle to have the greatest reaction. They felt that this was probably the result of the extension and contraction movement "invariably present in muscle". This study was designed therefore, to examine and quantitate this mechanical factor.

MATERIALS AND METHODS

The Sprague Dawley albino rat (250-300g) was chosen for this experiment. This animal is relatively inexpensive, easily handled and is hardy. More importantly, the details of its capsule formation as well as the structure of the final capsule have been studied, and have been shown to be very similar to that in humans (Vistnes *et al.*, 1978).

The implants were fabricated as hemispherically capped cylinders 1.6mm in diameter and 6.0mm in length, to minimize any increased irritation due to sharp edges, and to reduce the geometrically mediated dog-boning or clubbing effect (Wood *et al.*, 1970). A relatively reactive material, polyester (PE - Eastman 6P20, Prime Plastics, Barberton,Ohio) as well as a less reactive material (Harper ed., 1975), polyacetal (PA - polyformaldehyde "Delrin" acetal resin, Caddilac Plastics, King of Prussia,Pa.) were used to permit evaluation of chemical effects.

Twenty implants were placed, one per animal, at the minimal motion site (belly of the vastus lateralis), ten implants of polyacetal and ten of polyester. Twenty were also implanted at the maximal motion site (between the biceps femoris and the fasciae latae) again with ten animals implanted with polyacetal and ten with polyester.

The six remaining animals served as controls: three sham operated at the minimal motion site and three, at the maximal motion site.

The animals were anesthetized with .35cc of Sodium Pentobarbital (I.M.). Once this took effect, the left hind limb was shaven clean and an incision approximately 1-2 cm in length made directly above the site of implantation. With a pair of blunt ended scissors, the muscle fibers were teased apart (Coleman *et al.*, 1974a), to allow for implant insertion. In using blunt dissection, destruction of the muscle fibers was minimized. The pocket in the muscle was then closed with 5-0 (Tevdek) green braided suture and that in the skin, with 3-0 silk black braided suture. Aeroplast (Vibesate), was sprayed over the suture to prevent the animal from tearing the incision apart. The animals were caged and fed a laboratory diet and water ad libidum.

Of each group of 10 animals implanted with the different materials at the different sites, 3 were chosen randomly at 10 days and sacrificed. This was done as a general check on the progress of the soft tissue reaction, and to look for any signs of acute inflammation and/or infection. The remaining 7 animals from each group were sacrificed at 21 days (a time of relative maturity of the fibrous capsule) along with the controls.

At sacrifice, the muscles containing the implants were completely excised and fixed in formalin (10% buffered). Following a 5-7 day fixation period in the formalin, the implant was removed from the tissue. The capsule now had the characteristic stiffness of a formaldehyde-treated material, being changed very little upon the removal of the implant. Tissue blocks were carefully processed and mounted in paraffin, sectioned at 5μ perpendicular to the implant axis, and then stained with Van Giesson's stain (picric acid) for collagen, the main constituent of the fibrous capsule. The collagen appeared a brilliant red, thus allowing measurement of the capsule

thickness by light microscopy. The thicknesses were evaluated for
3 different cross sections, at 4 distinct locations on each section
(0°, 90°, 180° and 270°), and a mean value obtained. (It should be
pointed out that embedding the tissue in paraffin will cause some
shrinkage and subsequent gross artefacts. Therefore the absolute
capsule thicknesses will be changed. But the presumed uniformity
of the shrinkage will not alter the relative values.) The experiment
was later repeated in its entirety in order to verify its reproduce-
ability.

RESULTS

The mean capsule thicknesses, with the standard error of the mean,
are given in Tables 1 and 2, for both runs of the experiment. Table
3 presents the relative motion of the implant with that of the surrounding muscle tissue at the two surgical sites chosen, determined
by a modified stereo-radiographic technique of Stovall and Shalek
(1962). The degree of motion between the biceps femoris and the fasciae latae was significantly greater than that found at the minimal
motion site.

TABLE 1.   Results (A)

Material		Location	Capsule Thickness(Mean)$T_i (\overline{X} \pm$ SEM)	
1:	Polyester	Minimal Motion	24.3 ± 2.9 µm	n=5
2:	Polyester	Maximal Motion	31.4 ± 2.7 µm	n=3
3:	Polyacetal	Minimal Motion	14.4 ± 2.8 µm	n=2
4:	Polyacetal	Maximal Motion	25.1 ± 3.5 µm	n=3

TABLE 2.   Results (B)

Material		Location	Capsule Thickness(Mean)$T_i (\overline{X} \pm$ SEM	
1:	Polyester	Minimal Motion	16.5 ± 0.8 µm	n=5
2:	Polyester	Maximal Motion	24.1 ± 0.5 µm	n=3
3:	Polyacetal	Minimal Motion	12.4 ± 2.3 µm	n=4
4:	Polyacetal	Maximal Motion	21.6 ± 1.0 µm	n=3

TABLE 3.   Range of motion

Range* at minimal motion site	Range* at maximal motion site
0.00 ± 0.07 cm	0.18 ± 0.07 cm

*Motion between implant and tissue for full extension and full
flexion of the hip.

Figure 1 shows the typical appearance of 10 day implants. The
fibrous capsule, still in the process of maturation, lacks clarity,
making quantitative thickness measurements almost impossible. There
is evidence of the continued invasion of leukocytes into the area,
the nuclei of which are darkly stained. Cellular debris, muscle
bundles and the implant sites are all clearly visible.

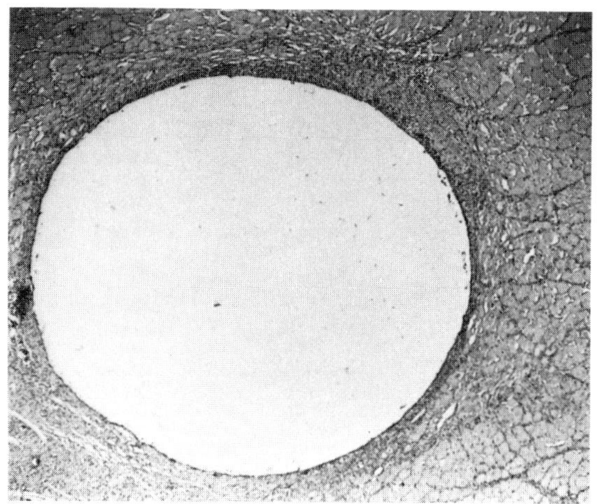

Fig. 1. Polyacetal (PA), Minimal Motion Site, 10 days.

Figures 2-5 are of typical 21 day implants, at a higher magnification. The well defined and uniform capsule is immediately obvious,
as compared to the 10 day specimens. Again, the implant site and
the muscle bundles are clearly visible. By contrast, Figure 6 shows
the appearance of the sham surgery site at 21 days. The blunt
incision line can be seen but the nearly complete absence of fibrosis
can be appreciated.

                    T. Kupp *et al.*

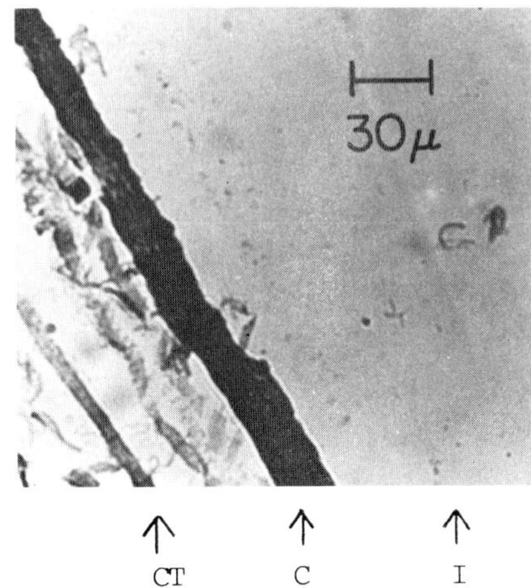

Fig. 2. Polyacetal (PA), Minimal Motion Site, 21 days.

Key for figures 2-5: C=fibrous capsule, CT=connective tissue
I=implant site, M=muscle bundles

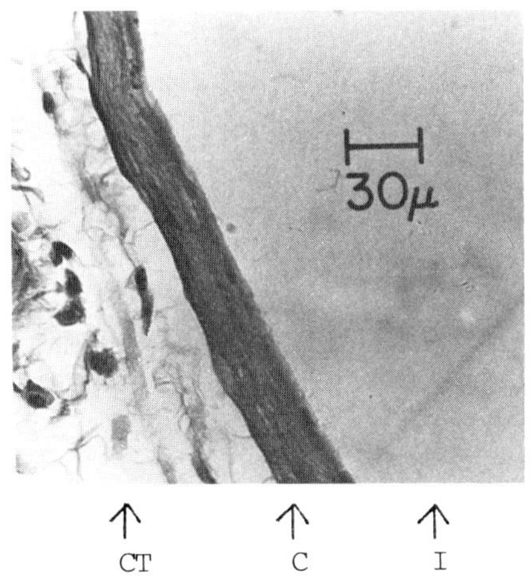

Fig. 3. Polyacetal (PA), Maximal Motion Site, 21 days.

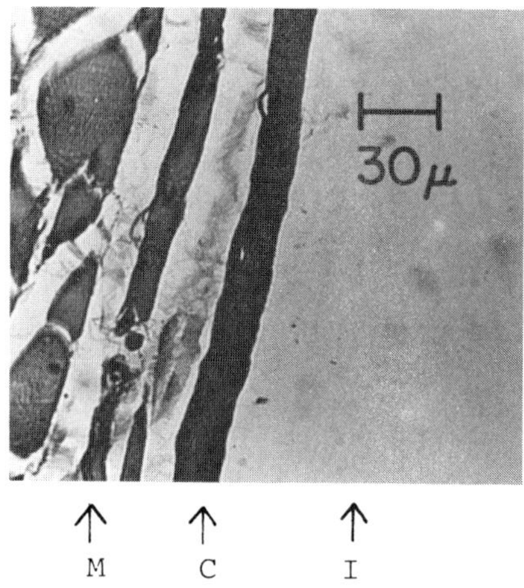

Fig. 4. Polyester (PE), Minimal Motion Site, 21 days.

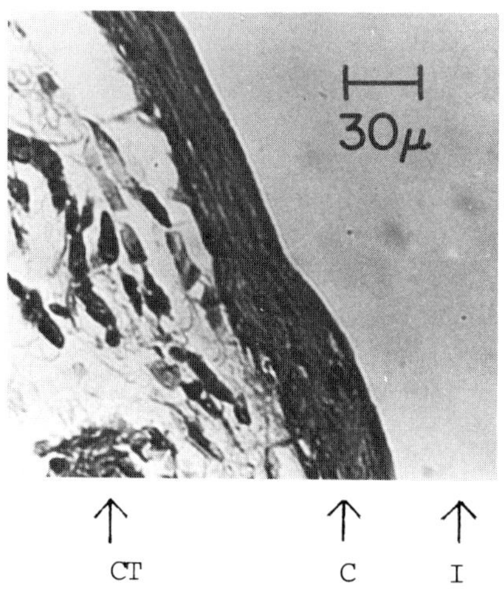

Fig. 5. Polyester (PE), Maximal Motion Site, 21 days.

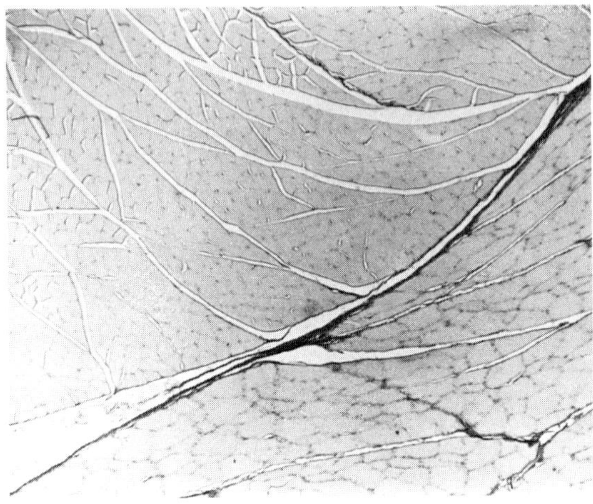

Fig. 6. Polyacetal (PA), Minimal Motion Site - Control
21 days.

DISCUSSION

Quantitatively, are there any significant differences between the
four experimental groups? Does the maximal motion site differ
significantly from the minimal motion site in the thickness of the
resultant fibrous capsule?

To test this hypothesis, a one-way analysis of the variance (ANOVA,
Table 4) was done. Any specimen in which the capsule was extensively
fragmented in histological preparation was discarded to avoid bias
in the measurement. Therefore, the analysis had to compensate for
different numbers of data points in each group.

The first hypothesis (H_1) tested whether or not the tissue response
to the polyester, the more chemically active polymer, was significantly different at the minimal motion site (24.3 $\pm$ 2.9 μm) from that
of the maximal motion site (31.4 $\pm$ 2.7 μm). Statistically, no difference was found (p>0.200). Yet when the minimal and maximal motion
sites were contrasted for the polyacetal implants (H_2), the more
chemically inert polymer of the two, a significant difference was
found (14.4 $\pm$ 2.8 μm vs. 25.1 $\pm$ 3.5 μm, p=0.125). From these con-
trasts it can be concluded that when the intrinsic chemical activity
is minimized by using a polymer such as polyacetal, the significant
effect of motion may be seen. However, when the relatively more

inflammatory material is used, motion differences are masked, due to an additive effect of a seemingly larger intrinsic chemical activity than the extrinsic mechanical activity.

Hypotheses H_3 and H_4 support these conclusions. When the motion was minimized, the different intrinsic chemical activities of the implants produced significantly different capsule thicknesses (24.3 ± 2.9 μm vs. 14.4 ± 2.8 μm, p=0.125). When motion was not controlled for, intrinsic chemical differences were not seen (H_4), again due to the addition effect (31.4 ± 2.7 μm vs. 25.1 ± 3.5 μm, p>0.500).

TABLE 4. Analysis (A)

Hypothesis	F	Significance
$H_1: \overline{T}_1 \neq \overline{T}_2$	2.05	ns, p>0.200
$H_2: \overline{T}_3 \neq \overline{T}_4$	3.07	s, p=0.125
$H_3: \overline{T}_1 \neq \overline{T}_3$	3.01	s, p=0.125
$H_4: \overline{T}_2 \neq \overline{T}_4$	0.60	ns, p>0.500

TABLE 5. Analysis (B)

Hypothesis	F	Significance
$H_1: \overline{T}_1 \neq \overline{T}_2$	11.10	s, p<0.010
$H_2: \overline{T}_3 \neq \overline{T}_4$	13.70	s, p<0.005
$H_3: \overline{T}_1 \neq \overline{T}_3$	3.07	s, p=0.125
$H_4: \overline{T}_2 \neq \overline{T}_4$	3.01	s, p=0.125

The controls, for both the maximal and minimal motion sites, showed no chronic infection and/or inflammatory response. No leukocytes were seen, nor any significant scar tissue, and the muscle bundles were intact.

The experiment was later repeated in its entirety producing some interesting differences in results (Tables 2 & 5). The mean capsule thicknesses all decreased as did the standard error of the mean for each group. This may be accounted for (Vistnes *et al.*, 1978) by a better surgical technique. What did not change though, was the rank of the mean capsule thickness of each group relative to the others.

The most important conclusion to be drawn from this experiment is that capsule thickness at 21 days appears to reflect the additive

response to two factors, an intrinsic chemical activity and an extrinsic mechanical activity. When the extrinsic factor is minimized, the
intrinsic difference between implant materials can be clearly seen.
On the other hand, when the intrinsic activity is held to a minimum,
the extrinsic mechanical effect can be clearly seen. But when either
factor is elevated, differences in the other factor may be masked,
especially in the presence of an unrefined surgical technique as seen
in the first experiment presented here (Tables 1 & 4).

The measurement of capsule thickness is only an indirect measure of
cellular response. Thus these studies should be extended to the
evaluation of the concentration and distribution of cellular enzymes
directly. But the implications of this experiment are that one
cannot ignore mechanical activities when looking at the soft tissue
response to an implant. Failure to control tissue-implant motion in
animal studies, may mask otherwise significantly different tissue
responses. It is therefore probable that variability in mechanical
as well as other extrinsic factors has adversely affected implant
evaluations of materials, and that past failures to consider them
may have resulted in erroneous quantitative conclusions on tissue
responses to various materials.

ACKNOWLEDGEMENTS

The authors gratefully acknowledge Gretchen Avery for her help with
the surgical technique, as well as Ann Eccleston and Carol Hayes
for their histological preparations.

REFERENCES

Bagnall, R.D. (1977) An approach to the soft tissue/synthetic
material interface. J. Biomed. Mater. Res., 11, 939-946.
Black, J. (1981) Materials in the Biological Environment, Marcel
Dekker, Inc., NY (in press).
Coleman, D.L., King, R.N., & Andrade, J.D. (1974a) The foreign
body reaction - an experimental protocol. J. Biomed. Mater. Res.
(Symp.), 5(1), 65-76.
Coleman, D.L., King, R.N., & Andrade, J.D. (1974b) The foreign
body reaction:a chronic inflammatory response. J. Biomed. Mater.
Res., 8, 199-211.
Handbook of Plastics and Elastomers (Ed., Harper), pp3-35 - 3-42,
4-8 - 4-42.McGraw-Hill, NY.
Homsy, C.A. (1970) Bio-compatibility in selection of materials
for implantation. J. Biomed. Mater. Res., 4, 341-356.
Kaminski, E.J., Oglesby, R.J., Wood, N.K., & Sandrik, J. (1968)
The behavior of biological materials at different sites of
implantation. J. Biomed. Mater. Res., 2, 81-88.
Matlaga, B.F., Yasenchak, L.P. & Salthouse, T.N. (1976) Tissue
response to implanted polymers:the significance of sample shape.
J. Biomed. Mater. Res., 10, 391-397.

Stoval, M. & Shalek, R. (1962) A study of the explicit distribution of radiation in interstitial implantations. Radiology, 78, 950-954.
Vistnes, L.M., Ksander, G.A., & Kosek, J. (1978) Study of encapsulation of silicone rubber implants in animals-a foreign-body reaction. Plast & Recon. Surg., 62(4), 580-588.
Wood, N.K., Kaminski, E.J., & Oglesby, R.J. (1970) The significance of implant shape in experimental testing of biological materials: disc vs. rod. J. Biomed. Mater. Res., 4, 1-12.

Biomaterials 1980
Edited by G. D. Winter, D. F. Gibbons, and H. Plenk, Jr.
© 1982 John Wiley and Sons Ltd.

ON THE ANTIGENICITY OF SYNTHETIC BIOMEDICAL POLYMERS

P.Y. Wang

Laboratory of Chemical Biology
Institute of Biomedical Engineering
Faculty of Medicine, University of Toronto
Canada M5S 1A8

SUMMARY

Previous studies of antigenicity on the molecular basis have shown that many proteins, synthetic homo- or heteropoly- peptides, nucleic acids, homo- or heteropolysaccharides can induce antibody production in many animal species. The essential requirement is a reasonably high molecular weight, while the nature and sequence of composing units are not always important. Accordingly, the possibility of immunological response to many synthetic polymers currently used as biomaterials cannot be completely excluded. My study showed that in 3 to 7 days, antibodies against sodium polystyrene sulfonate (PSS) and polyacrylic acid (PAA) were produced in C57BL mice, and against polyacrylamide (PAM) in SJL mice. The presence of humoral antibodies was detected by the hemagglutination method using polymer-sensitized sheep red blood cells. Maximum titres observed after 7 days to 6 weeks were -- PSS: 1/128, PAA: 1/32, and PAM: 1/16. None of these polymers was found to induce antibody production in A, BALB/c, and CBA mouse strains. The strain dependence indicates that immunological response to synthetic polymers is likely under genetic control. Failures in the past to induce antibody production readily in animals are attributed to the high tolerogenicity of these hydrocarbon polymers, which degrade very slowly <u>in vivo</u>.

INTRODUCTION

Recent advances in biomedical science have provided improved drugs, anesthetic and surgical techniques, and post-operative care. Consequently higher success rates are reported for organ transplants, correction of inborn defects and the repair of body parts damaged by injury or disease. However, the supply of homo- or xenografts is not unlimited. Often there are variations in quality and in host-donor tissue compatibility. The alternative is to meet the demands by using artificial parts made from synthetic polymers. In addition to availability and quality control of an artificial implant to meet set standards, the synthetic polymeric materials

themselves seem to be free from interaction with the natural
defense mechanism in the host body. There are occasional
references made to biocompatibility or foreign body reactions,
but they are usually not fully defined in the literature on
biomaterial studies.

Singer and his colleagues (Campbell 1957) appear to be among
the first to use synthetic vinyl polymers to evaluate the
molecular basis of immunological response to an antigen. Due
to the high immunizing doses used, the initial experiments
failed to produce detectable antibodies in rabbit. With the
phenomenon of immunological paralysis becoming more understood,
Gill and co-workers (Gill 1968) later used microgram doses, and
succeeded in demonstrating that several synthetic
non-biological polymers were indeed antigenic in rabbit.

The Immunological System. The understanding of this complex
and highly sophisticated system in the body is still far from
complete, although significant advances are being made.
Briefly, the mammalian immunological system is based
principally on the bone marrow derived B-lymphocytes and the
thymus derived T-lymphocytes. One class of antigens, such as
the high molecular weight dextran ($> 100,000$ daltons) can
interact with B-lymphocytes and stimulate them to produce
specific antibodies. These are called the T-independent
antigens, and their antigenicity is not usually subject to
species variations. Another example is polyvinylpyrrolidone
found in some proprietary ophthalmic medications. The second
group of macromolecules can induce the B-lymphocytes to produce
humoral antibodies only with the cooperation of the T-
lymphocytes (the helper cells). The synthetic
poly-L-aminoacids, which have been considered as candidates for
artificial skin (Schwope 1974), are typical T-dependent
antigens. In addition, there are occasions when a subgroup of
T-lymphocytes (the supressor cells) can block the production of
antibodies against T-dependent antigens. The response to
T-dependent antigens is under genetic control and variations
due to species are observed.

There are 5 main classes of antibodies - IgM, IgG, IgA, IgD,
and IgE. The initial response produces the high molecular
weight ($\sim$900,000 daltons) IgM, and they are readily detectable
in the serum 3 to 7 days after immunization. Thereafter, the
IgM's are replaced by IgG ($\sim$150,000 daltons), if the response
has been induced by a T-dependent antigen. The concentrations
of IgD, and IgE in an immune serum are much lower by
comparison. However, in cell mediated responses, such as organ
transplant, skin grafts, etc., the antibodies are cell bound
and not detectable in the serum. Further details of this
fascinating subject can be found in many texts (Kabat 1976;
Bach 1978).

<u>Features of Macromolecular Antigens</u>. The most frequently used antigens in immunological studies are natural (or haptenated) proteins and bacterial capsular polysaccharides. These are heteropolymers, but the production of humoral antibodies can also be induced by homopolyers such as the high molecular weight dextran, and the synthetic poly-L-lysine (antigenic in rabbit and guinea pig; not in mouse). Thus a complex molecular structure is not mandatory. The usual requirement seems to be a reasonably high molecular weight as demonstrated by the observation that dextran with a molecular weight less than 100,000 daltons is non-antigenic in man and can be used clinically as a plasma expander. However, tri-L-tyrosylarsanilate with a molecular weight of only 500 daltons can induce the production of antibodies in guinea pigs. Therefore, the antigenicity of a given substance is very difficult to predict, especially when there are interferences from suppressor cells and immunoparalysis. It is hoped that in future publications on biomaterials research, the term "non-antigenic" is referred to or quoted with caution.

<u>Some Antigenic Biomedical Polymers</u>. Many water-soluble polymers have been used clinically or used after insolubi- lization by further crosslinking (TABLE 1). Polymer bio- degradation is known to occur <u>in vivo</u> (Leininger 1965) and may result in dissolution of the parent biomedical polymer. In this report, I describe the testing of several polymers in 5 commonly available inbred mouse strains for antigenicity using standard immunochemical methods.

<u>MATERIALS AND METHODS</u>

Inbred mice of strains A, BALB/c, CBA, C57BL/6, and SJL were obtained from The Jackson Laboratory, Bar Harbor, MA, U.S.A. Sheep red blood cells (SRBC) in Alsevers solution and the normal rabbit serum used for dilution were supplied by Woodlyn Laboratories Limited, Guelph, Ontario, Canada. The biomedical polymers tested were polyvinylpyrrolidone (abbreviated henceforth as PVP; Mol. Wt. 360,000), sodium polystyrene sulfonate (PSS; Mol. Wt. 350,000), polyacrylic acid (PAA; Mol. Wt. 250,000), and polyacrylamide (PAM; Mol. Wt. 100,000). They were purchased from Polysciences, Inc., Warrington, PA, as highly purified materials with relatively narrow molecular weight distribution range and were sold as standards for the calibration of gel filtration chromatography columns. For immunization, a polymer was emulsified in Freund's complete adjuvant. After 3 to 6 days, and at weekly intervals thereafter, the immunized animal was bled by the orbital venous plexus using a blood collecting capillary. After rapid centrifugation to eliminate clots and cellular debris, the immune serum was decomplemented at 56°C for 30 min, and was further absorbed with SRBC to eliminate possible heterophile antibodies. In the case when the quantity of immune serum was low, this absorption step was replaced by a control assay using

normal serum from the same mouse strain collected before
immunization during the determination for specific antibodies.
For the detection of humoral antibodies, a 2% suspension of
SRBC was washed 3 times in phosphate buffered saline (PBS),
treated with an equal volume of 0.005% tannic acid solution in
PBS, and thoroughly washed. The tanned SRBC was sensitized by
mixing with a PBS solution containing 0.1 mg of a particular
antigen per ml, washed and adjusted to 2% SRBC (v/v). An
aliquot (0.025 ml) of the sensitized SRBC suspension was added
to each of the 12 wells in a horizontal row of the plastic
microtitre tray (Linbro Titertek, Flow Labs., Inc., Hamden,
CN.) containing a specific antiserum at progressive 1/2 fold
dilutions with 2% decomplemented normal rabbit serum. The
reciprocal of the highest dilution of antiserum still with some
antibodies which agglutinated the sensitized SRBC was taken as
the maximum titre for that assay.

RESULTS

As expected, the T-independent PVP was antigenic in all mouse
strains tested. The BALB/c strain was a high responder to this
polymer antigen (hemagglutination titre: 1/128), C57BL/6 and A
strains were intermediate (titre: 1/32), while CBA and SJL
strains were low responders (titre: 1/8). However, the other
three polymers produced antibodies in strains with certain
genetic background (TABLE 1). The antibody response was
observed to vary according to different immunizing dosages as
shown for PSS in TABLE 2. Another characteristic of the
polymer antigens tested was the lengthy period required to reach

TABLE 1   Antigenicity of some biomedical polymers

Mouse Strain	Antigen[1]	Max. Titre	Medical Uses
C57BL/6	PVP	32	Surgical antiseptic, Plasma expander
C57BL/6	PSS	128	Hyperpotassemia Treatment
C57BL/6	PAA	32	Bone & dental cements
SJL	PAM	16	Surgical sponge Wound dressing

[1]PVP = polyvinylpyrrolidone; PSS = polystyrene sulfonate
sodium salt; PAA = polyacrylic acid; PAM = polyacrylamide.

TABLE 2   Variation of serum antibody level in C57BL/6 mice with sodium polystyrene sulfonate doses

Dose (μg)	Max. Titre
0.05	16
0.1	128
0.2	32
0.5	4
1.0	2
5.0	2
10.0	0

The PSS in Freund's complete adjuvant was injected intraperitoneally and the antibody titres were measured by the hemagglutination method after 7 days to 6 weeks.

the maximum of primary response. After the first immunization, the humoral antibodies persisted for over 2 months. However, the secondary response (i.e. response to a "booster" injection) reached a maximum within 3 to 7 days as usually happens with protein antigens.

DISCUSSION

At present there is very little information available in the literature of biomaterials or immunology regarding the immunological response to biomaterials. However, some histological observations (Chvapil 1979) suggest that certain implant-tissue reactions may have an immunological origin. It is likely that other studies (Merritt and Brown, 1980) may yield important information and lead to a better understanding of this problem.

Immunological responses to artificial implants which degrade _in vivo_ to give water-soluble polymers, such as in controlled release drug delivery systems (Hellyer 1980), are much easier to evaluate by established immunochemical methods as already described. The results shown in TABLE 1 and 2 demonstrate that the response to polymers can vary greatly. Genetically controlled variations in human immunological response are more complex and not as well understood as in mice. Therefore, some implant materials previously referred to as non-antigenic may need to be re-evaluated.

The observations in this study further indicate that the assessment of biocompatibility of polymers _in vitro_ using cell culture techniques probably excludes a very important parameter, since the cell lines used in such tests do not possess immunological functions and thus, are not representative of the environment _in vivo_. With increasing uses of synthetic polymers in medicine and surgery, the immunological interaction of biomaterials should receive more emphasis in future research.

ACKNOWLEDGEMENT

I thank the Medical Research Council of Canada for a grant (MA-5666).

REFERENCES

Bach, J.F. (1978) Immunology, Wiley, Toronto.

Campbell, D.H. (1957) Some speculations on the significance of formation and persistence of antigen fragments in tissues of immunized animals. Blood, 12, 589-592

Chvapil, M., Chvapil, T.A., Owen, J.A., Kanton, M., Ulreich, J.B., and Eskelson, C. (1979) Reaction of vaginal tissue of rabbits to inserted sponges made of various materials. J. Biomed. Mater. Res., 13, 1-14.

Gill III, T.J., and Kunz, H.W. (1968) The immunogenicity of vinyl polymers. Proc. Nat. Acad. Sci., U.S.A., 61, 490-496.

Hellyer, J. (1980) Controlled release of biologically active compounds from bioerodible polymers. Biomaterials, 1, 51-57.

Kabat, E.A. (1976) Structural Concepts in Immunology and Immunochemistry, Holt, Rinehart and Winston, Toronto.

Leininger, R.I. (1965) Changes in properties of plastics during implantation, in Plastics in Surgical Implants, pp. 71-76. ASTM Special Technical Publication number 386, American Society for Testing and Materials, Philadelphia.

Merritt, K., and Brown, S.A. (1980). Sensitivity to metallic implants in experimental animals, Paper read at the First World Biomaterials Congress, Baden, April.

Biomaterials 1980
Edited by G. D. Winter, D. F. Gibbons, and H. Plenk, Jr.

USE OF A HUMAN EXCISED DONOR TISSUE CULTURE SYSTEM TO
EVALUATE THE SAFETY OF POLYDIMETHYLSILOXANE FOR OROFACIAL
PROSTHESIS

J. F. Lontz, M. D. Nadijcka, I. Mildan and N. E. Donacki

Maxillofacial Prosthetics Center, Veterans Administration
Center, Wilmington, Delaware, USA, 19805

SUMMARY

A comprehensive human excised donor (H E D) tissue culturing system
has been devised for regulatory qualification of polydimethyl siloxane elastomers developed specifically for orofacial prostheses. It
involves the assessment of toxicity and latent or potential tumorigenicity morphological, biochemical and biophysical parameters. The
H E D test system is intended as a supplement to conventional animal
toxicity and carcinogenicity screening, providing human relevance
devoid of a dependence on, or involvement of, animal models or their
seral components. Polydimethyl siloxane elastomers developed specially for fabricating soft, flexible orofacial prosthetic devices
have shown no inhibitive activity with a broad range of human tissues; whereas, several proprietary elastomer products have inhibited
growth of cultured tissue. Biochemical assessment was based on
selected enzymes. The amounts of acid and alkaline phosphatases and
lactic acid dehydrogenase were unaffected by the presence of test
material in the culture medium. Preliminary assessment based on conventional karyotype grouping showed no abnormal aberrations in cells
grown in contact with PDM siloxane.

INTRODUCTION

Orofacial prosthesis serve an important role in the treatment of dis-
figurements caused by accidents and surgery. Polydimethylsiloxane
formulations are attracting considerable attention for such implants
because they appear to be nontoxic (Lontz and Schweiger, 1977; Lontz
and Schweiger, 1978), when assessed by the human excised donor
(H E D) tissue culture technique which is appropriate for this type
of medical device (Horton, 1976). The objective of this study has
been to augment the short-term H E D morphological assessment with
biochemical and biophysical data as depicted in Fig. 1.

The overall assessment comprises three interdependent protocols,
namely: (a) morphological, for immediate short term assessment of
toxicity, (b) biochemical monitoring for enzyme and metabolite aberrations, and (c) biophysical, for long term monitoring of cell structures and chromosomes. The comprehensive H E D tissue culturing
technique is intended to supplement, or substitute for conventional

animal toxicity (Autian, 1973) and carcinogenicity screening (Ames, 1974; Ames, et al 1975).

MATERIALS AND METHODS

Polydimethyl (PDM) Siloxane Prosthesis Test Materials. Test sections of PDM siloxane were taken from flash-out sections of patient prostheses made in dental stone moldings cured by polymerization at $100 \pm 5^{\circ}C$. for 2 hours (Lontz and Schweiger, 1979). The flash-out was irregularly shaped and varied in thicknesses from approximately one-tenth to one millimeter. Cut out sections were disinfected with 5 percent sodium hypochloride (U.S.P.) by immersion for a minimum of 4 hours, followed by a generous rinse with sterile distilled water. For the H E D tissue culture testing, the irregular flash-out strips were cut into square, rectangular or triangular pieces with at least one centimeter in length and less than 1 mm in thickness. When pieces were 0.2 mm or less in thickness, fibroblasts rose and grew over the thin test pieces.

The PDM siloxane, being more dense (1.02-1.12) than the culture medium, lies on the bottom of culture vessels and adheres to the glass or plastic (polystyrene) surfaces. This obviates the need to use an agar culture method (Guess et al, 1956) which mitigates against normal aqueous diffusion and limits the test to 72 hours, beyond which the agar can itself inhibit growth.

Competitive Prosthetic Materials. Two types have been in general use for maxillofacial prosthesis, namely; (a) polyvinyl chloride (PVC) plastisol, Type III (Sweeny, 1972), coded T-121-23, (b) polyurethanes (Robeson, et al 1976; Gonzalez, 1978), coded L-124-91-A. Fabricated prosthetic forms made for patient wear have been sectioned into test pieces similar to that described above. The test pieces were sterilized in SEPHIRAN 1:500 dilution followed by sterile saline rinse prior to testing in tissue culturing.

Culture Media. In the initial phase of the H E D tissue culture testing we used the conventional minimum essential medium (MEM) with 5 to 20 percent fetal calf serum. We now use pooled human serum (PHS), supplemented with 1 percent glutamine and a mixture of 100 units of penicillin and 100 μg streptomycin. Further modifications are being made for optimal initiation and maintenance media of which there are innumerable variations (Paul, 1975) for specific cell types. These ongoing media modifications for uniform cell development, are applicable to low cell densities, 100 to 1000 cells/ml. The low cell population is purposely chosen to obviate the use of humidified carbon dioxide which is adequately supplied indigenously with the media-derivable carbon dioxide through metabolism. The cell growth is monitored every three to four days.

After the first passage, the cells are harvested and cultured on a series of cover slips in Leighton tubes, either with or without (control) a test sample. After a period of at least 7 days with periodic replenishment with fresh media every 3 to 4 days, the

microscope slides are withdrawn, fixed and appropriately stained for
morphological assessment. Photomicrographs at 100 and 200 magnifications are made for permanent recording with logged information on
tissue source, passage, media type, incubation periods, etc., along
with identification codes for prosthesis and source, as required by
the Federal Drug Administration (1978a, b).

For biochemical monitoring, samples of the initially prepared culture media as well as removed spent medium are frozen and saved for
enzyme and metabolite studies. Biophysical monitoring is to include
higher resolution of cell structures by transmission and scanning
electron microscopy and chromosomal characterizations.

Human Excised Donor Tissues - Source and Culturing. The principal
sources of human excised donor tissues are depicted in Figure 2.
From the surgical or biopsy sources, tissue samples, usually 1 to 2
millimeter, are placed in sterile saline and minced in MEM solution
with a sterile scalpel. Primary cultures are grown in 25 to 75 cm^2
culture flasks containing media augmented with the antibiotics and
selected serum these are grown to about two-thirds, fibroblast con-
fluency, which requires from one to four weeks depending upon cell
type and viability. The fibroblasts are harvested by trypsinization
and distributed into a series of replicate first passage culturing
flasks for both controls and test cultures. They are then cultured
for 7 to 28 days. The cells grown on cover slips are used for
direct visual examination and photomicrographic assessment of cell
structure and chromosomal characterization.

Photomicrographic Assessment. The stained tissue cells grown on
microscope slides in the presence of the prosthesis test sample are
viewed at 100x are taken such that one half of the field shows the
cover slip and the other half includes the test samples, so as to
demonstrate the nature of the growth of the cells in the immediate
area of the test samples.

Chromosomes are prepared by conventional methods, using colchicine
(Paul, 1975), photomicrographs are made at 600x magnification and
subsequently enlarged to 2500x and 5500x magnification for the preparation of idiograms.

RESULTS AND DISCUSSION

Toxicological Assessment. A typical series of H E D tissues grown
in the presence of several competitive maxillofacial prosthesis
materials are depicted in Figures 3, 4, and 5. The photomicrographs are displayed in such a manner as to show the test material
on the left and the control region on the right of the cultures
grown on cover slips placed on the bottom of the Leighton tubes.
Figure 3 shows the result of testing against cells derived from the
gingiva and nasal mucosa. The photomicrographs revealed equal
growth on the PDM siloxane test material side (left) and the control
side.

The polyvinyl chloride plastisol test material Figure 4 cultured
with the same gingiva and nasal mucosa tissues, caused a zone of
growth inhibition which suggests that toxic materials diffused from
the plastisol. Commercial formulations contain a number of low
molecular stabilizing additives, notably organotin mercaptides
(Struber, 1968) and these are known or suspect toxic compounds
(Christensen, Ed., 1978).

The polyurethane orofacial prostheses (Figure 5) caused pronounced
cell lysis in both test cultures and there was profuse cellular
debris presumably from initial rapid cell growth and mitotic division which was missed in the immediate visual observation.

The morphological assessment indicates that the PDM siloxane, developed and specified for orofacial prosthetics, should not impose any
deleterious, injurious or toxic effects when in direct contact with
human mucosal tissues. On the other hand, the present forms of
polyvinyl chloride plastisols and polyurethanes that have been
devised for maxillofacial prostheses are not biocompatible.

Biochemical Assessment. An independent assessment of biochemical
viability is considered important for corroboration of toxicity and
for ascertaining latent or potential tumorgenicity that may not necessarily be evident in the seemingly normal, non-inhibited cultured
growth such as was evident in the presence of the PDM siloxane. To
achieve this enzyme studies have been initiated as a means for demonstrating normal physiological values in vitro.

Since serum is an important component of the tissue culture media,
we have chosen to study serum enzymes, that have proved to be of
greatest interest in malignant diseases. These are the alkaline
and acid phosphatases and lactic acid dehydrogenases (Wilkinson,
1976). The acid and alkaline phosphatases also play an important
role in bone culture by determining or indicating the highly variable osteogenic cellular development (Shifrin, 1970). Therefore,
these three enzymes are under study in the H E D tissue culture test
system. We are attempting to (a) ascertain the normal enzyme values,
once cells have been removed from their in vivo physiology to the
isolated H E D system and (b) devise a standard set of media composition that would serve to discriminate the oncogenic from non-
oncogenic cells in order to determine the tumorigenic propensity of
materials in a tissue culture environment.

Table 1 summarizes our results to date on the range of extracellular
enzyme levels with typical Group I (Figure 2) orofacial tissues.
The data is intended to ascertain the levels from markedly different
tissue species, from which to derive the expected levels of enzyme
activities upon which to devise standardized culture media for (a)
short term 4 to 7 day toxicity assessment and (b) long term 7 to 28
day tumorigenic potential. It is evident that the alkaline and acid
phosphatase activities provide a broad range, adequate to encompass
all of the tissues such as listed in Table 1. The lactic acid dehydrogenase ranges thus far reveal two distinct levels of activities

that appear to differentiate the short term from the long term culturing periods. The long term results may be more representative of
matured, equilibrated lactic acid dehydrogenase activity, in vivo
and thus more suited to assessing toxic and tumorigenic effects of
prosthetic biomaterial.

Chromosomal Assessment. We believe that chromosomal assessment is
indispensible in the H E D tissue culture test system especially
since polymeric implants have had a long history of inducing tumor-
ous growth (Oppenheimer et al, 1955; Huepner, 1960), an indictment
that will long persist, despite contravening arguments. Our work,
which is in an early stage includes conventional characterization of
structural intra karyotype banding (Thompson and Thompson, 1980).
So far no significant deleterious chromosome distortions have been
found using PDM siloxane prosthesis test materials (Figure 4).

In conclusion, tissue culturing of living isolated cells using the
H E D tissue culture test system should serve to adjudicate risks of
toxicity and tumorgenicity with total or high human relevance devoid
of dependence on animal models, thus providing a means for assessing
safety of biomaterials.

ACKNOWLEDGEMENT

The authors are grateful for the support and encouragement accorded
by Dr. Vernon L. Nickel, Director, Veterans Administration Rehabili-
tative Engineering R & D Service, which has made possible the Contract V101(134) P-337 under which this work was performed.

Appreciation is extended to Dr. Ernest B. Mingledorff, School of
Dentistry, Temple University, which administers the Contract, and to
Dr. James W. Schweiger, Chief, Dental Service, Veterans Administration Center, Wilmington, Delaware, for coordinating the clinical
availability of the H E D tissues.

Special acknowledgement with much gratitude is expressed to Dr. W.
Hayman Behringer and Dr. James S. Reilly, formerly with the medical
staff at the Veterans Administration Center, Wilmington, Delaware,
for their assistance in providing H E D tissue biopsy sections incidental to their oral surgery and thereby making this work possible.

REFERENCES

Ames, B. (1974) A combined bacterial and liver test system for
detection and classification of carcinogens as mutagens. Genetics,
78, 91-95.
Ames, B., Mc Cann, J. & Yamasaki, E. (1975) Methods for detecting
carcinogens and mutagens with the salmonella/mammalian-microsome
mutagenicity test. Mutation Research, 31, 347-364.
Autian, J. (1973) A need for a more comprehensive toxicity testing
program for dental implants in Proceedings Symposium, Dental
Biomaterials-Research Priorities, DHEW Publication No. (NIH), pp.
183-195; note Table 1, p. 189.

Christensen, H. Editor. (1972) The toxic substances list. U.S.
Department of Health, Education and Welfare Publication, 513-514.
FDA, Federal Register (1978a) Nonclinical laboratory studies. Good
Laboratory Practice Regulations, Friday, December 22, 1978, Part II.
FDA, Federal Register (1978b) Manufacture, packing, etc. of medical
devices. Regulations Establishing Good Manufacturing Practices,
Friday, July 21, 1978, Part II.
Gonzolez, J. (1978) Polyurethane elastomers for facial prosthetics.
J. Prosth. Dent.. 39. 179-187.
Guess, W., Rosenbluth, S., Schmidt, B. and Autian, J. (1956) Agar
diffusion method for toxicity screening of plastics on cultured
monolayers. J. Pharm. Sci. 54, 1545-1547.
Horton, L. (1976) Medical Devices: Strengthening Consumer Protection, FDA Consumer, HEW Publication No. (FDA) 77.4005, October 1976.
Hueper, W. (1960) Experimental production of cancer by means of
implant polyurethane plastic. Am. J. Clin. Path., 34, 334-337.
Lontz, J. and Schweiger, J. (1977) Maxillofacial restorative biomaterials and techniques. Bull. Pros. Res., BPR 10-28 Fall 1977,
182-188.
Lontz, J. and Schweiger, J. (1978) Maxillofacial restoration bio-
materials and techniques. Bull Pros. Res., BPR 10-29 Spring 1978,
145-155.
Lontz, J. and Schweiger, J. (1979) Maxillofacial restoration bio-
materials and techniques. Bull Pros. Res., BPR 10-31 Fall 1979,
376-404.
Oppenheimer, B., Oppenheimer, E., Danishefsky, I., Stout, A. and
Eirich, F. (1955) Further studies on polymers as carcinogenic
agents in animals. Cancer Research, 15, 1957-1958.
Paul, J. (1975) Cell and tissue culture. Churchill Livingstone,
Edinburgh, London and New York.
Robeson, L., Saunders, W. and Chow, S. (1976) Development of
improved materials for extra extraoral maxillofacial prosthesis,
National Institute for Dental Research Contract, No. NO1-DE-42436.
Final Report.
Shifrin, L. (1970) Correlation of serum alkaline phosphatase with
bone formation rates, Clinical Orthopaedics and Related Research, 70,
212-215.
Struber, V. (1968) Theory and practise of vinyl compounding,
Chapter 7. Plastisol and Organosal Despersions, Argus Chemical
Corporation, New York.
Sweeney, W. (1972) Evaluation of improved maxillofacial prosthetic
materials, J. Prosth. Dent. 27, 297-305.
Thompson, J. and Thompson M. (1980) Genetics in Medicine, Chapter 2,
W.B. Saunders Company, Philadelphia.
Wilkinson, J. (1976) Chemistry of enzymes of diagnostic interest,
I. Oxidoreductases, pp. 46-54, The Principles and Practice of
Diagnostic Enzymology, Year Book Medical Publishers, Inc., New York.

TABLE 1. Summary of Ranges of Extracellular Enzyme Levels in H E D Tissue Culturing

H E D Tissue	Culture Period (Days)	Alkaline 10^3 BD Units	Acid 10^3 BD Units	Alkaline/ Acid Ratio	Lactic Acid Dehydrogenase Ranges (Relative Units)*
Skin	(a) 4-7	54 – 65	12 – 20	2.5 – 4.9	1.5 – 1.9
	(b) 7-28+	39 – 176	19 – 32	1.9 – 5.6	90 – 94
Lip	(a) 4-7	17 – 41	1 – 18	1.0 – 1.6	– – –
	(b) 7-28	– – –	– – –	– – –	29 – 95
Nasal mucosa	(a) 4-7	47 – 102	15 – 19	2.5 – 3.1	2.0 – 3.1
	(b) 7-28	– – –	– – –	– – –	– – –
Maxillo mucosa	(a) 4-7	48 – 162	20 – 37	1.2 – 6.0	– – –
	(b) 7-28	– – –	– – –	– – –	– – –
Larynx	(a) 4-7	9 – 30	41 – 104	1.5 – 6.6	1.6 – 6.1
	(b) 7-28	– – –	– – –	– – –	– – –

Nutrient   : MEM with 10% Fetal Calf Serum (being replaced with Pooled Human Serum).

Maintenance: Every $3\frac{1}{2}$ to 4 days replenishment with fresh nutrient stock

*Relative unit x 0.0073 = 1 IU Clinical; kinetic reaction extended to 30 mins.

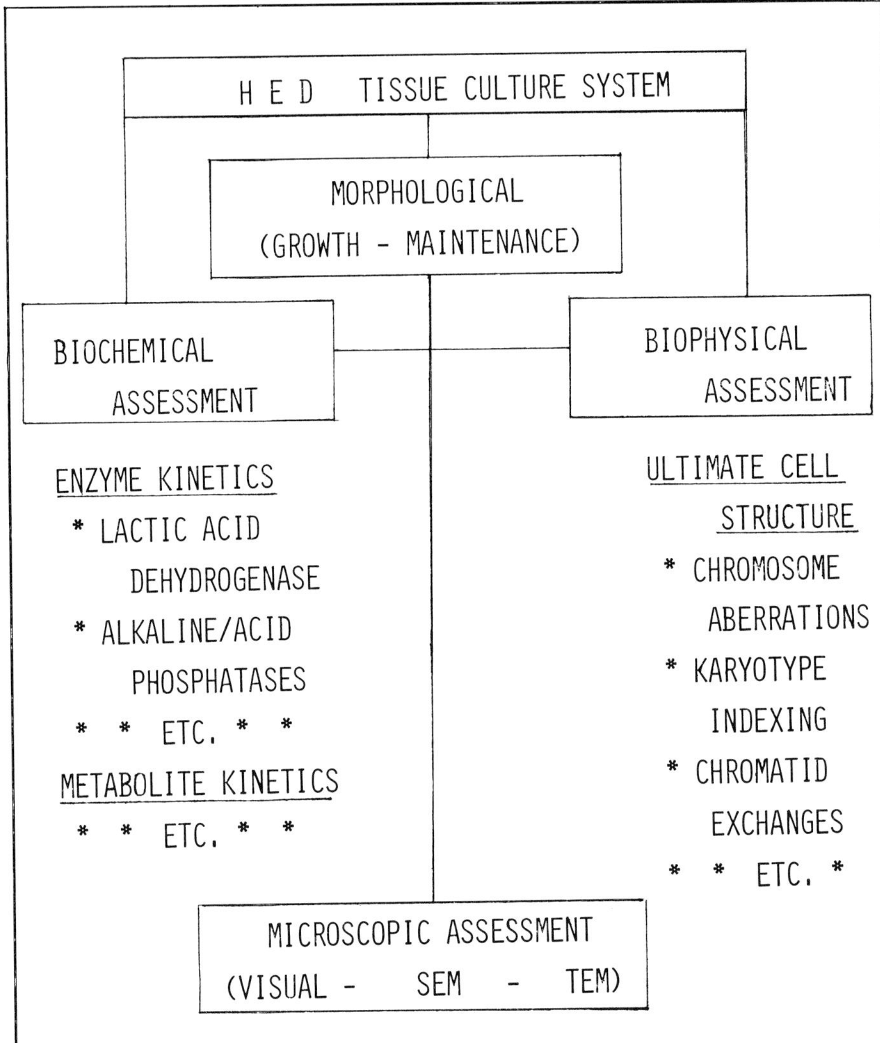

Figure 1. Comprehensive toxicity and potential tumorigenicity assessments of polydimethylsiloxane prostheses based on
human excised donor (H E D) tissue culture testing for demonstrating safe usage in contact with human tissues.

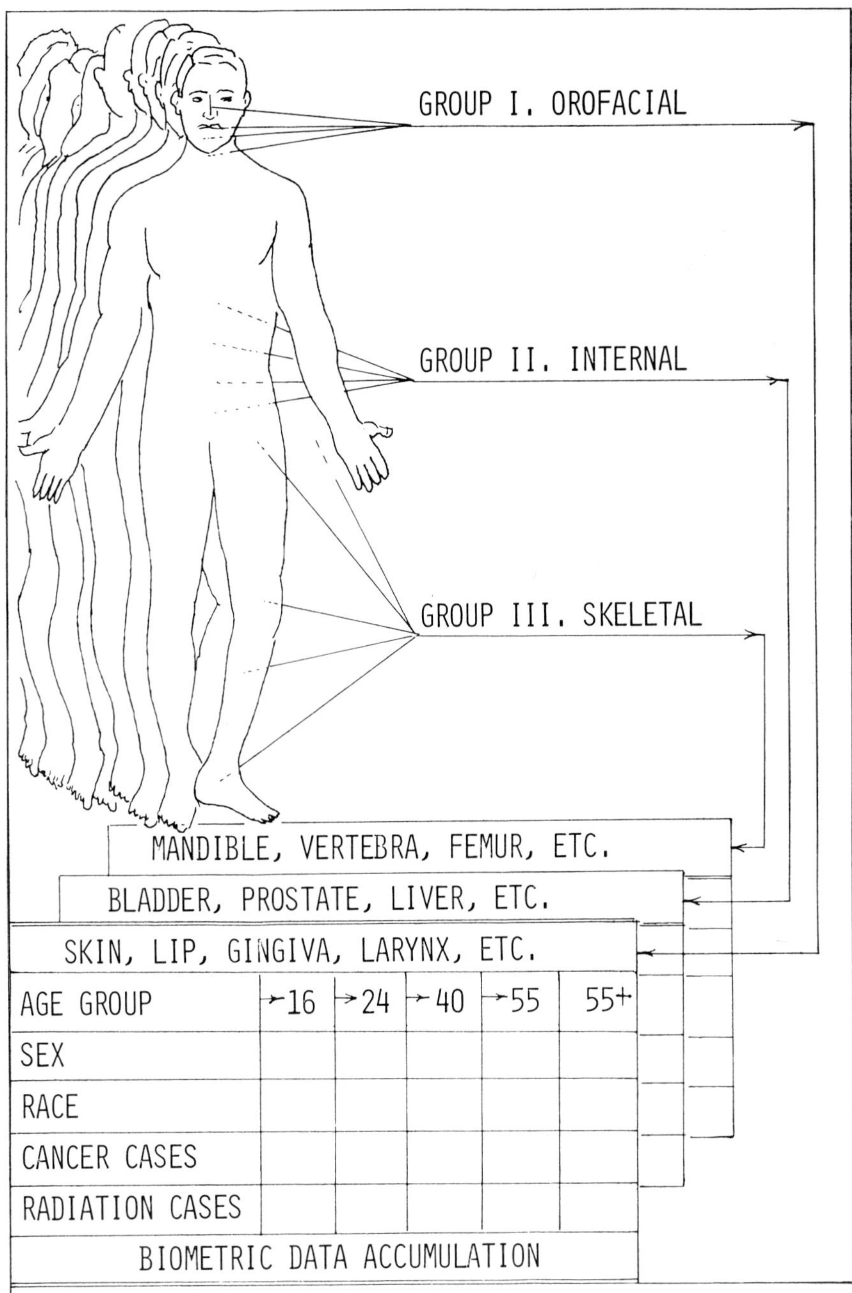

Figure 2. Principal sources and groups of human excised donor (H E D) tissue culturing for biometric data base to affirm non-toxicity and potential non-tumorigenicity of polydimethyl (PDM) siloxane for prostheses, implants, and medical devices.

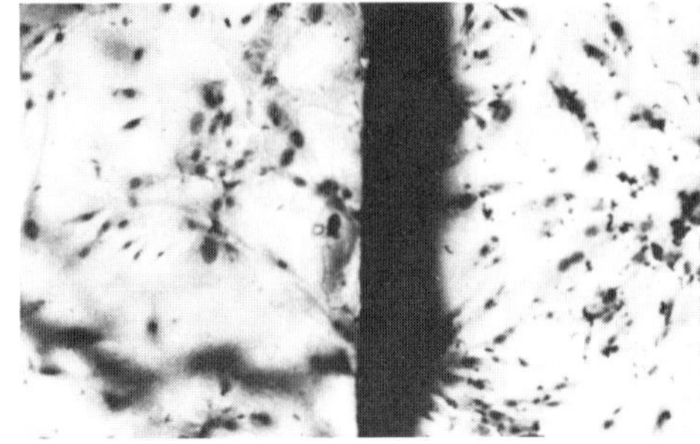

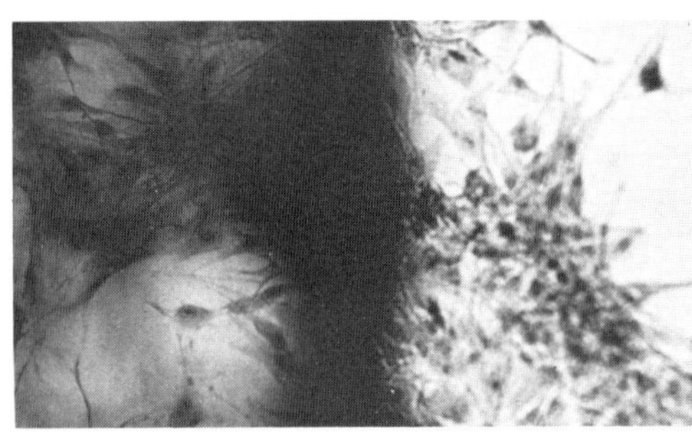

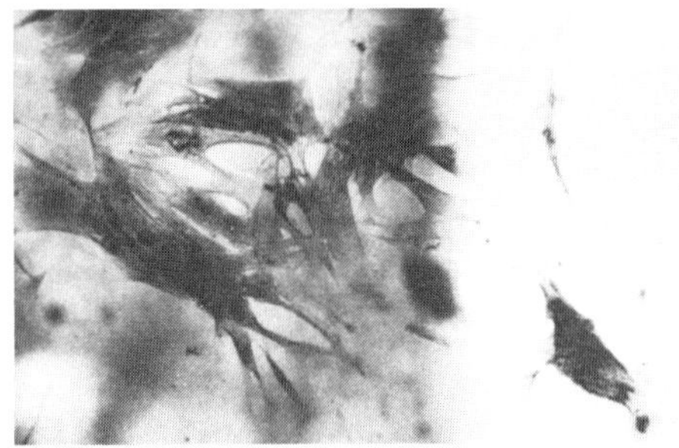

Figure 3. Tissue culture testing of orofacial prostheses
in presence of various human excised donor (H E D) tissues. (200X)

PDM SILOXANE: General Electric SE 4524U (Lot 256)(80 parts)
                Dow Corning DC 200 Fluid (20 parts)

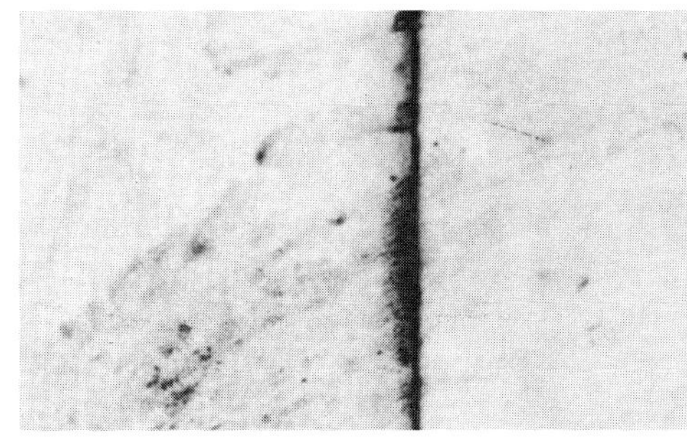

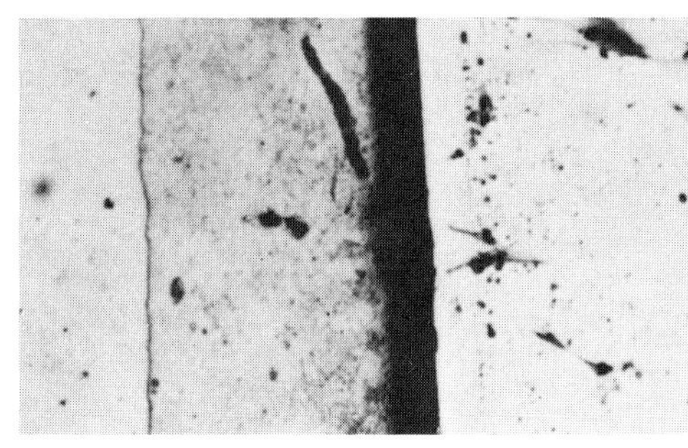

Figure 4. Tissue culture testing of polyvinyl chloride plastisols used in fabricating orofacial (maxillofacial) prosthetics.   (200X)

Sources: Upper test – Sweeney (1972)
         Lower test – VA Prosthetics Center (N.Y.)

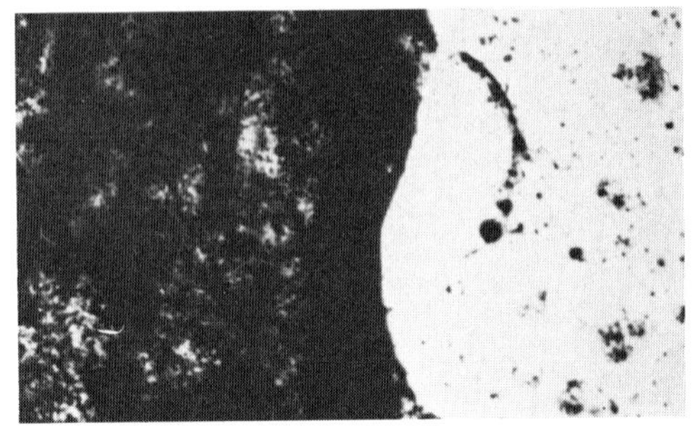

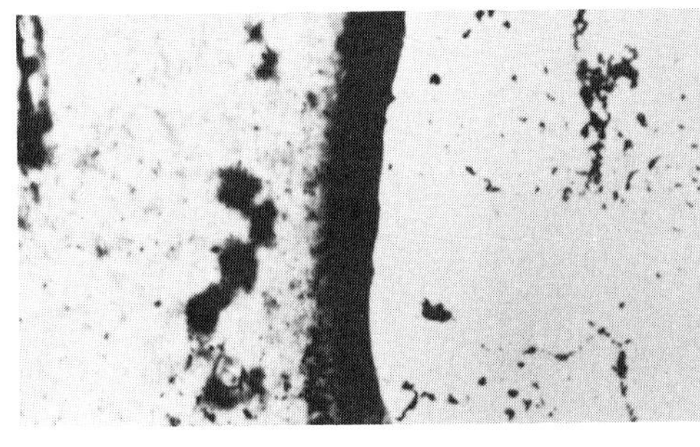

Figure 5. Tissue culture testing of polyurethane prosthesis test materials used in fabricating orofacial (maxillofacial) prosthetics.   (200X)

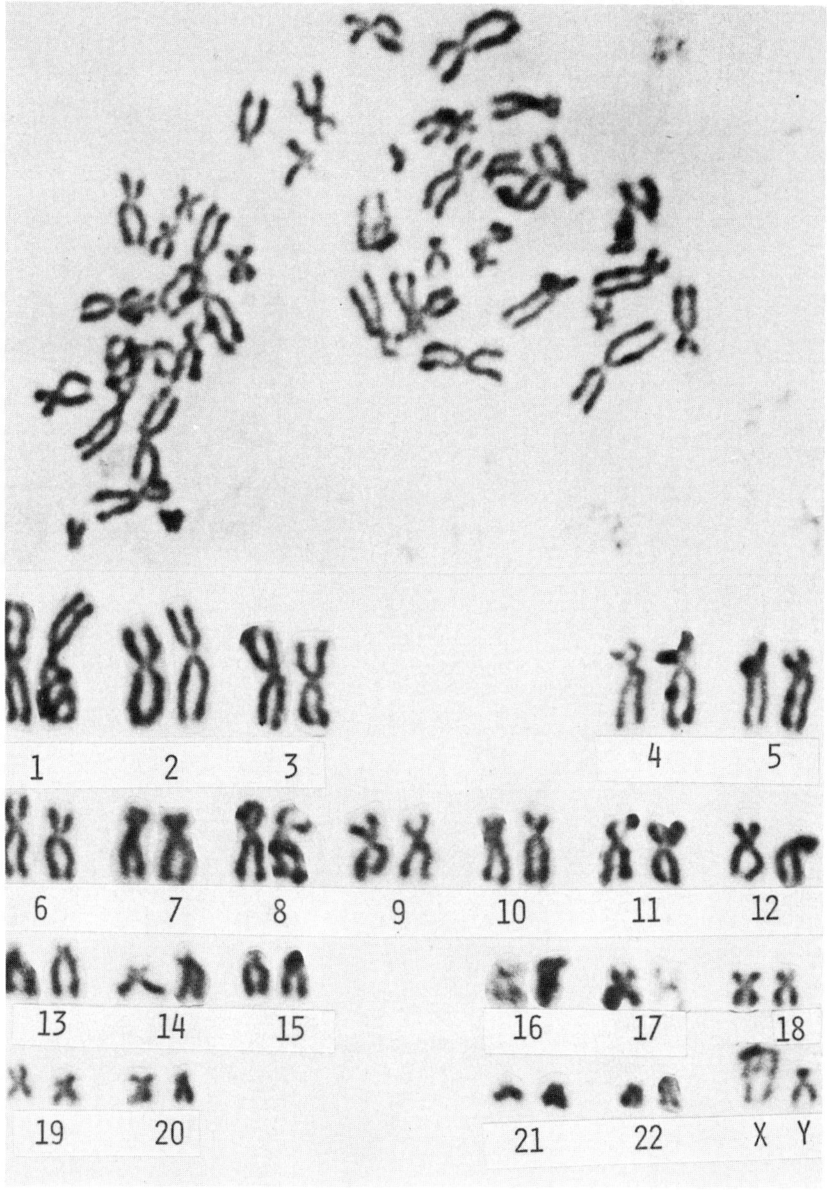

Figure 6. Chromosomal monitoring of human excised donor tissue (larynx, M/C/29/NC/NR) cultured in the presence of polydimethylsiloxane. Top section: chromosome spread. Lower section: idiogram array.

Biomaterials 1980
Edited by G. D. Winter, D. F. Gibbons, and H. Plenk, Jr.
© 1982 John Wiley and Sons Ltd.

TESTING OF IMPLANT MATERIALS FOR FOREIGN BODY CARCINOGENESIS

Inge Brand and K. Gerhard Brand

University of Minnesota Medical School, Department of
Microbiology, Minneapolis, MN., 55455, USA

SUMMARY

Case reports of human foreign body and scar-related cancers with
known latencies were collected. Over 25% had developed within 15
years, over 50% within 25 years. Millions of patients have been
carrying implants for 10 to 20 years. Since at least 25% of
cancers should have occurred by now, the low number observed
indicates that the incidence will remain low. This conclusion is
supported by in vitro studies on 27 specimens of chronic foreign
body reactions in man. The search for precancer cells was negative.
(In mice, which have a high foreign body tumor incidence, this test
is highly positive). While foreign body cancer incidence is low in
man, it is not zero. Therefore, the necessity of testing implant
materials for degree of carcinogenicity is often considered.
Procedural principles are proposed and exemplified by model experiments. These are: use of an animal strain with known susceptibility
for foreign body tumorigenesis; inclusion of a known carcinogenic
material for comparative evaluation; distinction of tumor "incidence"
and "latency" in the evaluation.

INTRODUCTION

Surgeons, technologists, manufacturers alike are very much aware of
the many possible hazards of artificial implants. Yet, one specific
concern may have not been adequately addressed: the concern regarding carcinogenicity. Granted, in most cases implants are of
vital necessity particularly in older patients; thus, the risk of
implant-associated cancers, which have exceedingly long latencies,
can justifiably be regarded as slight. However, today the number of
young implant-carriers is not small, and in many instances implantations have been performed solely for cosmetic reasons.

Cancer development from tissue-embedded foreign materials is a known
to occur phenomenon. In man, we see it especially in connection with
asbestosis and schistosomiasis (Brand 1979, 1980; Brand and Brand
1980). Implant-associated cancers, some with latencies of more than
50 years, have also been reported in the literature (Bischoff 1972;
Bischoff and Bryson 1964; Brand and Brand 1980; Ott 1970). Presently, many millions of people carry implants, although most of them for
only a relatively short time so far. Do we have to fear a wave of

implant-associated cancers as we approach the end of expected
latencies?

EVALUATION OF FOREIGN BODY AND SCAR-
RELATED CANCERS REPORTED IN THE LITERATURE

We have tried to assess the risk more precisely in two ways.
Firstly, we collected and evaluated case reports of foreign body-
associated cancers in man (Brand and Brand 1980a). The foreign
bodies were either accidentally acquired, for instance during
World War I, or they were implanted for medical reasons. We have
included only those cancers for which latencies, that is, the time
spans from implantation or injury until detection of the cancers,
are known. The solid columns in figure 1 illustrate the numbers of
foreign body-cancers arising after latencies indicated on the
abscissa. The broken columns give corresponding data for scar-
associated cancers which we and others consider to be closely
related to foreign body-induced cancers (Brand 1980; Ott 1970).
As the histogram shows, well over 25% of these cancers appeared
within 16 years, 50% within 24 to 28 years.

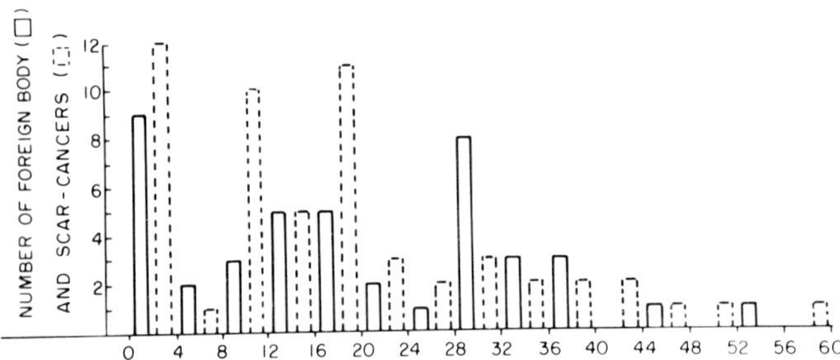

Fig. 1. Incidence and latencies of foreign body and scar-
associated cancers in man. The data were obtained from
several reports and surveys (Brand and Brand, 1980b).

The present upsurge of medical and cosmetic implantations began
about 20 years ago during the late 1950's and early 1960's. During
those years the number of implantations worldwide reached probably
into the hundred-thousands. The histogram tells us that at least
25% of implant-associated cancers should have emerged by now. This
would amount to several ten-thousand cases, if the incidence in man
approached 100% as it does in rats and mice. The fact is that
relatively few cases were reported in recent years, which provides
reasonable assurance, we believe, that the likelihood of implant-
associated cancers in man is small, although not zero.

IN VITRO SEARCH FOR PRECANCER CELLS IN HUMAN
FOREIGN BODY-REACTIVE TISSUES

An experimental investigation was undertaken, based on previous work
in our laboratory using a method for in vitro-culture of specific
preneoplastic cells from foreign body-reactive tissues of mice which
have carried subcutaneous plastic film implants for 3 or more months
(Buoen et al. 1975). The cultured preneoplastic cells differ from
normal cells by their growth behavior in vitro and by their morphology (Johnson et al. 1977). We have identified the cells as derivatives of mesenchymal stem cells of the microvasculature (Johnson et
al. 1973). Most importantly they are characterized by clone-specific
chromosomal abnormalities (Brand et al. 1967).

We have tried to detect preneoplastic cell types in foreign body-
reactive tissues of man (Brand and Brand 1980a). Twenty-seven
specimens were obtained from the surgical services of affiliated
hospitals. The implants comprised steel plates, staples, protheses,
steel mesh, pacemakers, plastic sponges, and silk sutures. The
materials had been in place for one to nineteen years. Despite
intensive technical efforts, none of the cultures yielded abnormal,
clonally aneuploid cells resembling the precancer cells of murine
foreign body reactions. Hence, the rarity of human, foreign body-
related cancers seems satisfactorily explained by the rare emergence
of precancer cells in human foreign body reactions.

RISK ASSESSMENT OF FOREIGN BODY-RELATED
CANCER IN MAN

We conclude that the low incidence of implant-induced cancers in man
presently observed will continue at this level. Latencies can reach
50 to 60 years, but an increase in frequency is not to be expected
in future years. We have now reached a point in time at which a
significant number of foreign body-cancers should have occurred if
the proneness of man to the development of such tumors is similar
to that in the mice we studied. Yet, it should be kept in mind that
the incidence is not zero. Therefore, the possibility of a neoplasm
developing in association with an implant, however remote, must not
be overlooked in the follow-up of any implant carrier.

TESTING OF IMPLANT MATERIALS FOR CARCINOGENICITY

For this same reason it may be deemed necessary to test prospective
implant materials for carcinogenicity in animals. In designing a
protocol and evaluating the results it is important to distinguish
between tumor incidence and latency. An implant material may have a
low capacity to evoke tumor originator cells in which case the tumor
incidence is truly low. Another material may cause delayed appearance of tumor originator cells, or it may decelerate tumor promotion;
then, tumor latency is prolonged. If the experiment is terminated
too early, the investigator would be wrong in claiming a low tumor
incidence. Thus, the question is: How long to observe? This

uncertainty can be eliminated by including a positive tumor control
in the investigation, i.e. a material with known tumorigenicity, for
example unplasticized monomer-free polyvinylchloride/acetate (Brand
et al. 1975). It should have the same size and shape as the test
implant.

A test protocol was developed and tried by comparing various experimental implant materials in groups of 20 female CBA/H-mice which
were 8 weeks old at the time of implantation. The incidence of
spontaneous fibrosarcomas in this particular mouse strain is zero
at the subcutaneous site. The materials were implanted subcutaneously as rectangular plates, 15 x 22 mm in size and 1 mm thick. In the
graph (figure 2), percent tumors as obtained in the various test
groups are cumulatively plotted against time in months after implantation.

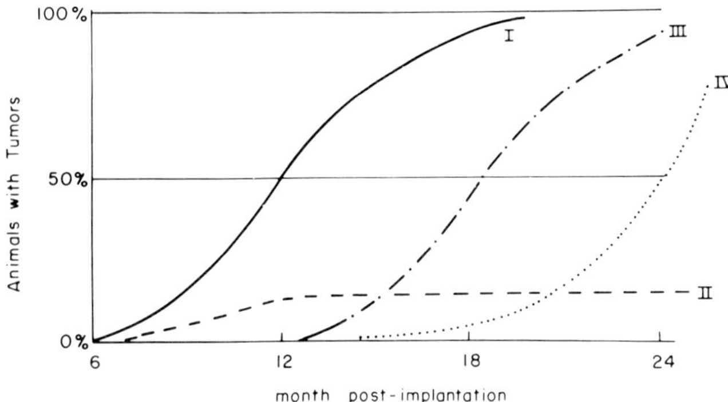

Fig. 2. Frequency and appearance time of foreign body
sarcomas in mice following implantation of (I) unplasticized polyvinylchloride/acetate, (II) porous polycarbonate,
(III) surface-textured polyvinylchloride/acetate, (IV)
polyethylene sponge with nonporous core. For further
methodological details see text.

Group I is the control group. Twenty mice received an implant of
polyvinylchloride/acetate. The degree of tumorigenicity of this
material in CBA/H-mice is known (Brand et al. 1977). As the graph
shows, 50% of the animals had developed fibrosarcomas at the implantation sites by the 11th month, 100% by month-18.

The 20 mice in group II received implants of a porous polycarbonate
material. About 80% of the animals remained tumor-free. This
result suggests that the material tested in group II has a low capacity to evoke tumor originator cells.

The 20 animals of group III received surface-textured polyvinyl-
chloride/acetate. The tumor curve runs parallel to the control curve

about 10 months behind. This result suggests that the material
delayed the appearance, but did not decrease the number of tumor
originator cells.

In group IV, a composite material of polyethylene sponge with a
fused nonporous core was implanted. Tumor appearance was sluggish
at first, but picked up during senescence of the animals. This
result suggests that preneoplastic cell maturation was slowed.

These model experiments demonstrate that certain conclusions can be
drawn from the timing, the shape, and the slope of the cumulative
tumor frequency curves. For practical purposes it is usually
sufficient to determine that the test material is significantly
less tumorigenic than the known control material. This can be
achieved relatively early in such an investigation by applying the
Student-t-Test to the tumor data as they are obtained (Brand et al.
1977). In the example given, a definite conclusion could have been
reached by the 12th month.

CONCLUSION

The incidence of implant-associated cancer in man is fortunately very
low, but it is not zero. Therefore, implant materials with minimal
tumorigenicity should be developed and selected. Some procedural
principles are proposed which facilitate comparative examination of
implant materials for tumorigenicity.

ACKNOWLEDGEMENTS

The research of the authors was supported by the U.S. Public Health
Service (grants (CA 10712 and ES 02101) and by the American Cancer
Society (grant IN-13-Q-34).

REFERENCES

Bischoff, F. (1972). Organic polymer biocompatibility and toxicology.
Clinical Chem., 18, 869-894.
Bischoff, F. & Bryson, G. (1964). Carcinogenesis through solid state
surfaces, Prog. Exp. Tumor Res., 5, (Karger, Basel, New York), 85-133.
Brand, I., Buoen, L.C. & Brand, K.G. (1977). Foreign-body tumors of
mice: Strain and sex differences in latency and incidence, J. Natl.
Cancer Inst., 58, 1443-1447.
Brand, K.G. (1979). Schistosomiasis-cancer: Etiological considera-
tions, Acta Tropica, 36, 203-214.
Brand, K.G. (1980). Cancer associated with asbestosis, schistosomi-
asis, foreign bodies, and scars, in Cancer, 2nd edition, vol. 1,
F.F. Becker, ed., Plenum Press, New York.
Brand, K.G. & Brand, I. (1980a) Risk assessment of carcinogenesis at
implantation sites. Plast. Reconstr. Surg., 66, 591-594.
Brand, K.G. & Brand, I. (1980b). Investigations and review of liter-
ature relating to carcinogenesis. Parts I, II, and III, Zbl. Bakt.,
I. Abt. Orig. B787.

Brand, K.G., Buoen, L.C. & Brand, I. (1967). Carcinogenesis from polymer implants: New aspects from chromosomal and transplantation studies during premalignancy, J. Natl. Cancer Inst., 39, 663-679.
Brand, K.G., Buoen, L.C. & Brand, I. (1975). Foreign-body tumorigenesis induced by glass and smooth and rough plastic. Comparative study of preneoplastic events. J. Natl. Cancer Inst., 55, 319-322.
Buoen, L.C., Brand, I. & Brand, K.G. (1975). Foreign-body tumorigenesis: In vitro isolation and expansion of preneoplastic clonal cell populations, J. Natl. Cancer Inst., 55, 721-723.
Johnson, K.H., Buoen, L.C. Brand, I. & Brand, K.G. (1977). Light-microscopic morphology of cell types cultured during preneoplasia from foreign body-reactive tissues and films, Cancer Res., 37, 3228-3237.
Johnson, K.H., Ghobrial, H.K.G., Buoen, L.C., Brand, I. & Brand, K.G. (1973). Nonfibroblastic origin of foreign body sarcomas implicated by histologic and electron microscopic studies, Cancer Res., 33, 3139-3154.
Ott, G. (1970). Fremdkörper sarkome, Exp. Med. Path. Klinik, Band 32, Springer, Berlin.

SUBJECT INDEX

828